# Advances in Preventing and Treating Violence and Aggression

**Series Editor**

Peter Sturmey
Queens College and The Graduate Center
City University of New York
Flushing, NY, USA

The series publishes books focused and developed across three domains. The first is understanding and explaining violence and aggression. Books in this domain address such subject matter as genetics, physiology, neurobiology, cultural evolution, biobehavioral, learning, cognitive, psychoanalytic, sociological and other explanations of violence. The second domain focuses on prevention and treatment for individuals and couples. Examples of books in this domain include cognitive behavioral, behavioral, counseling, psychopharmacological, psychosocial, couples, and family therapy approaches. They also explore extant treatment packages for individually focused treatments (e.g., mindfulness, cognitive analytic therapies). Within this domain, books focus on meeting the information needs of clinicians and professionals who work in youth facilities, emergency rooms, special education, criminal justice, and therapy settings. Finally, books in the third domain address prevention and treatment for groups and society, including topical focus on early intervention programs, school violence prevention programs, policing strategies, juvenile facility reform as well as socio-legal and ethical issues. Books in this series serve as must-have resources for researchers, academics, and upper-level undergraduate and graduate students in clinical child and school psychology, public health, criminology/criminal justice, developmental psychology, psychotherapy/counseling, psychiatry, social work, educational policy and politics, health psychology, nursing, and behavioral therapy/rehabilitation.

More information about this series at http://www.springer.com/series/15332

James McGuire • Emily Evans • Eddie Kane

# Evidence-Based Policing and Community Crime Prevention

Springer

James McGuire
University of Liverpool
Liverpool, UK

Eddie Kane
Centre for Health and Justice
University of Nottingham
Notttingham, UK

Emily Evans
Institute for Global Innovation
University of Birmingham
Birmingham, UK

Advances in Preventing and Treating Violence and Aggression
ISBN 978-3-030-76362-6    ISBN 978-3-030-76363-3 (eBook)
https://doi.org/10.1007/978-3-030-76363-3



This Springer imprint is published by the registered company Springer Nature Switzerland AG
The registered company address is: Gewerbestrasse 11, 6330 Cham, Switzerland

# Preface

Researchers, academics, and practitioners in many fields now readily embrace the concepts and principles of evidence-based practice. It might seem obvious that what professionals do in any area of applied work should be based on a sound body of knowledge derived from well-conducted research. But until not long ago, that was not the customary way to proceed, and even after proposals to do so were made, there was (and there continues to be) some resistance to following this route.

The movement towards adoption of a more scientifically grounded approach is widely understood to have begun in medicine, with the criticisms made by the British epidemiologist Archie Cochrane (1972) seen as pivotal in alerting medical doctors to the need for systematically accumulated research. This led to the foundation of the now worldwide Cochrane Collaboration (Chalmers et al., 1992). Parallel developments later arose in other disciplines, notably the Campbell Collaboration addressing the numerous unresolved issues in education, social work, criminal justice, and elsewhere.

It may have been inevitable, and perhaps it was only a matter of time before this innovation would reach policing. Equally, however, a case can be made that it had already emerged independently there. In 1972–73, a pioneering experiment was carried out in Kansas City, Missouri, to test the relative effectiveness of different levels of police car patrol (Kelling et al., 1974). Over a 12-month period, 15 police patrol beats, covering 32 square miles of the city, were matched on a number of crime-related variables and allocated to one of three conditions. In one set of areas ("reactive") there was no preventive patrol and police entered them only in response to calls for assistance. By contrast, in the second ("proactive") group, visible patrol was increased to two to three times its usual level. In the third ("control") set, the normal level of patrol was maintained.

This study, the Kansas City Preventive Patrol Experiment, has been described as a landmark of policing research (Braga, 2001). At the time, three-quarters (75%) of officers surveyed considered that patrol was the most important function of the police department. However, data analysis found no significant differences between the three patrol conditions in the level of crime, in citizens' attitudes toward police services, in their fear of crime, in police response times, or public satisfaction with them. The researchers concluded that "routine preventive patrol in marked police cars has little value in preventing crime or making citizens feel safe" (Kelling et al., 1974, p.vii).

Other studies concerned with police foot patrol have obtained similar findings, for example in Newark, New Jersey (Kelling, 1981), with no observable effect on crime, and a mixed pattern of effects on perceptions of police. Patrol has since been shown to have some positive effects, however, if directed at high crime locations ("hot spots") (Sherman & Weisburd, 1995).

It is important to note that discovering that some taken-for-granted police procedures are not reliably effective does not in itself provide an argument for reducing police resources. It could, on the contrary, suggest that policing benefits from more extensive community contacts – a step that might entail higher investment in personnel. To rephrase a motto often heard in Britain when police numbers are discussed, we may well need "more bobbies", but not necessarily "on the beat" unless there are clear indicators for the direction of this.

The specific issues of results here and their implications for practice are important; but perhaps still more fundamental is the idea that the questions raised over police operations and effectiveness can be answered by methodical research – the adoption and application of the scientific method, the development of guidelines for implementation, and the evaluation of practice, subsequently given a decisive impetus by Sherman (1998). Thus, the broader and more telling issue may not lie in the answer to specific questions about long-standing practices. Rather it is the more critical one of how we can find answers to questions by empirical testing of both these and other modes of operation.

In the Kansas City study, the researchers considered it a "distinct possibility that the police may more effectively deal with the problems of crime if they work more closely and systematically with their communities" (Kelling et al., 1974, p.40). Similarly, even in more recent studies on patrol and on police-public contacts, there is evidence that preventive or guardian-oriented approaches have better outcomes than those based on enforcement (Piza, 2018); they may also reinforce stronger links with communities (Peyton et al., 2019).

These two perspectives provide a foundation for the present book. The reviews reported in it were carried out within the framework and principles of evidence-based policing, with a particular focus on questions raised by police officers themselves about methods of working that entailed fuller interactions with other agencies and within the community.

## References

Braga, A. A. (2001). The effects of hot spots policing on crime. *Annals of the American Academy of Political and Social Science, 578*, 104–125.

Chalmers, I., Dickersin, K., & Chalmers, T. C. (1992). Getting to grips with Archie Cochrane's agenda. *British Medical Journal, 305*, 786–788.

Cochrane, A. L. (1972). *Effectiveness and Efficiency: Random Reflections on Health Services*. London: Nuffield Provincial Hospitals Trust.

Kelling, G. L. (1981). Conclusions. In *The Newark Foot Patrol Experiment*. pp. 111–129. Washington, DC: Police Foundation.

Kelling, G. L., Pate, T., Dieckman, D., & Brown, C. E. (1974). *The Kansas City Preventive Patrol experiment: A summary report*. Washington, DC: Police Foundation.

Peyton, K., Sierra-Arévalo, M. & Rand, D. G. (2019). A field experiment on community policing and police legitimacy. *Proceedings of the National Academy of Sciences*, *116*(40), 19894–19898. www.pnas.org/cgi/doi/10.1073/pnas.1910157116

Piza, E. L. (2018). The effect of various police enforcement actions on violent crime: Evidence from a saturation foot-patrol intervention. *Criminal Justice Policy Review*, *29*(6–7), 611–629.

Sherman, L. W. (1998). *Evidence-Based Policing*. Washington, DC: Police Foundation.

Sherman, L. W., & Weisburd, D. (1995). General deterrent effects of police patrol in crime "hot spots": A randomized controlled trial. *Justice Quarterly*, *12*(4), 625–648.

Liverpool, UK James McGuire
Birmingham, UK Emily Evans
Notttingham, UK Eddie Kane

# Acknowledgements

This book is the product of a research project jointly undertaken by staff of four Universities, of Birmingham, Liverpool, Nottingham and Suffolk, and two independent research and consultancy organizations, Crest Analytics and Skills for Justice, and carried out in the period 2014–2017. We thank the College of Policing, and the Higher Education Funding Council for England and Wales, for providing research funding to the project to the University of Nottingham as lead institution. We also thank Simon Bailey and Gareth Wilson, then Chief Constables, respectively, of Norfolk and Suffolk, and members of the project executive board, for steering the project objectives and identifying key areas towards which to direct the review work that is reported here, which formed just one part of the project as a whole.

We are very grateful to fellow members of the research team from the different organizations that were involved in the project work, and for the congenial and productive relationships that were established during its course. We particularly thank Jun Xia and her staff, of Review Solutions and the University of Nottingham, who designed several of the initial search strategies and carried out the associated electronic literature searches; Emily Garrod, of Suffolk Constabulary, who undertook screening of a portion of the records located; and Siddhartha Bandyopadhyay, of the University of Birmingham, for providing information on some of the follow-up work undertaken as part of the project.

March 2021

James McGuire
Emily Evans
Eddie Kane

# Contents

# About the Authors

**James McGuire, PhD** is emeritus professor of forensic clinical psychology at the University of Liverpool, where he was director of the Doctor of Clinical Psychology programme from 1995 to 2013. After an initial period in self-employment, he worked in learning disabilities services and then for several years in a high-security hospital. He has provided psycho-legal assessments and reports for Youth and Crown Courts, the Mental Health Tribunal, Parole Board, and Criminal Cases Review Commission and has conducted research in prisons, probation, addictions services, youth justice, and in policing. James was co-organizer of the What Works series of conferences in the UK in the 1990s, and has written or edited 15 books and numerous other publications on interventions to reduce reoffending and related issues. He has been an invited speaker in 21 countries and has engaged in a range of consultative work with criminal justice agencies in several parts of the world.

**Emily Evans, PhD** is a research fellow at the University of Birmingham. She has been researcher in the field of policing, criminal justice and community safety for over 15 years, primarily undertaking evaluations of interventions in these areas. She is based within the 21st Century Transnational Crime theme of the University's Institute of Global Innovation which delivers world-leading, multidisciplinary research to address the world's most pressing challenges. Emily holds a PhD from the University of Nottingham based on an evaluation of Integrated Offender Management and its potential to support desistance amongst prolific offenders.

**Eddie Kane, PhD** is director of the Centre for Health and Justice at the Institute of Mental Health, University of Nottingham. He leads teams delivering major national and international research programmes including Home Office and College of Policing grant funding programmes covering the development of evidence-based interventions at the health justice interface including violence reduction initiatives and mental health interventions in the justice system. Eddie is also a senior fellow in the Institute of Global Innovation at the University of Birmingham working on transnational crime research. He was formerly the national director of High Security Psychiatric Services. He also worked as the director of NHS performance and mental health for London and as director of mental health for the Northwest and West Midlands regions of England. Eddie has been an NHS Trust CEO and held board-level positions in a variety of public, private and voluntary organizations.

# Chapter 1
# Introduction and Background: Policing in Transition

## 1.1 Introduction and Overview

This book focuses on *evidence-based policing*, a major innovative development within police work involving a significant extension and strengthening of links between research and practice, directed to the task of increasing police effectiveness. Our main objective is to draw together the findings of research concerning a number of issues police officers face, to evaluate what has been learnt and to summarize the key practical messages that can be applied in police work, principally in the field of community crime prevention.

Policing is undergoing a significant transformation in many locations. For much of its history in many countries, the long-standing, traditional and central form it took was as a process essentially of reacting to events. The majority of those events were acts of crime, while another large proportion of them were disturbances of civil order. The customary mode of police activity consisted of responding to calls for assistance from the public, usually after being a victim of or witness to a crime. Thereafter the foremost focus was on crime detection, and in apprehending and prosecuting suspects, in an overall approach that has been characterized as reactive policing, incident-focused policing, the standard model of policing or more plainly as "crime fighting".

This is an over-simplification of course. Regular police work entails many different kinds of activities, and some of them contain a preventive element. They include recording information about crime that is then used in the production of local and national crime statistics. Another portion involves routine tasks such as security patrols and management of road traffic or of large crowds attending public events, from sports matches or festivals to demonstrations and protests. Some of it is undoubtedly very harrowing and hazardous, from attending fatal road accidents to arresting perpetrators of violent crimes or policing terrorist incidents. Policing is occasionally highly proactive, such as when there is a clampdown on a particular



J. McGuire et al., *Evidence-Based Policing and Community Crime Prevention*, Advances in Preventing and Treating Violence and Aggression,
https://doi.org/10.1007/978-3-030-76363-3_1

variety of crime. Investigating any violation of law requires interviewing victims, suspects and witnesses, assembly of evidence, presentation of it in court and the steady refinement of forensic and data-gathering techniques in support of this.

Over the last few decades however, the direction or the emphasis of policing has incrementally changed towards a position that places greater emphasis on crime prevention through more proactive and strategic approaches, drawing on analysis of crime data and relevant research evidence. By its nature much of this also relies on more intensive contact with the public. Alongside that development, there has also been a rapidly growing interest in collecting and utilizing evidence about police effectiveness and examining whether improvements can be made within it, what is familiarly portrayed as "what works" in policing.

That stance reflects similar changes that have occurred in many other areas of public service. Paralleling this, police forces have in addition been moving away from a stance in which the police were a somewhat insular agency with a uniquely sensitive role, functioning separately and often distantly from other public departments, to one that involves far more inter-agency cooperation and engagement with multiple services, indeed working in partnerships with them for particular purposes. That has been accompanied by greater complexity and sophistication in the models of practice that inform police strategies, and the modes of planning and operation that chief officers select and implement.

## 1.2 Setting the Scene: Policing Ancient and Modern

The present book seeks to adopt an international perspective on those developments and synthesizes recent research results from the USA, UK and many other countries, including systematic reviews of large bodies of evidence, to illuminate some of the most challenging issues currently faced by police forces worldwide. We will locate the research to be reviewed in the context of recent advances in models of policing and the expanding research base in outcome evaluation.

The objective of the present chapter is simply to provide a background and set the scene for the remainder of the book, by overviewing some of the main contemporary approaches to policing, and the evidence, where it is available, that illuminates their effectiveness or usefulness. We precede that with a brief sketch of the historical origins of policing, though again that is primarily for context-setting purposes. Policing has been carried out and organized in numerous different ways in many countries, sometimes with roots that stretch back over a period of many hundreds, even thousands of years.

Taking a long-term, global and big-picture view, some mode of policing is known to have existed in several societies since ancient times – "the concept of policing long predates the activities of state officers" (Zedner, 2006, p.82). As we might expect this followed different patterns according to the culture and epoch in which it arose.

Possibly the earliest known form of policing emerged in the eighteenth dynasty or New Kingdom of Egypt as long ago as 1570 BCE, under the pharaoh Ahmose I. Those appointed to the role guarded citizens and their property and patrolled markets and other public places to deter theft. But they also assisted in the collection of taxes, maintained the sanctity of temples and, at a later stage, protected tombs from robbery and looting. To help them pursue and detain miscreants, it is said they trained not only dogs but sometimes also monkeys (Mark, 2020). Much later, during the Ptolemaic period when Egypt was ruled by Greece, police duties widened to include that of investigating crimes (Bauschatz, 2007).

Similarly, in India from 600 BCE onwards, policing took a mixture of forms, including several kinds of watch duty to safeguard dwellings and other property but also as a means of deterring specific types of crime, including cattle theft, adultery and murder. At one stage, if they failed to recover items that were lost due to theft, police themselves were fined. Police officers were expected to be individuals with the highest personal qualities and were accountable to the community. Thus, they helped provide security to citizens but at times were also charged to "keep a close eye on their activities" (Sharma, 2004, p. 204). The tension between protecting the welfare of citizens while preserving the power of their rulers appears to have been embedded within police work from some time ago.

From the eighth century BCE onwards, China was governed through what is known as the *prefecture* system, a multi-layered mode of organization aspects which have remained intact until the present day. This was part of a lengthy hierarchical chain of accountability reaching from sub-prefects in local areas to prefects at roughly county level, to the magistrates who appointed them, then to provincial governors and thereby all the way to the emperor. It incorporated a role for policing, which served a range of functions. They included dealing with citizens' complaints of crimes and, in some places, investigation of them. The sub-prefects who policed localities were thus distant officers of the state. Amongst the techniques reputedly used at some stages was that of recruiting known thieves to assist in the entrapment of other thieves, in return for which the former would receive a lesser punishment (Zhang, 2019).

Within European nations too, there were major differences in how police forces originated and developed. In Anglo-Saxon England, communities were in many senses self-policing as there was a universal obligation for able-bodied citizens to take action when a crime occurred (Rawlings, 2008). In the centuries following the Norman conquest, this process was ratified in the 1285 Statute of Winchester, which instituted the legal role of night watch, and whereby anyone who became aware of a theft or robbery was required to raise the alarm and go in pursuit of the suspect in what was known as the "hue and cry". The local community (the *hundred*) had a responsibility to recompense the victim if the offender could not be caught (Joyce, 2011). Gradually over ensuing years, several other roles were formalized, including those of constable, justice of the peace (later magistrate) and coroner. The first of those was at that stage a part-time and voluntary role, with citizens undertaking it on a 12-month rotational basis (Zedner, 2006).

By contrast in medieval France, the system that developed was more highly centralized and was under the orders of senior officers of the French army. The resultant *maréchaussée* (marshalcy) existed from the early sixteenth century and had an intermittent political role in protecting the state. This was the predecessor of today's *gendarmerie* but is just one of several policing arrangements that exist in present-day France.

In the colonial American states prior to the war of independence, policing took a variety of forms. Informal arrangements including night watch arose in several cities in the seventeenth century - in Boston in 1636, in New York in 1657 and in Philadelphia in 1700. But officers worked only part time, and their commitment to their role appears to have been erratic, with some reported to be sleeping and drinking on duty (Waxman, 2017). In other states such as Virginia and North and South Carolina, a key policing task was to search for and recapture runaway slaves (Hadden, 1999, 2003). Such *slave patrols* were one forerunner of a culture thought to have had a far-reaching influence on some aspects of US policing, with consequences lasting right up to the present (Kapeller et al., 2020).

The principal drivers of the momentous changes that led to the emergence of modern policing in the late eighteenth and early nineteenth centuries were the twin forces of industrialization and urbanization. In Britain where these processes gathered pace very quickly, due to land enclosures and resultant loss of traditional livelihoods, coupled with a steeply rising demand for labour in the burgeoning factory system, there were massive migrations of population from rural areas into towns, transforming patterns of work and employment. The new industrial workforce was afflicted by widespread poverty, while others who made the journey never even found the work they expected and fell into destitution. At various stages this gave rise to widespread political agitation. These and other pressures of a rapidly changing economy and society gave rise to the inauguration of the first police services as a separate body employed by the courts.

As those changes unfolded, several initiatives were taken in various places to maintain order and react to crime. One was the advent of the Bow Street Runners, set up in London in 1749 by the novelist and magistrate Henry Fielding. This began as a group of six men and never numbered more than a few dozen, and due to other developments was disbanded in 1839. The City of Glasgow Police was established by an act of parliament in 1800, funded by a levy on local homes and business, and with an underlying ethos of crime prevention (Joyce, 2011, p. 19). But what is customarily referred to as the origin of modern policing in anglophone countries is usually traced to the year 1829 and the passing of the Metropolitan Police Act, steered into law by the then British Home Secretary Sir Robert Peel (Emsley, 2008). This created a new public role in London, officially employed preservers of order, wearing a blue uniform so as to be easily identifiable. The latter was done to ensure post-holders were not in a position to spy upon citizens or infiltrate their organizations, as police in continental Europe were, with some justification, believed to do. Though reputedly unpopular at first, and initially having a very high turnover rate amongst those recruited to the role, it was not long before this innovation was adopted in many other places.

In the USA, following a series of riots in major cities from 1835 onwards, full-time, publicly funded police forces were created in response, such that by the mid-1860s all larger cities and many smaller ones had organized police forces. But serious problems of inefficiency and corruption remained widespread for many decades. The modern era of policing is dated to the work of the National Commission on Law Observance and Enforcement, known as the Wickersham Commission, set up by President Herbert Hoover during the prohibition years (1920–1933). Its head, August Vollmer, Police Chief of Oakland, California, and its report published in 1931 played a key role in the advance towards legal and managerial reform and the professionalization of American policing (Kapeller et al., 2020).

Many countries in what is now called the global south, which during different periods were colonized by European powers, had police and other administrative systems imposed on them which resembled those of their respective colonizers (Mawby, 2008). Although there were divergent patterns within this, after independence some countries retained police forces organized along lines which reflected that segment of their history (e.g. Ayee, 2015).

In its initial stages after the establishment of a professional force in Britain, police activity was dominated by protection of property by means of regular patrol and did not typically involve evidence gathering or pursuit and arrest of suspected offenders. It was only after the launch of the Criminal Investigation Department (CID) as a branch of the Metropolitan Police in 1870 that these activities began to take shape and to form a larger component of policing, thereafter becoming a major plank of its agenda (Maguire, 2008, p. 432).

This is a very brief and selective outline of a complex history, designed mainly to illustrate the sheer multiplicity of paths that policing has taken. While there is a consensus on some aspects of that history, there are differing and sometimes polarized interpretations of the respective importance of different developments and processes within it. There are, for example, contrasts between what are labelled as orthodox and revisionist accounts of the nineteenth-century change from traditional to more modern forms of policing, and debates over the extent to which despite some differences there were also important continuities between them (Rowe, 2018). It would be difficult to write a history of policing that attracted universal acclaim.

## 1.3 Contemporary Policing

Today, countries differ considerably with respect to how their police are organized, administered and financed. While international comparisons are difficult to make reliably, what can be said unequivocally is that there is a very wide range in the absolute size of police services. Relevant information has been compiled and analysed by the European Institute for Crime Prevention and Control (HEUNI) and the United Nations Office on Drugs and Crime (UNODC). This shows, for example, that during the period 2000–2006, while Bangladesh and Kenya had respectively just 79.2 and 98.5 police personnel per 100,000 population, the corresponding numbers in Montenegro and Kuwait were by contrast 890.9 and 1065.2 per 100,000 (Harrendorf & Smit, 2010). The mean ratio across the 97 jurisdictions for which data were available was 341.8 per 100,000. Yet, notwithstanding the variations just noted, there was a very high correlation of 0.93 between police personnel levels and the size of a country's population. Police forces differ in size mainly because country populations do.

In some countries there are different divisions of police services with separate roles or distinct spheres of activity or areas of jurisdiction. Some are accountable to provincial, state or county authorities and deal with crime and community protection. Others are more centralized and may have a quasi-military role, for protection of key national assets or maintenance of public order in emergency situations. In many places there are specialized types of police forces, their composition varying between countries, such as transport, border or diplomatic police. Alongside these official organizations, there are many other security personnel serving specific functions for an array of private agencies. Finally, in addition to the internal arrangements within each country, there are also trans-national police organizations (Bowling & Sheptycki, 2012). They include the International Criminal Police Organization (Interpol), established in 1923; the ASEAN Association of Chiefs of Police (Aseanapol), founded in 1981; and the European Union Agency for Law Enforcement Cooperation (Europol), which became operational from 1999.

In the context of this remarkable variation, police structures and modes of organization have also evolved significantly over time. So too have the operational concepts that inform and influence how policing is carried out. Many recent developments represent a break from the predominantly responsive model depicted earlier. As regards the position and the role of police in society, this has been expressed in metaphorical terms as a move from being *warriors* to one more similar to that of *guardians* (McLean et al., 2019).

But the role of guardian is different from that in the past. We stated earlier that traditional policing was mostly reactive, dependent on requests for assistance, yet for much of its earlier history, a lot of policing included protection from crime, by direct physical presence or patrol. However, the method of providing it was highly labour-intensive and would be unsustainable today. Felson and Eckert (2019) give the example of the city of Austin, Texas, where to supply adequate everyday coverage of its 350,000 dwellings, each police officer would need to have a working day of 3200 hours. Calls to remedy that by increasing officer numbers are futile: "doubling in the number of police in a US city is doubling a drop in the bucket" (Felson & Eckert, 2019, p. 6). If crime prevention is to offer any prospect of success, it needs to be approached in some manner other than this.

The changes in the emphasis of policing that have occurred in recent times are almost all departures from both the idea of policing as continuous protection and the idea of reactive policing in which the police usually become involved only after a crime has been reported and then take action accordingly. Tilley (2008) has outlined three main forms those changes have taken: as community policing, problem-oriented policing and intelligence-led policing. Each entails movement towards a position in which police take anticipatory action, by adopting and enacting a broader approach to their objectives that will address underlying problems associated with the occurrence of crime, with the objective of reducing the prevalence or seriousness of those problems. To our knowledge, no one is sufficiently optimistic or naïve to imagine crime can be eradicated completely. But there is substantial evidence that the rate of it can be reduced by some kinds of preventive effort.

*Community policing* was influenced by a growing recognition that the relationship between police and the communities they served was often unsatisfactory and was driven by attempts to improve this to reduce the perceived distance between the two and improve levels of cooperation. While there was a coherent aspiration and philosophy underpinning this, in practice it took many diverse shapes. That was partly due to the amorphous definition of the term community which can encompass an enormous mix of ideas, and partly because however defined, communities themselves vary in numerous ways. Furthermore, those who attend community meetings to raise policing issues may not be representative of the population of a local area (Vitale, 2018). One aspect of redressing these imbalances involved a process of decentralization of police personnel, increasing local accessibility by, for example, installing sub-stations in dispersed areas or establishing neighbourhood teams. A different aspect involved police reaching out to other community-based organizations, creating more active connections with localized services, from public agencies such as schools, hospitals or social work departments, through charitable or third-sector organizations, to self-help neighbourhood groups. From the early 1990s onwards, community policing became increasingly popular and widely disseminated as an approach both in the USA and many other countries (Gill et al., 2014).

*Problem-oriented policing* by contrast took as its starting point the challenge that the demands on police often far exceed the resources available to meet them. In some localities or at some moments, police can be overwhelmed by the expectations placed on them. Rather than respond to problems when they arise as in reactive policing, the objective becomes being able to identify and address the underlying issues that produce them. This requires a more analytical and strategic conception of the policing task and clearer and more precise specification of the nature of problems that appear. Conceptually this makes use of the model of the *crime triangle*, a reciprocal or multidirectional dynamic interplay between offenders, victims and locations (Tilley, 2008). That is drawn from the *routine activity theory* of crime first articulated by Cohen and Felson (1979), where crime is understood as deriving from the convergence of "a likely offender, a suitable target, and the absence of a capable guardian against the offense" with the result that "opportunity is a root cause of crime" (Felson & Eckert, 2019, pp. 27, 36). This model is one of the foundations of the range of methods collectively known as *situational crime prevention*, for which Laycock (2017) enumerates a list of 25 different techniques.

Laycock (2017) also considers that the problem-oriented model of policing is in essence a translation of the scientific method into police work. As she has commented, "Policing has traditionally been a craft occupation led by something akin to an apprenticeship rather than being a profession supported by research-based knowledge with an ethical foundation" (Laycock, 2017, p. 533). As a policing strategy, first espoused by Goldstein (1979), problem-oriented policing was based on his suggestion that law enforcement, which many might see as the core task of policing, is a means to an end rather than an end in itself. If the objective is to have the law obeyed, the task of policing can be reconceptualized to focus on the problems which get in the way of that and find a means to solve them. But as Scott et al. (2017, p. 228) note, the ends of policing are "neither clear nor simple". Scott et al. provide a detailed account of the operation of problem-oriented policing which brings out the preventive nature of effective policing and how achieving its goals need not be dependent on the use of the criminal justice system as the only route to doing so.

*Intelligence-led policing* while overlapping with this has some additional features. In many respects this orientation is farthest removed from the responsive, event-focused mode of reactive policing where incidents are dealt with one at a time. It requires the systematic assembly and analysis of data on patterns of crime and criminal activity, on where and how the law is being broken, often focused on the identification of offender networks. Doing so then leads to the design and adoption of preventive measures, based on the intelligence that has been gathered (Carter & Carter, 2009; Maguire & John, 2006). Tilley (2008, p. 383) has characterized this as "a way of doing police business", and amongst other changes it has been instrumental in the UK in the establishment and dissemination of the National Intelligence Model. Formulated by the former Association of Chief Police Officers (ACPO, now the National Police Chief's Council), this was implemented in all police areas from 2000 onwards and is now an integral component of police practice, working to prescribed standards. As outlined by the College of Policing (2020), this is designed to generate a set of "core intelligence products" that can be used for tactical decision-making in police operations.

Achieving the objectives of both intelligence-led and problem-oriented policing relies on *crime analysis*, the collection and interpretation of data on the patterning of different types of law-breaking behaviour (Hirschfield, 2017). Recording and analysis of crime data contribute directly to shaping a potentially valuable preventive tool, as the first stage in accomplishing this is to understand the patterning of crime. For a clear picture of that, it is imperative to know *when* and *where* crime occurs, *how* it is carried out and *who* is likely to be involved. Answering the question *why* requires other levels of information. We can go some distance in reducing the likelihood of criminal events if we can assemble information on their occurrence. That would conform to the type of understanding that Tilley and Sidebottom (2017) class as theory light or even atheoretical. But if we seek to have an impact on the problems and related variables that have causal relationships to crime, we need an understanding of the mechanisms that are at work in its occurrence.

## 1.4 An Evidence Base for Policing

The concept of evidence-based policing, introduced by Sherman (1998, 2013, 2015), presents a different perspective on the possibilities for envisaging how police go about their work. It is one that applies across the entire spectrum of innovations in how to pursue the task of policing society. It is not a method of policing as such: rather it is an "overarching category" (Telep & Weisburd, 2016, p. 160) for helping to decide what policing can best consist of. Adopting a stance that has become influential, indeed pivotal, across virtually the whole field of human services, from medicine and healthcare to education, social work and other areas of criminal justice such as probation, an evidence-based approach is concerned with operational issues of what is done and how, but more fundamentally also addresses the question of why decisions are made to do some things rather than others. What are the choices we make informed by and based upon, if it is not a body of relevant knowledge generated by using the methods of empirical science?

In evidence-based policing, senior police managers review external research, or conduct or commission studies of their own, and then apply the best available evidence to inform the policies they adopt and the practices they implement. The approach may also be used to question and challenge existing practices that appear to have weak or non-existent effects, or to explore whether the same objective could be accomplished more efficiently in other ways. Regarding the attempt to gather evidence about the effectiveness of different kinds of police action, that may be done internally, that is, carried out by police research departments. Alternatively, or in addition, it can be facilitated by collaboration with external academic partners or other specialist agencies. We trust that the present volume is a useful illustration of the latter.

Research can serve two key purposes. The first, which might loosely be called basic research, is designed to generate an understanding of a problem, by mapping out the dimensions and patterning of it. That would include recording its response to changes in policing over time, or to other factors believed to influence it, with a view to determining possible causes – or hypotheses about them that can then be tested. Ideally the process is one of articulating "the conditions (or context) for the activation or deactivation of relevant causal mechanisms" (Tilley & Sidebottom, 2017, p. 5) and of testing the soundness of such ideas in empirical work. Doing this is a prerequisite of the second purpose, which focuses more on outcomes. Here the main concern is to examine the effects of a planned intervention. That could be done by studying the impact of a change in policing manoeuvres or in the evaluation of specialized services, such as crisis interventions teams, as was done, for example, by the Chicago Police Department in responding to crises in the lives of people with mental health problems (Watson, 2010). Going a step farther it could entail conducting carefully controlled field experiments of the impact of a particular innovation, such as the use of body-worn cameras (Ariel et al., 2014). Randomized experiments have been used in the evaluation of a number of policing innovations, although quasi-experiments, where allocation to different study conditions is not done randomly, are more frequent.

Focusing on the larger implications of adopting an evidence-based viewpoint, Weisburd and Neyroud (2011) considered that in the past the relationship between policing and science was disconnected. They advocated an objective of building and strengthening that association, part of which would require improving links between police and other bodies such as universities. But beyond this, they proposed the nurturing of a new paradigm, in which police services themselves took ownership of police science and of a scientific orientation to their task. The weak linkages that have been the norm in the past are of course partly manifestations of the significantly lower amounts of funding made available to research in criminal justice compared to the sums spent in other fields. But rather than regarding science as a luxury, police should strive to have a closer affiliation with it and to embrace science-based policing.

As has happened in healthcare and other settings where evidence-based practice has come to the fore, the word *evidence* ought not to be used uncritically. The value of research findings can be placed in a hierarchy according to the level of confidence that we are able to place in them. That is usually a function of several factors, notably the nature and clarity of the question that has been asked, followed by the appropriateness and the quality or robustness of the methodology used to conduct the inquiry. It is also related simply to the amount of work that has been done on a given question and, once that achieves a certain critical mass, on how it can be integrated and interpreted through research review.

The standard route to knowledge-building follows an agreed series of steps. Separate pieces of research or individual projects are called *primary studies*. Many different forms or *designs* of research can be used for the purpose of evaluating interventions, and examples of several of them can be found in the reports that are summarized in the chapters of this book. The most important and most frequently encountered are the following.

***Randomized controlled trial (RCT).*** In this type of design, a set of units (usually individuals) is divided randomly with one portion being delivered the planned intervention (the experimental or treatment condition) and another not (the comparison or control condition). The two conditions are then statistically compared. In a *cluster RCT*, groups of individuals or separate sites (like schools, neighbourhoods) are randomized. More elaborate RCTs can be designed to compare different active treatments alongside each other.

***Quasi-experimental or non-equivalent design*** Where allocation to conditions cannot be done on a random basis, for organizational or ethical reasons, two or more conditions can be compared with each other and statistical adjustments made to take account of other likely pre-existing differences between them.

***Before-and-after design*** Where no relevant comparison condition is available or feasible, measures can simply be made before and after a change is introduced to test for differences, sometimes with the addition of follow-up measurement at some later point to test if an observed change has been maintained.

***Interrupted time-series design*** In a time-series design, data are collected at many measurement points (e.g. daily, weekly) to examine the trend in some variable. In an *interrupted* version of this, tests are made to evaluate the impact of a change that is introduced. This is similar to a before-and after design but involves many more data collection points, allowing greater sensitivity to the effect of change when it occurs.

***Qualitative research studies*** While less directly focused on outcomes, studies using qualitative methods, such as detailed, in-depth interviews or group discussions, can reveal aspects of beliefs or perceptions or identify processes that influence change, in ways that are not generally accessible in quantitative evaluation research.

Once an adequate number of primary studies has been amassed relating to a given question, they can be gathered together to test whether it can be answered or to what extent a pattern emerges that points to a likely answer. It is widely accepted that, while primary research is obviously indispensable, it is a mistake to draw conclusions from any single study without taking account of the results of other studies that have investigated the same question. That process is called research review, and a formal set of procedures has been developed for it, known as *systematic review*. In some circumstances it is possible to combine and integrate the data from several primary studies and carry out a statistical review or *meta-analysis*. At an even higher level, the findings of multiple reviews can be brought together to assemble a larger picture of the state of knowledge on a given question, producing "reviews of reviews". If sufficiently coherent they can be used for *translational* purposes, that is, in the format of *practice guidelines*, sets of statements which can help shape approaches to problems, practitioner training and management decisions. We will encounter examples of each of these in later chapters of the book. The process of research review and how it can contribute to policing is described by Bowers et al. (2017), and Lum and Koper (2017) outline a framework for *translational criminology* whereby research-based knowledge can be used to develop "operationally useful guidance for police agencies" (p. 276).

If several well-designed experiments unanimously point towards a particular finding, conclusions will be easier to draw. As most police and other researchers know however, that is a rare occurrence, given the complexity of the issues to be addressed in law and criminal justice. In the reverse scenario, where there is little formal research or perhaps none at all, other evidence such as expert opinion or a consensus of professional experience can be taken as a provisional guideline until more systematic data become available. In the more common intermediate position, where some findings appear to be at odds with others, the differences could be and often are due to variations in context. There may be no general answer to the question that has been asked, and any solution may have to be adapted to the environments and circumstances prevailing in separate places or at discrete times.

A substantial quantity of research has now been conducted applying an evidence-based lens, examining the outcomes of different policing approaches to crime in general and to specific types of it. The multiplicity of available methods is such that some overarching framework can be helpful for organizing this conceptually, to bring coherence to it. Weisburd and Eck (2004) proposed a typology of advances in police practices, classifying them in terms of two dimensions. One pertained to the *diversity of approach*, which referred to the content of policing methods, where traditional law enforcement (the previously outlined standard model) represented the simplest method with one strategy predominant, while community policing utilized a range of strategies. The other was concerned with the *level of focus*, meaning the extent of targeting of police activities.

Subsequently Lum et al. (2011) devised a framework for systematizing the steadily enlarging assortment of methods that can be deployed in policing and located them in a three-dimensional space. The *crime prevention matrix* categorizes police interventions in terms of (a) the breadth of their selected target, from individuals via micro-places and neighbourhoods all the way to the entire nation, (b) the level of specificity of the prevention mechanisms they are designed to activate and (c) where they stand on a continuum with respect to their level of reactivity versus proactivity. Lum et al. then populated the three-dimensional space with results from 97 evaluation studies. They are divided into groups according to their effect on crime: whether they had a significant positive effect, a non-significant effect, mixed effects or a significant negative or counter-productive *backfire* effect. The resultant configuration of results showed that "proactive, focused, place-based interventions are more likely to reduce crime and disorder than strategies concentrating on individuals, or those that are reactive and/or general in nature" (Lum et al., 2011, p. 20). The matrix was designed to have the advantage of being open-ended so that new studies could be inserted as they appeared.

## 1.5 Evaluating Police Effectiveness

There have now been numerous reviews of the overall effectiveness of police practices as a means of achieving crime prevention or ensuring public safety, and as we will see later it has become a central concern of police services to monitor this aspect of their performance. But in one sense it could seem puzzling that such a question can be asked. Surely the police must be effective, or society would be overrun by criminality, and in a permanent state of disorder. We are confronted with grim scenes of that kind when there is a general breakdown of law and order in some locations, with widespread looting, mayhem and violence. These are usually caused by major ruptures, from calamities such as earthquakes, cyclones or tsunamis to civil wars, insurrections or *coups d'états*.

But even following extreme events, whether or not there is an upsurge in crime depends on a large number of variables. Historical analysis of incidents such as police strikes and work slowdowns (go-slows), which are highly unusual but have happened at times, does not support the expectation, sometimes called the *thin blue line hypothesis*, that there will inevitably be societal breakdown and chaos as a result. Analyses of such events in the USA and in Finland have found that in most cases the absence of police on its own, when other conditions remained stable, had no more than a marginal effect on the volume of crime (Chandrasekher, 2016; Makinen & Takala, 1980; Pfuhl, 1983). Where more serious disorder did occur, it was precipitated by economic or political disruption outside the control of the police (White, 1988). These counter-intuitive findings may be explicable not in terms of most citizens' fears of legal sanction if they break the law, but of their respect for its legitimacy and attendant willingness to comply with its edicts the majority of the time (McAdams, 2017; Tyler, 2006). This also connects to the view of Scott et al. (2017) outlined earlier, to the effect that notwithstanding its massive power, the criminal justice system is only one amongst many influences on people's behaviour.

Concerning the reverse scenario, Sherman (1990) reviewed 18 studies in which police imposed crackdowns on particular sorts of crimes. These combined three tactical elements, which were announced to the public: increased officer presence, greater usage of sanctions, and threats of increased sanction certainty. In five of six studies of short-term crackdowns (<6 months) on vehicle-related offences, residual effects were observed: that is, the effect continued after the police back off from the exercise. But in 12 longer-term experiments focused on more serious offences such as drug sales and trafficking, only 2 studies obtained residual effects. In another two, there was disturbing evidence that other groups of crimes had increased, including homicides associated with illegal drug markets.

Alongside this, many hundreds of studies have been reported that examine the relationship between different policing indicators such as the numbers of police personnel or amounts of money spent on policing and crime rates. The assembled evidence pertaining to this, obtained by a variety of methods, shows a perplexing mix of findings. In the best attempt to date to resolve such discrepancies, Carriaga and Worrall (2015) carried out a systematic review of 24 well-designed studies, of which it was possible to conduct a meta-analysis of 12. The policing variable was either the number of sworn officers per capita or some measure of spending per capita for the population in the respective administrative district (city, county or state). Crime rate per 100,000 people was based on the FBI Uniform Crime Reports. The relationship between the two sets of variables was calculated for total crime, violent crime, property crime and seven index offences – homicide, rape, robbery, assault, burglary, larceny and motor vehicle theft. The relationship was examined over time, not cross-sectionally (i.e. comparing places at a single point in time).

For crime overall, there was a statistically significant but comparatively small inverse association between police variables and the crime rate. Broadly therefore, more police personnel or money spent on policing was correlated with a lower rate of crime. However, none of the associations was significant for any other crime variable. All were very close to zero and for two – homicide and rape – the association was positive rather than the other way around, that is, with numbers of offences increasing. While there is evidence of a connection here, it is relatively weak given the taken-for-granted assumption that crime is only kept at bay due to the relentless efforts of the police.

Whether or not policing automatically achieves the results that the public assume are attributable to it therefore becomes an open question. That having been said, detailed examination of the effects of police strategies and practices does demonstrate significant positive outcomes. Broadly speaking, the results of evidence-based policing research show almost consistently better outcomes for the newer forms of policing summarized above than for the traditional crime-fighting format it had for many decades before. Conversely, the concept of good policing as consisting of increased officer presence through routine patrol and surveillance does not receive a great deal of empirical support.

For example, Mazerolle et al. (2006) reported a series of meta-analyses of 14 studies that compared different policing approaches to the problem of street-level drug crime. They used the framework developed by Weisburd and Eck (2004) outlined earlier. Each of the approaches showed some benefits, but problem-oriented policing that involved forging partnerships with third parties yielded more positive outcomes than unfocused law enforcement with simple increased presence. Sullivan and O'Keefe (2017) found effects that challenged earlier enthusiasm for the well-known "fixing broken windows" formula that had been relied on for some years by the New York Police Department (NYPD). This entailed an extensive use of arrest for low-level offending and other tactics compatible with proactive, aggressive policing, founded on the principle that reducing the rate of minor crimes would through a chain of events also lower the rate of more serious ones. The opportunity to evaluate the validity of this arose in late 2014 when the NYPD had a police slowdown as part of a dispute between employers and unions. The effect on complaints of serious crimes was the opposite of what was expected. Taking account of other factors that may have influenced the observed change, the impact of the slowdown in policing of low-level events was a fall in reports of more serious ones.

Similar findings have emerged both from overall policing effectiveness research and from evaluations more closely targeted on specific methods and practices. Telep and Weisburd (2012, 2016; see also Weisburd et al. 2017) reported a large and wide-ranging overview of 17 systematic reviews of police work encompassing numerous approaches to it. They included street-level drug enforcement, community policing, problem-oriented policing and several other initiatives. The pattern of outcomes indicated that the police are "most effective when they focus on high-activity people and places", when they "focus in particular on proactive problem-solving" and when they do not "rely exclusively on law enforcement and arrest" (Weisburd et al., 2016, p. 164). They are more likely to obtain superior results when they metaphorically expand the toolbox by fostering collaborative alliances with other community agencies.

Findings that parallel these have been obtained in other reviews that have compared policing methods. Braga et al. (2015), for example, located 28 studies that were concerned with policing disorderly localities, varying in size from single buildings to whole police precincts. Across the 30 statistical comparisons that could be made, there were "noteworthy crime control gains" (p. 580) in reducing violent, property, disorder and drug-related crimes. Policing interventions were grouped into two types, one consisting of community problem-solving programmes, the other aggressive order-maintenance programmes. The former outperformed the latter by a large margin, and the mean effect was statistically significant, whereas for the latter it was not.

The procedures that compose community policing are less well defined and its effects are more diffuse than for other policing approaches. Perhaps more importantly, its success depends on aspects of communities which vary in the services they require. This makes it more difficult to evaluate than policing methods that have a more precise focus. Hence, when Gill et al. (2014) carried out a systematic review of its effects, they examined a variety of outcomes. They surveyed results from 25 studies that between them reported a total of 65 tests of comparative outcomes, and were able to conduct a meta-analysis of 37 of the latter. Their degree of success varied by category of outcome. Percentages of studies showing effective outcomes were as follows: for citizen satisfaction 78%, for perceived legitimacy of police 60%, but for fear of crime 44% and official records of crime, 36%. When the last of these was analysed statistically, the effect on crime was only significant for violent and not for property crimes, and the former effect was very small.

With regard to community policing therefore, "findings are ambiguous" (Gill et al., 2014, p. 419). But while the approach performs more weakly than other more precisely directed strategies for crime reduction, it has strengths in promoting positive perceptions of police. Crowl (2017) reviewed a set of 27 studies containing a total of 70 independent comparisons. This found the strongest evidence for citizen satisfaction with police, and perceptions of police legitimacy, but a more varied pattern for effects on fear of crime, and job satisfaction amongst police officers, and only very limited evidence of impact on officially recorded crime.

Ranging widely over the spectrum of issues linked to community policing, Kapeller et al. (2020) considered its respective benefits and challenges. While its direct effects in relation to crime reduction were uncertain, it appeared important for maintaining healthy police-community relations. Kapeller et al. (2020) were firm in dispelling impressions that the approach was in any sense soft on crime as good police-community links were associated with overall better crime control, but the parameters of this had not yet been clarified in specific ways.

The specific effectiveness of the problem-oriented policing (POP) approach has also been appraised. In an initial review Weisburd et al. (2010) located ten studies, four of them randomized experiments, and found a positive and statistically significant, but modest effect of problem-oriented strategies. Amongst a separate set of 45 pre-post or before-and-after uncontrolled studies, that is with no comparison condition, there was an overwhelming support for the effectiveness of POP: on average a 44% decrease in measures of crime or disorder. However, those are regarded as weaker research designs.

A later, updated and larger review by Hinkle et al. (2020) added a further 24 experimental studies to those found by Weisburd et al. (2010), making a total of 34. This review found an impressive mean reduction of almost 34% in rates of crime and disorder in POP areas as compared to control areas. The authors concluded that their findings "support the notion that proactive policing strategies that identify specific problems, conduct analyses to determine underlying causes, and develop and deliver tailor-made responses, are more effective in reducing crime and disorder than standard, reactive methods of policing" (Hinkle et al., 2020, p. 3). The findings showed considerable heterogeneity, but this is not surprising given the range of problems addressed and the differing contexts in which the work was done. Results related to secondary outcomes such as fear of crime were fewer in number, but of eight studies that examined this, most found no impact. Another eight studies that undertook cost-benefit calculations found that problem-oriented policing "was associated with a substantial costs savings" (Hinkle et al., 2020, p. 42).

There is a caveat to interpretation of these findings, concerning the fidelity of implementation of problem-oriented policing interventions. A study by Hassell and Lovell (2015) inside one police department found that despite official claims, the problem-solving approach was not being properly employed. Weisburd et al. (2010) had noted this problem in some of the studies they reviewed, but Hinkle et al. (2020) were able to check this more fully and did not report it as a concern. It is a rudimentary but crucial question in all evaluation research as to whether a method supposedly being tested is genuinely being delivered, and whether that is happening as intended.

One specialized variant, a synthesis of the intelligence-led and problem-oriented approaches, is *hot spots* or *place-based* policing, in which attention is concentrated on specific locations where there have been high frequencies of crime. In a series of reviews, Braga and his colleagues have drawn together evaluations of this approach (Braga, 2005; Braga et al., 2014; Braga et al., 2019). Their largest review collated 65 studies, including 27 randomized controlled trials and 38 quasi-experiments. They came from 9 countries, producing 78 tests of the effectiveness of hot spot interventions. The overall result was positive in terms of crime reduction, though the effect size was not large. There were statistically significant reductions in violent, property and drug crimes and in public disorder. The positive outcomes of this are thought to derive in part from the restriction in crime opportunities that occurs, and deterrence through perceived heightened likelihood of arrest. Once again, problem-oriented policing interventions produced "a modestly larger overall mean effect" (p. 303) than that found for traditional policing methods.

A recurring issue over localized interventions such as this is whether a problem at one spot decreases because criminal activity has simply transferred elsewhere, the problem of *displacement*. The review by Braga et al. (2019, p. 300) found instead that there was a small, but statistically significant "diffusion of crime control benefits" effect. Other reviews of research on crime displacement patterns (Bowers et al., 2011; Johnson et al., 2014) have also found that displacement to nearby catchment areas, usually neighbourhoods surrounding the initial hot spot, is by no means inevitable, and a spread of crime reduction effects is just as common.

On a broader level, it is reassuring to discover, as Welsh et al. (2012) have reported, that there is no evidence that the predilections or preferences of researchers involved in the evaluation of police work have an impact on the findings they report. The phenomenon of *evaluator influence* is known to arise in intervention outcome or evaluation research, particularly when researchers are appraising proposals or methods they themselves have devised. This is an example of what is known as *confirmation bias*, one of several types of bias that can confound the interpretation of research results. It is rarely a matter of blatant dishonesty, such as by massaging or manufacturing data, though that is not entirely unknown. More often it occurs through subtle judgemental processes that are not palpable to the researchers involved, for example, when they allegedly become too invested in a particular outcome. Nevertheless, its existence has led to a certain level of cynicism when reviews are collated, a position which Welsh and colleagues endeavoured to check.

Welsh et al. analysed 42 pieces of research concerned with police-based crime prevention measures, consisting of 9 randomized controlled trials and 33 quasi-experiments (between-group comparisons in which group membership is not allotted on a random basis). In most of them (34/42) an external evaluator was working with the police. Evaluators differed in the extent to which they had been involved in the development of the interventions being tested. While there was a slight tendency for internal police researchers to find larger effects, this was not statistically significant, and overall, there was no discernible association between the intensity of involvement of researchers in any particular outcome and the magnitude of the outcomes that were observed.

As this brief overview indicates, there is now a plethora of ideas concerning how the task of policing can be carried out, and an accumulated body of evidence that supports its efficacy. Given the impetus of many changes in approach that have been adopted by police departments in recent years, and with the added advantages of evidence-based procedures at their disposal, the prospect appears highly favourable of there being significant further enhancements in policing methods and systems. The importance of this is signified in that in England and Wales, *effectiveness* is one of the features of police forces assessed annually by the Inspectorate of Constabulary and Fire and Rescue Services (HMICFRS, 2019), alongside *efficiency* and *legitimacy*. There is every indication that the evidence-based approach has become firmly indeed centrally embedded in modern policing practice.

## 1.6 Advances and Reversals?

Police departments in many respects have been exemplary in adopting useful technological innovations as they have appeared. Historically, that included methods of improving key processes, such as the use of motorized patrol, of two-way radio and of access via telephone calls, all of which have now been construed as standard for many years. More recently this could be seen almost as a distinct definition of the use of an evidence base in policing, in that it involves drawing on results from forensic science (Williams, 2008). This has achieved numerous advances in techniques of detection, from fingerprinting or crime scene photography to electrostatic deposition analysis, DNA matching or genetic fingerprinting, behavioural analysis of crime scenes and tracking of encoded Internet communications. For the criminal investigation components of policing, the value of such research is inestimable and seems unlikely to be questioned. But in addition to the contribution that physical, biological and medical sciences can make to policing, over the past 50 years or so, there have also been major influences from social sciences, including criminology, psychology, social work and allied areas, on other parts of the police's role.

However, notwithstanding the numerous advances that have been made, in some countries and in some critical respects, policing is currently going through a period of acute crisis. It is facing significant challenges and controversies on a number of levels and has been the focus of a degree of concern and criticism that is perhaps unprecedented. A central issue has been that of the often severely strained relationship between police forces and ethnic minority communities, particularly in the USA. Amongst the many dimensions of this was the stark statistic that between the beginning of January 2015 and the end of October 2020, a total of 5740 people were shot dead by US police, with the rate for Black people more than twice that for Whites (Washington Post, 2020). As Vitale (2018) has noted, in the 10 years prior to that, also during which thousands were killed, only 54 police officers were charged as being responsible, of whom just 11 were convicted, serving an average sentence of 4 years (Washington Post, 2015). Adding to the deep and simmering resentment that these and other circumstances created, there followed several highly distressing and lethal incidents in 2020, most notoriously the killing of a black citizen, George Floyd, by a police officer in Minneapolis, that was made instantly visible by mobile telephone images that spread round the world. The subsequent level of protest was such that reactions rapidly became highly politicized and bitterly polarized.

Amongst the calls that emanated from this was one for police departments to be "defunded". This has been interpreted in several ways, the most uncompromising position meaning that police departments should be abolished, or services disbanded, and their entire budgets reassigned to other sectors of public service, such as education or social welfare agencies. That perception and its accompanying anger and fear led to further escalation in conflict. Another interpretation of defunding however renders it not very different from a set of proposals that have been discussed for some time, with more in-depth reviews undertaken in periods of lesser turmoil than of the kind that erupted in 2020.

*Justice reinvestment* refers to a process of re-balancing of expenditure between different sectors of the criminal justice and penal system. In most jurisdictions, most money is spent at what we might call the front end of the system, for example, in England and Wales in 2018–2019 the proportion reserved for policing was 58% (Ford, 2019). There have been intermittent recommendations that there should be a re-balancing of spending priorities, chiefly to reduce the numbers of people incarcerated, but also such that a portion of the policing budget should be re-allocated to preventive services such as social welfare, family support, youth services or more widely in education or mental health. Doing so would allow some of the agencies with whom the police have partnerships to have more resources at their disposal, better enabling them to help achieve policing and broader community goals.

Parallel propositions have been forwarded by researchers who have studied the comparative amounts of spending on different stages of the criminal justice process (Brown et al., 2016), and in the UK the concept of reinvestment has been endorsed by the parliamentary Justice Committee (House of Commons, 2010). There is empirical evidence supporting the proposition that moving in such a direction could potentially lead to a significant reduction in crime. Placing this in a broader context, a report by the White House (Council of Economic Advisers, 2016) reviews evidence that affording wage increases to those at economic disadvantage could have a proportionately larger impact in this respect than spending the money in other ways, such as increasing imprisonment rates or extending sentence lengths. A comprehensive revision of the contours of public investment could result in more appropriate ways to address crime and its relation to other economic and social factors. Perhaps police are being used to in response to problems that are beyond the capacity of their role to solve.

Such an argument has been reinforced and amplified by Vitale (2018) who portrays a picture of both the history and the role of modern policing that differs radically from the conventional, widely accepted one. In the nineteenth century, in Britain and America alike, the prime role of police was "…not fighting crime, but managing disorder and protecting propertied classes from the rabble" (Vitale, 2018, p. 35). That their main objective was and continues to be the first of those is a liberal myth. The police have been used as a response to threats to social order in a way that does not resolve any of the underlying problems, but merely preserves hierarchy in ways that benefit some people far more than others. Vitale proposes not reforms with the nature of a "technocratic fix" but ones that form part of a larger vision that redefines the basic mission of the police (p. 221). He argues that greater public safety and security would be more effectively provided through creation of employment opportunities and investment in decent and affordable housing, education and community services.

Given the formidable challenges of these tasks and the expectations of the public regarding many different aspects of police performance, there have been a number of high-level analyses and re-appraisals undertaken to identify the key objectives of police work and to make recommendations concerning how it can most effectively and most efficiently be pursued in the context of current challenges.

At the time of writing, such a goal is currently being pursued in England and Wales. One expression of this is in the *Strategic Review of Policing 2020*, a response to the numerous multilevel changes that have taken place over recent years both in police services and in society. The police are widely considered to require radical reform, and there is recognition that the process of doing this should itself be evidence-led. Preliminary documents for the *Review* state its objective as being to set a long-term strategic direction for twenty-first-century policing (Barber, 2020). For example, most calls to the police are not related to crime (College of Policing, 2015), and there is increasing momentum to move still further beyond reactive policing to problem-oriented and other approaches to the task and the role. Documents also propose that the police should engage with the arguments behind the defund movement. It is acknowledged that police services have lost substantial funding over the period 2010–2020, without that having been invested anywhere in preventive services, as supporters of defunding would have sought. The first phase of the review was scheduled for completion by the middle of 2021.

## 1.7 The Present Volume

We began this chapter by emphasizing the uneven evolution of police work, sometimes rapid and disorderly, at other times more gradual and measured. As one of the markers of further recent change in the UK, following the creation of the new roles of Police and Crime Commissioners (PCCs) in 2012, another new agency was also established – the College of Policing, formed from the National Police Improvement Agency (which had been founded in 2007). Part of the remit of the College since its inception has been to work with research agencies, including the Higher Education Funding Council for England and Wales, to commission research projects from academic partners.

To place this volume in the context in which the work was done, it formed part of two inter-related research projects of this kind, carried out by a consortium of universities and independent research organizations for two police forces, respectively, in the counties of Norfolk and Suffolk. It is one of the products of a 3-year research programme involving a collaboration between four academic organizations, the universities of Nottingham, Birmingham, Liverpool and Suffolk, and two independent research organizations, CREST Analytics and Skills for Justice.

The activities that comprised the project were allocated into a series of work packages, one of which involved conducting a series of evidence reviews and preparation of reports. These addressed topics identified by police services themselves, through a project Executive Board that included Chief Constables and other senior staff and service-based police researchers. That portion of the project was undertaken by the authors of the present book, and over the course of the research, a total of 13 such reviews was completed. The contents of the book therefore consist of a summation of the major part of that work, incorporating a series of research reports (all originally in a similar format), edited into book form. As three of the research reviews retrieved relatively little evidence in the designated areas, the book consists of ten chapters based on the reviews that located more primary studies (original pieces of research) and yielded fuller sets of results. The present, introductory chapter was designed to explain the background to the work and to outline several key models of policing. In the succeeding chapters therefore, we address a series of ten sets of problems that were given priority in the research project just described. To conclude the book, a final closing chapter then draws out key lessons from the findings and seeks to highlight potential future directions and developments.

Chapters adopt a similar format resembling the structure of a research report, but with some elements removed to fit better with the requirements of a book. Each of the areas identified is approached first by defining the key questions to be addressed. Davies (2011) emphasizes that, for evidence-based practice purposes, a vital starting point centres on the importance of being able to state clear questions. We then proceed by describing how the relevant research material was located. The latter included collating any previously published reviews of the area in focus, followed by collation and review of the findings of primary studies published subsequently. There are some recurrent limitations within this that reappear throughout. Notably, we were able only to review research available in English or translated into English, and we also excluded unpublished research dissertations. Other kinds of limitations vary from area to area depending on the quantity and quality of research that has been published. In each area, where relevant information was accessible, we report an appraisal of the methodological rigour of the research that we locate. For some areas however, the heterogeneity of research methods was such that meaningful comparisons were difficult to make.

We then draw both pre-existing reviews and new primary studies together to construct the best body of evidence that can inform police work pertaining to the area in question. As far as possible this process was guided by use of the PICO model, employed in other areas of research review. This involves specifying the kinds of information to be collected and analysed under four headings: the *Population* (or participants) to be studied, the *Intervention* (or indicator) to be investigated, the *Comparison* (or control) alongside which it can be meaningfully evaluated and the *Outcomes* that have been measured or recorded.

In most cases, outcomes (findings or results) are presented in tabular form, extracting and reporting key information from the located studies. Finally, efforts are made to summarize the pattern of results and highlight key points that can be concluded from the review, taking specific account of the level of confidence that can be placed in each conclusion.

The reviews that formed part of the research project were undertaken consecutively in the period 2014–2017. One, which forms the content of Chap. 11, took the form of a *scoping* review, which is a more limited process used in surveying areas where there is relatively less formal research and no review has been published previously. In other areas that were more fully researched, for the purpose of converting this to book format, it was not possible to follow the detailed review procedures employed during the project itself. Instead, a less extensive method of updating was adopted, confined to the databases that had generated most material in the initial reviews, using a more restricted set of search terms, and designed to locate research reviews and empirical evaluations of interventions that had involved the police.

Accompanying this, as an additional check a search was carried out of the tables of contents of nine leading police research journals for the 6-year period 2015–2020. The journals were *Cambridge Journal of Evidence-Based Policing*, *International Journal of Police Science and Management*, *Journal of Police and Criminal Psychology*, *Policing: A Journal of Policy and Practice*, *Policing: An International Journal of Police Strategies & Management*, *Policing and Society: An International Journal of Research and Policy*, *Police Practice and Research: An International Journal*, *Policing Quarterly* and *The Police Journal*. This process located a total of

87 articles that appeared relevant to one or more of the areas covered in the book, though on screening the number reduced in most areas.

Applying this model, the volume examines implications for policing of the results obtained in relation to the challenges to be faced, and those fell into three broad areas. The first is directly connected to different aspects or contexts of the focus of this book series, the problem of violence – in the night-time economy, in family homes, between intimate partners or occurring in schools and in the prospects for early intervention to reduce the likelihood of more serious crimes at later stages. The second addresses issues that arise in dealing with people who manifest different kinds of vulnerability such as mental health problems or who are in need of safeguarding. The third is concerned with victims and witnesses of crime: in the provision of support to them and in seeking to ensure their participation in the criminal justice process as cases proceed toward court hearings. While some of the latter areas may have a less immediate link with violence, they are closely associated with its consequences or with broader approaches to preventing its recurrence.

The book is designed as a sourcebook or reference resource which we hope will prove informative for the practice of policing. Clearly however, the demands made upon police forces are immense, covering almost any area of activity that is regulated by law. The selection of areas covered herein was determined by the practical, operational policing priorities of two police departments in England. The contents of the book thus genuinely reflect ongoing concerns of police officers. In relation to some questions that were raised, there was very little evidence discovered that could be sufficient to inform police practice and decision-making, and these have been omitted from the book. Other areas could potentially have been included, but the limits of any commissioned project are such that not everything that either police or researchers would like to do can be done. We are aware of empirical work in several areas not considered here and hope that further volumes may draw that evidence together making it available for use in book form.

To complete the book, a closing chapter attempts to summarize some general conclusions we believe can be drawn taking the material reviewed here as a whole, and we attempt to identify some key lessons learnt from the process and from the findings overall. On that basis we also suggest potential next steps in the process of consolidating and expanding the knowledge base, but more broadly we reflect on what implications this may have for policing viewed from an evidence-based perspective.

As authors we hope that the book will be a useful, accessible and valuable resource for senior police managers, police officers, researchers, academics, practitioners and advisors, as well as graduate students in the fields of police science, criminology, criminal justice studies, law, forensic psychology, social work and community development.

## References


Ariel, B., Farrar, W. A., & Sutherland, A. (2014). The effect of police body-worn cameras on use of force and citizens' complaints against the police: A randomized controlled trial. *Journal of Quantitative Criminology, 31*, 509–535.

Ayee, J. R. A. (2015). Ghana: Reducing police corruption and promoting police professionalism through reforms. In K. R. Hope (Ed.), *Police corruption and police reforms in developing societies* (pp. 65–84). CRC Press.

Barber, M. (2020). *Public safety and security in the 21st century: The first report of the strategic review of policing in England and Wales*. The Police Foundation.

Bauschatz, J. (2007). The strong arm of the law? Police corruption in Ptolemaic Egypt. *The Classical Journal, 103*(1), 13–19.

Bowers, K., Johnson, S., Guerette, R. T., Summers, L., & Poynton, S. (2011). Spatial displacement and diffusion of benefits among geographically focused policing initiatives: A meta-analytical review. *Journal of Experimental Criminology, 7*(4), 347–374.

Bowers, K., Tompson, L., Sidebottom, A., Bullock, K., & Johnson, S. D. (2017). Reviewing evidence for evidence-based policing. pp. 98–116. In J. Knutsson & L. Tompson (Eds.), *Advances in evidence-based policing*. Routledge.

Bowling, B., & Sheptycki, J. (2012). *Global policing*. Sage Publications.

Braga, A. A. (2005). Hot spots policing and crime prevention: A systematic review of randomized controlled trials. *Journal of Experimental Criminology, 1*, 317–342.

Braga, A. A., Papachristos, A. V., & Hureau, D. M. (2014). The effects of hot spots policing on crime: An updated systematic review and meta-analysis. *Justice Quarterly, 31*(4), 633–663.

Braga, A. A., Turchan, B. S., Papachristos, A. V., & Hureau, D. M. (2019). Hot spots policing and crime reduction: An update of an ongoing systematic review and meta-analysis. *Journal of Experimental Criminology, 15*, 289–311.

Braga, A. A., Welsh, B. C., & Schnell, C. (2015). Can policing disorder reduce crime? A systematic review and meta-analysis. *Journal of Research on Crime and Delinquency, 52*, 567–588.

Brown, D., Cuneen, C., Schwartz, M., Stubbs, J., & Young, C. (2016). *Justice reinvestment: Winding Back imprisonment*. Palgrave Macmillan.

Carriaga, M. L., & Worrall, J. L. (2015). Police levels and crime: A systematic review and meta-analysis. *Police Journal: Theory, Practice and Principles, 88*(4), 315–333.

Carter, D. L., & Carter, J. G. (2009). Intelligence-led policing: Conceptual and functional considerations for public policy. *Criminal Justice Policy Review, 20*(3), 310–325.

Chandrasekher, A. C. (2016). The effect of police slowdowns on crime. *American Law and Economics Review, 18*(2), 385–437.

Cohen, L. E., & Felson, M. (1979). Social change and crime rate trends: A routine activity approach. *American Sociological Review, 44*, 588–608.

College of Policing (2015). *College of policing analysis: Estimating demand on the police service*. https://www.college.police.uk/About/Pages/Demand-Analysis-Report.aspx

College of Policing (2020). *Intelligence management*. https://www.app.college.police.uk/app-content/intelligence-management/analysis/intelligence-products/

Council of Economic Advisers. (2016). *Economic perspectives on incarceration and the criminal justice system*. Council of Economic Advisers, Executive Office of the President of the United States.

Crowl, J. N. (2017). The effect of community policing on fear and crime reduction, police legitimacy and job satisfaction: An empirical review of the evidence. *Police Practice and Research, 18*(5), 449–462.

Davies, K. S. (2011). Formulating the evidence based practice question: A review of the frameworks. *Evidence Based Library and Information Practice, 6*(2), 75–80.

Emsley, C. (2008). The birth and development of the police. In T. Newburn (Ed.), *Handbook of policing* (2nd ed., pp. 72–89). Willan Publishing.

Felson, M., & Eckert, M. A. (2019). *Crime and everyday life: A brief introduction* (6th ed.). Sage.

Ford, M. (2019). *Trends in criminal justice spending, staffing and populations 2008–2009 to 2017–2018*. UK Justice Policy Review Focus, Issues 5. London: Centre for Crime and Justice Studies.

Gill, C., Weisburd, D., Telep, C. W., Vitter, Z., & Bennett, T. (2014). Community-oriented policing to reduce crime, disorder and fear and increase satisfaction and legitimacy among citizens: A systematic review. *Journal of Experimental Criminology, 10*, 399–428.

Goldstein, H. (1979). Improving policing: A problem-oriented approach. *Crime and Delinquency, 25*, 236–258.

Hadden, S. E. (1999). Colonial and revolutionary era slave patrols in Virginia. In M. A. Bellesiles (Ed.), *Lethal imagination: Violence and brutality in American history* (pp. 69–85). New York University Press.

Hadden, S. E. (2003). *Slave patrols: Law and violence in Virginia and the Carolinas*. Harvard University Press.

Harrendorf, S., & Smit, P. (2010). Attributes of criminal justice systems: Resources, performance and punitivity. In S. Harrendorf, M. Heiskanen, & S. Malby (Eds.), *International statistics on crime and justice* (pp. 113–151). HEUNI Publication Series No. 64. Helsinki and Vienna: European Institute for Crime Prevention and Control (HEUNI) and the United Nations Office on Drugs and Crime (UNODC).

Hassell, K. D., & Lovell, R. D. (2015). Fidelity of implementation: Important considerations for policing scholars. *Policing and Society, 25*(5), 504–520.

Her Majesty's Inspectorate of Constabulary and Fire and Rescue Services (HMICFRS). (2019). *PEEL assessments 2018/2019*. https://www.justiceinspectorates.gov.uk/hmicfrs/peel-assessments/peel-2018/

Hinkle, J. C., Weisburd, D., Telep, C. W., & Petersen, K. (2020). Problem-oriented policing for reducing crime and disorder: An updated systematic review and meta-analysis. *Campbell Systematic Reviews, 16*, e1089.

Hirschfield, A. (2017). Analysis for intervention. In N. Tilley & A. Sidebottom (Eds.), *Handbook of crime prevention and community safety* (2nd ed., pp. 491–515). Routledge.

House of Commons Justice Committee (2010). *Cutting crime: the case for justice reinvestment*. First report of session 2009–2010. London: The Stationery Office Limited.

Johnson, S. D., Guerette, R. T., & Bowers, K. (2014). Crime displacement: What we know, what we don't know, and what it means for crime reduction. *Journal of Experimental Criminology, 10*, 549–571.

Joyce, P. (2011). *Policing: Development & Contemporary Practice*. Sage Publications.

Kapeller, V. E., Gaines, L. K., & Schaefer, B. P. (2020). *Community policing: A contemporary perspective* (8th ed.). Routledge/Taylor and Francis.

Laycock, G. (2017). Deciding what to do: Adopting a problem-oriented approach. In N. Tilley & A. Sidebottom (Eds.), *Handbook of crime prevention and community safety* (2nd ed., pp. 516–535). Routledge.

Lum, C., & Koper, C. S. (2017). *Evidence-based policing: Translating research into practice*. Oxford University Press.

Lum, C., Koper, C. S., & Telep, C. W. (2011). The evidence-based policing matrix. *Journal of Experimental Criminology, 7*, 3–26.

Maguire, M. (2008). Criminal investigation and crime control. In T. Newburn (Ed.), *Handbook of policing* (2nd ed., pp. 430–464). Willan Publishing.

Maguire, M., & John, T. (2006). Intelligence led policing, managerialism and community engagement: Competing priorities and the role of the National Intelligence Model in the UK. *Policing and Society, 16*(1), 67–85.

Makinen, T., & Takala, H. (1980). 1976 police strike in Finland. In R. Hauge (Ed.), *Policing Scandinavia*. Universitetsforlaget.

Mark, J. R. (2020). Policing in ancient Egypt. *Ancient History Encyclopedia*, located at: https://brewminate.com/police-in-ancient-egypt/

Mawby, R. I. (2008). Models of policing. In T. Newburn (Ed.), *Handbook of policing* (2nd ed., pp. 14–46). Willan Publishing.

Mazerolle, L., Soole, D. W., & Rombouts, S. (2006). Street-level drug law enforcement: A meta-analytic review. *Journal of Experimental Criminology, 2*, 409–435.

McAdams, R. H. (2017). *The expressive powers of law: Theories and limits*. Harvard University Press.

McLean, K., Wolfe, S. E., Rojek, J., Alpert, G. P., & Smith, M. R. (2019). Police officers as warriors or guardians: Empirical reality or intriguing rhetoric? *Justice Quarterly*. https://doi.org/10.1080/07418825.2018.1533031

Pfuhl, E. H. (1983). Police strikes and conventional crime – A look at the data. *Criminology, 21*(4), 489–504.

Rawlings, P. (2008). Policing before the police. In T. Newburn (Ed.), *Handbook of policing* (2nd ed., pp. 47–71). Willan Publishing.

Rowe, M. (2018). *Introduction to policing* (3rd ed.). Sage Publications.

Scott, M. S., Eck, J. E., Knutsson, J., & Goldstein, H. (2017). Problem-oriented policing. In R. Wortey & M. Townsley (Eds.), *Environmental criminology and crime analysis* (2nd ed., pp. 227–258). Routledge.

Sharma, A. (2004). Police in ancient India. *Indian Journal of Political Science, 65*(1), 101–110. https://www.jstor.org/stable/41855800

Sherman, L. W. (1990). Police crackdowns: Initial and residual deterrence. *Crime and Justice: A Review of Research, 12*, 1–48.

Sherman, L. W. (1998). *Evidence based policing*. Police Foundation.

Sherman, L. W. (2013). The rise of evidence-based policing; targeting, testing, and tracking. *Crime and Justice, 42*(1), 377–451.

Sherman, L. W. (2015). A tipping point for "totally evidenced policing": Ten ideas for building an evidence-based police agency. *International Criminal Justice Review, 25*(1), 11–29.

Sullivan, C. M., & O'Keefe, Z. P. (2017). Evidence that curtailing proactive policing can reduce major crime. *Nature Human Behaviour, 1*, 737–737.

Telep, C. W., & Weisburd, D. (2012). What is known about the effectiveness of police practices in reducing crime and disorder? *Police Quarterly, 15*(4), 331–357.

Telep, C. W., & Weisburd, D. (2016). Policing. In D. Weisburd, D. P. Farrington, & C. Gill (Eds.), *What works in crime prevention and rehabilitation: Lessons from systematic reviews* (pp. 137–168). Springer.

Tilley, N. (2008). Modern approaches to policing: Community, problem-oriented, and intelligence-led. In T. Newburn (Ed.), *Handbook of policing* (2nd ed., pp. 373–403). Willan Publishing.

Tilley, N., & Sidebottom, A. (2017). Theory for crime prevention. In N. Tilley & A. Sidebottom (Eds.), *Handbook of crime prevention and community safety* (2nd ed., pp. 3–21). Routledge.

Tyler, T. R. (2006). *Why people obey the law*. Princeton University Press.

Vitale, A. S. (2018). *The end of policing*. Verso.

*Washington Post* (11 April, 2015). 'Thousands dead, few prosecuted'. https://www.washingtonpost.com/sf/investigative/2015/04/11/thousands-dead-few-prosecuted/

*Washington Post* (30 October, 2020). 'Fatal force: 994 people have been shot and killed by police in the past year'. https://www.washingtonpost.com/graphics/investigations/police-shootings-database/

Watson, A. C. (2010). Research in the real world: Studying Chicago Police Department's crisis intervention team program. *Research on Social Work Practice, 20*(5), 536–543.

Waxman, O. B. (2017). How the U.S. got its police force. *Time*, 18th May.

Weisburd, D., & Eck, J. E. (2004). What can police do to reduce crime, disorder, and fear? *Annals of the American Academy of Political and Social Science, 593*, 42–65.

Weisburd, D., Farrington, D. P., & Gill, C. (Eds.). (2016). *What works in crime prevention and rehabilitation: Lessons from systematic reviews*. Springer.

Weisburd, D., Farrington, D. P., Gill, C., Ajzenstadt, M., Bennett, T., Bowers, K., Caudy, M. S., Holloway, K., Johnson, S., Lösel, F., Mallender, J., Perry, A., Tang, L. L., Taxman, F., Telep, C., Tierney, R., Ttofi, M. M., Watson, C., Wilson, D. B., & Wooditch, A. (2017). What works in crime prevention and rehabilitation: An assessment of systematic reviews. *Criminology & Public Policy, 16*, 415–449.

Weisburd, D., & Neyroud, P. (2011). *Police science: Toward a new paradigm.* Harvard University Press.
Weisburd, D., Telep, C. W., Hinkle, J. C., & Eck, J. E. (2010). Is problem-oriented policing effective in reducing crime and disorder? *Criminology and Public Policy, 9*, 139–172.
Welsh, B. C., Braga, A. A., & Hollis-Peel, M. E. (2012). Can "disciplined passion" overcome the cynical view? An empirical inquiry of evaluator influence on police crime prevention program outcomes. *Journal of Experimental Criminology, 8*, 415–431.
White, J. R. (1988). Violence during the 1919 Boston police strike: An analysis of the crime control myth. *Criminal Justice Review, 13*, 61–68.
Williams, R. (2008). Policing and forensic science. In T. Newburn (Ed.), *Handbook of Policing* (2nd ed., pp. 760–793). Willan Publishing.
Zedner, L. (2006). Policing before and after the police: The historical antecedents of contemporary crime control. *British Journal of Criminology, 46*, 78–96.
Zhang, Y. (2019). *The book of swindles*. Columbia University Press.

# Chapter 2
# Policing the Night-Time Economy: A Systematic Review of Evidence-Based Practice

## 2.1 Research Question and Review Objectives

The key questioned posed in this review was: what strategies and interventions through policing, or in combination with other agencies, can reduce crime and increase public safety in the night-time economy (NTE)? A principal driver of concern over this and of senior police managers' interest in it was the significant expenditures police were incurring in night-time patrol of city and town centres, without any measurable effect on rates of several types of crime. Chief Constables therefore requested a review of evidence that would enable them to compare different strategies and select potentially more effective methods of policing.

Our objectives therefore were to conduct an evidence review and prepare a report summarizing what is known about effective strategies and interventions concerning the above, and to identify possible approaches to addressing the issues more effectively. As a starting point for conducting the review, the Population, Intervention, Comparison, Outcome (PICO) framework was used to outline and develop an approach, specifying key features as shown in Table 2.1.

## 2.2 Background

It is important first to examine what is meant by the "night-time economy" (NTE). This is a relatively new concept and according to accounts by sociologists and criminologists began to be used in the UK from approximately the mid-1990s onwards. The phrase refers to a changing pattern of daily routines and activities in the lifestyles of a large number of people, particularly though not exclusively young adults and those in the early adult years (approximately 18 to 35 years). The NTE is associated with the entertainment industry and with districts of towns and cities where



J. McGuire et al., *Evidence-Based Policing and Community Crime Prevention*, Advances in Preventing and Treating Violence and Aggression,
https://doi.org/10.1007/978-3-030-76363-3_2

**Table 2.1** PICO framework as applied to the literature search strategy for evidence-based policing strategies for the night-time economy

| | |
|---|---|
| Population/ participants | Citizens, youth, public, customers of bars, restaurants, clubs, casinos<br>Bar staff, waiters, door staff, taxi drivers, other night workers<br>Emergency staff, ambulance workers, accident and emergency (A&E) departments<br>Youth workers, other agencies engaging target groups (e.g. homeless) and police |
| Intervention/ indicator | Alterations at a number of levels that have been tested in situational crime prevention, environmental design, street lighting, closed-circuit television (CCTV), pedestrian and traffic management, signage, transport links; in law and regulation, alcohol/gaming licences, hours of operation; police presence, patrols, contact points and availability |
| Comparison/ control | Compare areas with and without specific interventions, or with different interventions or combinations of them, in identified hot spots or in more widely selected districts with approximately equivalent features<br>Evaluation using either cross-sectional group comparisons or time-series or multiple-baseline designs |
| Outcome(s) | Measurement of activity levels, footfall, traffic flows; recording of crime, licence violations, drunkenness, drug abuse and trafficking, criminal damage, assaults, fighting, sexual offences, sex industry; surveys of public perceptions, noise, nuisance, feedback, news reporting; and benefit-cost or cost-efficiency calculations for different interventions |

there is a concentration of venues that remain open in the late evening, early morning or throughout the night. As such it has a close connection with restaurants, pubs, bars, nightclubs, casinos and an almost inextricable link with alcohol consumption and sometimes also with other drug use. The problems of crime and disorder that arise from it, and that are of primary concern to the police and public, emanate first and foremost from that aspect of it, though other elements are also involved. That pattern however changes over time: for example, according to the UK Association of Licensed Multiple Retailers over the 10 years up to August 2015, the number of nightclubs in Britain declined markedly, from 3144 to 1733. During the COVID pandemic restrictions of 2020, many such venues closed temporarily and some permanently, having a massive impact on the rate of several kinds of crime.

Several factors are thought to have influenced the evolution of the NTE into the pattern it exhibits today (Winlow, 2010). They included altering patterns of work and leisure in the British economy, which had a particular impact on town and city centres in terms of property availability, attempts at regeneration and the ways in which different sectors of towns were used. In addition, there were cultural changes that reflected attitudes in other parts of the world. Alongside these developments, the price of alcohol relative to other consumer items steadily fell over a number of years, giving rise to what was perceived as a worrying if not alarming pattern of binge drinking, notably amongst young adults. Whatever their exact origins, the net effect of these changes, which has been widely recognized, was that a larger number of people than before were awake, socially active and drinking in public for extended periods after nightfall, especially at weekends. Despite generally declining crime rates, specific problems arose at particular locations that became recognized as hot spots for crime and disorder. Addressing the problem of antisocial behaviour, crime and public safety in the NTE raises a complex set of issues regarding how crime events in themselves are a function of changing social trends and patterns of activity. Many of the latter, perfectly legal in themselves and sought after by many citizens, nevertheless generate new situations in which there can be unforeseen risks, including the emergence of new crime opportunities.

It has of course always been the case that a proportion of crimes (in some cases, the majority) are committed during night-time hours, when darkness affords some anonymity to an offender and lowers the chances of being detected or recognized, when property may be unprotected or insecure, and when unsuspecting victims may be at their most vulnerable. The NTE does not however refer to this, but to crime and disorder that flows from nightlife activities and primarily from the consumption of alcohol. This is linked to a variety of offences, from breaches of licensing or gaming laws, to public drunkenness, drink-driving, theft, property damage, violence and sexual crimes. Research by the UK Home Office (Finney, 2004) found that the peak time for violent offending is weekend nights and that the peak location is in or near pubs and clubs. Most incidents involve drinking by the offender, victim or both; and a proportion of street violence is associated with congregations of people outside drinking venues. Some researchers have investigated the patterning of these offences at specific locations (e.g. in Cardiff and Worcester: Nelson et al., 2001), while others have analysed the causal factors involved in giving rise to such aggression at an individual (McNally, 2004; Miller et al., 2016) and group level (Levine et al., 2012). Nevertheless, it is also claimed that the relations between different factors and how they influence each other remain poorly understood (Newton & Hirschfield, 2009). For that position to improve, perhaps a central issue is that of how best to capture the parameters of NTE violence and analyse the interactions between them. In that connection, Philpot et al. (2019) provided a useful review and critique of different methodologies for researching and analysing violence in the NTE.

Numerous research studies have examined variations in the amounts of crime or of hospital injury admissions in relation to changes in the alcohol licensing hours. Humphreys et al. (2013) reported an analysis of this following the introduction of all-night opening after the implementation of the Licensing Act 2003. While that was not found to have a substantially adverse effect, elsewhere increases in licensing hours have been found to result in significant rises in the rates of assault (e.g. Rossow & Norström, 2011).

Many other aspects of the NTE have been researched. They include the dynamics of interactions between bar staff and customers (Graham et al., 2005, 2011) and the extent to which bars can be stopped from providing drink to customers who are already heavily intoxicated (Buvik & Rossow, 2015; Hughes et al., 2014). Research has also focused on the ambience of different drinking venues, and different patterns of governance of them by managers (Byrnes et al., 2014; Cozens & Grieve, 2014), and also on the implicit interactional rules that permit fighting or even make it obligatory under some sets of circumstances (Copes et al., 2013). There have been studies of the particular roles of door staff (bouncers), who are themselves at risk of assault (Monaghan, 2003; Tutenges et al., 2015), but who may block some customers from entry, or eject unruly patrons who then add to disturbance on the street. There have also been studies of additional challenges such as pre-loading (drinking cheaply at home before going out at night) (Barton & Husk, 2012) and of mixing alcohol with other drugs such as stimulants (Pennay et al., 2014) or cocaine (Ayres & Treadwell, 2011). Other elements of the NTE, such as the growth of the strip industry (Sanders & Hardy, 2012), have been comparatively neglected by comparison with the alcohol-related aspects. A similar pattern was found in the updating searches. Sex trafficking is also linked to the NTE in many large cities, but here too the amount of available research is very limited (Couture et al., 2016).

Clearly, overall, there are multiple questions to be answered if the factors involved in the NTE are to be better understood, and the challenges for effective policing are undoubtedly immense. In contemporary policing, there is an accelerating movement away from a reactive stance towards crime events, which is leading to more extensive use of research intelligence, and an adoption of proactive, inter-agency and community-wide efforts to address the causes of problems. Success in achieving this would yield undoubted advantages, including greater community safety, fewer crimes and reduced costs of policing and other criminal justice agencies. A review of interventions that can address problems associated with the NTE could form part of such developments.

## 2.3 Method

To begin the review, search terms were developed from the PICO framework (Table 2.1) and search strategies devised to locate both published and unpublished evaluations of policing and other initiatives that have had or potentially could have desired impacts on outcome targets. A first step within this was to locate previous reviews of the topic or of adjoining areas, to discover what has been learnt to date.

### *2.3.1 Previous Reviews*

No review was found that covered exactly the area being focused on here. Several reviews, however, were very closely related and there have been reviews of adjacent areas or of related aspects of the general issue of crime and safety in the NTE. Nine potentially relevant reviews were found. Table 2.2 provides a brief summary of each of them. Another study (Middleton et al., 2010), related to that by Hahn et al. (2010) and conducted by the same research group, was excluded from this table as it dealt with entire daytime availability of alcohol for sale, rather than just portions of the day covering the hours of darkness.

The research literature reviews listed in Table 2.2 show that a great variety of approaches have been evaluated in seeking to address the problem of crime and

**Table 2.2** Previous reviews of areas related to policing the night-time economy

| Review | Focus | Number of studies | Findings |
|---|---|---|---|
| Adams (2003) | Juvenile curfews and crime prevention | 10 | Many local authorities in the USA have 10:00 or 11:00 pm curfews for persons under 17 or 18 years. This review of evaluations showed they had no impact in reducing crime, though a more recent study (Kline, 2012) found more positive results |
| Bolier et al. (2011) | Experimental studies on prevention of alcohol and drug use in nightlife settings | 17 | Community interventions obtained positive results and showed potential to reduce substance-related harm; working with bar staff had more mixed results; educational and policy initiatives had small effects. Combining different approaches with enforcement offered the most promising prospects |
| Droste et al. (2014) | Feasibility and effectiveness of community interventions based on emergency data sharing | 8 | All studies demonstrated that data sharing is a valuable process with substantial reductions in assaults and emergency department attendances |
| Farrington and Welsh (2002) | Improved street lighting and crime prevention | 13 | In eight US studies the results were mixed but in five UK studies results were positive, with an overall 20% reduction in crime. However, reductions were also found in daytime crime, suggesting some factors other than lighting in itself produced the results |
| Hahn et al. (2010) | Effects of increasing hours of alcohol sales in on-premises drinking outlets | 16 | Amongst ten studies where opening hours were increased by ≥2 hours, six found increases in alcohol-related harms, two the reverse and two mixed effects. In six studies where the increase was <2 hours, no clear conclusions could be drawn |
| Jones et al. (2011) | Effective approaches to reducing harm in drinking environments. Included studies on server training, policing/enforcement, community interventions | 28 | Many studies had inadequate designs. However, the clearest indicators of positive effects were from seven studies of multi-component programmes with community mobilization, bar staff training and strict enforcement of licensing laws |

(continued)

**Table 2.2** (continued)

| Review | Focus | Number of studies | Findings |
|---|---|---|---|
| Liu et al. (2016) | Effect of policing methods to reduce alcohol-related violence in the night-time economy in Australia | 10 studies of 15 tests | Located studies of 15 police interventions focused on licensed premises in a range of cities and rural districts, comparing areas with and without interventions, which relied on either monitoring/enforcement strategies or collaborative partnerships. Seven of ten studies were rated overall methodologically as weak and only one (a randomized controlled trial) was rated as strong. Did not find any "convincing evidence" of the effectiveness of the approaches used |
| Stockwell and Chikritzhs (2009) | Impact of changes to permitted hours of drinking | 14 | Of 49 studies located only 14 had adequate datasets; amongst them, 11 showed an association between increased availability of alcohol and increased harms; the remaining three found no effect or a reverse association |
| Taylor et al. (2018) | Mapping review of alcohol restrictions in night-time entertainment precincts in six countries; majority of located studies used police datasets | 35 studies 13 reviews | Narrative/qualitative synthesis of results of studies of interventions, including changes in trading hours, use of lockouts, drink restrictions, patron bans, control of outlet density and price increases. Most methods resulted in some reduction in alcohol-related harms. The authors were critical of the studies on the basis that they lacked modelling of causal relationships, i.e. when large-scale changes are introduced, it is not possible to discern the relative effects of each element |

disorder at night. Interventions covered in these reviews show remarkable variety. Examples include (1) legal and policy changes at local level: alterations in hours or days of alcohol sales and juvenile curfews; (2) enforcement-oriented methods (patrols, police visits to licensed venues, blood alcohol testing, sobriety checkpoints, policing high-risk premises); (3) engagement and consultation with stakeholders such as licensees, staff and consumers (alcohol education, brief interventions, driver awareness and bar staff training, e.g. responsible beverage service (RBS) training); (4) collaborative multi-agency initiatives (with hospital emergency departments, information-sharing arrangements, liaison with local authorities); and (5) multi-component and community-wide interventions incorporating media campaigns, community mobilization, codes of practice for venue management and other initiatives carried out in parallel.

Outcome variables amongst the studies included in these reviews also showed considerable variety. They included numbers of road deaths and of other serious accidents, rates of different types of crime (violence, drunkenness, driving while intoxicated), levels of inebriation (blood alcohol), numbers of visits to hospital emergency departments, rates of serious injury and numbers of telephone calls to police contact centres. It has to be kept in mind, however, that the quality of the research found in these reviews is very variable. There are frequent criticisms made by reviewers, to the effect that many studies have weak research designs, rendering the drawing of clear conclusions difficult. For example, in some cases changes are introduced and an attempt made to measure them in the absence of any pre-intervention data. Another recurrent problem is that often the changes that are the subject of an investigation are introduced at the same time as other changes are also taking place in that locality. Thus, it was often hard, if not impossible, to discern which factors had been the cause of any changes observed in the outcome variable.

### 2.3.2 Search Strategy

Tracking down research relevant to the objectives of the present review was done in a series of steps. First, a pilot, exploratory search of the PsycINFO database was carried out using the simple terms *night-time economy* and *polic**. This yielded a total of only 38 items but was useful in developing the PICO framework and in giving a preliminary indication of the range and types of study that might be discovered in a fuller review. Subsequently the following five databases were searched using a fully developed and comprehensive search strategy: EMBASE (*Excerpta Medica database*), Web of Science, Scopus, National Criminal Justice Reference Service (NCJRS, US Department of Justice) and the Netherlands Institute for the Study of Criminality and Law Enforcement (NISCALE). Initial electronic searches of these were carried out in July 2015 at the University of Nottingham. The timeframe for EMBASE searches was 1974 to 2015. The first three resources listed above are large-scale electronic literature databases that incorporate many other more specialized databases across the fields of medicine and healthcare and the social, physical, and biological sciences. The latter two are specifically run by major criminal justice agencies and collate research work carried on by government departments.

A more detailed list of search terms was prepared involving permutations of different terms designating several types of crime, and variant forms of relevant words denoting types of policing interventions. Given the objectives of this review, studies were retained for final analysis if they met the following inclusion criteria: (1) The study described an intervention either through policing alone or by other agencies in collaboration with the police. (2) The intervention addressed an issue associated with the NTE and activities in the period from 10:00 pm till early morning. (3) Data were collected on patterns of offences, public disorder or injuries or on public perceptions of safety. (4) An evaluation was conducted, reporting either quantitative or qualitative data (or both), testing the effectiveness of the intervention.

Studies also had to be published in English, as timescales and resources did not permit the possibility of translation. Studies were excluded if they examined large-scale changes that were expected as a result of legal or policy frameworks, such as the introduction and implementation of the Licensing Act 2003 (e.g. Humphreys et al., 2013), or if they focused on the effects of changes in alcohol pricing (e.g. Booth et al., 2011). The process of selection with numbers of items discarded and retained at each phase is presented in Fig. 2.1.

The initial searches located many thousands of research articles and other documents which after de-duplication resulted in a total of 1055 hits which were saved in an *Endnote* file. Those studies eligible for full review were then identified through a two-stage selection process. In Stage 1, titles and where necessary abstracts were read for relevance to the review objectives, resulting in a narrowing down to 157 items, for example, by removing studies that were found of night vision equipment. In Stage 2, abstracts and in some cases electronic documents were read in more detail, to identify research on the NTE as defined for the review, yielding 66 items. Numerous research studies were found on factors influencing crime and disorder in the NTE, but only those entailing an intervention that had been methodically evaluated were retained for full review, resulting in a final set of 20 studies. For example, some studies were eliminated that had only preliminary, pilot data that was inconclusive, with further research planned (e.g. Pointing et al., 2012). In supplementary searches covering the period 2015–2020, a further 11 studies were located, one of which was a continuation of a study included earlier (Kypri et al., 2016).

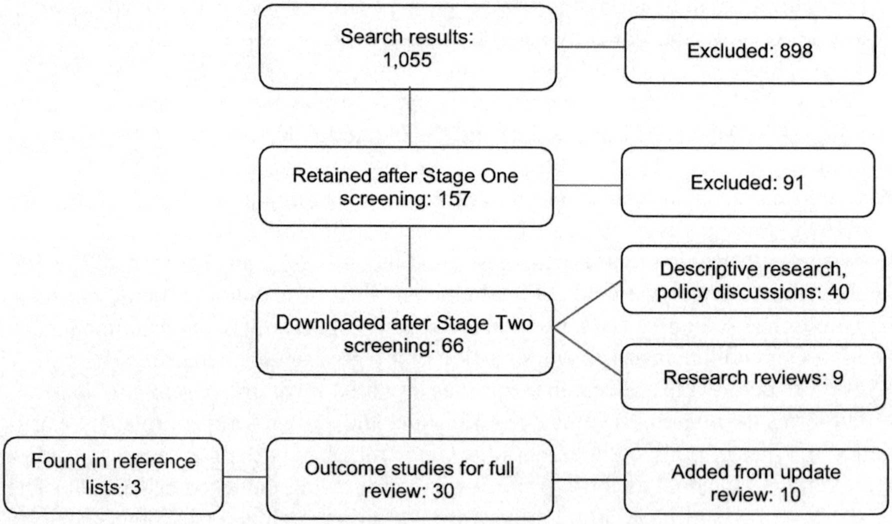


**Fig. 2.1** Flowchart of search results for policing and the night-time economy

## 2.4 Results

The locations of the 30 studies by country were Australia (11), the UK (7), the USA (4), Brazil (3), Sweden (2) and one each from Canada, Finland and Germany. As Table 2.3 shows they included a wide variety of interventions and employed a range of evaluation research designs. The interventions can be placed in a number of major categories. Note that police departments played some role in all but two of the interventions, but that role varied considerably. The two non-police interventions were on university campuses. The studies retained were as follows.

- *Police patrol interventions* (one study): hot spots police patrols (Frogner et al., 2013)
- *Design against crime* (one study): pedestrianization of a Gay Village neighbourhood (Marselle et al., 2012)
- *Safer Bars project* (one study): intervention involving risk assessment and bar staff training in Toronto (Graham et al., 2004)
- *College-based initiatives* (two studies): 21st birthday card and late-night activity programme (LaBrie et al., 2010; Patrick et al., 2010)
- *Information sharing* (two studies): both in the UK (Cardiff), involving exchange of information between hospital emergency departments and police who responded with specific actions at high-risk locations (Florence et al., 2011; Warburton & Shepherd, 2006)
- *Restricting availability of alcohol* or access of customers to licensed venues (six studies): licensing hour restrictions, lockouts, graduated driving license procedures (Fell et al., 2011; Kypri et al., 2010, 2016; Marcus & Siedler, 2015; Miller et al., 2011; Palk et al., 2010, 2012)
- *Multilevel community projects* (seven studies): with varying permutations of ingredients that included police, licensees, licensing authorities, schools, local government, general practitioners, pharmacies, hospitals, media outlets, etc. (Maguire & Nettleton, 2003; Miller et al., 2014; Navarro et al., 2013; Nottinghamshire Police, 2002; Shakeshaft et al., 2014; Wallin et al., 2003; Warpenius et al., 2010)

Some of the studies are separate outputs from the same long-term project, but in each case, they reported independent data. The study by Palk et al. (2012) can be seen as a replication of the findings from the Palk et al. (2010) study. That is, it was carried out to evaluate whether an intervention that was found to be effective in one locality could be transferred to other places. These authors also cite an earlier evaluation of a lockout experiment in the city of Ballarat, Victoria, which was reported to have positive effects. The documents pertaining to it, however, were unpublished and despite efforts to do so could not be retrieved.

In some respects, this is an impressive array of research outputs. Many of them involved very complex interventions that will have required extensive consultations between a number of agencies. Many were run over periods of several years. The research designs are mostly of reasonably rigorous quality, with several employing

**Table 2.3** Individual studies evaluating a variety of interventions to prevent or reduce crime related to the night-time economy.

| Study (country) | Focus | Methodology | Samples/data sources | Intervention and outcomes |
|---|---|---|---|---|
| Baldin et al. (2018) (Brazil) | Evaluation of a web-based intervention that provided "personalized normative" feedback | RCT | From a survey of 31 nightclubs in São Paulo: 465 customers assessed by the *Alcohol Use Disorders Identification Test* (AUDIT) as problem drinkers and "high risk" | Participants were randomized into experimental and controls. The former was exposed to a web-based intervention that provided feedback on harms associated with the amount of alcohol they were consuming. The outcome variable was extent of binge drinking. Groups were matched at outset. At 6-month follow-up the experimental group reported 38% lower binge drinking than at baseline ($p = 0.026$), while change in the controls was non-significant. However, there was a high level of attrition at the follow-up point (only 50% of baseline groups remaining) |

(continued)

**Table 2.3** (continued)

| Study (country) | Focus | Methodology | Samples/data sources | Intervention and outcomes |
|---|---|---|---|---|
| Byrnes et al. (2019) (USA) | Evaluation of a group-based mobile intervention | RCT: groups entering nightclubs randomly allocated to intervention and control conditions | 352 groups (of 2260 approached) containing 959 young people visiting San Francisco nightclubs. Outcome data were levels of use of strategies and levels of alcohol and drugs assayed by fluid and breath samples on venue entry and exit | Evaluated the use of *Nightlife Safety Plans* in which groups are given skills for identifying high-risk behaviours associated with overuse of alcohol or drugs, through a tablet-based app taking 5–6 minutes to view, and select an agreed strategy to employ if these problems arose. On exiting venues, intervention condition participants used significantly more protective actions to keep group members safe, and had significantly lower blood alcohol concentration, but not lower levels of other drugs |
| De Andrade et al. (2016) (Australia) | Lockout process in licensed premises in Surfers Paradise | Single-cohort pilot study, linear regression analysis | Data were collected on total crime, violent crime, injuries, assaults, ambulance attendances, reported incidents of intoxication or overdose, up to a 36-month period | Lockout is a regulation in which individuals who leave a venue after a certain time (here 3:00 am) are not allowed to return, though those who remain inside can continue drinking until the venue closes (here 5:00 am). The study monitored rates and "hot spot" locations of several kinds of incident in the period before and after the introduction of the lockout. Analysis found no significant pre-post lockout rates on any outcome variable |

(continued)

**Table 2.3** (continued)

| Study (country) | Focus | Methodology | Samples/data sources | Intervention and outcomes |
|---|---|---|---|---|
| Duailibi et al. (2007) (Brazil) | Examination of the effect of restricting opening hours | Single-cohort, time-series analysis study | Monthly counts of homicides and assaults against women in the city of Diadema over a 10-year period (1995–2005) | Investigated the impact of introducing a closing-time regulation on the expectation that reducing alcohol availability and thereby consumption would also lead to a reduction in alcohol-related violence. The regulation closing bars at 11:00 pm took effect in mid-2002. There was a 44% decline in homicides; assaults against women also fell but the extent of this was harder to calculate because of considerable variability in the monthly data |
| Fell et al. (2011) (USA) | Graduated license night-time restrictions | Panel study, comparing different states over time | American states which introduced "graduated driving licences" in different years between 1996 and 2008 | Many American states have Graduated Driver Licensing systems which limit an individual in what he/she can do before certain ages. The study examined whether numbers of fatalities of young drivers changed as different states introduced night-time Graduated Driver Licensing restrictions on drivers below a specified age. The introduction of midnight restrictions was associated with a significant drop in alcohol-related accidents and fatalities |

(continued)

**Table 2.3** (continued)

| Study (country) | Focus | Methodology | Samples/data sources | Intervention and outcomes |
|---|---|---|---|---|
| Florence et al. (2011) (UK) | Information sharing | Non-equivalent experimental study and time-series analysis | Comparison between Cardiff and 14 other UK cities designated similar, over the period 2000–2008 (84 months) | Evaluated the impact of an information-sharing procedure on violent assaults involving police, local government, licensing authorities and hospital emergency department staff. Data were collected from injured persons and used to inform police activity over the weekends including patrol routes. There was a significant drop in assault hospitalizations: after implementation of the programme, total assault fell to 79% and wounding to 68% of its previous levels; no such reductions showed in comparison cities |
| Frogner et al. (2013) (Sweden) | Directed hot spot patrols | Before-and-after group comparison | Focused on crime hot spots for night-time street violence in the town of Örebro (pop. 140,000) | Eight pairs of two private security guards, monitored by the police, patrolled at pre-arranged times between 8:00 pm and 4:00 am at violence hot spots. Applied over June to September weekends comparing 2008–2009 with 2010–2011 (total 68 weekends). There was a decrease of 23.6% in reported street violence, but this was not statistically significant |

(continued)

**Table 2.3** (continued)

| Study (country) | Focus | Methodology | Samples/data sources | Intervention and outcomes |
|---|---|---|---|---|
| Garius et al. (2020) (UK) | Evaluation of the effects of an alcohol awareness initiative | Mixed-methods comparison of monthly violent and sexual crime rates | Analysis of police-recorded crime data before and after the alcohol awareness intervention in three NTE venues in two cities | Evaluation of *Drinkaware Crew*, an initiative of an alcohol awareness charity to reduce alcohol-related crime and other harms in the NTE. In one city, the venue where the initiative was introduced was compared with a control area; in the other city, periods before and after were compared at two sites. Results were inconclusive for the first venue and showed a negative effect in the other two venue studies. It was thought that the unexpected results might be spurious due to external influences on the data |
| Graham et al. (2004) (Canada) | Reducing bar violence | Randomized controlled trial with time-series analysis | Evaluation of the *Safer Bars* programme in Toronto | *Safer Bars* had two components, a risk assessment workbook and a 3-hour training session for bar staff. Bars were randomly allocated to an experimental group (18 bars) and a control group (12 bars). Monitored over 734 nights. There was a significant impact in reducing levels of severe aggression and moderate aggression with intent. Overall levels of aggression were however low and the findings are regarded as promising only |

(continued)

**Table 2.3** (continued)

| Study (country) | Focus | Methodology | Samples/data sources | Intervention and outcomes |
|---|---|---|---|---|
| Hoffman et al. (2017) (Australia) | Changes in law to impose last drinks and lockout rules | Retrospective cohort study of the period 2003–2015 | Evaluation of the impact of 2008 legislative changes limiting hours for sale of alcohol. Recorded numbers presenting with injury between 18:00 on Friday and 06:00 on Sunday | Study conducted within a maxillofacial surgery unit, analysing rates of change in injuries due to assault before and after the implementation of new laws. Over the study period, on average there were 152 patient attendances for assault each weekend. In the period before the change rates of injury increased on average by 14% per annum. In the period following, injuries decrease at a rate of 21% per annum. Similar patterns emerged in different sub-samples analysed separately |
| Kypri et al. (2010, 2016) (Australia) | Restricting pub closing times | Non-equivalent, quasi-experimental design | Compared police-recorded assaults in the towns of Newcastle and Hamilton, NSW | Pubs were compelled to close at 3:00 am in Newcastle but no restriction was imposed in Hamilton. Over an 8-year period (2001–2009) recorded assaults fell in Newcastle by 34%, while there was a small increase of 2% in Hamilton. Over a further follow-up period covering 2013–2015, assaults in Newcastle continued to fall till they were 50% of the rate at outset. There was also a fall in Hamilton but it was not statistically significant |

(continued)

**Table 2.3** (continued)

| Study (country) | Focus | Methodology | Samples/data sources | Intervention and outcomes |
|---|---|---|---|---|
| LaBrie et al. (2010) (USA) | Student 21st birthday card | Non-equivalent, quasi-experimental design | Students resident in college halls at Loyola Marymount University, Los Angeles; basis of allocation to groups is unclear | Students approaching their 21st birthday who were planning to celebrate by drinking were divided into two groups. One received a birthday card containing advice on safe drinking, the others did not. The former consumed significantly fewer drinks than the latter (for males, 23.4% reduction; for females, 40.2% reduction). Blood alcohol levels showed corresponding reductions |
| Maguire and Nettleton (2003) (UK) | Multiple-level community interventions | Before-and-after design | Recorded rates of violence in 12 months before and 2 months after commencement of the Tackling Alcohol-related Street Crime project | Evaluation of the Tackling Alcohol-related Street Crime project in Cardiff and Cardiff Bay. A multifaceted project employing a range of intervention and research methods. Found an overall decrease of 4% in alcohol-related assault, against a background of 10% increases in comparable areas. But there was also an increase of 49% in incidents of alcohol-related disorder, though the rate declined over the course of 12 months |

(continued)

**Table 2.3** (continued)

| Study (country) | Focus | Methodology | Samples/data sources | Intervention and outcomes |
|---|---|---|---|---|
| Marcus and Siedler (2015) (UK) | Ban on late-night alcohol sales (Germany) | Time-series analysis | Random sample of data on hospital admissions throughout Germany for the years 2007–2011 | Investigated the effect of a ban on late-night off-premises alcohol sales in the state of Baden-Württemberg, to reduce binge drinking and alcohol-related violence, comparing it with the rest of Germany. Over 60 months, there was a significant reduction in alcohol-related hospital admissions amongst adolescents and young adults (e.g. by 20% amongst 20–24-year-olds, though less in other groups). The study includes numerous checks on the robustness of the results |
| Marselle et al. (2012) (UK) | Design-against-crime intervention | Case study methodology | Manchester Gay Village, violent incidents + pedestrian survey | Describes work of the Manchester Crime and Disorder Partnership (police and local authority) to pedestrianize streets in the Gay Village in Manchester city centre. The number of violent incidents was too low for statistical evaluation but remained stable, while increases were noted in other localities. Analysis of public survey data showed a high level of support for the change and perceptions of improved safety |

(continued)

**Table 2.3** (continued)

| Study (country) | Focus | Methodology | Samples/data sources | Intervention and outcomes |
|---|---|---|---|---|
| Menéndez et al. (2015) (Australia) | Restricting pub closing and alcohol purchasing times | Time-series analysis of trends comparing areas | Central areas of Sydney compared with regional New South Wales. Rates of non-domestic assault over a 6-year period (2009–2014) | Evaluated the effect of January 2014 legislative reforms which introduced 1:30 am lockouts from drinking venues and a 10:00 pm ban on take-away alcohol sales. Analysis showed large and statistically significant reductions in assaults in target areas (26—40%) and smaller but also significant reductions elsewhere (9%). Tested whether there had been a displacement effect on adjacent areas but observed reductions rather than increases, except near one venue with a 24-hour liquor licence |
| Miller et al. (2011) (Australia) | Comparison of regulatory and voluntary licensing | Non-equivalent control group design with time-series analysis | Data on alcohol-related injuries in the period 12:00–6:00 am in the cities of Newcastle, NSW and Geelong, VIC | Describes the Dealing with Alcohol-related problems in the night-time economy project. Compares two forms of licensing conditions, regulated (Newcastle) and voluntary (Geelong). While the latter had no effect on injury levels, the former was associated with a significant decline in injuries, equivalent to preventing 344 emergency department admissions per year |

(continued)

**Table 2.3** (continued)

| Study (country) | Focus | Methodology | Samples/data sources | Intervention and outcomes |
|---|---|---|---|---|
| Miller et al. (2014) (Australia) | Multiple-level community interventions | Time-series analysis | Alcohol-related attendance at Geelong Hospital in the period 2005–2009 | Describes the Dealing with Alcohol-related problems in the NTE project focusing in this study on the introduction of a multilevel community-based intervention in Geelong, Victoria. This included a newspaper "'Just Think" campaign; ID scanners in venues; increased police presence, including both high-visibility patrols and undercover license checks; and other components. However, none of the interventions was associated with a decline in alcohol-related hospital attendances |

(continued)

**Table 2.3** (continued)

| Study (country) | Focus | Methodology | Samples/data sources | Intervention and outcomes |
|---|---|---|---|---|
| Moore et al. (2017) (UK) | Effectiveness of a venue-based intervention to reduce alcohol-related violence | Two studies: RCT with alcohol outlets as units of analysis, intention-to-treat analysis; + non-randomized study | Licensed premises in Wales where there had been at least one violent incident. In RCT: 208 received intervention 245 control In non-randomized study: 285 received intervention 321 control | The intervention *Safety Management in the Licensed Environment* consisted of visits to premises by environmental health practitioners who undertook a "risk audit" and provided feedback to venue managers on risks for violence and advise on how to address them. Control venues received "usual practice" only. Monitored police records of further violence over 455 days from start of the intervention. Results were the reverse of expectations with intervention venues reporting: "the intervention was associated with a sustained increase in police recorded violence" (p.1904). It is possible the additional scrutiny in experimental venues increased the police ascertainment rate of violence. For a small number of venues that had follow-up visits, there was a significant reduction in violent incidents |

(continued)

**Table 2.3** (continued)

| Study (country) | Focus | Methodology | Samples/data sources | Intervention and outcomes |
|---|---|---|---|---|
| Navarro et al. (2013) (Australia) | Multi-component intervention | Randomized controlled trial with matched pairs of locations | 20 Australian locations allocated to experimental or control conditions; data collected on recorded crimes at high-risk times for the period 2001–2009 | Coordinated programme involving police, local councils, local media and licensees in each experimental community. Compared weekends designated as "problematic" and "non-problematic". Found a statistically significant reduction of 64% in sexual assaults in the former and of 19% in other assaults in the latter. Reported a cost-benefit analysis showing the reduction in sexual assaults led to a saving of AU $3.9 million during the study period and a benefit-cost ratio of 22:1 |
| Nottinghamshire Police (2002) (UK) | Multiple-level community interventions | Before-and-after design | Nottingham city centre, police-recorded data on violent crime/ disorder in the periods April 2000–2001 and April 2002–2002 | Data showed a growth of 60% in NTE venues in Nottingham in the period 1994–2000. Appointed "'Licensing Officers" with a specialized role in visiting licensed premises; also adding high-visibility patrols, CCTV, an education and media campaign, door supervisor training. Found reductions in alcohol-related assaults (18%) and alcohol-related disorder (22%). A cost-benefit analysis was to be undertaken but is not reported |

(continued)

**Table 2.3** (continued)

| Study (country) | Focus | Methodology | Samples/data sources | Intervention and outcomes |
|---|---|---|---|---|
| Palk et al. (2010) (Australia) | Lockout policy | Before-and-after design | Nightclubs in the Gold Coast, Queensland: data collected for 4 weeks before and 5 weeks after the intervention began | Part of a larger programme of research: The Alcohol and Drugs Incident Management Survey. Nightclubs with a closing time of 5:00 am were asked to apply a lockout rule where no one could be admitted after 3:00 am and anyone leaving after then could not re-enter. This was associated with significant reductions in several offences in the participating nightclubs: for alcohol-related disturbances 6.2%, for street disturbances 12.3% and for sexual offences 33.7%. Largest reductions were in the periods midnight to 3:00 am and 3:00–6:00 am |
| Palk et al. (2012) (Australia) | Lockout policy | Before-and-after design | Nightclubs in three locations in Queensland; data on various offences before and after the lockout was introduced | Generalization test by extension of the previous study by Palk et al. (2010) to two other areas, the centre of Brisbane and the district of Fortitude Valley, 4 weeks before and 4 weeks after the introduction of the same lockout procedure. Results were mixed for these two areas, with only a few marginally positive effects which may have been attributable to the lockout as they were mainly for the period 3:00–6:00 am. The study also included a qualitative component comprising interviews with 20 stakeholders |

(continued)

**Table 2.3** (continued)

| Study (country) | Focus | Methodology | Samples/data sources | Intervention and outcomes |
|---|---|---|---|---|
| Patrick et al. (2010) (USA) | Late-night alcohol-free programming | Longitudinal design | Stratified random sample of 689 students (age <21) at Pennsylvania State University | Students recorded daily levels of drinking for a baseline period, then over 14 daily surveys, on a web-based survey. Research tested the effect of taking part in an alcohol-free late-night entertainment programme (9:00 pm–2:00 am at weekends). Participants drank 40% fewer drinks on evenings they took part (and 74% fewer when they stayed in) than on evenings they went out. Odds of binge drinking were 79% lower on attending the programme. Effects were larger for females than males |
| Sanchez and Sanudo (2018) (Brazil) | Differential effects of a web-based intervention | Survey linked to RCT: From a survey of 31 nightclubs: 1057 customers assessed by the AUDIT | Interviews on nightclub entry, exit, + completion of online survey: 515 intervention group 542 control group | Study associated with Baldin et al. (2018, see entry above). Participants were followed up at 3, 6 and 12 months after initial assessment. Data collected on extent of binge drinking. There was no overall treatment effect of the intervention, but there was a significant reduction in binge drinking for those with high AUDIT scores but increases in binge drinking for those with low AUDIT scores. However, there was a high rate of attrition by the end-point |

(continued)

**Table 2.3** (continued)

| Study (country) | Focus | Methodology | Samples/data sources | Intervention and outcomes |
|---|---|---|---|---|
| Shakeshaft et al. (2014) (Australia) | Community action programme | Cluster randomized controlled trial + longitudinal design | 20 communities in Australia with populations in the range 5000–20,000. Studied for a baseline period (2001–2004), intervention (2005), post-intervention (2006–2009) | Communities were randomly allocated to experimental or control conditions. The intervention had 13 components, involving multiple agencies (general practitioners, media, school-based intervention, workplace policies, sports programme, brief interventions, etc.). However, the response rate was unsatisfactory (only 24% at post-intervention). While some significant differences were noted between experimental and control samples, it was concluded that no evidence was obtained that community action had been effective. Some components were fairly limited in content |
| Wallin et al. (2003) (Sweden) | Community alcohol prevention programme | Quasi-experimental design with time-series analysis | Police-recorded violent crimes in Stockholm City centre and a comparison area over 44 months pre-intervention and 33 months post-intervention | Evaluation of the Stockholm Prevents Alcohol and Drug Problems project, a multi-component programme including community mobilization, responsible beverage service training and more effective enforcement of licensing laws. There was a significant reduction of 29% in reported violent crimes in the intervention area, while violent crimes in the control area (Södermalm) and nationally in Sweden slightly rose |

(continued)

**Table 2.3** (continued)

| Study (country) | Focus | Methodology | Samples/data sources | Intervention and outcomes |
|---|---|---|---|---|
| Warburton and Shepherd (2006) (UK) | Combined police and hospital intervention | Longitudinal intervention | Data on assaults in licensed premises and street assaults in Cardiff over three 9-month periods in 1999–2000–2001 | Evaluation of the Tackling Alcohol-related Street Crime project in Cardiff. Entailed liaison between hospital emergency departments and police who had two levels of intervention, low (establishing contacts with licensed premises, regular monitoring) and high (more intensive redeployment of police resources with both high visibility and covert operations). Despite overall rise in premises capacity and in violence (12%), high-risk premises showed 22–69% reductions in violence |
| Warpenius et al. (2010) (Finland) | Multilevel intervention programme | Before-and-after quasi-experimental group comparison | Compared two towns (Jyväskylä – experimental + control area) on rates at which intoxicated persons were refused service, in the period 2004–2007 | An intervention was devised with four components: stricter law enforcement, local campaigns, media advocacy and training for bar staff in refusing drinks to customers who were already intoxicated. The outcome variable was the numbers of times actors pretending to be drunk were refused service. There were significant increases in the rates of refusal in the experimental but not the control area, in bars and pubs, but not nightclubs |

(continued)

randomized controlled trial (RCT) formats or time-series analysis and some had both. Where quasi-experiments were conducted (i.e. experimental and control conditions were not equivalent), care was taken to ensure the comparisons were as appropriate as possible.

The studies reported a wide range of outcomes, but the general trend amongst the results is positive. Although some studies found no beneficial effects, the majority (20/30) did, and some achieved remarkable levels of success. Ideally, for firm conclusions to be drawn from a review, a larger set of studies would be needed, as some of the findings obtained in this set are at odds with one another, making clear interpretation difficult. For example, some of the multilevel community interventions were effective, while others were not. The difference may be due to the particular combination of elements that each contained, but in any intervention that involves multiple components, discerning the discrete effect of each one can be very difficult to do, unless (for example) they were introduced in a phased sequence, with changes occurring at each stage being carefully monitored.

There have been studies of the extent to which people visiting busy and potentially risky venues in the NTE are assured by the presence of others, including police officers. In a survey in the Netherlands, Brands and van Doorn (2020) found that the police are trusted more than privately employed security personnel such as door staff and more than the use of closed-circuit television (CCTV). In a quite different innovation in part of Wales, Swann et al. (2015) reported a survey of perceptions of Christian street pastors operating in the NTE offering help to those who appeared to be in distress. These are not interventions as such and had no outcome evaluation, so were not included in Table 2.3. Nevertheless, they produce useful information in considering approaches to lowering anxiety in the NTE.

Three of the 30 studies did not show positive effects: the multilevel community intervention used in Geelong, Australia (Miller et al., 2014); the attempt by Palk et al. (2012) to extend the intervention they had tested in Australia's Gold Coast to parts of the city of Brisbane; and the community action programme described by Shakeshaft et al. (2014) which had apparently promising results but where the response rate was too low for any firm conclusions to be drawn. It may also be that in that study, some parts of the intervention were comparatively weak, e.g. a school-based programme on alcohol risks that formed part of the intervention consisted of a single hour's input only. In a fourth study (Maguire & Nettleton, 2003), while there were some positive effects, other findings were mixed; and in a fifth (Marselle et al., 2012) findings on crime levels were inconclusive but public reactions were positive.

The most effective interventions appear to have been of three main kinds. The first was the restriction of alcohol sales, through reducing hours of opening or limiting access through lockout periods. That this should be effective is consistent with the findings of many studies on the relationship between variations in opening times and levels of crime and disorder, cited previously. However, without specific justifications such as incidents of violence or disorder, this may be difficult to apply, and in some studies licensees were reluctant to participate in experiments that limited their times of opening. While some portions of the community would probably welcome such changes, others might have the opposite reaction, and there are risks of displacement of activity from a legal status to one of illegality (thereby driving the problem underground). The second form of effective intervention was the data exchange procedures involving collaboration between the police force and hospital emergency departments. The studies conducted in Cardiff involved focusing police attention on high-risk venues based on information obtained from assault victims, and this was complemented by the involvement of hospital doctors in meeting licensees and other stakeholders with a focus on preventing injury. Researchers have outlined the considerable possibilities of making more extensive use of emergency department data for prevention targeting (Bellis et al., 2012). The third type of intervention with positive outcomes consisted of some of the multilevel community interventions. As mentioned earlier, because there are some contradictions in this subset of evidence, the relationships between the components and the effects are not wholly clear. One key element appears to be enforcement of licensing laws: projects that do not include this were less effective than ones that do. Other useful elements include community information campaigns, specific forms of training for bar staff and door staff and police engagement of licensees in considering aspects of bar management that can reduce risks.

The two university-campus-based studies also reported positive results, and as students may be a significant fraction of those participating in the NTE, these could be useful results if there was to be liaison between police and local colleges. It is less easy, however, to translate these results into police-led initiatives in NTE locations where there may be problems of disorder and/or violence.

Also retrieved in the literature searches, but not retained for final review, were several reports of an ongoing, very extensive evaluation study being conducted in Wales but which at the time of writing was still in progress. Moore et al. (2007) and Moore et al. (2011) reported survey studies on the prevalence of alcohol use in the NTE and also research in which it proved possible to combine hospital and police data to identify violent premises. On the basis of these and other observations, the Violence Research Group at Cardiff University designed a protocol for a randomized controlled trial (Moore et al., 2010) which was first conducted in an exploratory form (Moore et al., 2012) but encountered several obstacles due to the unwillingness of licensees to participate voluntarily. The research group concluded that a trial was necessary on a far larger scale, involving numerous establishments and enforced participation, and a new study was designed. The All-Wales Licensed Premises Intervention (Moore et al., 2014) was begun, and the entire project incorporating the planned follow-up period ran from 2012 to 2016. The project involved close collaboration between hospital emergency staff and police throughout 22 local authorities in Wales. Disappointingly however, the final project results did not support the hoped-for outcome of reducing violence in the NTE (Moore et al., 2017).

Only one of the studies included for final review incorporated a benefit-cost evaluation. The study by Navarro et al. (2013) reported a very favourable ratio of 22:1 in relation to the impact of the intervention they evaluated in reducing sexual assaults. That is a very impressive figure and one of the highest reported in criminal justice research. If figures such as this can be reproduced with interventions at other places, seemingly high initial costs of embarking on new developments could be justified by longer-term financial savings. This however remains an isolated figure in the present review.

### 2.4.1 *Other Studies*

The preceding sections have described the findings of a literature search and review of studies located that met specified inclusion criteria. A number of other studies that did not meet those formal criteria, however, are also of interest and could provide possible indicators for future actions. They include work on the effects of banning glassware in bars in Glasgow (Forsyth, 2008), which, although an observational study only, suggested this was complied with and had beneficial effects. In a separate strand, work by Brands and Schwanen (2014) in the Netherlands has examined the advantages and disadvantages of different practices in the use of CCTV and police on-street patrols, and the reactions evoked by each amongst those pursuing entertainment in the NTE.

## 2.5 Discussion

On the basis of the present review, generally it can be concluded that police-led, multilevel interventions that include several components, delivered methodically on an inter-agency basis, while not guaranteed to work, stand the greatest chance of success. The most effective programmes entail a process of engagement with various stakeholders combined with enforcement. That is, where license holders and owners of outlets share the police objective of bringing down crime in the NTE, maintain environmental standards, provide staff training and adhere to the provisions of the law, levels of disorder and violence are likely to be lower than in locations that do not follow those practices.

In response to the findings of this review, some changes were made to police deployment in the two commissioning police areas, and a new partnership between police, nightclub owners and licensing magistrates was established, supported by funding from the Chief Constables' *Dragon's Den* fund. In addition, further work was commissioned to research the impact of these new approaches: in particular the use of data from nightclub entry control systems. This proved to be particularly effective in reducing overall NTE incidents but also led to several more serious crimes (including rape) being solved and perpetrators brought to justice. This also led to the conduct of an empirical study of a specialized ID scanning technology, *Scannet*, which was piloted and followed up in one of the police commissioning areas and two others in different parts of England (Bandyopadhyay et al., 2019). There were however mixed effects, appearing to be moderated by people's willingness to report crimes according to the likelihood that suspects would be identified and apprehended.

### 2.5.1 *Limitations*

The present review like any work of its kind has some limitations. One is that no attempt was made to ensure access to the grey literature (unpublished reports or other documents produced by agencies at work in a given field but who do not see their role as generating research). On the plus side, however, that also means that almost all the included studies had been subject to peer review. That does not, however, confirm that relevant and potentially well-conducted studies may have been carried out but have not been found. Another issue is that the extraction of information from the located studies was done by one person only, and ideally a proportion would be checked to ensure fidelity in terms of how findings were summarized. That is not however a major issue when the number of located studies is fairly small as was the case here.

Compared to what was anticipated when the PICO framework was prepared for this review, there was a dearth of research found on aspects of the NTE less directly associated with alcohol. The overwhelming majority of studies were on one or other aspect of drinking and its relation to disorder. Obviously, that is a principal concern, but it is to be hoped that the investigation of the NTE will expand to cover other problem areas in addition. As briefly mentioned earlier, for example, while there is evidence that the NTE is also a conduit for other types of criminality such as sex trafficking, no empirical studies were located that indicated how this could be addressed as part of NTE policing. Wider or further reaching initiatives are required, focusing on the market structures that create opportunities for and drive those activities.

Crime outside urban areas, in predominantly rural areas or ones with medium-sized centres of population (often county towns) and a dispersed network of smaller communities, shows different patterns from that found in large metropolitan districts (Mawby & Jones, 2004). The contextual differences between the two may be quite large, to the extent that interventions that are effective in one type of location may prove not to be in another. Several of the studies examined here, however, were carried out in centres of population not dissimilar in size to the main regional centres of many parts of the UK, and medium-sized towns in many countries, and the interventions described here could potentially be adapted and applied in those settings.

## References

Adams, K. (2003). The effectiveness of juvenile curfews at crime prevention. *Annals of the American Academy of Political and Social Science, 587*, 136–159.

Ayres, T. C., & Treadwell, J. (2011). Bars, drugs and football thugs: Alcohol, cocaine and violence in the night-time economy among English football firms. *Criminology and Criminal Justice, 12*, 83–100.

Baldin, Y. C., Sanudo, A., & Sanchez, Z. M. (2018). Effectiveness of a web-based intervention in reducing binge drinking among nightclub patrons. *Revista de Saúde Pública, 52*(2), 1–11. https://doi.org/10.11606/S1518-8787.2018052000281

Bandyopadhyay, S., Davies, K., & Matsa, A. (2019). *Scannet report: Using ID scanning technology to manage and prevent crime and anti-social behaviour in the night-time economy*. Norfolk and Suffolk Constabularies and the Better Policing Collaborative.

Barton, A., & Husk, K. (2012). Controlling pre-loaders: Alcohol related violence in an English night-time economy. *Drugs and Alcohol Today, 12*, 89–97.

Bellis, M. A., Leckenby, N., Hughes, K., Luke, C., Wyke, S., & Quigg, Z. (2012). Nighttime assaults: Using a national emergency department monitoring system to predict occurrence, target prevention and plan services. *BMC Public Health, 12*, 746. www.biomedcentral.com/1471-2458/12/746

Bolier, L., Voorham, L., Monshouwer, K., van Hasselt, N., & Bellis, M. (2011). Alcohol and drug prevention in nightlife settings: A review of experimental studies. *Substance Use and Misuse, 46*, 1569–1591.

Booth, A., Meier, P., Shapland, J., Wong, R., & Paisley, S. (2011). *Alcohol pricing and criminal harm: a rapid evidence assessment of the published research literature*. School of Health and Related Research, University of Sheffield.

Brands, J., & Schwanen, T. (2014). Experiencing and governing safety in the night-time economy: Nurturing the state of being carefree. *Emotion, Space and Society, 11*, 67–78.

Brands, J., & van Doorn, J. (2020). Policing nightlife areas: Comparing youths' trust in police, door staff and CCTV. *Policing and Society: An International Journal of Research and Policy, 30*(4), 429–445.

Buvik, K., & Rossow, I. (2015). Factors associated with over-serving at drinking establishments. *Addiction, 110*(4), 602–609.

Byrnes, H. F., Miller, B. A., Bourdeau, B., Johnson, M. B., Buller, D. B., Berteletti, J., & Rogers, V. A. (2019). Prevention of alcohol and other drug overuse among nightclub patrons: A randomized trial of a group-based mobile intervention at nightclubs. *Journal of Studies on Alcohol and Drugs, 80*, 423–430.

Byrnes, H. F., Miller, B. A., Johnson, M. B., & Voas, R. B. (2014). Indicators of club management practices and biological measurement of patron's drug and alcohol use. *Substance Use & Misuse, 49*, 1878–1887.

Copes, H., Hochstetler, A., & Forsyth, C. J. (2013). Peaceful warriors: Codes for violence among adult male bar fighters. *Criminology, 51*(3), 761–794.

Couture, T., Kimball, J., Jakiel, S., Sorenson, K., Cook, M. L., Romero, K., & Folwer, M. (2016). *More than drinks for sale: Exposing sex trafficking in Cantinas and Bars in the U.S*. Polaris project.

Cozens, P., & Grieve, S. (2014). Situational crime prevention at nightclub entrances in Perth, Western Australia: Exploring micro-level crime precipitators. *Crime Prevention and Community Safety, 16*, 54–70.

De Andrade, D., Jomel, R., & Townsley, M. (2016). Trouble in paradise: The crime and health outcomes of the Surfers Paradise licensed venue lockout. *Drug and Alcohol Review, 35*, 564–572.

Droste, N., Miller, P., & Baker, T. (2014). Review article: Emergency department data sharing to reduce alcohol-related violence: A systematic review of the feasibility and effectiveness of community level interventions. *Emergency Medicine Australasia, 26*, 326–335.

Duailibi, S., Ponicki, W., Grube, J., Pinsky, I., Laranjeira, R., & Raw, M. (2007). The effect of restricting opening hours on alcohol-related violence. *American Journal of Public Health, 97*(12), 2276–2280.

Farrington, D. P., & Welsh, B. C. (2002). Improved street lighting and crime prevention. *Justice Quarterly, 19*, 313–342.

Fell, J. C., Todd, M., & Voas, R. B. (2011). A national evaluation of the nighttime and passenger restriction components of graduated driver licensing. *Journal of Safety Research, 42*, 283–290.

Finney, A. (2004). *Violence in the night-time economy: key findings from the research*. Findings 214. London: Home Office, Research, Development and Statistics Directorate.

Florence, C., Shepherd, J., Brennan, I., & Simon, T. (2011). Effectiveness of anonymised information sharing and use in health service, police, and local government partnership for preventing violence related injury: Experimental study and time series analysis. *British Medical Journal, 342*, d3313.

Forsyth, A. J. M. (2008). Banning glassware from nightclubs in Glasgow (Scotland): Observed impacts, compliance and patron's views. *Alcohol and Alcoholism, 43*, 111–117.

Frogner, L., Andershed, H., Lindberg, O., & Johansson, M. (2013). Directed patrol for preventing city centre street violence in Sweden – a hot spot policing intervention. *European Journal of Criminal Policy Research, 19*, 333–350.

Garius, L., Ward, B., Teague, K., & Tseloni, A. (2020). Evaluating harm-reduction initiatives in a night-time economy and music festival context. *International Journal of Comparative and Applied Criminal Justice, 44*(4), 321–333.

Graham, K., Bernards, S., Osgood, D. W., Homel, R., & Purcell, J. (2005). Guardians and handlers: The role of bar staff in preventing and managing aggression. *Addiction, 100*, 755–766.

Graham, K., Bernards, S., Wells, S., Osgood, D. W., Abbey, A., Felson, R. B., & Saltz, R. F. (2011). Behavioural indicators of motives for barroom aggression: Implications for preventing bar violence. *Drug and Alcohol Review, 30*, 554–563.

Graham, K., Osgood, D. W., Zibrowski, E., Purcell, J., Gliksman, L., Leonard, K., Pernanen, K., Saltz, R. F., & Toomey, T. L. (2004). The effect of the Safer Bars programme on physical aggression in bars: Results of a randomized controlled trial. *Drug and Alcohol Review, 23*, 31–41.

Hahn, R. A., Kuzara, J. L., Elder, R., Brewer, R., Chattopadhyay, S., Fielding, J., Naimi, T. S., Toomey, T., Middleton, J. C., Lawrence, B., & the Task Force on Community Preventive Services. (2010). Effectiveness of policies restricting hours of alcohol sales in preventing excessive alcohol consumption and related harms. *American Journal of Preventive Medicine, 39*, 590–605.

Hoffman, G. R., Palazzi, K., Oteng Boateng, B. K., & Oldmeadow, C. (2017). Liquor legislation, last drinks, and lockouts: The Newcastle (Australia) solution. *International Journal of Oral and Maxillofacial Surgery, 46*, 740–745.

Hughes, K., Bellis, M. A., Leckenby, N., Quigg, Z., Hardcastle, K., Sharples, O., & Llewellyn, D. J. (2014). Does legislation to prevent alcohol sales to drunk individuals work? Measuring the propensity for night-time sales to drunks in a UK city. *Journal of Epidemiology and Community Health, 68*, 453–456.

Humphreys, D. K., Eisner, M. P., & Wiebe, D. J. (2013). Evaluating the impact of flexible alcohol trading hours on violence: An interrupted time series analysis. *PLoS One, 8*(2), e5551. https://doi.org/10.1371/journal.pone.0055581

Jones, L., Hughes, K., Atkinson, A. M., & Bellis, M. A. (2011). Reducing harm in drinking environments: A systematic review of effective approaches. *Health & Place, 17*, 508–518.

Kline, P. (2012). The impact of juvenile curfew laws on arrests of youth and adults. *American Law and Economics Review, 14*, 44–67. https://doi.org/10.1093/aler/ahr011

Kypri, K., Jones, C., McElduff, P., & Barker, D. (2010). Effects of restricting pub closing times on night-time assaults in an Australian City. *Addiction, 106*, 303–310.

Kypri, K., McElduff, P., & Miller, P. (2016). Night-time assaults in Newcastle 6–7 years after trading hour restrictions. *Drug and Alcohol Review, 35*, E1–E2.

LaBrie, J. W., Migliuri, S., & Cail, J. (2010). A night to remember: A harm-reduction birthday card intervention reduces high-risk drinking during 21st birthday celebrations. *Journal of American College Health, 57*, 659–663.

Levine, M., Lowe, R., Best, R., & Heim, D. (2012). "We police it ourselves": Group processes in the escalation and regulation of violence in the night-time economy. *European Journal of Social Psychology, 42*, 924–932.

Liu, T., Ferris, J., Higginson, A., & Lynham, A. (2016). Systematic review of Australian policing interventions to reduce alcohol-related violence — A maxillofacial perspective. *Addictive Behaviors Reports, 4*, 1–12. https://doi.org/10.1016/j.abrep.2016.05.002

Maguire, M., & Nettleton, H. (2003). *Reducing alcohol-related violence and disorder: an evaluation of the 'TASC' project*. Home Office Research Study 265. London: Home Office Research, Development and Statistics Directorate.

Marcus, J., & Siedler, T. (2015). Reducing binge drinking? The effect of a ban on late-night off-premise alcohol sales on alcohol-related hospital stays in Germany. *Journal of Public Economics, 123*, 55–77.

Marselle, M., Wootton, A. B., & Hamilton, M. G. (2012). A design against crime intervention to reduce violence in the night-time economy. *Security Journal, 25*, 116–133.

Mawby, R. I., & Jones, C. (2004). Explaining patterns of victimization within a rural county of England. *International Criminal Justice Review, 14*, 99–123.

McNally, I. M. (2004). Causal factors in weekend city center aggression. *Journal of Police and Criminal Psychology, 19*, 45–57.

Menéndez, P., Weatherburn, D., Kypri, P. & Fitzgerald, J. (2015). *Lockouts and last drinks: The impact of the 2014 liquor license reforms on assaults in NSW, Australia*. Crime and Justice Bulletin No. 183. Sydney: NSW Bureau of Crime Statistics and Research.

Middleton, J. C., Hahn, R. A., Kuzara, J. L., Elder, R., Brewer, R., Chattopadhyay, S., Fielding, J., Naimi, T. S., Toomey, T., Lawrence, B., & the Task Force on Community Preventive Services. (2010). Effectiveness of policies restricting hours of alcohol sales in preventing excessive alcohol consumption and related harms. *American Journal of Preventive Medicine, 39*, 575–589.

Miller, P., Curtis, A., Palmer, D., Busija, L., Tindall, J., Droste, N., Gillham, K., Coomber, K., & Wiggers, J. (2014). Changes in injury-related hospital emergency department presentations associated with the imposition of regulatory versus voluntary licensing conditions on licensed venues in two cities. *Drug and Alcohol Review, 33*, 314–322.

Miller, P., Sønderlund, A., Coomber, K., Palmer, D., Gillham, K., Tindall, J., & Wiggers, J. (2011). Do community interventions targeting licensed venues reduce alcohol-related emergency department presentations? *Drug and Alcohol Review, 30*, 546–553.

Miller, P., Zinkiewicz, L., Hayley, A., Sønderlund, A., Litherland, S., Medew-Ewen, T., Ewells, S., & Graham, K. (2016). Barroom aggression among Australian men: Associations with heavy episodic drinking, conformity to masculine norms, and personal and perceived peer approval of barroom aggression. *Journal of Studies on Alcohol and Drugs, 77*, 421–430.

Monaghan, L. F. (2003). Danger on the doors: Bodily risk in a demonised occupation. *Health, Risk and Society, 5*, 11–31.

Moore, S. C., Brennan, I., & Murphy, S. (2011). Predicting and measuring premises-level harm in the night-time economy. *Alcohol and Alcoholism, 46*, 357–363.

Moore, S. C., Brennan, I. R., Murphy, S., Byrne, E., Moore, S. N., Shepherd, J. P., & Moore, L. (2010). The reduction of intoxication and disorder in premises licensed to serve alcohol: An exploratory randomised controlled trial. *BMC Public Health, 10*, 607. http://www.biomedcentral.com/1471-2458/10/607

Moore, S. C., Fasihul Alam, M., Heikkinen, M., Hood, K., Huang, C., Moore, L., Murphy, S., Playle, R., Shepherd, J., Shovelton, C., Sivarajasingam, V., & Williams, A. (2017). The effectiveness of an intervention to reduce alcohol-related violence in premises licensed for the sale and on-site consumption of alcohol: A randomized controlled trial. *Addiction, 112*, 1898–1906.

Moore, S., Murphy, S., Moore, S. M., Brennan, I., Byrne, E., Shepherd, J., & Moore, L. (2012). An exploratory randomised controlled trial of a premises-level intervention to reduce alcohol related harm including violence in the United Kingdom. *BMC Public Health, 12*(1) http://www.biomedcentral.com/1471-2458/12/412

Moore, S., O'Brien, C., Alam, M. F., Coihen, D., Hood, K., Huang, C., Moore, L., Murpohy, S., Playle, R., Sivarajasingam, V., Spasic, I., Williams, A., & Shepherd, J. (2014). All-Wales licensed premises intervention (AWLPI): a randomised controlled trial to reduce alcohol-related violence. *BMC Public Health, 14*, 21. http://www.biomedcentral.com/1471-2458/14/21

Moore, S., Shepherd, J., Perham, N., & Cusens, B. (2007). The prevalence of alcohol intoxication in the night-time economy. *Alcohol and Alcoholism, 42*, 629–634.

Navarro, H. J., Shakeshaft, A., Doran, C. M., & Petrie, D. J. (2013). Does increasing community and liquor licensee's awareness, police activity, and feedback reduce alcohol-related violent crime? A benefit-cost analysis. *International Journal of Environmental Research and Public Health, 10*, 5490–5506. https://doi.org/10.3390/ijerph10115490

Nelson, A. L., Bromley, R. D. F., & Thomas, C. J. (2001). Identifying micro-spatial and temporal patterns of violent crime and disorder in the British city centre. *Applied Geography, 21*, 249–274.

Newton, A., & Hirschfield, A. (2009). Measuring violence in and around licensed premises: The need for a better evidence base. *Crime Prevention and Community Safety, 11*, 171–188.

Nottinghamshire Police. (2002). *The alcohol related violence: Crime reduction project*. Dangerous Persons Management Unit, Nottinghamshire Police.

Palk, G. R. M., Davey, J. D., & Freeman, J. E. (2010). The impact of a lockout policy on levels of alcohol-related incidents in and around licensed premises. *Police Practice and Research: An International Journal, 11*, 5–15.

Palk, G., Davey, J. D., Freeman, J. E., & Morgan, H. (2012). Perspectives on the effectiveness of the late night liquor trading lockout legislative provision. *Criminal Justice Policy Review, 23*, 465–492.

Patrick, M. E., Maggas, J. L., & Osgood, D. W. (2010). LateNight Penn State alcohol-free programming: Students drink less on days they participate. *Prevention Science, 11*, 155–162.

Pennay, A., Miller, P., Busija, L., Jenkinson, R., Droste, N., Quinn, B., Jones, S. C., & Lubman, D. I. (2014). 'Wide-awake drunkenness'? Investigating the association between alcohol intoxication and stimulant use in the night-time economy. *Addiction, 110*, 356–365.

Philpot, R., Liebst, L. S., Møller, K. K., Lindegaard, M. R., & Levine, M. (2019). Capturing violence in the night-time economy: A review of established and emerging methodologies. *Aggression and Violent Behavior, 46*, 56–65.

Pointing, S., Hayes-Jonkers, C., Bohanna, I., & Clough, A. (2012). The role of an open-space CCTV system in limiting alcohol-related assault injuries in a late-night entertainment precinct in a tropical Queensland city, Australia. *Injury Prevention, 18*, 58–61.

Rossow, I., & Norström, T. (2011). The impact of small changes in bar closing hours on violence. The Norwegian experience from 18 cities. *Addiction, 107*, 530–537.

Sanchez, Z. M., & Sanudo, A. (2018). Web-based alcohol intervention for nightclub patrons: Opposite effects according to baseline alcohol use disorder classification. *Substance Abuse, 39*(3), 361–370.

Sanders, T., & Hardy, K. (2012). Devalued, deskilled and diversified: Explaining the proliferation of the strip industry in the UK. *British Journal of Sociology, 63*, 513–532.

Shakeshaft, A., Doran, C., Petrie, D., Breen, C., Havard, A., Abudeen, A., Harwood, E., Clifford, A., D'Este, C., Gilmour, S., & Sanson-Fisher, R. (2014). The effectiveness of community action in reducing risky alcohol consumption and harm: A cluster randomised controlled trial. *PLoS Medicine, 11*(3), e1001617. https://doi.org/10.1371/journal.pmed.1001617

Stockwell, T., & Chikritzhs, T. (2009). Do relaxed trading hours for bars and clubs mean more relaxed drinking? A review of international research on the impacts of changes to permitted hours for drinking. *Crime Prevention and Community Safety, 11*, 153–170.

Swann, R., Green, A., Johns, N., & Sloan, L. (2015). Street pastors as substitutes for trust in the context of plural policing. *Safer Communities, 14*(4), 168–182.

Taylor, N., Miller, P., Coomber, K., Mayshak, R., Zahnow, R., Patafio, B., Burn, M., & Ferris, J. (2018). A mapping review of evaluations of alcohol policy restrictions targeting alcohol-related harm in night-time entertainment precincts. *International Journal of Drug Policy, 62*, 1–13.

Tutenges, S., Søgaard, T. F., Krøll, L. T., Bloomfield, K., & Hesse, M. (2015). Violent work environments: A survey of bouncers and their experiences of violence, stress and other work-related problems. *International Journal of Workplace Health Management, 8*, 129–141.

Wallin, E., Nortsröm, T., & Adreasson, S. (2003). Alcohol prevention targeting licensed premises: A study of effects on violence. *Journal of Studies on Alcohol, 64*, 270–277.

Warburton, A. L., & Shepherd, J. P. (2006). Tackling alcohol related violence in city centres: Effect of emergency medicine and police intervention. *Emergency Medical Journal, 23*, 12–17.

Warpenius, K., Holmila, M., & Mustonen, H. (2010). Effects of a community intervention to reduce the serving of alcohol to intoxicated patrons. *Addiction, 105*, 1032–1040.

Winlow, S. (2010). Violence in the night-time economy. In F. Brookman, M. Maguire, H. Pierpoint, & T. Bennett (Eds.), *Handbook on crime* (pp. 331–350). Willan Publishing.

# Chapter 3
# Managing Sex Offenders on Licence: Effectiveness of Registration and Notification Procedures

## 3.1 Question to Be Addressed and Overall Objectives

What general approaches and specific methods can be applied by the police in the safe supervision and monitoring of convicted sex offenders on licence conditions to avoid re-offending or relapse? Our objective was to conduct an evidence review and prepare a report summarizing what is known about effective policing methods and practices in carrying out the task of monitoring convicted sex offenders on licence. Given the awareness that senior police managers had of the complexities of these tasks, it was hoped that research may be able to identify possible approaches to conducting licence and parole supervision as effectively as possible. As a preliminary strategy and starting point for conducting the review, the PICO framework was used to outline and develop an approach, specifying key features as shown in Table 3.1.

## 3.2 Background

Research by the Ministry of Justice (2013) analysing survey data over a 3-year period indicated that there was an estimated average of 430,000 to 517,000 sexual offences committed each year in England and Wales. Given that many sexual crimes are not reported, perhaps more so than for most other types of offence, and that many victims do not contact the police, the number of officially recorded sexual offences then was a far lower figure at 54,310 (a 3-year average), which included 15,670 rapes. The rate of detection and of subsequent court proceedings is lower still, to such an extent that the numbers of convictions for sexual offences and for rape respectively were 5620 and 1070 (again based on a 3-year average). We will revisit these issues in Chap. 9 when we consider some of the reasons why



J. McGuire et al., *Evidence-Based Policing and Community Crime Prevention*, Advances in Preventing and Treating Violence and Aggression,
https://doi.org/10.1007/978-3-030-76363-3_3

**Table 3.1** PICO framework: managing sex offenders on licence

| | |
|---|---|
| Population/ participants | Persons convicted of sexual offences who have been released on licence from prison (target population)<br>Members of the community in a range of roles: parents, teachers, employers<br>Partner agencies: probation, social services, community mental health teams, forensic outpatient units<br>Police officers involved in supervision and monitoring procedures |
| Intervention/ indicator | Conduct of pre-release risk assessment; communication of parole reports and other information to police, probation and allied agencies<br>Establishing and maintaining systems of multi-agency team coordination<br>Development and implementation of action plans for monitoring of required reporting levels, ensuring appropriate engagement and reviewing the functioning and wellbeing of licensees<br>Use of electronic monitoring and computer e-safety monitoring processes |
| Comparison/ control | It is unlikely that any adapted forms of licence monitoring can be evaluated in a case-control study design; however, parallel comparisons of different procedures (comparing multiple treatments) may be feasible. The alternative would be time-series (before-and-after) comparisons. Studies are already known that have used each of these approaches |
| Outcome(s) | Maintenance of improved public safety; reduced rates of sexual offences<br>Public perceptions of safety and confidence in police actions and arrangements<br>Increased self-confidence and self-management skills development of licensees; reduced use of illicit websites or chatrooms, etc.<br>Impact on workloads, cost-efficiency of different monitoring strategies |

prosecutions are often not carried through to their conclusion. A more recent Crime Survey for England and Wales (Office for National Statistics, 2018, p.8) "estimated that approximately 700,000 adults aged 16 to 59 had experienced sexual assault in the 12 months prior to interview". Although sexual offences constitute only a small proportion of total police-recorded crime, by their nature and the harm they do, they are the source of marked distress and of continuing public concern.

Sexual offending, its occurrence and society's response to it are highly emotive subjects. The harm caused by sexual victimization and the portrayal of those who perpetrate it give rise to considerable revulsion and alarm, not solely because of the events themselves but also because they appear to touch on sensitivities close to many citizens' deepest concerns. It has been suggested that sexual offending produces reactions beyond those caused by other types of crime because it "…corrupts what in other contexts should be the most intimate and tender of human encounters" (Miller, 2014, p. 68). Such reactions become more powerful still when the victims of offences are children, and those who commit offences of that kind possibly generate more antipathy and anathema than virtually any other group.

There have been attempts to regulate those who commit serious violent or sexual crimes for many years (Thomas, 2011). The development of the present range of legal sanctions and the restrictions placed on those who have been found guilty of sexual offences are often traced to particularly horrific sexual assaults and murders of children that took placed in the 1990s. In the USA, where most of the research collected for the present report was carried out, the abduction and disappearance of

Jacob Wetterling and the murder of Megan Kanka and later of Adam Walsh had a massive impact on public opinion, leading to calls for tighter controls to be placed particularly upon those who were sentenced to prison and later returned to the community. The offences just mentioned were all committed by men who had previous records of sexual assaults against children. In response to the ensuing media attention and public outcry, there were numerous developments. The results were the passage in 1994 by the US Congress of the *Jacob Wetterling Crimes Against Children and Sexually Violent Offender Registration Act* (Levenson, 2018) and the establishment in many jurisdictions of registers of sex offenders, coupled in some cases with processes for notifying local communities when a convicted sex offender who had been released from prison was living nearby, and with restrictions placed on where such individuals were allowed to reside. Sex offender registration and notification (SORN) laws were introduced in all American states in the period 1990–1999 (dates for each were tabulated by Vasquez et al. (2008)).

In the UK, several new laws and practices were successively introduced, including the Sex Offenders Act 1997, which codified the process of placing specific requirements on sexual offenders, and the establishment of the Multi-Agency Public Protection Arrangements (Ministry of Justice, 2015), which became operational from 2000 onwards, with several measures consolidated in the Sexual Offences Act 2003. Subsequently other processes were introduced including the Violent and Sexual Offender Register (ViSOR) from 2005 onwards (Thomas, 2011).

Do these laws achieve their planned objectives? One challenge in answering this is that there are multiple objectives of registers: to ensure information contained in the Police National Computer is kept up to date, to help identify possible suspects after a crime, to deter individuals already convicted of such crimes from potential re-offending and to have a broader use in the general prevention of such crimes in the community. Most evaluation studies focus on the deterrence and crime prevention objectives and mainly on the specific effects on those persons placed on the register. Evaluation of effects that might be occurring in the context of the numerous factors that influence any type of criminal activity is not an easy type of research to conduct in a way that can lead to drawing clear or definitive conclusions. That these issues remain unresolved underpins the considerable controversies that still arise concerning the possible introduction of SORN in other places, for example, in Canada (Lussier & Mathesius, 2019).

Some other approaches to managing sex offenders in the community are basically similar to those proposed and tested for use with any group of offenders considered to present a possible risk to others. They include spatial tracking by means of the Global Positioning System (GPS) and radio-frequency monitoring. They can be used to impose curfews on individuals requiring them to return to a specific location by a specified time each day, to remain within certain geographical confines or to exclude them from certain others. Although GPS uses advanced satellite-based technology, its use in this context has sometimes been difficult to implement as a result of technical problems.

## 3.3 Review Objectives

The following more specific objectives were set for the present review: (1) to carry out a literature search using selected terms to locate studies focused on evaluating the effectiveness of different methods of police supervision and monitoring of individuals convicted of sexual offences and placed under licence conditions and (2) to summarize the findings from the located studies, with a view to identifying possible options for action that could be taken to develop and enhance the supervision and monitoring process.

Throughout this report, the term sex (or sexual) offender is used frequently. This is difficult to avoid as it is a standard terminology in criminology, psychology, policing and elsewhere for individuals convicted of crimes with a sexual element. It is recognized that this has additional overtones beyond those usually associated with other words used to refer to individuals who have broken other types of laws and can have pejorative and often counter-productive effects. The fact that an individual has committed a sexual offence is often taken to indicate many other attributes, and it thus has a pervasive effect on how such an individual is perceived. Despite these ramifications, unfortunately no other form of words is easily usable for discussing the issues to be addressed in this review.

## 3.4 Previous Reviews

As far as could be ascertained, there are no previous reviews of research covering the precise area designated for the present work. Neither the initial nor the updated searches reported here found reviews with that exact focus. There are however reviews of adjacent areas of activity relevant to this work, and these will be briefly described and summarized. There is a very large literature on the nature of sexual offending, on assessment and treatment of those who perpetrate it, on risk assessment and on evaluation of treatment outcomes (see, e.g. Boer et al., 2011; Craig et al., 2008; Laws & O'Donohue, 2008). For present purposes use was also made of two books covering the broader topic of the community management of persons who have committed sexual offences, incorporating both analysis and discussion of legal frameworks and reviews of research on monitoring and supervision arrangements (Thomas, 2011; Wright, 2015).

### *3.4.1 Treatment of Sex Offenders*

A first issue that might arise in connection with this is that of whether sexual recidivism can be reduced. There are numerous outcome studies on the effectiveness of treatment with this group of offenders, and it is an area that has been reviewed on a number of occasions. There is evidence of positive treatment outcome effects with adults (Alexander, 1999; Hall, 1995; Hanson et al., 2002; Gallagher et al., 1999; Lösel & Schmucker, 2005; Polizzi et al., 1999; Schmucker & Lösel, 2008, 2015, 2017) and with adolescents (Reitzel & Carbonell, 2006; Walker et al., 2004) who have sexually offended, and also with sexually aggressive adults assessed as showing psychopathic features (Doren & Yates, 2008). There is, furthermore, evidence showing that treatment can be cost-effective (Prentky & Burgess, 1990). It has been argued that essentially the same principles as are applied with many other types of offending, based on an approach to intervention known as the *risk-need-responsivity* model (Bonta & Andrews, 2017), are also applicable to those who have committed sexual offences (Hanson et al., 2009).

However, the methodology of many outcome studies in this area is rather weak, and some authors have expressed criticism concerning the robustness of the findings (Bilby et al., 2006; Brooks-Gordon et al., 2006). Given that only a small proportion of the outcome research that has been published has involved well-designed evaluations, some reviewers have remained sceptical regarding the extent and durability of any reported change. When more robust evaluation studies (randomized controlled trials only) have been reviewed, evidence of treatment effects has been less convincing, and more research has been called for (Dennis et al., 2012). Furthermore, prison-based sex offender treatment programmes, while they have shown some benefits, have sometimes been found to be only marginally effective if at all in group comparison studies (Friendship et al., 2003; Grady et al., 2015), and sometimes to be actually counter-productive (Mews et al., 2017). Nevertheless, in large sample studies of prison-based sex offender treatment comparing predicted with actual rates of reconviction, strong effects have been found (Travers et al., 2014). Similarly, positive results have also been obtained from an evaluation of community-based sex offender treatment (Hollis, 2007).

### 3.4.2 Risk Assessment

Many aspects of the treatment and management of those who have committed sexual offences, especially when they have a history of such offending, are predicated on the possibility of being able to evaluate risk of further re-offending with some degree of accuracy. The field of sexual offending risk assessment is quite highly developed. There has been a large volume of work, and many separate instruments have been devised and a sizeable volume of information collected in attempts to validate them. It is possible to make predictions of the likelihood of further offending at levels of accuracy well above chance. However, there appears to be a ceiling of predictive power such that beyond a certain level further increments in predictive accuracy for violence may prove to be unobtainable (Whittington et al., 2013). The portfolio of sex offending risk assessments presently available has limited power in predicting recidivism by offence type (Parent et al., 2011). It is also unclear to what extent relapse prevention plans, self-management and self-monitoring, support services, and liaison and coordination between community partner agencies have an aggregate effect in reducing risk.

The degree of success in managing sex offenders on licence is likely to be partly dependent on the extent to which individuals have participated in treatment while in prison, on their overall level of risk of relapse and recidivism and on the specific factors that influence their sexual behaviour and their conduct in other respects. It is also likely to be a function of the services available to support the reintegration and rehabilitation process once an individual is released from prison.

Several other aspects of community-based management of sexual offenders have been examined in other previous reviews. Table 3.2 lists a series of six that were found as part of the present evidence assessment.

The overall impression emerging from the above reviews is that the introduction of laws regulating the lives of sexual offenders following release from custody has not resulted in any major or consistent benefits. While a few studies have found a measurable impact on re-arrest or re-offending rates, the majority have not. While offenders themselves have agreed with the need for such laws, many have experienced negative consequences as a result of them, both for themselves and for their relatives. While the public at large reportedly welcome the inception of such laws, it is not clear to what extent they use the information made available through them, and the impact on feelings of safety is sometimes negative rather than positive.

## 3.5 Method

Preliminary scoping searches identified a number of sources of relevant evidence in this area and located reports on specially designed projects; although the number of high-quality evaluations seemed very limited, there appeared to be a sizeable number of quasi-experimental evaluations from the USA, Canada, Australia, New Zealand and elsewhere, and there were several developments occurring in the UK.

### 3.5.1 *Search Strategy*

Search terms were developed from the PICO framework (Table 3.1) and from the articles that had already been located in preliminary scoping searches. Fuller search strategies were initially designed to survey published and unpublished evaluations of policing and other initiatives that have had or potentially could have desired impacts on outcome targets. Databases searched included the Campbell and Cochrane libraries, EMBASE, MEDLINE, the National Criminal Justice Reference Service (NCJRS, USA), the National Police Library Catalogue, OpenGrey, ProQuest, PsycINFO, PubMed, Scopus and Web of Science. For the updating review however (2016–2020), searches were confined to studies directly connected

**Table 3.2** Previous reviews of areas related to sex offender licence management

| Review | Focus | Number of studies | Findings |
|---|---|---|---|
| Clarke et al. (2015) | Circles of support and accountability | 15 | Evaluated the effect of a specific intervention developed for working with individuals who have committed sexual offences. Re-offending rates amongst both Circle Members and control groups were low. There was a trend towards lower rates amongst Circle Members but only a few significant differences were found. Only one study employed an RCT design |
| Drake and Aos (2009) | Sex offender registration and notification | 9 | No statistically significant effect was found in terms of *specific deterrence*, i.e. reduced rate of re-offending amongst offenders made subject to registration and notification laws. Two studies showed some indication of a wider *general deterrence* effect, i.e. reduced rates of offending in the community as a whole. Overall findings were too variable and based on too small samples to draw firm conclusions. All studies were quasi-experiments (there were no RCTs) |
| Elliott and Völlm (2018) | Systematic review of studies of the post-conviction usage of the polygraph test with sex offenders | 19 | Evaluation of whether the polygraph led to higher levels of disclosure of risk-relevant information on sexual offences. Most studies used before-and-after designs with only four including a comparison group. Differing numbers of studies (from 2 to 7 of 19) reported higher levels of disclosure of aspects of offences. However, there were substantial dropout rates and in 13 studies participants were also receiving some form of psychological therapy |
| Lasher and McGrath (2012) | Impact of sexual offender laws on community reintegration | 8 | Respondents ($N = 1503$ across all studies) reported negative effects including loss of jobs or accommodation, being harassed or threatened. They also reported positive effects including being motivated to prevent themselves from re-offending |
| Pawson (2002) | Impact of "Megan's Law" | na | Although titled a "systematic review", this monograph adopts a different method and is instead an analysis of theories that inform the procedures involved in applying "Megan's Law". It does not contain a summary of findings as such |
| Socia and Stamatel (2010) | Impact of sex offender laws | 35 | Review article in three sections. The first reviewed eight studies on whether registration and notification laws achieved their set goals: two studies found those subject to notification had lower arrest rates. The second reviewed 18 studies of collateral effects of laws. The third reviewed nine studies of effects of the laws on the public. Only a small number of citizens made use of notification, and its effects were mixed, sometimes producing increased fear |

with the use of and effectiveness of registration and notification procedures, as those are the activities most pivotal within police work.

Searches thus covered the period from 1990 to 2020. They were not limited by language or publication type or with respect to whether or not they were published or unpublished. Due to the large number of records retrieved however, only publications available in full text in English, and that were published, were retained following the initial screening process. In total, 6678 records were identified through database searches. From them 1602 duplicates were removed, leaving 5076 records that were then screened for relevance to the objectives of the review. Two researchers divided this set of studies approximately in half and screened in the region of 2500 records each. Comparisons were made and discussions held regarding inclusion/exclusion decisions for 26 records, details of which were initially retained in a separate file for fuller scrutiny. In due course an initial set of 73 reports was selected for downloading. Fuller inspection resulted in 15 of these being removed, yielding 58 reports considered most closely relevant to the study aims. A further 13 were added from the update review giving a final total of 71 reports on 67 studies. These were categorized in specified areas considered relevant to the review objectives. However, no studies were identified which fully met the criteria for the review, in evaluating the specific role of policing in sex offender supervision. The final set of studies retained for full download was arrived at through application of a number of inclusion and exclusion criteria as below.

### 3.5.2 *Inclusion and Exclusion Criteria*

The following criteria were set for making decisions regarding inclusion or exclusion of items located through searches. Reports were sought which present empirical data from a research study which examined some aspect of the management of sex offenders in the community after release from prison. Searches were designed to locate studies of the role of policing in that process. The outcomes were to include information on relapse or recidivism, which could be measured in terms of re-arrest, reconviction or recall to prison. Studies were also sought which evaluated the effects of management strategies on community perceptions of safety or levels of fear, as well as their effects on offenders' own perceptions of their impact on community reintegration following discharge from prison. Both quantitative and qualitative studies were to be included, and studies of both juvenile and adult offenders were retained.

The volume of material collected in searches was considerable, and as noted earlier it was decided to exclude documents where the main text was in languages other than English, research dissertations or other unpublished reports and discussion or polemical items analysing legal, ethical or other dimensions of sex offender management. Basic research on sexual offending (concerning its origins, development, manifestations, relationship to sexuality in general, theoretical accounts of it or its relationship to some mental disorders) was also outside the scope of the review, as were studies of the mental health or wellbeing of offenders.

Unfortunately, no studies were found which directly addressed the question posed for this review, regarding evaluation of the effectiveness of specific policing practices on management of sex offenders, on rates of re-offending or on comparative costs of different approaches. However, several studies were found in adjacent areas of interest, and given that they are closely associated with police work or that effective policing may be strengthened through an awareness of them, these areas will be described in the present report. This will however be done in less detail that would be the format in a standard systematic review where studies directly relevant to the review objectives had been located. Figure 3.1 presents a flowchart of the numbers of items located, excluded or retained at successive phases of the search, screening and downloading decision-making process.

Studies were not included if they consisted solely of a survey at a single time point of perceptions of or attitudes towards the use of a sex offender registration or notification scheme, unless they contained information about responses to the changes that had resulted in those who were being managed by them. Several studies have been undertaken of general attitudes to SORN, covering many different groups including police officers (Masters & Kebbell, 2019), the general public (Bartels et al., 2020), policy makers (Jung et al., 2020) and offenders themselves

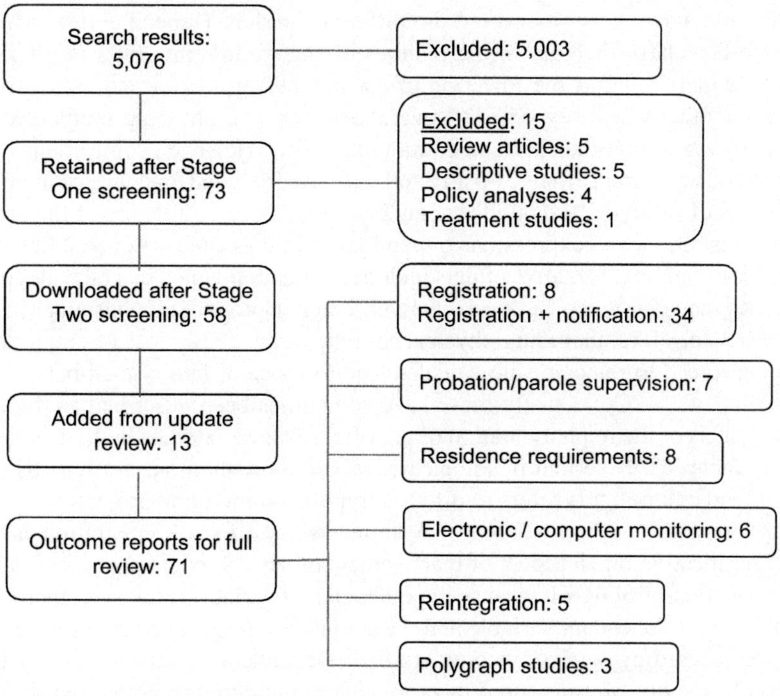


**Fig. 3.1** Flowchart of search results on sex offender licensing and notification

(Kemshall et al., 2012). Most find that there are many misconceptions concerning the frequency, likelihood or location of sexual offences in community samples and also concerning why an individual would be placed on a sex offender register or website (Taylor, 2017).

## 3.6 Results

There are several areas of work that are of varying levels of relevance to the central question which this review was intended to address. The 71 reports that were retained have been grouped into several categories which will be described in sequence.

### *3.6.1 Registration and Notification*

The largest single batch of studies focused on the direct and indirect effects of the application of sex offender registration and notification laws. Direct effects that have been researched include the extent to which registered sexual offenders desisted from crime; therefore, rates of re-arrest, recall, reconviction or re-incarceration have been measured in different studies ("specific deterrence"). Indirect effects have included wider patterns of change in crime rates (both sexual and non-sexual), such as the lowering of the number of new offenders relative to what would otherwise be expected ("general deterrence"). Thus, a principal emphasis in many evaluations has been on community safety. However, some studies have examined other indirect effects. Positive effects have included evidence of increased perceptions of safety by the public, or endorsement by sex offenders of the usefulness of registration, and expressions of confidence in it as a means of enabling them to avoid re-offending. Negative effects include vilification which can take numerous forms. Stigmatization can have adverse and counter-productive consequences for offenders themselves, including physical assault, verbal abuse, loss of employment and being forced to relocate, and can also lead to abuse of family members (Evans & Cubellis, 2015). Collectively these have sometimes been described as the "collateral" effects of the implementation of sex offender laws. Studies in these areas are listed in Table 3.3. Note that in some cases where more than one study is listed in the left-hand column, this refers to different reports on the same project.

All the research studies in Table 3.3 examined some effect of registration or community notification on an aspect of management of sex offenders or responses to it; the introduction of SORN laws was the independent variable. However, there were several types of dependent variable and the studies can be grouped into several subcategories according to the outcome studied. Dependent variables were of three main kinds: recidivism (measured in various ways including re-arrest, reconviction or re-incarceration), effects on community perceptions or effects on the lives of

**Table 3.3** Studies of registration and community notification (42 reports on 38 studies)

| Study | Methodology | Samples/data sources | Focus and findings |
|---|---|---|---|
| *Registration only* | | | |
| Brewster et al. (2012) | Descriptive, content analysis study | Data from all 50 US states + DC | Undertook a content analysis of sex offender registries by examining and classifying the variables recorded in them, to examine similarities and differences between them. Reports and tabulates the kinds of data found in different registries |
| Burchfield and Mingus (2014) | Survey-based study | 333 offenders in 2 phases, 2007 and 2008 | Investigated sex offenders' perceptions of levels of community support in their local neighbourhoods. Statistical model showed social ties, neighbour behaviour and neighbourhood attachment were linked to feelings of support |
| Caldwell and Dickinson (2009) | Group comparison and follow-up study | 106 registered 66 unregistered Juvenile sex offenders | Compared two groups of discharged youthful sex offenders, one registered, the other not, in terms of level of assessed risk and new offences over a 4-year period. Group membership did not predict sexual or violent re-offending; few differences of any kind emerged between the groups. No evidence that registration had an impact at follow-up |
| Duwe and Donnay (2010) | Retrospective quasi-experimental design | Two groups of offenders one with ($N = 126{,}270$) and one without FTR convictions ($N = 1391$) | Studied the effect of offenders' failing to register (FTR) as legally required on their subsequent rates of conviction. FTR offenders were more often from ethnic minorities, had prior supervision failures and more previous convictions and used more force in sex offences. Both FTR groups had significantly higher rates of FTR and general recidivism |

(continued)

**Table 3.3** (continued)

| Study | Methodology | Samples/data sources | Focus and findings |
|---|---|---|---|
| Harris and Cudmore (2018) | Survey of usage of sex offender registers | Stratified sample of 1000 US adults | Surveyed the extent of and reasons for use of the register, alongside demographic and social attitude information as correlates. Most (55%) respondents had never accessed it. Most who did had done so only 1–2 times. Only 7.4% had accessed it >5 times. Doing so more often was associated with having young children and with conservative ideology. Most said the register had no effect on feelings of safety. High-level users reported feeling less safe |
| Kernsmith et al. (2009) | Computer-assisted telephone survey | 733 randomly sampled residents of Michigan | Investigated the level of awareness of sexual offence registers amongst the public. Almost all respondents knew the register existed and was publicly available, but only 37% had ever looked at it. Reasons for not doing so are analysed in relation to other variables |
| Letourneau, et al. (2018a) | Between-group comparison of registered and non-registered offenders | 251 boys (aged 12–17) receiving treatment for sexually harmful or inappropriate behaviour | 73 of 251 (29%) children had been placed on sexual offender registers. Data collected on offence histories, mental health, social support and other variables. Registered children had higher suicide risk and poorer mental health outcomes, but more social support than non-registered children. They also felt less safe and were more likely to have been sexually assaulted or molested |
| Tewkesbury (2005) | Anonymous postal survey | 121 offenders on the Kentucky Sex Offender Registry | Examined the effects of sexual offence registration on individuals' lives. Survey had a potential pool of 2408 individuals; thus, the response rate was 15.4%. Major problems reported included loss of friendships, jobs, and places to live; being harassed and assaulted; and being threatened by phone or mail |

(continued)

**Table 3.3** (continued)

| Study | Methodology | Samples/data sources | Focus and findings |
|---|---|---|---|
| *Registration + notification* | | | |
| Anderson and Sample (2008) | Telephone survey-based study, gathered both quantitative and qualitative data | 1821 adult residents of Nebraska | The objective of the study was to seek views on citizens' knowledge of registration and notification laws and perceptions of safety due to accessing the registry. Most (89.8%) knew the registry existed, but only 34.8% ever accessed it. Of these only one-third took any preventative or coping action |
| Beck and Travis III (2004) | Postal survey-based study with two-group comparison | 97 residences notified<br>139 residences not notified | Compared reactions and perceptions of residents in two conditions, one notified and the other not notified of sex offenders living nearby. Statistical analysis showed that notification group influenced levels of personal fear, but gender and education were stronger predictors. Notification was unrelated to altruistic fear (concern for members of one's household) |
| Beck and Travis III (2006) | Group (county) comparison design using survey data | Two samples of residents in each of two counties ($N = 87, 109, 149, 115$) | Different states and US counties employ different procedures for community notification, some more "proactive" and others more "passive". This study compared two counties with different practices. The former succeeded in conveying information to a higher proportion of residents. There were however no observed differences in reported fear or perceived risk of victimization |
| Blasko et al. (2011) | Group comparison study | 76 prisoners in 2 groups: 20 classified as sexually violent predators, 56 not so classified | The study tested whether there were specific features of prisoners classified as requiring enhanced registration and notification following release. However, no differences were found between the two groups, and suggested allocation decisions were not properly evidence based |
| Bouffard and Askew (2019) | Interrupted time-series analysis of sexual and non-sexual offending data (1977–2012) | NeuLaw Criminal Records Database of Harris County/ Houston, Texas | Analysed rates of different offences over periods since SORN laws were introduced (1991) and modified (1997, 2005). There were increasing trends for all crimes, after controlling for other population variables, not affected by the initiation of SORN laws or by modifications expanding those laws |

(continued)

**Table 3.3** (continued)

| Study | Methodology | Samples/data sources | Focus and findings |
|---|---|---|---|
| Brannon et al. (2007) | Survey of attitudes, group comparison | 125 sexual offenders and 193 members of the public | Compared attitudes to registration and notification laws and practices. More offenders considered laws were applied unfairly (70% vs 22%), were ineffective (42% vs 10%) and reported a higher level of vigilante attacks than members of the public were aware of |
| Caputo and Brodsky (2004) | Telephone survey | 250 residents who had been notified of a sex offender living locally | Notification predicted increased fear, especially amongst those who attached more importance to it, but was not associated with increased use of specific coping strategies for reducing risk of victimization |
| Cubellis et al. (2018) | Mixed-methods study: In-depth interviews and statistical analysis of correlates | Interviews with 105 law enforcement officers + survey of 1156 enforcement staff from 49 states | Focused on the "collateral impacts" of SORN and examined the extent to which police and other enforcement personnel were concerned about these. Respondents mainly viewed SORN as effective and "did not express great concern for the possible collateral impacts" (p.1093). A small group working most closely in SORN showed greater awareness of those impacts |
| Duwe and Donnay (2008) | Retrospective quasi-experimental design | Three groups of sex offenders released from prison | Compared 155 high-risk offenders subject to notification after it was introduced, with 155 not subject to it and 125 released from prison before notification laws were introduced. The first group had lower 3-year recidivism than the other two, with largest differences for sexual offences |
| Elbogen et al. (2003) | Survey of forensic in-patients guilty of sex offences | 40 offenders detained in a forensic mental health unit | Study investigated relationships between offenders' knowledge of notification laws, attitudes to them and willingness to comply with them. Most (72%) saw the laws as a major incentive not to re-offend but considered many aspects of them as unfair |

(continued)

**Table 3.3** (continued)

| Study | Methodology | Samples/data sources | Focus and findings |
|---|---|---|---|
| Harris et al. (2010) | Comparison of two American states with respect to the impact of SORN laws | Ohio: 24,994<br>Oklahoma: 10,197 offenders in prisons or community | Examined changes in sex offender classification in two states following the passage of the 2006 Child Protection and Safety Act in the USA. There was a significant upward shift in classified risk levels in both states, with most offenders placed in upper tiers (Ohio, 56%; Oklahoma, 82%) |
| Harris et al. (2018) | Mixed-methods study with interviews + national online survey | Interviews with 105 law enforcement officers + survey of 1374 personnel | Interviewees collectively identified five main functions of SORN policies. The majority saw them as being effective or very effective in all five areas, although the lowest rate was for reducing re-offending. Interview and survey data generated numerous issues on the challenges of applying SORN and how its implementation could be improved |
| Hughes and Kadleck (2008) | Spatial mapping study | 975 offenders (Nebraska)<br>5163 offenders (Oklahoma) | Examined the effects of SORN laws in areas of two states on the numbers of sex offenders living in different census tracts. In both states, neighbourhood disadvantage was related significantly to the number of resident sex offenders and negatively related to affluence |
| Jennings et al. (2012) | Group comparison | 247 sex offenders<br>250 non-sex offenders | Compared post-release recidivism of two cohorts of parolees under SORN requirements. Offending patterns were very similar in both groups. There were five times more high-risk non-sex than sex offenders. Living conditions for sex offenders were more difficult than for non-sex offenders |
| Kemshall et al. (2010, 2012) | Qualitative process study | 186 interviews: 82 police or offender managers;<br>43 applicants; 61 registered sex offenders | UK study investigating process of implementing procedures of enabling citizens to apply for disclosure of information on persons working with children, piloted in four police areas from 2007. The number of applicants was lower than expected. Most were satisfied with the process. Practitioners thought the new arrangements clarified processes. No changes were reported in offender behaviour |

(continued)

**Table 3.3** (continued)

| Study | Methodology | Samples/data sources | Focus and findings |
|---|---|---|---|
| Letourneau et al. (2010a) | Time-series analysis | All charges against males aged 14–17 in the period 1991–2004 | Studied the effects of SORN policies on sex crimes by juveniles in South Carolina. Tested whether changes in the law in 1995 and 1999 were followed by changes in sex crimes, non-sexual assaults and robberies. There were some apparent trends but analyses suggested there were no significant effects. SORN had no effect in deterring sex crimes |
| Letourneau et al. (2010b, 2010c) | Time-series analysis | 205,197 arrests of 194,575 arrestees in the period 1990–2005 | Tracked rates of arrest for sex crimes, assault or robbery of those aged ≥18 over a 16-year period in South Carolina. Following inception of SORN policies (1995), there was an 11% drop in arrests for sex crimes but not in the other offences. No effect was observed for the inception of online registration (1999) |
| Letourneau, et al. (2018b, 2019) | Time-series analysis of offence rates before and after enacting SORN laws | Rates of new charges and convictions for sexual and other offences (NIBRS data) | Evaluated extent of general and specific deterrence from use of SORN with juvenile sex offenders. Detailed analysis of trends over periods up to 19 years found no evidence that SORN had any effect on deterring sexual offences or offending in general, despite variations in the implementation process across states |
| Levenson and Tewkesbury (2009) | Online survey | 584 family members of registered offenders (80% female) | Explored the impact of SORN laws on the families of registered sex offenders. A substantial proportion reported adverse effects including having been threatened or harassed, financial hardship and other problems, for themselves and for their children |
| Maurelli and Ronan (2013) | Interrupted time-series design | Data on 50 US states over the period 1960–2008 | Compared rates of rape in 50 states of the USA before and after the introduction of sex offender laws. A significant drop was found in 17 states, no change in 32 states (data for 1 state could not be analysed) |

(continued)

**Table 3.3** (continued)

| Study | Methodology | Samples/data sources | Focus and findings |
|---|---|---|---|
| McCartan (2013) | Qualitative focus group and content analysis | 35 members of the public in Wales and Northern Ireland (3 groups each) | Analysis of focus group discussions discovered that participants believed they should be given information on sex offenders living in their areas, but became divided and conflicted when considering aspects of this. Results revealed a sizeable level of suspicion of the disclosure scheme and mistrust of authorities' management of the issues |
| Prescott and Rockoff (2011) | Statistical analysis of a large dataset of crime events (328,260 sex offences) | Data from the US NIBRS | Analysed the impact of SORN laws on the numbers of sex offences. Registration reduced the frequency of reported sex offences against victims known to offenders but not against strangers. Notification deterred non-registered sex offenders but on balance slightly increased recidivism in registered sex offenders |
| Sandler et al. (2008) | Time-series analysis | Rates of sexual and other types of offence in New York State in 1986–2006 | Analysed the impact of introducing registration laws on the rate of sexual crimes amongst 160,000 offenders. No effect was found on the rates of sexual crime but there was a possible reduction in crimes of robbery. There were no effects on any types of crime by non-sex offenders |
| Sandler et al. (2017) | Analysis of crime incident reports before and after start of registration laws | NIBRS data | Analysed data on crime rates (for 8 types of sexual + 36 types of nonsexual offence) by juveniles following the introduction of sex offender registers in 4 US states. The enactment of a juvenile sex offender registration policy did not yield a reduction in sexual offences in any state and a reduction in only one offence type in one state |
| Tewkesbury and Jennings (2010) | Time-series analysis | 5019 persons on sex offender registry in Iowa | Studied patterns of sexual offending 5 years before and 5 years after introduction of SORN laws. 87.4% showed no recidivism, 9.7% a low rate and 2.9% a high rate. This did not notably differ from the pre-SORN pattern. Most post-SORN re-offending took place in the first year of release |

(continued)

**Table 3.3** (continued)

| Study | Methodology | Samples/data sources | Focus and findings |
|---|---|---|---|
| Vasquez et al. (2008) | Time-series analysis | Data on rape rates for ten US states for the period 1990–2000 | Compared monthly rates of rape in ten states in the period before and after introducing sex offender laws. Five states experienced reductions, and in three this was statistically significant. Five states experienced increases and in one this was statistically significant. The overall pattern of findings was regarded as inconclusive |
| Whitting et al. (2016, 2017) | Mixed-methods study; in-depth interviews + analysis of information in police databases | Police ($N = 21$) managing a SORN scheme in 1 state of Australia + file information on 2047 offenders | Evaluated police perceptions of a register and notification Scheme 6 months after its introduction, alongside information on 125 registered offenders. After a large number of inquiries and high workload when the system was launched, this later reduced. No incidents of vigilantism were recorded. There was no clear evidence of an impact on offender compliance |
| Zevitz (2006) | Follow-up (4.5 years) and group comparison study | Sex offenders released from prison in Wisconsin | Compared two groups of released prisoners, one ($N = 47$) subject to extensive notification, the other ($N = 166$) to a more limited form. Rates of return to prison were very similar for the two groups (48.9%, 49.3%), but most recalls were not for sexual offences |
| Zgoba and Bachar (2009) | Before-and-after study | Data from 21 counties in New Jersey and on 550 sex offenders | Evaluated aspects of the effect of introducing Megan's Law in New Jersey. There was no reduction in the number of rearrests for sex offences. Sentence lengths were reduced, but the numbers given parole fell (The largest drop in sex offence rates in NJ took place prior to the change in law.) |

(continued)

**Table 3.3** (continued)

| Study | Methodology | Samples/data sources | Focus and findings |
|---|---|---|---|
| Zgoba et al. (2010) | Before-and- after study | 550 offenders, 50 per year over an 11-year period (1990–2000) | More detailed report on the above evaluation. Compared the offence patterns following the release of 275 offenders from a Diagnostic and Treatment Center and with 275 from the general prison population, each 5 years before and 5 years after the implementation of Megan's Law. There was a significant reduction in arrest rates for general offending, but with other variables controlled, the effect was not found. There was no observed change in arrest rate for sexual crimes |

*SORN* sex offender registration and notification, *NIBRS* National Incident-Based Reporting System

offenders. Amongst those studies that examined some form of recidivism, three found positive effects (Duwe & Donnay, 2008, 2010; Letourneau et al., 2010b, 2010c). In addition, Bouffard and Askew (2019) cite an unpublished report which could not be located which, drawing on data from all 50 American states, found that the introduction of registration laws resulted in a small (2%) but significant reduction in the number of rapes reported to the police. In two other studies there was a mixture of effects, with positive impact on some variables but no effect on others (Maurelli & Ronan, 2013; Prescott & Rockoff, 2011). Most however, a total of nine evaluations, found the introduction of SORN arrangements made no difference to re-offending outcomes (Caldwell & Dickinson, 2009; Jennings et al., 2012; Letourneau et al., 2010a; Sandler et al., 2008; Tewkesbury & Jennings, 2010; Vasquez et al., 2008; Zevitz, 2006; Zgoba & Bachar, 2009; Zgoba et al., 2010).

Studies of how SORN laws were perceived can be further sub-divided into two groups, those reporting reactions of communities and those reporting reactions of offenders. Investigation of how community perceptions were influenced by the introduction of registration and notification obtained a broadly similar pattern of findings. All found that community respondents were aware of the establishment of registration and notification procedures, but that relatively few citizens directly accessed information or made use of it (Anderson & Sample, 2008; Kemshall et al., 2010; Kemshall et al., 2012; Kernsmith et al., 2009). Thus, it was not clear that communities' reactions to these arrangements were such that they used information in a constructive way (Beck & Travis III, 2004; Caputo & Brodsky, 2004; McCartan, 2013). Offenders understood and accepted the rationales for the inception of SORN laws and appeared to consider that they could reinforce their wish to avoid further offending (Brannon et al., 2007). However, they considered that the laws were unfairly applied and too many individuals were unnecessarily made subject to them (Elbogen et al., 2003). There was evidence from four studies that there were different patterns in how the policies were implemented (Beck & Travis III, 2006; Blasko et al., 2011; Harris et al., 2010; Hughes & Kadleck, 2008), and the impact of registration and notification depended to some extent on who was allocated to registers and how communities were informed. Three studies of the "collateral effects" of implementing SORN laws found that they had quite damaging consequences for offenders themselves (Tewkesbury, 2005; Brannon et al., 2007; Elbogen et al., 2003) and one found there were also deleterious effects on their families (Levenson & Tewkesbury, 2009).

### *3.6.2 Probation/Parole Supervision*

A second focus of research was on the processes and the impact of supervision. For most sex offenders, this entails inter-agency collaboration, and several writers have commented on aspects of this (Alexander, 2010; Palmiotto & MacNichol, 2010; Payne & DiMichele, 2010a; Pimentel & Muller, 2010). However, apart from registration and/or reporting to police where that is mandatory, most routine direct supervisory contact with offenders is done by probation officers (and in Australia, Canada and the USA, parole officers). Research placed under this heading is listed in Table 3.4.

The above studies focus partly on how risk factors for re-offending emerged as being associated with relapse or other difficulties arising while under supervision (Harris & Hanson, 2003; Johnson, 2006). Two studies illustrated processes that appeared to be helpful in strengthening the supervision process (Ryan et al., 2014; Wilson et al., 2000), and one reported the negative effect on supervision of housing patterns of offenders and the distance needed to travel to supervision centres (Sloas et al., 2012). Severson and Pettus-Davis (2013) described the challenging nature of supervision of this group and noted that some staff experienced "secondary trauma" as a result of doing so.

### *3.6.3 Residence Requirements*

In some jurisdictions there are laws governing where individuals who have been convicted of sexual offences are allowed to live following their release from prison. This is founded on the concept that in order to minimize risk they should, for example, be kept away from potential victims and thus should not live near schools, playgrounds or day-care centres with minimum distances sometimes being prescribed. Their daily routines should be arranged such that they are not presented with opportunities to re-offend. This group of studies consists of evaluations of the effects of imposing restrictions on where adjudicated sex offenders can reside in the community. The overall pattern of findings to emerge from these studies is that the risks of proximity may be over-estimated, and the effect of imposing restrictions may prove to be counter-productive. For example, it may mean individuals are

**Table 3.4** Studies of probation and/or parole supervision (seven studies)

| Study | Methodology | Samples/data sources | Intervention and outcomes |
|---|---|---|---|
| Harris and Hanson (2003) | Descriptive account of progress on a project | >1000 sex offenders in 16 jurisdictions in Canada and the USA | Describes findings of the Dynamic Supervision Project involving repeated assessments of sex offenders under community supervision. Work includes assessment of risk factors and monitoring change every 6 months |
| Johnson (2006) | Descriptive study on demographic and case history data | 7339 offenders under US federal probation in 1999–2005 | Analysed factors associated with revocation of parole in a large sample of offenders under federal probation supervision. Identified principal influences such as unemployment, prior convictions and Risk Prediction Index scores. Does not discuss registration or notification |
| Mercado et al. (2011) | Description and analysis of database | Archival data on 3168 offenders in New Jersey in 1996–2007 | Reported analysis of one state's database on sex offenders over a 12-year period. Assessed factors predicting placement in a treatment facility; doing so was linked to a lower rate of *general* recidivism than not (25% vs 51.7%). Only 5% of offenders were convicted of a new sexual offence over an average of 6.5 years. However, treated and untreated groups showed no difference in *sexual* recidivism |
| Ryan et al. (2014) | Descriptive and statistical study | 182 offenders assessed for extended supervision | Describes "psychological health assessment" of persons placed on Extended Supervision Orders (ESO) for sexual offenders in New Zealand. Examined possible improvements in selection procedures. Placement under ESO was most closely associated with the presence of a higher number of dynamic risk factors, such as sexual deviance and poor self-regulation |
| Severson and Pettus-Davis (2013) | Qualitative focus group study | 49 parole officers in 5 groups | Part of a large study exploring sex offender management procedures and outcomes. The focus was on examining secondary trauma experienced by professionals working with sex offenders (parole officers and supervisors). Many participants described emotional effects of their work similar to clinical descriptions of secondary trauma |

(continued)

**Table 3.4** (continued)

| Study | Methodology | Samples/data sources | Intervention and outcomes |
|---|---|---|---|
| Sloas et al. (2012) | Spatial mapping study | 53 providers of treatment; 1074 sex offenders | Investigated factors associated with time taken to travel to treatment centres in the community. Established that most sex offenders in Kentucky are concentrated in low-income urban areas but had very disparate travel times to treatment facilities. Long travel times are associated with adverse effects including isolation |
| Wilson et al. (2000) | Programme evaluation of community | 107 offenders released to community maintenance services in Canada | Study retained as it illustrates the combination of a treatment programme with the process of supervision in community management of sex offenders. A high-risk programme was delivered in a forensic mental health unit, but was complemented by a maintenance programme administered by correctional staff. Mean re-offence rate was 3.7% at 3½ years |

placed under other pressures that could be destabilizing, that result in them having very lengthy or circuitous journeys to and from workplaces, that lead to them finding it difficult to access treatment or support or that give them no choice other than to live in impoverished neighbourhoods. Cumulatively, this could also result in a concentration of registered sex offenders in certain areas, an effect not envisaged or planned when placing restrictions. Table 3.5 summarizes research located on this issue.

The above studies almost uniformly reported problematic effects of placing residence restrictions on sex offenders in the community. Findings included increased levels of hardship amongst offenders, with the associated possibility of decreasing individuals' coping capacities (Barnes et al., 2009; Levenson, 2008). One unforeseen result of residence requirements was a concentration of offenders in particular areas, usually ones of deprivation and disadvantage (Hughes & Burchfield, 2008; Mustaine & Tewkesbury, 2011). Overall, these requirements appeared to achieve no meaningful benefits for either communities or offenders and often had counterproductive effects whereby the net outcome was an elevation in risk of re-offending (Duwe et al., 2008; Socia, 2012; Zandbergen et al., 2010).

### *3.6.4 Electronic and Computer Monitoring*

GPS technology has been introduced as a possible means of managing several types of high-risk offender in the community. It is often viewed in principle as an attractive option in allowing offenders to remain living at home or other designated location, while still being kept under control but at far lower cost than if given a custodial sentence (Padgett et al., 2006). In common with registration and notification

**Table 3.5** Studies of the effects of residence requirements (eight studies)

| Study | Methodology | Samples/data sources | Intervention and outcomes |
|---|---|---|---|
| Barnes et al. (2009) | Spatial analysis | 246 registered sex offenders from 4 counties in South Carolina | Used geographical mapping to investigate the distribution of sex offenders with different residence requirements imposed (e.g. to live a minimum distance from schools). Studies the effect of these restrictions on choices over where offenders can live and work, finding that the resultant increased hardship may increase risk levels, restrict access to treatment or may also result in them all being concentrated in specific undesirable areas |
| Duwe et al. (2008) | Follow-up single-cohort study | 224 released prisoners returned to prison (Minnesota) | Sample regarded as the most serious cases. The majority (79%) offended against someone they knew. There was no evidence that residence restrictions would have prevented most crimes |
| Hughes and Burchfield (2008) | Spatial mapping and statistical analysis | 872 local neighbourhoods and 2025 child sex offenders | Analysed data on registered sex offenders living in Chicago in relation to data on locations of community landmarks, facilities and socio-economic characteristics of neighbourhoods. Offenders were concentrated in disadvantaged areas. The study illustrated that the use of residence laws can have unintended effects |
| Levenson (2008) | Survey using questionnaire | 109 from pool of 160 offenders receiving outpatient treatment | Large proportions of the study sample reported negative effects of residence restrictions. Few reported that restrictions made them less likely to re-offend, the majority stating they could have re-offended despite them |
| Mustaine and Tewkesbury (2011) | Regression analysis of file data | Census data for a single US county for the years 2004–2006 | Analysed factors predicting the rate per 1000 population of sexual offenders living in localities. Higher rates were associated with great social disadvantage and higher rates of other serious crimes |
| Socia (2012, 2015) | Quasi-experimental longitudinal design (two interrelated studies) | Analysis of rates of rape first in New York, then in 49 states of the USA + DC in 1990–2008 | Statistical models developed to predict rate of rape and changes in it over a 19-year period. States with residence restrictions for sexual offenders had higher rates of rape than those which did not. There was no decrease in rapes when restriction policies were present |

(continued)

**Table 3.5** (continued)

| Study | Methodology | Samples/data sources | Intervention and outcomes |
|---|---|---|---|
| Zandbergen et al. (2010) | Group comparison design using spatial analysis (geocoding) | 330 offenders in two matched groups, recidivist and non-recidivist | Tested whether sexual recidivism was associated with living close to a school or day-care centre. Both groups were located throughout the state (Florida) and there was no concentration in a single area. Both groups lived at very similar distances from schools. Sex offenders who lived in close proximity to schools were not more likely to re-offend than those who lived farther away |

however, the GPS approach too has been found to produce some unanticipated consequences, such as the occurrence of high technical error rates, the gaining of a false sense of security or compromising the balance between enforcement, surveillance and treatment (Payne & DiMichele, 2011). Note that several of the studies included here are connected in that they are evaluations of the effectiveness of GPS monitoring in California (Bulman, 2013; Gies et al., 2012; Omori & Turner, 2012; Turner et al., 2015). Only one study was found of the use of computer software for detection of indicators of Internet-based sexual offending, such as accessing child pornography or attempting to groom potential victims (Elliott et al., 2010). This and the studies of GPS monitoring are summarized in Table 3.6.

A mixed picture emerges from studies of these methods of working. Technical problems including false alarms have been repeatedly reported as a problem in some studies (Armstrong & Freeman, 2011; Turner et al., 2015; Turner, Chamberlain). However, one set of studies has reported positive outcomes (Bulman, 2013; Gies et al., 2012) with sex offender populations. This is in contrast to earlier results with non-sex offenders which yielded no evidence of positive benefits from the use of electronic monitoring (see, e.g. the results of Bonta et al., 2000, who also reviewed earlier research on this area). Where the costs of GPS or other monitoring methods have been compared with other conditions, they are usually found to be higher and that it also results in increased workload where the opposite might have been expected (Omori & Turner, 2012; Payne & DiMichele, 2010b). Additional costs would probably be seen as justified if the preventive effects were significant, but the relationship between increased costs and payoffs in terms of beneficial results remains uncertain.

### 3.6.5 Reintegration

This category consists of studies focused on the impact of applying sex offender laws on the process and outcomes of community reintegration for sex offenders, and the course of rehabilitation, after discharge from prison. The collateral consequences

**Table 3.6** Evaluation of electronic and computer monitoring (six studies)

| Study | Methodology | Samples/data sources | Intervention and outcomes |
|---|---|---|---|
| Armstrong and Freeman (2011) | Descriptive study | 154 offenders convicted of a sexual crime against children | Examined "alerts" in a cohort of offenders placed on mandatory GPS monitoring in Arizona over a 2½-year period. Classified reasons for alerts (e.g. violating inclusion or exclusion area, curfew violation, tampering with equipment, technical failure). As a large proportion of alerts were not due to violation, it was concluded there are unexpected time and staff costs in the use of GPS technology |
| Bulman (2013), Gies et al. (2012) | Quasi-experimental design group comparison and follow-up study | 516 high-risk parolees, half monitored by GPS, half not | Compared offenders on GPS monitoring with others on traditional supervision in California. The latter commit more new offences and were returned to custody at a rate 38% higher than the former. Costs of GPS monitoring were higher ($8.51 per day), but as it resulted in 12 percentage points lower arrest rate, overall costs were lower. There was evidence of laxity in ensuring that offenders maintained treatment attendance |
| Elliott et al. (2010) | Pilot study, descriptive data | 11 offenders (incl. 1 female) supervised by Surrey Police | UK 6-month pilot study of remote monitoring of computer use by sex offenders, employing specially designed software installed on home PCs. Only a small number of violations occurred. Offenders reported that the process enabled them to demonstrate cooperativeness. Police (Risk Management Officers) also gave positive feedback. Participation was voluntary |
| Omori and Turner (2012) | Quasi-experimental two-group comparison | GPS-monitored offenders: 93 Comparison sample: 88 | A cost-effectiveness evaluation of GPS monitoring in California; average cost of parole using GPS was US $4600 more than that for those placed on standard supervision. GPS offenders had lower rates of new crimes, but the difference arose mainly from not reporting to the sex offender register |
| Payne and DiMichele (2010b) | Survey of practitioners | 228 probation and parole officers | A study of the workloads and work patterns of personnel involved in GPS-based supervision of sex offenders. Staff in this role made more home visits and employment checks than non-GPS staff, and made more use of polygraphs, plethysmographs and mandated treatment |
| Turner et al. (2015) | Quasi-experimental two-group comparison | GPS-monitored offenders: 94 Comparison sample: 91 | Evaluation of the use of GPS monitoring in California. Offenders made subject to GPS had a lower rate of new offences (19%) than a non-GPS comparison group (35%). Comparison group members were three times more likely to abscond or to fail to register their sex offender status |

found in most surveys of sex offenders subject to notification laws included a wide range of difficulties, and many considered the laws were applied to too wide a range of offenders. However, many also considered that they generated motivation to avoid re-offending. The studies found are listed in Table 3.7.

For this category and the next, the number of located studies was relatively small. Regarding research on reintegration however, there are some consistent findings that emerge from the studies found. It seems clear that the process of return to the community is a difficult one for those with a history of sexual offending, with many, sometimes serious, adverse events occurring (Levenson & Cotter, 2005; Levenson

**Table 3.7** Research on community reintegration of sex offenders on licence (five studies)

| Study | Methodology | Samples/data sources | Intervention and outcomes |
|---|---|---|---|
| Levenson and Cotter (2005) | Questionnaire-based survey study | 183 convicted male sex offenders from two counselling centres | Examined the effect of community notification on the process of community re-entry for sex offenders in Florida. Although physical attacks were rare, roughly one-third of the sample reported other "dire events" such as losing a job or home, and most reported stress, isolation, loss and negative feelings |
| Levenson et al. (2007) | Questionnaire-based survey study | 239 offenders attending counselling centres | Examined the effect of community notification on the process of community re-entry for sex offenders in Connecticut ($n = 91$) and Indiana ($N = 148$). 10% had been assaulted; many endured job loss, threats, harassment, property damage and suffering of household members, and the majority reported psychosocial stress and feelings of isolation, shame and hopelessness |
| Lussier and Gress (2014) | Quasi-experimental longitudinal design | 169 prisoners, comparing 2 different types of post-release supervision in British Columbia | Risk status (high/medium/low) was a significant predictor of rates of technical violation of supervisory conditions and of general recidivism. Negative social influence was also a significant predictor but could be mitigated by intensive supervision and outreach work |
| Scoones et al. (2012) | Follow-up study of released prisoners | 196 prisoners convicted of child molesting, released from a treatment unit in New Zealand | Prisoners discharged from Kia Marama Unit were followed for a mean of 11 years. Adding details of features of release planning increased predictive accuracy of risk assessments and was associated with a reduced likelihood of re-offending |
| Willis and Grace (2009) | Follow-up and group comparison study | Compared 30 recidivist with 30 non-recidivist ex-prisoners in New Zealand | The quality of reintegration planning was measured with reference to practical details concerning accommodation, social support, employment and other issues. The quality was poorer for child molesters who re-offended than for those who did not |

et al., 2007). Encouragingly however, there is evidence that the quality of pre-release planning and the kinds of support provided through supervision are associated with better chances of success in achieving integration while avoiding relapse or re-offending (Lussier & Gress, 2014; Scoones, Willis & Grace, 2012; Willis & Grace, 2009). This is an area from which potential lessons might be drawn for making policing and supervision more effective.

### 3.6.6 Polygraph Testing

Although several studies were found on this, only a small proportion of them dealt with its use in the context of registration and notification arrangements supervised by police. As a potential component of such supervision, it was thought that this warranted retention in the review and merited a separate category as it does not belong neatly elsewhere.

There is a large amount of research on polygraph testing ("lie detection") in general terms. While it is approved for specified purposes in some jurisdictions, it is not permitted in others, and its status remains controversial in many more. The original concept of the polygraph as a method of detecting deception has been assimilated into present-day folklore. But considered evaluation of relevant research has cast significant doubt on its efficacy. Notably, the National Research Council of the US National Academy of Sciences published a major review of studies in 2003, a task later updated by Iacono and Ben-Shakar (2019). Both drew similarly critical conclusions regarding the polygraph's validity.

Nevertheless, some practitioners and researchers have advocated its value in clinical and risk assessment. Grubin (2008) and Wilcox (2008) discussed several aspects of polygraph testing in the context of supervision of sexual offenders. A study by Gannon et al. (2007) indicated that men who had molested children were less likely to conceal cognitive distortions or to engage in impression management – both usually assessed via questionnaires – when they believed it possible that their dishonesty would be detected by a machine. This study was not included in the present review as it did not employ an actual polygraph measure.

It may be recalled from the systematic review of 19 studies by Elliott and Völlm (2018) cited earlier (Table 3.2) that there is some evidence that polygraph use can result in persons convicted of sexual offences revealing more information than they might otherwise do about their past offences or about risk-related behaviour (e.g. admitting masturbation to deviant fantasies). Located studies not included in the Elliott and Völlm (2018) systematic review or in one case published since then are listed in Table 3.8.

All three studies listed in Table 3.8 found that the use of polygraph testing was either associated with increased levels of risk-related divulgence or suggestive of its usefulness for that purpose. The value of the disclosures made was not entirely clear however. For example, in the study by Wood et al. (2020), while police officers and offender managers regarded the disclosures as useful, there is only minimal

**Table 3.8** Research on the use of the polygraph in monitoring sexual offenders (three studies)

| Study | Methodology | Samples/data sources | Intervention and outcomes |
|---|---|---|---|
| Konopasek (2015) | Single-cohort correlational design + 5-year follow-up | 192 sexual offenders on probation or parole | Obtained tentative evidence that polygraph testing as a means of eliciting sexual history was associated with successful completion of treatment. However, there was no association between polygraph disclosure and recidivism |
| Wilcox et al. (1999) | Case study summary | Five offenders on probation | Describes some findings from the West Midlands Polygraph Trials but provided only case summaries and did not include original data. The authors concluded that the polygraph has potential utility as part of supervision |
| Wood et al. (2020) | Controlled experimental study in six police areas in England | 557 police supervisees<br>142 suspects<br>104 applicants for removal of notification | Within each of the three samples, individuals were randomly allocated to polygraph testing or to comparison groups. The outcome variable was the number of risk-relevant disclosures made by each group. It was found that polygraph testing increased the likelihood of individuals making risk-relevant disclosures, though more were prior to and after than during polygraph sessions. Police officers and offender managers had generally very favourable views on the use of the polygraph |

information given on how that occurred or what it meant in terms of the action taken. Reference is made to steps taken towards greater public protection but no detail is given on what this entailed. Similarly, there is no evidence given that it was associated with recorded changes in subsequent levels of recidivism. It may also be important that the polygraph-tested groups had a significantly higher level of contact with their offender managers during the course of this research study. Hence, questions remain over the validity of such revelations as indicators of the likelihood of further offending (Rosky, 2013, 2016).

The research by Wood et al. (2020) is the most recent in a series of studies reported by the University of Kent, of which previous studies have been conducted mainly in probation service settings (Gannon et al., 2014; Spruin et al., 2018). In both of the earlier studies, offender managers described the polygraph as useful in supervision and reported making use of the information obtained. The later study by Wood et al. (2020) also reports the results of a public survey ($N = 2091$) conducted by the poll organization Ipsos MORI. This showed that a sizeable majority of those surveyed (66.7%) supported the police use of the polygraph (strongly agreed or tended to agree). Paradoxically however, 41% of those surveyed said they knew nothing about polygraphs, and 50.4% said they were aware of them but not in great detail. Despite these figures, 57.9% thought the polygraph was fairly, very or extremely accurate.

Notwithstanding these positive reports and perceptions, the use of the polygraph for this purpose remains highly contentious. The method has been widely used by police and probation services for the purposes under discussion here, and at the time of writing its use was being incorporated into a forthcoming Parliamentary Bill. However, both scientists (Meijer et al., 2008) and lawyers (Kotsoglou & Oswald, 2020) have expressed strong reservations and criticisms in relation to the use of the polygraph for this purpose.

It is argued by proponents that the objective of testing in this context is different: it is not to uncover deception but to elicit information that would otherwise be withheld (Grubin, 2008; Grubin et al., 2019). Conversely however, it has also been claimed that with only a minimal amount of training or preparation, individuals taking a polygraph can learn to simulate their responses in a manner that may make all the results uninterpretable. More fundamentally, the association between any material that individuals disclose and independent validity data such as their likelihood of re-offending remains unclear.

## 3.7 Discussion

The general pattern of findings that has emerged from the studies included in the present review is essentially similar to that found in the review studies discussed earlier and listed in Table 3.2. There is a modicum of evidence of benefits in terms of reduced recidivism and increased community safety from some patterns of sex offender management in the community. The use of registers on the present scale appears to be an innovation that would be difficult to put into reverse and it can have some beneficial outcomes. But the obtained effects are comparatively weak, and the findings of research reviewed here indicate that the empirical basis for the procedure is far from convincing. A majority of studies found no significant effects on key outcome variables. Findings for community notification and for the placing of residence restrictions on sex offenders are weaker still and in fact often fundamentally backfire, producing more negative than positive effects (Zgoba, 2011). There are some potentially useful findings with regard to what enables supervision to be more effective. Results from studies of electronic monitoring are essentially inconclusive, and those on use of the polygraph, while viewed positively by police officers, are difficult to evaluate in the absence of a separate indicator of their validity.

Managed carefully, the messages from this research can prove beneficial. Partly on the basis of the findings reported here, but also as a result of other initiatives, a Public Protection Unit officer was located HM Prison Bure, a prison with a high proportion of those convicted of sexual crimes, following a joint decision by the Norfolk Chief Constable and Prison Governor. The objectives of the role were to facilitate and enhance working relationships and cooperation between the prison and the police. The role subsequently expanded to include Registered Sex Offenders (RSOs) held in a second neighbouring prison.

The assigned responsibilities of the Public Protection Unit officer included (1) meeting with registered sex offenders shortly before release to gather intelligence and provide information on release conditions and the role of their supervisors; (2) multi-agency working and information sharing with all agencies within the prison, including prison officers, probation staff, the chaplaincy and police Prison Liaison Officer; (3) updating the Violent and Sex Offenders Register (*ViSOR*, the Multi-Agency Public Protection Arrangements database) with relevant information and intelligence on offenders to be released; and (4) other activities in support of these, such as preparing and organizing training for prison, probation and police staff.

The nature of the new role was evaluated through a series of interviews conducted with both practitioners (including the Public Protection Unit officer, police Prison Liaison Officer, Prison Probation Officer, the Unit Governor and others) and a small number of prisoners whose transition to the community would be managed by the post-holder.

This evaluation of a newly established Public Protection Unit officer role within the prison setting demonstrated a number of benefits and potential positive effects of the introduction of the role, regarding intelligence development, safeguarding, offender management and multi-agency working. The role faced a number of practical obstacles, to which solutions have largely been found, and has continued to balance the at times competing demands and priorities of the different agencies based within the prison. However, all practitioners interviewed, and offenders themselves, reported the role to be beneficial.

The way in which the role operates in the designated prison is unique: the equivalent role in the second prison has developed somewhat differently as a result of contextual factors. Expansion of such roles to other establishments would therefore need to identify the best pattern of working to achieve the benefits summarized here.

On the basis of this evidence review, other possible suggestions can be made for experimental or other research work that could be carried out. But first, to decide in what ways the evidence found in this review could most usefully be applied, it would be important to set it alongside data on patterns of residence of registered sex offenders in a given local area, and in addition the locations of those at different levels of Multi-Agency Public Protection Arrangements or other statutory monitoring processes.

One possibility then would be to conduct an interview-based survey or qualitative study asking offenders on licence to describe the patterns of support they perceive, and what aspects of lifestyles they find challenging and that potentially place them at risk of re-offending. A second would be to undertake an audit of the kinds of information that are provided to the police when sex offenders are released from prison, or a process or decision-focused study to examine the different pathways from prison to community, and the sequences of decisions made in allocating individuals to different licence requirements. The objective of such studies would be to identify the parameters of effective supervision of this offender population, in ways that are constructive and not counter-productive, to avoid placing at risk the progress that was made to enable them to be released.

## References


Alexander, M. A. (1999). Sexual offender treatment efficacy revisited. *Sexual Abuse: Journal of Research and Treatment, 11*, 101–116.

Alexander, R. (2010). Collaborative supervision strategies for sex offender community management. *Federal Probation, 74*, 16–19.

Anderson, A. L., & Sample, L. L. (2008). Public awareness and action resulting from sex offender community notification laws. *Criminal Justice Policy Review, 19*, 371–396.

Armstrong, G. S., & Freeman, B. C. (2011). Examining GPS monitoring alerts triggered by sex offenders: The divergence of legislative goals and practical application in community corrections. *Journal of Criminal Justice, 39*, 175–182.

Barnes, J. C., Dukes, T., Tewkesbury, R., & De Troye, T. M. (2009). Analyzing the impact of statewide residence restriction law on South Caroline sex offenders. *Criminal Justice Policy Review, 20*, 21–43.

Bartels, L., Gelb, K., Spiranovic, C., Warner, K., Roberts, L., & David, J. (2020). What does the public think about sex offender registers? Findings from a national Australian study. *Psychiatry, Psychology and Law*. https://doi.org/10.1080/13218719.2020.1805813

Beck, V. S., & Travis, L. F., III. (2004). Sex offender notification and fear of victimization. *Journal of Criminal Justice, 32*, 455–463.

Beck, V. S., & Travis, L. F., III. (2006). Sex offender notification: An exploratory assessment of state variation in notification processes. *Journal of Criminal Justice, 34*, 51–55.

Bilby, C., Brooks-Gordon, B., & Wells, H. (2006). A systematic review of psychological interventions for sexual offenders II: Quasi-experimental and qualitative data. *Journal of Forensic Psychiatry & Psychology, 17*, 467–484.

Blasko, B. L., Jeglic, E. L., & Mercado, C. C. (2011). Are actuarial risk data used to make determinations of sex offender risk classification? An examination of sex offenders selected for enhanced registration and notification. *International Journal of Offender Therapy and Comparative Criminology, 55*, 676–692.

Boer, D. P., Eher, R., Craig, L. A., Miner, M. H., & Pfäfflin, F. (Eds.). (2011). *International perspectives on the assessment and treatment of sexual offenders: Theory, practice and research*. Wiley-Blackwell.

Bonta, J. & Andrews, D. A. (2017). *The psychology of criminal conduct*. (6th ed.). Routledge.

Bonta, J., Wallace-Capretta, S., & Rooney, J. (2000). Can electronic monitoring make a difference? An evaluation of three Canadian programs. *Crime & Delinquency, 46*, 61–75.

Bouffard, J. A., & Askew, L. N. (2019). Time-series analyses of the impact of sex offender registration and notification law implementation and subsequent modifications on rates of sexual offenses. *Crime & Delinquency, 65*(11), 1483–1512.

Brannon, Y. N., Levenson, J. S., Fortney, T., & Baker, J. N. (2007). Attitudes about community notification: A comparison of sexual offenders and the non-offending public. *Sexual Abuse, 19*, 369–379.

Brewster, M. P., DeLong, P. A., & Moloney, J. T. (2012). Sex offender registries: A content analysis. *Criminal Justice Policy Review, 24*, 695–715.

Brooks-Gordon, B., Bilby, C., & Wells, H. (2006). A systematic review of psychological interventions for sexual offenders I: Randomised control trials. *Journal of Forensic Psychiatry & Psychology, 17*, 442–466.

Bulman, P. (2013). Sex offenders monitored by GPS found to commit fewer crimes. *National Institute of Justice Journal, 271*, 22–25.

Burchfield, K. B., & Mingus, W. (2014). Sex offender reintegration: Consequences of the local neighbourhood context. *American Journal of Criminal Justice, 38*, 109–124.

Caldwell, M. F., & Dickinson, C. (2009). Sex offender registration and recidivism risk in juvenile sexual offenders. *Behavioral Sciences & the Law, 27*, 941–956.

Caputo, A. A., & Brodsky, S. L. (2004). Citizen coping with community notification of released sex offenders. *Behavioral Sciences & the Law, 22*, 239–252.

Clarke, M., Brown, S., & Völlm, B. (2015). Circles of support and accountability for sex offenders: A systematic review of outcomes. *Sexual Abuse: A Journal of Research and Treatment, 26*. https://doi.org/10.1177/1079063215603691

Craig, L. A., Browne, K. D., & Beech, A. R. (Eds.). (2008). *Assessing risk in sex offenders: A practitioners' guide*. Wiley.

Cubellis, M. A., Walfield, S. M., & Harris, A. J. (2018). Collateral consequences and effectiveness of sex offender registration and notification: Law enforcement perspectives. *International Journal of Offender Therapy and Comparative Criminology, 62*(4), 1080–1106.

Dennis, J. A., Khan, O., Ferriter, M., Huband, N., Powney, M. J., & Duggan, C. (2012). Psychological interventions for adults who have sexually offended or are at risk of offending. *Cochrane Database of Systematic Reviews, 12*. https://doi.org/10.1002/14651858.CD007507.pub2

Doren, D. M., & Yates, P. M. (2008). Effectiveness of sex offender treatment for psychopathic sexual offenders. *International Journal of Offender Therapy and Comparative Criminology, 52*, 234–245.

Drake, E. K., & Aos, S. (2009). *Does sex offender registration and notification reduce crime? A systematic review of the research literature*. Washington State Institute for Public Policy.

Duwe, G., & Donnay, W. (2008). The impact of Megan's law on sex offender recidivism: The Minnesota experience. *Criminology, 46*, 411–446.

Duwe, G., & Donnay, W. (2010). The effects of failure to register on sex offender recidivism. *Criminal Justice and Behavior, 37*, 520–536.

Duwe, G., Donnay, W., & Tewkesbury, R. (2008). Does residential proximity matter? A geographical analysis of sex offense recidivism. *Criminal Justice and Behavior, 35*, 484–504.

Elbogen, E. B., Patry, M., & Scalora, M. J. (2003). The impact of community notification laws on sex offender treatment attitudes. *International Journal of Law and Psychiatry, 26*, 207–219.

Elliott, I. A., Findlater, D., & Hughes, T. (2010). Practice report: A review of e-Safety remote computer monitoring for UK sex offenders. *Journal of Sexual Aggression, 16*, 237–248.

Elliott, E. & Völlm, B. (2018). The utility of post-conviction polygraph testing among sexual offenders. *Sexual Abuse, 30*(4), 367–392.

Evans, D. N., & Cubellis, M. A. (2015). Coping with stigma: How registered sex offenders manage their public identities. *American Journal of Criminal Justice, 40*, 593–619.

Friendship, C., Mann, R. E., & Beech, A. R. (2003). Evaluation of a national prison-based treatment program for sexual offenders in England and Wales. *Journal of Interpersonal Violence, 18*, 744–759.

Gallagher, C. A., Wilson, D. B., Hirschfield, P., Coggeshall, M. B., & MacKenzie, D. L. (1999). A quantitative review of the effects of sexual offender treatment on sexual reoffending. *Corrections Management Quarterly, 3*, 19–29.

Gannon, T. A., Keown, K., & Polaschek, D. L. L. (2007). Increasing honest responding on cognitive distortions in child molesters: The bogus pipeline revisited. *Sexual Abuse: Journal of Research and Treatment, 19*(1), 5–22. https://doi.org/10.1007/s11194-006-9033-0

Gannon, T. A., Wood, J. L., Pina, A., Tyler, N., Barnoux, M. F. L., & Vasquez, E. A. (2014). An evaluation of mandatory polygraph testing for sexual offenders in the United Kingdom. *Sexual Abuse: A Journal of Research and Treatment, 26*, 178–203.

Gies, S. V., Gainey, R. Cohen, M. I., Healy, E., Duplantier, D., Yeide, M., Bekelman, A., Bobnis, A., & Hopps, M. (2012). *Monitoring high-risk sex offenders with GPS technology: An evaluation of the California Supervision Program. Final report*. Bethesda, MD: Office of Research and Evaluation, National Institute of Justice.

Grady, M. D., Edwards, D., & Pettus-Davis, C. (2015). A longitudinal outcome evaluation of a prison-based sex offender treatment program. *Sexual Abuse: A Journal of Research and Treatment*, online first. https://doi.org/10.1177/1079063215585731

Grubin, D. (2008). The case for polygraph testing of sex offenders. *Legal and Criminological Psychology, 13*, 177–189.

Grubin, D., Kamenskov, M., Dwyer, R. G., & Stephenson, T. (2019). Post-conviction polygraph testing of sex offenders. *International Review of Psychiatry, 31*(2), 141–148.

Hall, G. C. N. (1995). Sexual offender recidivism revisited: A meta-analysis of recent treatment studies. *Journal of Consulting and Clinical Psychology, 63*, 802–809.

Hanson, R. K., Gordon, A., Harris, A. J. R., Marques, J. K., Murphy, W., Quinsey, V. L., & Seto, M. C. (2002). First report of the Collaborative Outcome Data Project on the effectiveness of psychological treatment for sex offenders. *Sexual Abuse: A Journal of Research and Treatment, 14*, 169–194.

Hanson, R. K., Bourgon, G., Helmus, L., & Hodgson, S. (2009). The principles of effective correctional treatment also apply to sexual offenders: A meta-analysis. *Criminal Justice and Behavior, 36*, 865–891.

Harris, A. J., & Cudmore, R. (2018). Community experience with public sex offender registries in the United States: A national survey. *Criminal Justice Policy Review, 29*(3), 258–279.

Harris, A., & Hanson, R. K. (2003). The Dynamic Supervision Project: Improving the community supervision of sex offenders. *Corrections Today*, August, 60–64.

Harris, A. J., Lobanov-Rostovsky, C., & Levenson, J. S. (2010). Widening the net: The effects of transitioning to the Adam Walsh Act's federally mandated sex offender classification system. *Criminal Justice and Behavior, 37*, 503–519.

Harris, A. J., Levenson, J. S., Lobanov-Rostovsky, C., & Walfield, S. M. (2018). Law enforcement perspectives on sex offender registration and notification: Effectiveness, challenges, and policy priorities. *Criminal Justice Policy Review, 29*(4), 391–420.

Hollis, V. (2007). *Reconviction analysis of Interim Accredited Programmes Software (IAPS) data*. Research Development Statistics, National Offender Management Service.

Hughes, L. A., & Burchfield, K. B. (2008). Sex offender residence restrictions in Chicago: An environmental injustice? *Justice Quarterly, 25*, 647–673.

Hughes, L. A., & Kadleck, C. (2008). Sex offender community notification and community stratification. *Justice Quarterly, 25*, 469–495.

Iacono, W. G., & Ben-Shakar, B. (2019). Current status of forensic lie detection with the comparison question technique: An update of the 2003 National Academy of Sciences report on polygraph testing. *Law and Human Behavior, 43*(1), 86–98.

Jennings, W. G., Zgoba, K. M., & Tewkesbury, R. (2012). A comparative longitudinal analysis of recidivism trajectories and collateral consequences for sex and non-sex offenders released since the implementation of sex offender registration and community notification. *Journal of Crime and Justice, 35*, 356–364.

Johnson, J. L. (2006). Sex offenders on federal community supervision: Factors that influence revocation. *Federal Probation, 70*, 18–32.

Jung, S., Allison, M., Toop, C., & Martin, E. (2020). Sex offender registries: Exploring the attitudes and knowledge of political decision-makers. *Psychiatry, Psychology and Law, 27*(3), 478–492.

Kemshall, H., Wood, J., Westwood, S., Stout, B., Wilkinson, B. Kelly, G., & Mackenzie, G. (2010). *Child Sex Offender review (CSOR) public disclosure pilots: a process evaluation* - 2nd edition. Research report 32. London: Home Office Research, Development and Statistics Directorate.

Kemshall, H., Dominey, J., & Hilder, S. (2012). Public disclosure: Sex offenders' perceptions of the pilot scheme in England. Compliance, legitimacy and living a "Good Life". *Journal of Sexual Aggression, 18*, 311–324.

Kernsmith, P. D., Comartin, E., Craun, S. W., & Kernsmith, R. M. (2009). The relationship between sex offender registry utilization and awareness. *Sexual Abuse: A Journal of Research and Treatment, 21*, 181–193.

Konopasek, J. E. (2015). Expeditious disclosure of sexual history via polygraph testing: Treatment outcome and sex offense recidivism. *Journal of Offender Rehabilitation, 54*, 194–211.

Kotsoglou, K. N., & Oswald, M. (2020). Not 'Very English' – on the use of the polygraph by the penal system in England and Wales. *The Journal of Criminal Law*. https://doi.org/10.1177/0022018320976284

Lasher, M. P., & McGrath, R. J. (2012). The impact of community notification on sex offender registration: A quantitative review of the research literature. *International Journal of Offender Therapy and Comparative Criminology, 56*, 6–28.

Laws, D. R., & O'Donohue, W. T. (2008). *Sexual deviance: Theory, assessment, and treatment* (2nd ed.). Guilford Press.

Letourneau, E. J., Bandyopadhyay, D., Armstrong, K. S., & Sinha, D. (2010a). Do sex offender registration and notification requirements deter juvenile crimes? *Criminal Justice and Behavior, 37*, 553–569.

Letourneau, E. J., Levenson, J., Bandyopadhyay, D., Armstrong, K. S., & Sinha, D. (2010b). Effects of South Carolina's sex offender registration and notification policy on deterrence of adult sex crimes. *Criminal Justice and Behavior, 37*, 537–552.

Letourneau, E, J., Levenson, J., Bandyopadhyay, D., Sinha, D. & Armstrong, K. S. (2010c). *Evaluating the effectiveness of sex offender registration and notification policies for reducing sexual violence against women. Final Report*. National Institute of Justice.

Letourneau, E. J., Harris, A. J., Shields, R. T., Walfield, S. M., Ruzicka, A. E., Buckman, C., Kahn, G., & Nair, R. (2018a). Effects of juvenile sex offender registration on adolescent well-being: An empirical examination. *Psychology, Public Policy, and Law, 24*(1), 105–117.

Letourneau, E. J., Sandler, J. C., Vandiver, D. M., Shields, R. T., Nair, R. (2018b). *Juvenile registration and notification policy effects: A multistate evaluation project*. Final Technical report. Washington, DC: US Department of Justice, Office of Justice Programs.

Letourneau, E. J., Shields, R. T., Nair, R., Kahn, G., Sandler, J. C., & Vandiver, D. M. (2019). Juvenile registration and notification policies fail to prevent first-time sexual offenses: An extension of findings to two new states. *Criminal Justice Policy Review, 30*(7), 1109–1123.

Levenson, J. (2008). Collateral consequences of sex offender residence restrictions. *Criminal Justice Studies, 21*, 153–166.

Levenson, J. S. (2018). Sex offender management policies and evidence-based recommendations for registry reform. *Current Psychiatry Reports, 20*. https://doi.org/10.1007/s11920-018-0884-0

Levenson, J., & Cotter, L. P. (2005). The effect of Megan's Law on sex offender reintegration. *Journal of Contemporary Criminal Justice, 21*, 49–66.

Levenson, J., & Tewkesbury, R. (2009). Collateral damage: Family members of registered sex offenders. *American Journal of Criminal Justice, 34*, 54–68.

Levenson, J., Amore, D. A., & Hern, A. L. (2007). Megan's Law and its impact on community re-entry for sex offenders. *Behavioral Sciences & the Law, 25*, 587–602.

Lösel, F., & Schmucker, M. (2005). The effectiveness of treatment for sexual offenders: A comprehensive meta-analysis. *Journal of Experimental Criminology, 1*, 117–146.

Lussier, P., & Gress, C. L. Z. (2014). Community re-entry and the path towards desistance: A quasi-experimental longitudinal study of dynamic factors and community risk management of adult sex offenders. *Journal of Criminal Justice, 42*, 111–122.

Lussier, P., & Mathesius, J. (2019). Not in my backyard: Public sex offender registries and public notification laws. *Canadian Journal of Criminology and Criminal Justice / Revue canadienne de criminologie et de justice pénale, 61*(1), 105–116.

Masters, K. B., & Kebbell, M. R. (2019). Police officers' perceptions of a sex offender registration scheme: Identifying and responding to risk. *Psychiatry, Psychology and Law, 26*(3), 396–413.

Maurelli, K., & Ronan, G. (2013). A time-series analysis of the effectiveness of sex offender notification laws in the USA. *Journal of Forensic Psychiatry and Psychology, 24*, 128–143.

McCartan, K. (2013). From a lack of engagement and mistrust to partnership? Public attitudes to the disclosure of sex offender information. *International Journal of Police Science and Management, 15*, 219–236.

Meijer, E. H., Verschuere, B., Merckelback, H. L. G. J., & Crombez, G. (2008). Sex offender management using the polygraph: A critical review. *International Journal of Law and Psychiatry, 31*, 423–429.

Mercado, C. C., Jeglic, E., & Markus, K. (2011). *Sex offender management, treatment, and civil commitment: An evidence based analysis aimed at reducing sexual violence*. Department of Psychology, John Jay College of Criminal Justice.

Mews, A., Di Bella, L. & Purver, M. (2017). *Impact evaluation of the prison-based core Sex Offender Treatment Programme*. Ministry of Justice.

Miller, L. (2014). Rape: Sex crime, act of violence, or naturalistic adaptation? *Aggression and Violent Behavior, 19*, 67–81.

Ministry of Justice. (2013). *An overview of sexual offending in England and Wales*. Statistics Bulletin. London: Ministry of Justice, Home Office and Office for National Statistics.

Ministry of Justice. (2015). *Multi-agency public protection arrangements: Annual report 2014/15*. Statistics Bulletin. London: Ministry of Justice and Office for National Statistics.

Mustaine, E. E., & Tewkesbury, R. (2011). Residential relegation of registered sex offenders. *American Journal of Criminal Justice, 36*, 44–57.

National Research Council of the National Academy of Sciences. (2003). *The polygraph and lie detection*. The National Academies Press.

Office for National Statistics. (2018). *Sexual offending: Victimization and the path through the criminal justice system*. Office for National Statistics.

Omori, M. K., & Turner, S. F. (2012). Assessing the cost of electronically monitoring high-risk sex offenders. *Crime & Delinquency, 61*, 873–894.

Padgett, K. G., Bales, W. D., & Bloomberg, T. G. (2006). Under surveillance: An empirical test of the effectiveness and consequences of electronic monitoring. *Criminology and Public Policy, 5*, 61–91.

Palmiotto, M., & MacNichol, S. (2010). Supervision of sex offenders: A multi-faceted and collaborative approach. *Federal Probation, 74*, 27–30.

Parent, G., Guay, J.-P., & Knight, R. A. (2011). An assessment of long-term risk of recidivism by adult sex offenders: One size doesn't fit all. *Criminal Justice and Behavior, 38*, 188–209.

Pawson, R. (2002). *Does Megan's Law Work? A theory-driven systematic review*. ESRC UK Centre for Evidence Based Policy and Practice.

Payne, B. K., & DiMichele, M. (2010a). The role of probation and parole officers in the collaborative response to sex offenders. *Federal Probation, 74*, 23–27.

Payne, B. K., & DiMichele, M. (2010b). Electronic supervision for sex offenders: Implications for work load, supervision goals, versatility, and policymaking. *Journal of Criminal Justice, 38*, 276–281.

Payne, B. K., & DiMichele, M. (2011). Sex offender policies: Considering unanticipated consequences of GPS sex offender monitoring. *Aggression and Violent Behavior, 16*, 177–187.

Pimentel, R., & Muller, J. (2010). The containment approach to managing defendants charged with sex offenses. *Federal Probation, 74*, 24–26.

Polizzi, D. M., MacKenzie, D. L., & Hickman, L. J. (1999). What works in adult sex offender treatment? A review of prison- and non-prison-based treatment programs. *International Journal of Offender Therapy and Comparative Criminology, 43*, 357–374.

Prentky, R. A., & Burgess, A. W. (1990). Rehabilitation of child molesters: A cost-benefit analysis. *American Journal of Orthopsychiatry, 60*, 108–117.

Prescott, J. J., & Rockoff, J. E. (2011). Do sex offender registration and notification laws affect criminal behavior? *Journal of Law and Economics, 54*, 161–206.

Reitzel, L. R., & Carbonell, J. L. (2006). The effectiveness of sexual offender treatment for juveniles as measured by recidivism: A meta-analysis. *Sexual Abuse: A Journal of Research and Treatment, 18*, 401–421.

Rosky, J. W. (2013). The (f)utility of post-conviction polygraph testing. *Sexual Abuse: A Journal of Research and Treatment, 25*(3), 259–281.

Rosky, J. W. (2016). More polygraph utility: A comment on Jensen, Shafer, Roby and Roby (2015). *Journal of Interpersonal Violence, 31*(10), 1956–1970.

Ryan, J., Wilson, N., Kilgour, G., & Reynolds, N. (2014). Balancing efficiency and accuracy: Guidelines for the psychological assessment of extended supervision orders for child sex offenders in New Zealand. *Psychiatry, Psychology and Law, 21*, 139–157.

Sandler, J. C., Freeman, N. J., & Socia, K. M. (2008). Does a watched pot boil? A time-series analysis of New York State's sex offender and notification law. *Psychology, Public Policy, and Law, 14*, 284–302.

Sandler, J. C., Letourneau, E. J., Vandiver, D. M., Shields, R. T., & Chaffin, M. (2017). Juvenile sexual crime reporting rates are not influenced by juvenile sex offender registration policies. *Psychology, Public Policy, and Law, 23*(2), 131–140.

Schmucker, M., & Lösel, F. (2008). Does sexual offender treatment work? A systematic review of outcome evaluations. *Psicothema, 20*, 10–19.

Schmucker, M., & Lösel, F. (2015). The effects of sexual offender treatment on recidivism: an international meta-analysis of sound quality evaluations. *Journal of Experimental Criminology, 11*, 597–630.

Schmucker, M., & Lösel, F. (2017). Sexual offender treatment for reducing recidivism among convicted sex offenders: a systematic review and meta-analysis. *Campbell Systematic Reviews*, 2017:8. https://doi.org/10.4073/csr.2017.8

Scoones, C. D., Willis, G. M., & Grace, R. C. (2012). Beyond static and dynamic risk factors: The incremental validity of release planning for predicting sex offender recidivism. *Journal of Interpersonal Violence, 27*, 222–238.

Severson, M., & Pettus-Davis, C. (2013). Parole officers' experiences of the symptoms of secondary trauma in the supervision of sex offenders. *International Journal of Offender Therapy and Comparative Criminology, 57*, 5–24.

Sloas, L. B., Steele, P. D., & Hare, T. S. (2012). Geographical access to treatment for sex offenders under community supervision in Kentucky. *Journal of Sexual Aggression, 18*, 294–310.

Socia, K. M. (2012). The efficacy of county-level sex offender residence restriction in New York. *Crime & Delinquency, 58*, 612–642.

Socia, K. M. (2015). State residence restrictions and forcible rape rates: A multistate quasi-experimental analysis of UCR data. *Sexual Abuse: A Journal of Research and Treatment, 27*, 205–227.

Socia, K. M., & Stamatel, J. P. (2010). Assumptions and evidence behind sex offender laws: Registration, community notification, and residence restrictions. *Sociology Compass, 4/1*. https://doi.org/10.1111/j.1751-9020.2009.00251.x

Spruin, E., Wood, J. L., Gannon, T. A., & Tyler, N. (2018). Sexual offender's experiences of polygraph testing: A thematic study in three probation trusts. *Journal of Sexual Aggression, 24*(1), 12–12.

Taylor, S. C. (2017). Community perceptions of a public sex offender registry introduced in Western Australia. *Police Practice and Research, 18*(3), 275–290.

Tewkesbury, R. (2005). Collateral consequences of sex offender registration. *Journal of Contemporary Criminal Justice, 21*, 67–81.

Tewkesbury, R., & Jennings, W. G. (2010). Assessing the impact of sex offender registration and community notification on sex-offending trajectories. *Criminal Justice and Behavior, 37*, 570–582.

Thomas, T. (2011). *The registration and monitoring of sex offenders: A comparative study*. Routledge.

Travers, R., Mann, R. E., & Hollin, C. R. (2014). Who benefits from cognitive skills programs? Differential impact by risk and offense type. *Criminal Justice and Behavior, 41*, 1103–1129.

Turner, S., Chamberlain, A. W., Jannetta, J., & Hess, J. (2015). Does GPS improve recidivism among high risk sex offenders? Outcomes for California's GPS pilot for high risk sex offender parolees. *Victims & Offenders, 10*. https://doi.org/10.1080/15564886.2014.953236

Vasquez, B. E., Maddan, S., & Walker, J. T. (2008). The influence of sex offender registration and notification laws in the United States. *Crime & Delinquency, 54*, 175–192.

Walker, D. F., McGovern, S. K., Poey, E. L., & Otis, K. E. (2004). Treatment effectiveness for male adolescent sexual offenders: A meta-analysis and review. *Journal of Child Sexual Abuse, 13*, 281–293.

Whitting, L., Day, A., & Powell, M. (2016). Police officer perspectives on the implementation of a sex offender community notification scheme. *International Journal of Police Science & Management, 18*(4), 261–272.

Whitting, L., Day, A., & Powell, M. (2017). An evaluation of the impact of Australia's first community notification scheme. *Psychiatry, Psychology and Law, 24*(3), 339–355.

Whittington, R., Hockenhull, J. C., McGuire, J., Leitner, M., Barr, W., Cherry, M. G., Flentje, R., Quinn, B., Dundar, Y., & Dickson, R. (2013). A systematic review of risk assessment strategies for populations at high risk of engaging in violent behaviour: Update 2002-8. *Health Technology Assessment, 17*(50), 1–128.

Wilcox, D. T. (2008). Application of the clinical polygraph examination to the assessment, treatment and monitoring of sex offenders. *Journal of Sexual Aggression, 5*, 134–152.

Wilcox, D. T., Sosnowski, D., & Middleton, D. (1999). The use of the polygraph in the community supervision of sex offenders. *Probation Journal, 46*, 234–240.

Willis, G. M., & Grace, R. C. (2009). Assessment of community reintegration planning for sex offenders: Poor planning predicts recidivism. *Criminal Justice and Behavior, 36*, 494–512.

Wilson, R. J., Stewart, L., Stirpe, T., Barrett, M., & Cripps, J. E. (2000). Community-based sex offender management: Combining parole supervision and treatment to reduce recidivism. *Canadian Journal of Criminology, 42*, 177–188.

Wood, J. J., Alleyne, E. O., Ciardha, C., & Gannon, T. A. (2020). *An Evaluation of Polygraph Testing by Police to Manage Individuals Convicted or Suspected of Sexual Offending*. University of Kent, Centre of Research and Education in Forensic Psychology.

Wright, R. G. (Ed.). (2015). *Sex Offender Laws: Failed policies, new directions* (2nd ed.). Springer.

Zandbergen, P. A., Levenson, J. S., & Hart, T. C. (2010). Residential proximity to schools and daycares: An empirical analysis of sex offense recidivism. *Criminal Justice and Behavior, 37*, 482–502.

Zevitz, R. G. (2006). Sex offender community notification: Its role in recidivism and offender reintegration. *Criminal Justice Studies, 19*, 193–208.

Zgoba, K. M. (2011). Residence restriction buffer zones and the banishment of sex offenders: Have we gone one step too far? *Criminology and Public Policy, 10*, 391–400.

Zgoba, K. M., & Bachar, K. (2009). *Sex offender registration and notification: Limited effects in New Jersey*. Office of Justice Programs, National Institute of Justice.

Zgoba, K. M., Veysey, B. M., & Dalessandro, M. (2010). An analysis of the effectiveness of community notification and registration: Do the best intentions predict the best practices? *Justice Quarterly, 27*, 667–691.

# Chapter 4
# Domestic Abuse and Intimate Partner Violence: A Review of Police-Led and Multi-agency Interventions

## 4.1 Question to Be Addressed and Overall Aim

Our key question in this chapter is: what general approaches and specific methods can be applied in work with those who have committed domestic abuse to reduce the likelihood of the behaviour recurring? To address that question a Rapid Evidence Review was undertaken of relevant research literature. This had the integrated aim of identifying possible approaches to addressing these issues more effectively through policing. Doing so entailed identifying a series of terms and combinations of them in order to carry out searches of a number of key electronic databases likely to contain material with a bearing on the question. A set of inclusion and exclusion criteria was devised to narrow the focus, given the expectation that a large number of potentially relevant studies would initially be identified. The PICO framework, a standard format used as guidance for conducting evidence reviews, was developed for this specific search question and is as shown in Table 4.1.

## 4.2 Background

Abuse of one family member by another has at different times been known by several names, including domestic abuse (DA), domestic violence (DV), family violence, partner abuse, partner violence, intimate partner violence (IPV), spousal assault and battering. They are often used interchangeably though in many respects they refer to slightly different patterns depending on whether there is a single victim (usually a spouse or partner) or multiple victims (other family members in addition such as children or older parents). The term violence in its narrow sense refers specifically to physical assaults, but is also often used more widely to refer to other aspects of domination of one partner by the other within a close relationship, and so



J. McGuire et al., *Evidence-Based Policing and Community Crime Prevention*, Advances in Preventing and Treating Violence and Aggression,
https://doi.org/10.1007/978-3-030-76363-3_4

**Table 4.1** PICO framework: domestic abuse and IPV

| | |
|---|---|
| Population/ participants | Persons convicted of violence in which the victim was a partner or close family member; persons convicted of fraud against older adults.<br>Victims of domestic abuse.<br>Partner agencies: probation, social services, staff of women's support or refuge agencies.<br>Police officers involved in investigation, assessment and monitoring procedures |
| Intervention/ indicator | Follow-up data on offenders released from prison or who are under probation supervision or have completed periods of probation.<br>Follow-up of individuals supervised by forensic mental health services in secure units or in the community.<br>Evaluations of domestic violence programmes in the UK and internationally.<br>Analysis of the impact of arrest, warnings or other police actions.<br>Evaluation of changes in other moderator variables, e.g. alcohol consumption, control of movement of victims |
| Comparison/ control | Comparisons between outcomes of different sentences.<br>Where possible, extracting information from randomized controlled trials or quasi-experimental trials of interventions |
| Outcome(s) | Recorded or self-reported rates of abuse incidents.<br>Re-arrest, reconviction, severity of penalties imposed.<br>Partner reports, third-party reports where available.<br>Feedback from support agency staff.<br>Psychological assessment of change, use of specially devised measures, e.g. Conflict Tactics Scales, attitude scales |

may include sexual, emotional, financial and other forms of coercion and control. The term abuse has been used to include all forms of behaviour where one individual causes harm to or violates the rights of another.

In England and Wales some of these terms have recently been given more formal and exact definitions for the purposes of recording by the police and for data collection and analysis by the Office for National Statistics (ONS). At the time the current review was begun, the ONS employed the term *domestic abuse* to refer to four types of behaviour which are against the law and which are recorded in the Crime Survey for England and Wales (Office for National Statistics, 2016a). The category *domestic abuse* includes non-sexual partner abuse, non-sexual family abuse, sexual assault and stalking carried out by a current or former partner or other family member. Domestic abuse incidents are defined as "…any incidence of threatening behaviour, violence or abuse (psychological, physical, sexual, financial or emotional) between adults, aged 16 and over, who are or have been intimate partners or family members, regardless of gender or sexuality" (Office for National Statistics, 2016a, p. 8).

For a range of reasons, partly deriving from how crimes have traditionally been defined and partly as a function of long-standing social attitudes, there are strong indications that many of these forms of behaviour do not come to the attention of the police: "It is known that only a small proportion of domestic abuse incidents are reported to the police" (Office for National Statistics, 2016a, p. 8). This is in many senses often a hidden type of offence and according to one estimate (Garside, 2006) in numerical terms may even be the commonest form of crime, exceeding in frequency what are usually regarded as the more typical "volume crimes", such as theft and other acquisitive offences.

### 4.2.1 Prevalence

According to the January 2016 report from the Crime Survey for England and Wales, during the year ending March 2015 the police recorded 943,628 incidents of domestic abuse (Office for National Statistics, 2016a). As Her Majesty's Inspectorate of Constabulary noted in its report published in December 2015 (HMIC, 2015), that figure corresponds to receiving an average of over 100 calls an hour concerning this type of offence. During that year, 8.2% of women and 4% of men reported being victims of domestic abuse on one or more occasion, while 5.8% of women and 2.6% of men reported having been victims of non-sexual partner abuse. The corresponding figures for long-term experience of victimization (ages 16–59) were as follows: for any domestic abuse 27.1% for women and 13.2% for men and for non-sexual partner abuse 20.7% for women and 8.6% for men. For the year 2014–2015, domestic abuse-related crime formed 10% of all recorded crime and a third of all recorded assaults resulting in injury (HMIC, 2015).

In a new departure, covering the 6-month period May to September 2015, the Office for National Statistics (ONS) piloted experimental recording by police of incidents that were flagged as "domestic abuse related" (ONS, 2016b). This found that one-third of offences of violence against the person fell into this category. The largest single group of victims of DA were women in the age range 20–34. In addition to assaults, the figures include other types of offences considered by police officers to be linked to domestic abuse, for example: threat or possession with intent to commit criminal damage (31%), public order offences (23%), perverting the course of justice (18%) and criminal damage to a dwelling (14%) or to a vehicle (3%). The percentages in brackets are of all offences of that type that were classed as related to DA.

These figures can be compared with others from European and worldwide data sources. Alhabib et al. (2010) collated results from a total of 134 studies on the prevalence of domestic violence (physical, sexual or emotional) against women from 50 countries across all major world regions, published in the period 1995–2006. They found considerable variation in prevalence rates, ranging from 1.9% to 70% with those extremes both occurring within one country (the USA). Esquivel-Santoveña and Dixon (2012) and Esquivel-Santoveña et al. (2013) sought to establish a true rate of IPV against either women or men by collating data from 11 surveys conducted mainly in the USA but with others in Mexico, Ukraine and South Africa. In a later review focused on violence against women in low- and lower-middle-income countries, Semahegn et al. (2019) combined results from 57 studies, of which 33 could be included in a meta-analysis. This found a pooled prevalence of lifetime partner violence of 55%, with corresponding figures for different kinds of violence of 39% physical, 45% psychological and 20% sexual violence.

In Europe, surveys of violence against women have been conducted by the European Union Agency for Fundamental Rights, across all (then) 28 EU member countries (FRA, 2014). This found an average reported rate since the age of 15 for either physical or sexual violence by a partner of 22%. The lowest rate of 13% was in Austria, Croatia, Poland, Slovenia and Spain, while the highest at 32% was in Denmark and Latvia. The corresponding figure for the UK was 29%. Several regional and global surveys have been conducted under the auspices of international bodies such as the World Health Organization (2013) and other composite agencies of the United Nations (UN) (García-Moreno et al., 2013; Stöckl et al., 2013). These have found relatively lower rates in the high-income countries of the European region and Japan (23.2% and 24.6%, respectively), but higher rates for the African, Eastern Mediterranean and Southeast Asian regions (respectively 36.6%, 37% and 37.7%).

A portion of IPV is fatal, and it has been reported that approximately 14% of homicides occur in partner relationships (39% of femicides and 6% of killings of men). Not surprisingly, the lethality rate rises when there are firearms accessible (Zeoli et al., 2016). Corradi and Stöckl (2014) analysed patterns of intimate partner homicide in ten European countries including the UK. Over the period 2000–2011, there were 2559 female and 5530 male homicides in the UK, of which respectively 1076 (42%) and 306 (5.5%) were committed by intimate partners. While overall there are more male victims of homicide, most are killed by other men and a large fraction of female victims are killed by male partners.

The problem of partner violence is not solely domestic, in other words occurring only in couples who co-habit the same household, but also arises in other close relationships. Straus (2008) summarized data from the International Dating Violence Study, a survey involving a total of 13,601 participants in 32 countries. In a survey of respondents from this sample who had been in a relationship for at least 1 month, Straus (2008) found a mean reported rate of assault within their relationships during the previous 12 months of 31.2%, with a range from 16.6% in Portugal to 77.1% in Iran. Data from studies of this type have given rise to a set of frequently debated issues in the study of domestic abuse/intimate partner violence (DA/IPV).

One is the question of the relative proportions of DA/IPV that are committed by males against females, by females against males or in same-sex couples. This raises highly sensitive issues as part of the explanation of domestic abuse is considered by some to derive from patriarchal power structures (male dominance). On that basis the first of the patterns just mentioned would be expected to be more common. Police and victim survey statistics suggest that this is indeed the case, but other survey data concerning the scale of the difference are more variable. Thus, there is acknowledged to be *bi-directionality*, i.e. there are perpetrators in both genders.

A second, related question is whether there is gender *symmetry*: i.e. do men assault women and women assault men at similar rates, or is the former more prevalent? That the number and proportion committed by males would be higher accords with the general picture regarding crime as a whole, and violent and sexual offences in particular, including homicides. Some researchers have however contended that symmetry or even mutuality is the more customary pattern but that this is unrecognized, even denied, by other workers in the field (Straus, 2010, 2014). One interpretation is that violence by men towards women is more frequent at all levels of seriousness, but while the difference may be marginal at the lowest levels of aggression, sometimes called ordinary or situational partner violence, it becomes far larger with increasing levels of seriousness, and in relation to grievous harm and to murder, the difference is very pronounced. An alternative interpretation is that there is symmetry at most levels of severity, other than a small proportion of cases where there is extreme violence which is driven by clinical factors. A comprehensive review integrating 48 studies provides more support for the bi-directionality perspective (Langhinrichsen-Rohling et al., 2012).

A third dispute that emerges from this is the extent to which female violence towards males is reactive, i.e. not initiated by a woman but more typically a defensive response to male aggression. Evidence indicates that while this occurs in a proportion of cases, there is also violence that is instigated by females that is not solely a response to that of males.

Notwithstanding these disputes it is universally accepted that DA/IPV can have a number of serious consequences in terms of the health of victims. The World Health Organization prevalence studies (García-Moreno et al., 2013) document a range of sequelae for women including increased rates of depression and other mental health problems, elevated suicide risk (Devries et al., 2011) and increased likelihood of having an abortion or of giving birth to a low-weight baby. IPV also has a significant impact on children who witness it (and who may be used by some men against female partners: Beeble et al., 2007), such as later elevated risks of behaviour problems and of deficits in cognitive and social functioning. But there is also considerable variability in the effects of exposure to it, influenced by a number of other factors (Hungerford et al., 2012).

### 4.2.2 Explaining Domestic Abuse and Partner Violence

Many factors are considered to play a contributory role in the occurrence of domestic abuse, and research investigations have found numerous variables associated with it. Ali and Naylor (2013a, b) have reviewed the major categories of factors – biological, psychological, feminist, social and ecological – that have been found to play a part in the occurrence and patterning of IPV and the principal theories that have been offered to account for how they operate. Some authors argue however that it can be understood using the same constructs applied to other kinds of violent offending (Felson & Lane, 2010).

Based on a household survey carried out in both urban and rural locations in ten countries, Abramsky et al. (2011) found that despite sizeable variations in prevalence, there were some consistent associations between domestic violence towards women and a number of risk and protective factors. The former included alcohol abuse, cohabitation status, younger age, attitudes supportive of spouse abuse, sexual partners outside the relationship, prior child abuse and exposure to DA. The latter included secondary education, high socio-economic status and official marriage. However, there is not a straightforward link between multiple deprivation and rates of DA/IPV, even when investigated in a single area (the city of São Paulo, Brazil: Kiss et al., 2012).

In a review of 17 carefully selected studies published in the period 2000–2010, VanderEnde et al. (2012) examined the associations between DA and a number of community-level variables such as indicators of social disorganization, neighbourhood cohesion, socio-economic status, levels of other forms of violence and norms for behaviour between males and females. Levels of DA/IPV were not uniformly a direct function of concentrated disadvantage. While this was reliably found in some large cities, the link failed to emerge in other settings. In some societies, widespread acceptance of partner mistreatment amongst both perpetrators and victims appears to be a stronger influencing factor than poverty and associated hardships. The World Health Organization has issued "a call to action" for all nation-states to address the specific and endemic problem of violence against women as a vital aspect of ongoing global development (García-Moreno et al., 2015).

At present however there is no satisfactorily unified account regarding how potential contributory factors interconnect (Bell & Naugle, 2008; Dixon & Graham-Kevan, 2011). It is beyond the scope of this chapter to synthesize the very wide range of information concerning this or to develop a comprehensive account. What does seem clear is that in order to encompass the breadth of influences that appear to be directly or indirectly involved, several sets of factors, operating on different levels, need to be included in an integrative framework. A potentially useful way of conceptualizing this is in terms of an ecological model of the type forwarded by Heise (1998, see also Beyer, Wallis & Hamberger, 2015) illustrated as shown in Fig. 4.1 (adapted from McGuire & Duff, 2018).

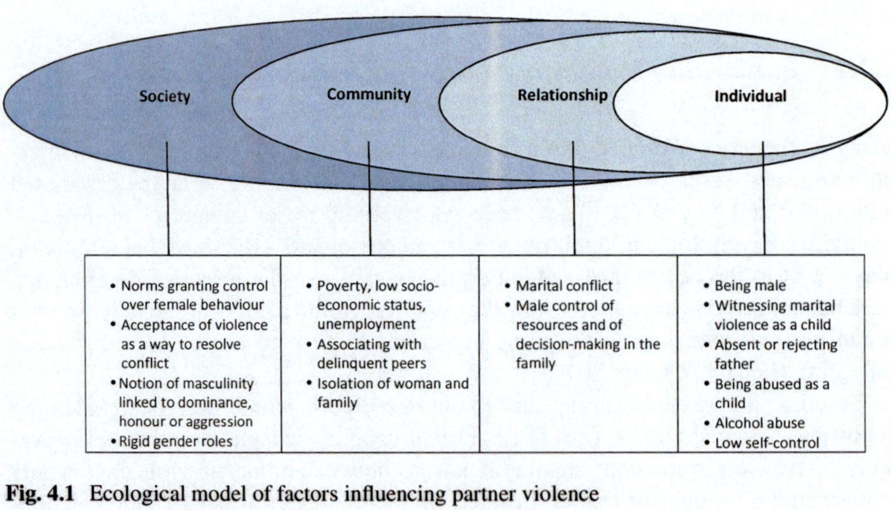


**Fig. 4.1** Ecological model of factors influencing partner violence

At an individual level, perpetrators show considerable heterogeneity (Dixon & Browne, 2003; Dixon & Graham-Kevan, 2011). That is manifested in several variables such as impulsivity or in features of anger (Birkley & Eckhardt, 2015; Eckhardt et al., 2008; Norlander & Eckhardt, 2005) and in overall level of risk which is thought to remain comparatively stable over time (Cavanaugh & Gelles, 2005). Several typologies or attempts at classification have been offered, for example, dividing IPV perpetrators into generalists who have committed other types of violent offences versus specialists who have not (Herrero et al., 2016; Huss & Ralston, 2008). Other approaches have identified varying levels of criminality and psychopathology linked to lethal violence (Dixon et al., 2008).

Moving leftwards to other elements of the schematic framework in Fig. 4.1, there are different patterns of dynamics within relationships, which may be egalitarian or may be marked by the exercise of power by one partner over another (Straus, 2008). Violence may be triggered by specific events and situations in the course of the relationship (Wilkinson & Hamerschlag, 2005). Johnson (2008) combined individual and relational features according to the level to which violence is used as a means of control. This enabled him to distinguish four patterns of conflict: situational violent incidents, mutual violent control, violent resistance and "intimate terrorism". Note however that this is just one of several approaches to classifying IPV that have been developed (Ali et al., 2016). Many of the correlates of abuse in same-sex couples parallel those found in heterosexual relationships (Bartholomew et al., 2008), but there is evidence that the overall level of violence is higher (Badenes-Ribera et al., 2015), and differences have also been reported, for example, in patterns of jealousy (Barelds & Dijkstra, 2005). The community surrounding the couple may be characterized by features often associated with higher levels of family stress and dysfunction (Beyer et al., 2015; VanderEnde et al., 2012). For transgender individuals in close relationships, a review of 85 studies by Peitzmeier et al. (2020) indicated that they were 1.7 times more likely to experience IPV of some kind than cisgender individuals; for physical and sexual violence, the odds were 2.2 and 2.5 times greater.

Finally, the cultural norms within the society as a whole may permit or even instil dominance and inequity between females and males with associated links to rates of relationship violence (Yodanis, 2004). Reporting a meta-synthesis of 12 studies of factors that influence partner violence in African countries, Okeke-Ihejirika, Salami and Amodu (2019, p. 104) suggested that culture in many places supported a paradoxical set of attitudes of males towards females. This drew on a "dual-identity discourse, which mirrors a cycle of episodic honeymoon behaviour and violent episodes". In the latter parts of this, men felt justified in acting violently either as an expression of male vigour or heroic energy or a sense of an "emasculated self that lost control to a manipulative wife".

Some variables cannot of course be located in a single category only. Attitudes, for example, are held by individuals, but are shaped by the culture in which they develop. Gracia et al. (2020) integrated findings from 62 studies of attitudes carried out in 11 member countries of the European Union, with a combined study sample of over 109,000. Some aspects of attitudes were drawn from the legitimation and acceptability of particular views, notably sexism which is extensively supported by many culturally normative processes, some tacit, others explicit, even in places where the opposite is proclaimed.

## 4.3 Specific Objectives

The specific objectives of this evidence review were: (1) to locate studies of general approaches and specific methods applied in response to domestic abuse where there had been some evaluation of their effect and (2) to identify which approaches if any have generated evidence of effectiveness in reducing the frequency or severity of DA/IPV. In order to accomplish these goals, a literature search was carried out, the findings of which are summarized in what follows.

Although the problems of domestic abuse and partner violence have been known for a long time, there is broad agreement amongst experts that in a manner similar to child sexual abuse, the extent of them has only come to be realized in the relatively recent past. Even today our knowledge appears far from adequate. In a historical review of the area, Barner and Carney (2011) describe the emergence of legislation designed to address the problem of spousal abuse in the USA and recount the origins of the first women's refuges. There are now reportedly over 1200 such shelters in the UK, the first having been established in 1972 (Corradi & Stöckl, 2014). From that period onwards there has been steadily widening recognition of the extent of DA/IPV as a major social problem, resulting in a series of changes in the law and in policing.

Where it is clear that domestic abuse has happened, as with any other assault conventional criminal justice processing will follow. But in many contexts, it can be very difficult to establish what may or may not have occurred. As a result, a variety of responses have emerged in working with possible or suspected DA/IPV. The principal patterns of action taken have included arrest, which may or may not be followed by charge and prosecution; a number of other police or multi-agency responses, some mandated through court procedures; and a wide spectrum of treatment or intervention programmes focused either on the DA perpetrator or in some cases on working with the couple as a unit.

## 4.4 Method

### *4.4.1 Search Strategy*

An initial, fairly brief pilot search was carried out to locate major reviews as a form of scoping exercise, to ascertain whether there were any recent reports covering the area and also to identify likely useful search terms. This was also used to devise the

PICO framework (Table 4.1). A formal list of search terms was then developed from the framework and from the articles that had already been located in the preliminary scoping search. Fuller search strategies were initially designed to locate published and unpublished evaluations of policing and other initiatives that have had or potentially could have desired impacts on outcome targets. Searches were carried out in the following nine electronic databases: *PsycINFO* (EMBASE), the *National Criminal Justice Reference Service* (NCJRS, Washington DC), *Web of Science, Scopus, Criminal Justice Abstracts, Psychology and Behavioral Sciences Collection* (EBSCO), *Australian Institute of Criminology, Swedish National Council for Crime Prevention* (Brå, Stockholm) and the *Netherlands Institute for the Study of Criminality and Law Enforcement* (NISCALE, Leiden University).

### *4.4.2 Inclusion and Exclusion Criteria*

Initial searches covering the period from January 2000 to December 2015 located a total of 3832 records entered for screening into an Endnote file. However, in common with other areas covered in the book searches were later updated, though in a less extensive way, to November 2020. They were not initially limited by language or publication type or with respect to whether or not they were published or unpublished. However, following perusal of the Endnote file, several decisions were made regarding the material obtained. A number of inclusion and exclusion criteria were set and applied in making decisions about individual records.

A decision was made to exclude research dissertations. These would usually be included in a full systematic review, but that is a larger scale exercise than the present one and there was insufficient time to include them. The Endnote file contained a large number of doctoral dissertations, of which a total of 66 appeared relevant to the review. In addition, there were 18 published papers in languages other than English (15 Spanish, 3 French). Due to limitations of time and absence of resources for translation, these studies were excluded from further consideration but were retained in a separate file for future reference.

During the screening and data extraction process, 63 additional studies were found from the reference lists of the initial records located or from lists generated by publisher databases (e.g. ScienceDirect, SAGE journals, Ex Libris). The majority of studies (3353) were excluded at first stage screening. A set consisting of 542 studies was retained for fuller screening, of which 428 were excluded for a range of reasons, for example, that they were descriptive only (36), were studies of risk and predictive factors (32), examined the effects of court or legal decisions (30), investigated variables contributing to domestic abuse (28) and so on for a total of 27 categories. The selection process incorporating the updating review followed a pathway as shown in Fig. 4.2.

With respect to content, as already noted family violence can take several forms and has been classified a number of ways, first and foremost according to who is the victim. As there is a large amount of research on family violence, to keep the present

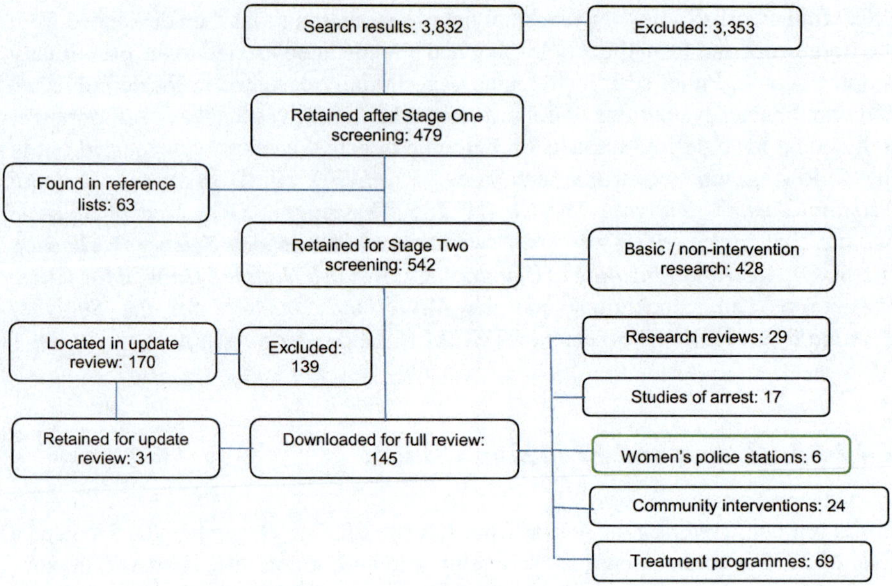


**Fig. 4.2** Flowchart of search and selection process on DA/IPV

review within manageable limits, it excluded child abuse and elder abuse. The focus is on partner abuse, meaning conflict between spouses or other intimate partners, whether in heterosexual or same-sex relationships. The review also excludes sexual abuse. This is a difficult distinction to sustain as sexual assault (including rape) can be a function of a variety of motives, some of them non-sexual, and because during the course of some physical assaults, attackers may also act in a sexually abusive or degrading manner. However, there is a very large and to some extent specialized literature on sexual assault, and a separate set of procedures surrounding the policing of sexual offences. In addition, the volume of work in the review could have become unwieldy if sexual aggression was also included in searches. The numbers of items excluded or retained at successive phases of the process were as shown in Fig. 4.2.

The 145 downloaded reports were divided into 5 groups. Twenty-nine of them were previous reviews of relevant research and will be described first. Across the two phases of the review (initial and update), a total of 32 other articles were also examined which contained partial review material but were not formal review studies as such. The four other sets of studies respectively consisted of research on the effectiveness of arrest (17), of community-based interventions led by or involving police (24), of the establishment of women's police stations (6) and of IPV or batterer treatment and other types of intervention programmes (69).

## 4.5 Previous Reviews

There is a large quantity of research on the problem of personal violence in general and on that of domestic abuse and IPV more specifically. There are therefore large numbers of studies and of research reviews with potential relevance to the objectives of the present work. Before considering the results of the present searches, in this section several previous reviews of aspects of the problem to be addressed will be briefly discussed.

Often a proportion of those who have committed domestic abuse have also committed other types of crime, including offences of violence against the person. In addition, and as already noted, there is often evidence of the presence of substance abuse problems and of anger disturbances and of loss of self-control amongst perpetrators of domestic abuse. Larsen and Hamberger (2015) reported a review of the experiences of males and females who are either perpetrators or victims of IPV. There are meta-analyses of the link between domestic violence and alcohol and other drug abuse (Foran & O'Leary, 2008; Langenderfer, 2013; Moore et al., 2008) and of its relationship to anger and hostility (Birkley & Eckhardt, 2015; Norlander & Eckhardt, 2005). In addition to those review studies, there have been overviews of other closely related topics, such as the usefulness of perpetrator typologies (Boxall et al., 2015; Cavanaugh & Gelles, 2005), risk factors for DA/IPV (e.g. Capaldi et al., 2012; Cattaneo & Goodman, 2005; Yakubovich et al., 2018) and the usefulness of risk assessment (e.g. Bowen, 2011a; Hilton & Harris, 2005). A review of the last of these areas found that, despite the existence of several structured methods for approaching this, police staff were often not trained in their use or relied on their own tacit knowledge ("gut feeling") when assessing IPV risk (Svalin & Levander, 2020).

Given such findings, evidence of the effectiveness of some other kinds of intervention is also potentially relevant to the question of how to work with those who have committed domestic abuse. There are several reviews with a direct bearing on this. There are broad-ranging reviews of interventions for the reduction of violent offending (McGuire, 2008; Whittington & McGuire, 2020). There are also more specific meta-analyses of (a) interventions designed to reduce violent offending by adults (Jolliffe & Farrington, 2007), (b) treatment of self-control problems (Piquero et al., 2009) and (c) interventions to improve anger management using CBT-informed approaches, that is, the ones influenced by the models of cognitive-behavioural therapy (Henwood et al., 2015). However, as these reviews do not focus on the problem of DA/IPV in itself, they are not considered in detail here.

There are several overviews of the field taking a narrative and discursive approach rather than a formal, focused one employing standard literature review procedures (e.g. Aldarondo, 2010; Barner & Carney, 2011). These can be helpful in setting research studies and their results in a wider context. Hamilton et al. (2012) surveyed provision of domestic violence programmes in Europe. They obtained information on 54 programmes being delivered by a variety of agencies in 19 countries;

however, they noted that the standard of evaluation was poor. They found very little sound evidence that could be used as a basis for informing practice or policy.

Another large-scale review was carried out and reported by Lilley-Walker et al. (2018) as part of *IMPACT: Evaluation of European Perpetrator Programmes project*. These authors located 60 evaluation reports of programmes for the treatment of domestic violence perpetrators from 12 European countries. The principal objective of the review was to examine and compare the research methodologies that were employed, and led to a set of proposals for improved evaluation designs and more consistent data collection and reporting principles. The review quotes the findings of some intervention studies but does not contain any summary with a systematic, integrated account of results nor any statistical analysis or comparison of outcomes or trends. This review was therefore not included in Table 4.2.

The searches reported here found 29 published systematic or meta-analytic reviews of evaluation research, listed in Table 4.2 (some published in more than one form, hence the multiple references in some cases). In addition, as noted there were 24 further narrative or other non-quantitative reviews of parts of the field of DA/IPV treatment intervention. We were also fortunate in being allowed access to draft reports being written for the College of Policing (Schucan-Bird et al., undated; Vigurs et al., undated).

The review by MacMillan et al. (2001, Wathen et al., 2003) covered several aspects of screening women for risk of IPV victimization in primary care settings but also included a review of batterer interventions. The review by Stith et al. (2003) of the effectiveness of couples therapy for reducing IPV was followed by a further review of the same area (McCollum & Stith, 2008), but it adds relatively little to the initial report and therefore was not dealt with separately in this list. Another wide-ranging review by Sartin et al. (2006) was also excluded.

The overall pattern of findings that emerges from the review studies listed in Table 4.2 lends itself to one broad and fairly straightforward but unfortunately not very useful conclusion. To date, there is not enough convincing evidence on any individual-level response to DA, or any approach to working with DA perpetrators to be able to make confident statements or offer definitive recommendations about the best course of action to follow. Given that only a small proportion of the studies employed robust experimental designs, and that there are often high levels of drop-out, there are relatively few findings with enough consistency to allow any generalizations to be made. This is a very difficult area to research and the use of high-quality research designs is not easy to implement. The most widely used programme in this area based on the long-standing Duluth model has not reliably yielded positive effects.

Nevertheless, there are some indications of possible routes to improved results. Some types of programmes have obtained more positive outcomes, though they are not especially consistent, for example, from CBT programmes or with interventions also focusing on substance abuse treatment, as found in the Miller et al. (2013a) review. They also emerged from work with lower-risk cases. But where based on more recently developed interventions, they are as a result still very few in number.

**Table 4.2** Previous reviews of aspects of domestic abuse/intimate partner violence intervention (29 reviews)

| Review | Focus | Number of studies | Findings |
|---|---|---|---|
| Akoensi et al. (2012) | Effectiveness of DV intervention programmes in six European countries | 12 | Extended the work of Hamilton et al. (2012) surveying DV programmes in Europe. Only one study had an equivalent-group comparison. There were high levels of attrition. All programmes involved a mixed model. No clear conclusions could be drawn from the review regarding effective interventions |
| An and Choi (2017) | Narrative review of interventions linked to training in non-medical settings | 16 | Interventions were based in child welfare and other agencies, but three were focused mainly on police participants and three others included police officers. Changes were found in knowledge levels, longer time spent at IPV scenes and increases in arrest rates. Studies were classed by quality as good (4), fair (4) and poor (8) |
| Aos et al. (2006) | General review of adult corrections programmes | 11 | In a broad-ranging review of correctional programmes, included nine evaluations of educational or cognitive-behavioural interventions for DV offenders and two evaluations of domestic violence courts. Mean effect sizes for both sets of studies were zero |
| Arce et al. (2020); *see also* Arias et al. (2013) | Batterer intervention programmes | 25 (62 effect sizes) | Reviewed studies with a total sample size of 20,860. There was a mean overall effect size of 0.43. Recidivism reported by couples was significantly higher than official rates. Most evaluations were of the Duluth model, but its mean effect size (0.37) was lower than for cognitive-behavioural programmes (0.88) and other types of intervention (0.63). There was no significant effect of short interventions (<16 weeks) but a positive and significant effect for longer interventions. It was estimated that overall, there was a 21% reduction in recidivism for "intervened" versus "non-intervened" batterers. However, because of variations within each programme type, no conclusions were drawn that can be considered generalizable |

(continued)

**Table 4.2** (continued)

| Review | Focus | Number of studies | Findings |
|---|---|---|---|
| Armenti and Babcock (2016) | Review of studies of conjoint (couples-based) treatment of situational partner violence | 12 | Reviewed studies in which violence is not a direct result of the attempts by one partner to control the other. Found results that are superior to those found for individual therapy with abusive males, but applicable only with some couples. The review does not report mean effect sizes or statistical comparisons with other approaches |
| Babcock et al. (2004) | Batterer intervention programmes | 22 | Found 17 quasi-experimental designs and 5 randomized experiments. Used both police and partner reports as outcomes. Found on average an effect size of $d = 0.34$ which shows a modest improvement for treated samples, but taking other factors into account the effect was estimated to be lower than this |
| Bourey et al. (2015) | Systematic review of interventions to reduce IPV in low- and middle-income countries | 16 studies from 9 countries: 20 reports | Reviewed evaluations of structural interventions, which focus on altering economic, political, legal, physical or environmental factors associated with violence risk. There were 13 RCTs with a mean follow-up of 2 years. 13 of 16 studies obtained evidence of statistically significant reductions in at least one form of IPV, though few showed a direct effect on physical or sexual violence or impacted on multiple outcome variables. However, significant effects were found on other (non-IPV) outcome variables |
| Cluss and Bodea (2011) | Effectiveness of batterer intervention programmes | 22 | Reviews a series of studies by quality level (high, medium, low) but includes both reviews and separate intervention studies at each level. Does not report statistical integration of findings. Concludes that there is very little or no empirically demonstrated effectiveness of the widely available group interventions (p. 15) |
| Davis et al. (2008) | Effects of second responder programmes | 10 | Evaluated programmes in which a police officer or a victim advocate makes a follow-up contact after the initial police response. Found a small increase in reporting of second incidents but no effect on reports of new abuse incidents |

(continued)

**Table 4.2** (continued)

| Review | Focus | Number of studies | Findings |
|---|---|---|---|
| De Koker et al. (2014) | Preventing adolescent IPV | 6 | Reviewed nine studies based on six RCTs from the USA, Canada and South Africa on prevention programmes for adolescents to reduce risks of IPV perpetration or victimization. Four of the programmes had significant beneficial effects over some long-term follow-up periods, two shorter programmes did not |
| Dowling et al. (2018) | Wide-ranging review of the effects of policing on different aspects of domestic violence | 346 | Very extensive review of several aspects of police responses to domestic violence. Authors searched 10 databases up to 2016, locating a total of 346 relevant reports, grouped into 6 areas: (a) the impact of workforce development, notably practice-oriented training; (b) interventions to increase rates of reporting IPV; (c) the effects of first response, including arrest; (d) preventing repetition of IPV; (e) factors influencing investigative outcomes; and (f) police decisions to lay charges |
| Eckhardt et al. (2013) | Intervention programmes for perpetrators and victims | 61 | Total sample size 20,829. There were 20 studies of "traditional" Duluth or CBT-based batterer interventions, 10 of "alternative" approaches, 16 of brief victim-focused methods and 15 of extended victim interventions. Results from perpetrator interventions were equivocal though there were some significant results. There were more encouraging outcomes from studies that took account of motivation and readiness to change, and from counselling interventions with DA/IPV victims |
| Feder and Wilson (2005); Feder et al. (2008) | Court-mandated batterer intervention programmes | 10 | Reviewed six quasi-experimental evaluations and four RCTs of psycho-educational or CBT programmes which misdemeanour (low-risk) offenders were mandated to attend. Effect size from RCTs was $d = 0.26$, statistically significant. Quasi-experimental studies were less robust and results more mixed. Suggested more trials needed |
| Jewell and Wormith (2010) | Attrition from domestic violence treatment programmes | 30 | Review of factors influencing attrition from DV intervention programmes. Tested for differences between completers and dropouts. The former was linked to being older, having a job, court-mandated, less likely to have previous DV or other offences, or drug use. Similar factors predicted dropout and re-offending |

(continued)

**Table 4.2** (continued)

| Review | Focus | Number of studies | Findings |
|---|---|---|---|
| MacMillan et al. (2001); Wathen et al. (2003) | Broad review of screening for IPV in primary care, but including a review of batterer interventions | 10 | From studies published in the period 1986–2000, found conflicting evidence regarding the effectiveness of batterer interventions in reducing rates of further domestic violence |
| Maxwell and Garner (2012); Garner and Maxwell (2011) | Compares crime control effects of sanctions | 31 | Compared the effects of prosecution, conviction and severity of penalties on repeat offending in IPV. Conducted 143 tests within the obtained studies. Findings were diverse and inconsistent and no firm pattern emerged, but the dominant finding was one of "no effect" (p.489). This was thought possibly due to lack of statistical power, selection biases and missing data |
| Maxwell et al. (2002) | Pooled data from the *Spousal Assault Replication Program* studies (see next section on arrest) | 5 | Analysed 4032 incidents of spousal assault across 5 sites. Multivariate analysis indicated modest, but consistent reductions in subsequent prevalence of new victimizations. Depending on the outcome variable measured, this ranged from 4% (official arrest data) to 30% (victim report data) |
| Miller et al. (2013a) | Meta-analysis of intervention studies | 9 | Applied strict criteria to initial set of 34 studies and retained 9 with 11 effect sizes. Evaluations of Duluth programmes had an effect size close to zero. Evaluations of other programmes (4 types) showed better results (33% reduction in DV recidivism) |
| Nesset et al. (2019) | Systematic review of cognitive-behavioural group programmes with IPV perpetrators | 6 (4 RCTs, 2 non-random) | Mixed results with three of four RCT studies reporting a significant reduction in IPV after treatment, but neither of the quasi-experimental studies doing so. There was a risk of bias in several studies and it was concluded that the evidence base for group CBT remains inconclusive |
| Rivas et al. (2016) | Advocacy interventions | 13 | Combined studies had a sample size of 2141. Advocacy involved direct work or inter-agency work with IPV victims. Several kinds of impact were evaluated, and some positive effects found, but they were fairly minor and variable. Many studies were statistically underpowered |

(continued)

**Table 4.2** (continued)

| Review | Focus | Number of studies | Findings |
|---|---|---|---|
| Santirso et al. (2020) | Interventions for IPV that included motivational strategies using RCT designs | Review: 12 Meta-analysis: 7 | Evaluated a range of effects including treatment dropout and self-reported physical and psychological violence. All trends showed treatment gains but some only marginally. Recidivism was analysed in only 3/12 trials showing a mean odds ratio of 1.46, a statistically non-significant but favourable trend. The authors concluded that interventions with motivational strategies were significantly more effective for sustaining attendance than those without |
| Sheehan et al. (2012) | A review of evidence concerning "turning points" in treatment of IPV perpetrators | 6 | Review of qualitative studies based on interview or observation data with small samples of male IPV perpetrators. Identified some common themes within "incidents, factors or circumstances" (p. 31) that engender processes of change in how they view violence and abuse in their relationships |
| Smedslund et al. (2011) | CBT for physically abusive men | 6 | Cochrane Collaboration Systematic Review, RCTs only, four included in meta-analysis. The results were inconclusive, with only a small effect size and mainly equivocal results |
| Stith et al. (2003); McCollum and Stith (2008) | Effectiveness of couples therapy for reducing violence | 15 | Reviewed six experimental, one quasi-experimental and eight pre-post evaluations of joint treatment (couples therapy). Found some encouraging results but the review contains no quantitative synthesis |
| Stover et al. (2009a) | Review of the effect of interventions on perpetrators, victims, couples and witnesses | 21 | Compared effects of different interventions by "primary treatment focus": batterers (7), victims (6), couples (5) and child witnesses (4). Some studies had multiple measures across the four domains. Interventions for batterers showed high dropout and were described as having "meagre" effects. Each category contained a diverse mix of interventions making results difficult to interpret |
| Subirana-Malaret et al. (2019) | Scoping review of IPV intervention research | 0 | Review designed to locate studies evaluating interventions specific to sexual orientation and gender minoritized populations. Located 75 studies that met inclusion criteria but none described programmes specific to sexual orientation and gender minoritized groups |

(continued)

**Table 4.2** (continued)

| Review | Focus | Number of studies | Findings |
|---|---|---|---|
| Walker et al. (2013) | Process of desistance from IPV | 15 | Entailed features of systematic review but reports no quantitative synthesis. Reported associations between features of IPV stability and prevalence, of couple dynamics, of individual perpetrators and of behaviour change processes and the likelihood of desistance from IPV |
| Whitaker et al. (2013) | Primary prevention of partner violence | 19 | Reviewed studies of interventions designed to stop IPV before it begins. Most studies (13) were conducted in schools; 15 were randomized studies, 4 quasi-experiments. Follow-up from 1–60 months but only 6 studies had follow-up >12 months. Outcomes were "IPV-related" behaviour. Several studies showed positive effects but others nil effects |
| Zeoli et al. (2016) | Studies of legal interventions to reduce firearm possession by IPV perpetrators | 4 | Review of research on the risk of fatality where firearms are present in IPV; partly focused on interventions. Legal statutes to prohibit purchase of firearms by those under DV restraining orders (DVROs) reduced the risk of lethality in 3/3 studies; a fourth study showed reduction in nonfatal IPV |

The most promising findings are those where interventions were delivered at the social or structural rather than the individual level, applying the framework from Fig. 4.1. As described by Bourey et al. (2015, pp. 2–3), these interventions "aim to change structural factors, which are aspects of the economic, politico-legal, physical, and social environment that produce and reproduce risk… such interventions modify systems, structures, and processes at the highest level of the social ecology in order to affect risk at multiple levels". The review by Bourey et al. also incorporated a very extensive search strategy and a thorough analysis of risk of bias and addressed multiple-level influences on IPV.

Also impressive are the results of De Koker et al. (2014) and Whitaker et al. (2013) on preventive interventions with adolescents, an encouraging set of results given the possibility of enabling participants to avoid becoming DA/IPV perpetrators or victims as they grow towards adult life. These programmes also contain possible messages for policing as the interventions were based in schools or other community agencies and drew on other professional groups as contributors in their delivery.

## 4.6 Results: Evidence Review on Policing and IPV

The studies identified for inclusion in the present review are classified in three areas: (a) the use of arrest, (b) other police-led or collaborative, multi-agency responses and (c) treatment interventions for DA/IPV perpetrators which are provided by a variety of agencies in which delivery often requires liaison between providers and police services. The studies that were located under each of these headings will be considered in turn.

### *4.6.1 Arrest*

The importance attached to the arrest of DA perpetrators derives from a seminal study published over 30 years ago, the Minneapolis Domestic Violence Experiment (MDVE) (Sherman & Berk, 1984). Traditionally, the police had been reluctant to make arrests for domestic violence, unless victims demanded they do so or the situation became difficult to manage otherwise. They occasionally became involved in dispute resolution or asked one of the parties to leave the scene for a short period. In a formal experimental arrangement, three different interventions were compared with each other in their effects. They were arrest of the alleged perpetrator, provision of advice to the couple or temporarily separating the couple. Over a period of approximately 18 months, 330 cases were randomly allocated to 1 of the 3 conditions. Arrest resulted in a statistically significant reduction in the number of recurrences of domestic violence as compared to the other two interventions.

The MDVE had considerable research and public impact and over ensuing years a number of US cities and states implemented arrest practices. There was also a series of five trials conducted to test the reliability of the finding in other locations, the *Spousal Assault Replication Program* (SARP). This produced what at first appeared to be an inconsistent set of findings, although it was commented that some of the replication studies were not very accurate reflections of the original MDVE design. At a later stage however, data from several evaluations of the SARP experiments were combined in integrative reviews (Garner et al., 1995; Garner & Maxwell, 2000; Sugarman & Boney-McCoy, 2000). As summarized earlier in Table 4.2, Maxwell et al. (2002) used multivariate statistics and showed that when other variables were taken into account, there was evidence of an effect of arrest on reducing IPV recidivism. However, the perpetrator's prior arrest record was a stronger predictor, and in most cases there was a decline in the number of assaults committed over time which appeared to be independent of external influences. Some studies in Table 4.3 also involved re-analysis (secondary analysis) of the SARP data.

Despite these complexities research has continued on the role of arrest as a potentially effective intervention for reducing IPV, and in the present review 17 studies of it were located that were published in the period 2000–2020. They are listed in Table 4.3.

**Table 4.3** Studies of arrest (17 studies)

| Study | Methodology | Samples/data sources | Intervention and outcomes |
|---|---|---|---|
| Broidy et al. (2016) | Cross-sectional comparison of types of intervention | Analysis of all 1709 IPV cases in New Mexico in 2002, tracking outcomes up to 2006 | The rate of IPV in New Mexico was reportedly 3× the US national average. Study compared three forms of intervention: arrest, civil protection order and both combined. Analysis found no difference in re-offending outcomes between the three approaches. Perpetrator age and offence history were best predictors for the 23% involved in further incidents |
| Cho and Wilke (2010) | Analysis of National Crime Victimization Survey (USA) data, interview-based study | 2462 female and 298 male victims | The female-to-male gender ratio of being an IPV victim was 8:1. At 1-year follow-up, arrest of male perpetrators reduced rates of re-victimization of female partners by 45%. Arrest of female perpetrators did not reduce the rates of re-victimization of male partners |
| Davis et al. (2001) | Analysis of district attorney case files in Milwaukee | 237 general court cases, 190 DV court cases | Found a small, non-significant reduction in new assaults at serious level (felonies) but an increase at less serious level (misdemeanours). There was no effect of the change to DV court |
| Felson et al. (2005) | Longitudinal analysis of National Crime Victimization Survey (USA) data | 2564 victims of DA/IPV; 145 in same-sex couples | Found that reporting to police had a strong deterrent effect but arrest did not. Failure to report was associated with an 89% increase in odds of re-victimization. Found no evidence of retaliation by perpetrators after victim complaints to police |
| Gerstenberger and Williams (2012) | Arrests for DV in Connecticut, Feb–Mar 2007 | IPV in 2155 heterosexual partners | Compared effects of single and dual arrest on IPV recidivism at 18 months. There were more dual arrests where perpetrators were female. Dual arrest was associated with a 29% reduction in recidivism, independently of gender of perpetrator |
| Hilton et al. (2007) | Archival study of arrest data in Ontario | 522 cases of wife assault recorded in electronic files | Based on analysis of predictors, there was no evidence that arrest affected wife assault recidivism. There was evidence of the usefulness of a risk assessment, Ontario Domestic Assault Risk Assessment, for identifying higher-risk cases |

(continued)

**Table 4.3** (continued)

| Study | Methodology | Samples/data sources | Intervention and outcomes |
|---|---|---|---|
| Hirschel (2008) | Survey of the use and effects of dual arrest using the NIBRS[a] | US-wide arrest data + detailed study of 25 police departments | Dual arrest is used when police cannot determine which partner is at fault (therefore both are arrested), occurring in 1.9% of cases involving IPV. No evidence was found that its use affected subsequent re-arrest rates |
| Johnson and Goodlin-Fahncke (2015) | Secondary analysis of the SARP data, comparing sub-groups | 2412 heterosexual male batterers | Assessment classified 95% of IPV offenders into 3 clusters. Arrest had no deterrent effect but increased recidivism amongst two groups called the generally violent/antisocial and low-level antisocial groups. Suggested that for arrest to have an effect, it needed to be followed by other types of action |
| Klein and Tobin (2008) | Longitudinal study: 10-year follow-up | 342 men convicted of DV in Massachusetts | Though only 32% committed DA again within 1 year, over 10 years 60% did so and were either re-arrested or subject to restraining orders. The majority were arrested multiple times. Concluded that short-term indicators were not useful for predicting long-term risk |
| Mears et al. (2001) | Regression and survival analyses to investigate predictors of IPV recidivism | 336 IPV cases in Texas, in 3 groups: arrest only = 126 restraining order (PO) only = 83 both = 127 | Investigated whether age, race/ethnicity, prior convictions, drug use and socio-economic context predicted recidivism; also evaluated the impact of type of legal intervention. There was no difference found between groups in the prevalence of re-victimization or in time (number of days) for it to occur |
| Miller (2003) | Interview based study | 595 victims from the SARP study in Miami, 385 at 6-month follow-up | There was an association between partner arrest and reported feelings of safety by victims, but this appeared to depend on the level of legal power victims perceived themselves as having as a result of the abuser being arrested |

(continued)

**Table 4.3** (continued)

| Study | Methodology | Samples/data sources | Intervention and outcomes |
|---|---|---|---|
| Morrow et al. (2016) | Impact of body-worn cameras on IPV arrest and case process | Analysis of outcomes in 2063 calls for service to IPV incidents in 2012–2014 in Phoenix, Arizona | Compared IPV cases in two police squad areas, before and after introduction of body-worn cameras in one of the areas. Cases where body-worn cameras were used were significantly more likely to result in an arrest (40.9 vs 34.3%), to have charges filed (37.7 vs 26%), for cases to be furthered (12.7 vs 6.2%), for there to be a guilty plea (4.4 vs 1.2%) and guilty verdict (4.4 vs 0.9%) |
| Oehme et al. (2016) | Survey of police officer responses to IPV before and after web-based training | 852 police officers provided an online training package to address officer-involved domestic violence (OIDV) | Evaluation of Module 1 of the *National Prevention Toolkit* online training concerned with Ontario Domestic Assault Risk Assessment, focused on understanding IPV using case scenarios. Officers reported large increases in the likelihood of arrest, despite difficulties in doing so with a fellow police officer. There were increases in the willingness to intervene and to advise couples to seek help |
| Natarajan (2016) | Case study of usefulness of mobile phones in responding to IPV | 994 officers from the Metropolitan Police given training in use of specialized mobile handsets | Evaluated the use of specialized mobile phone technology which enables IPV victims to contact police using a speed dial facility. The study reports demographic profiles of 742 individuals who were issued handsets, and details of 7 cases of life-threatening situations. Use of the phones increased the rate of perpetrator arrest and other benefits, e.g. reduced fear and improved quality of life |
| Piquero et al. (2005, 2006) | Secondary analysis of the SARP data | Total of 4095 DA offenders across 4 locations | Found that there were sub-groups within the SARP samples that had different trajectories: escalators whose offences became more serious, de-escalators whose path was the opposite and others with stable patterns of low- or high-level aggression |

(continued)

**Table 4.3** (continued)

| Study | Methodology | Samples/data sources | Intervention and outcomes |
|---|---|---|---|
| Sherman and Harris (2015) | Long-term follow-up of RCT participants | 1125 DV victims in the Milwaukee DV experiment | Examined death rates amongst victims of DV 23 years after participation in an RCT on the effectiveness of arrest. Found that arrest was associated with increased mortality, very highly amongst African-American but only marginally amongst Caucasian victims |
| Siddique (2013) | Secondary analysis of the MDVE data | Data from Sherman and Berk (1984) | Re-analysed the original data from the Minnesota experiment but applied a more elaborate, highly technical statistical analysis which the author claims showed the effects of arrest were larger than originally concluded |

[a]National Incident-Based Reporting System (USA)

Concerning effects of arrest, the review by Dowling et al. (2018) located 137 studies. However, "the most common research design was the inferential analysis of relationships between variables" (p. 113). There were 86 studies of this type, comprising 61% of all those located, whereas only 13% (19 studies) were the ones that permitted evaluation of outcomes, either researcher-manipulated, involving experimental or quasi-experimental designs, or naturally occurring before-and-after or between-group comparisons.

The studies included in Table 4.3 show different directions of effects. Based on a re-analysis of the SARP projects, Siddique (2013) suggested the effectiveness of arrest has been under-estimated in the past. Cho and Wilke (2010) found a large effect of arrest on reducing IPV by men, and Gerstenberger and Williams (2012) found a sizeable effect for dual arrest. On the other hand, there were several studies that found no effect (Davis et al., 2001; Felson et al., 2005; Hirschel, 2008; Hilton et al., 2007), one which suggested short-term effects can be misleading as to longer-term outcomes (Klein & Tobin, 2008), and two which suggest there may be differential effects according to the pattern of an individual's DA history and other kinds of offending (Johnson & Goodlin-Fahncke, 2015; Piquero et al., 2005). In contrast, there is a finding that the reporting of DA to police, and the sense of power that a victim so gains, can be a more potent influence on reducing its recurrence than arrest (Miller, 2003). Moreover, when perpetrators are arrested, it may not be that itself which has an effect, but what happens afterwards in terms of prosecution, processing and treatment. Finally, there is the worrying implication that arrest may be associated with deleterious effects on victims far later, including premature death (Sherman & Harris, 2015).

Methodologically, these studies are not strong and the majority involve single cohorts only, although three involved long-term follow-ups of the SARP experiments and others made use of large-scale survey data. In other respects, they are a fairly diverse mixture in terms of both their specific objectives and research designs. It is difficult to conclude from them that arrest, which at one stage appeared to offer prospects of a notable impact on DA/IPV, is well supported by the accumulated evidence. At the same time there is a possibility that it may have an effect on a subgroup of those who commit IPV, if that group can be successfully identified. Doing so could involve a combination of risk assessment and examination of abuser type. But these would be difficult decisions to make at the scene following a contact unless the perpetrator or partner were already known to the police.

### 4.6.2 Coordinated Community Response

The second set of 24 studies located in the review were concerned with other types of response to DA/IPV, of a more elaborate nature and involving more than one agency. In some cases, these were police-led; in others they entail joint, collaborative action, for example, through domestic violence response teams (DVRTs) or domestic violence units (DVUs), or systems of coordinated community response (CCR). Findings from them are summarized in Table 4.4.

As found with research on arrest, there is no definitive pattern of results emerging from these 24 studies. Part of the reason for that resides in the studies having focused on a variety of interventions, which despite having some features in common also differ in important ways. Most can be grouped into one of three main categories: (a) the use of specialist domestic violence response teams or units (DVRTs, DVUs); (b) Domestic Violence Home Visit Intervention (DVHVI), involving joint home visit procedures by police and another agency; and (c) coordinated community response (CCR), a form of public education or awareness campaign. Some trends emerge in favour of the use of DVRTs/DVUs. They deal with more serious cases, though perhaps with the result that prosecutions can be more difficult to obtain (Friday et al., 2006). They are perceived positively (Corcoran et al., 2001), and there is tentative evidence that they can have significant effects on DA recidivism (Exum et al., 2014; Whetstone 2001). The study by Exum et al. (2014) yielded the largest effect in support of a specialized police DV Unit. The one they evaluated, in Charlotte, North Carolina, consisted of a sergeant, four detectives, an administrative assistant, four counsellors and a group of citizen volunteers. The unit pursued intensive investigation of DA/IPV cases and undertook preparation of materials for court, in combination with provision of victim assistance.

The DVHVI involves specialist training for police officers who are paired with victim support advocates. The four studies by Stover and her colleagues (Stover, 2012; Stover et al., 2008, 2009b, 2010) reported evaluations of different aspects of these services and found they led to improved relationship of victims to police. However, findings on other effects are more equivocal. Second responder schemes, sometimes used as part of them, show mixed outcomes, but the recent study by Scott et al. (2015) found very encouraging effects. Where agencies work together,

**Table 4.4** Studies of other community-based, police-led and collaborative interventions (24 studies)

| Study | Methodology | Samples/data sources | Intervention and outcomes |
|---|---|---|---|
| Corcoran et al. (2001) | Interview-based survey in one locality | 219 police officers | Examined police perceptions of a DVRT involving social workers and volunteers. 79% thought the response team was helpful in DV incidents either in supporting police actions or in providing other services to the victims |
| Davis et al. (2007, 2010) | RCT | Three conditions:<br>24 hours: $N = 75$<br>7 days: $N = 77$<br>No response: $N = 148$ | Evaluated a second responder programme which involves following an initial contact with a second one within a specified period. Compared 24 hour, 7 days and no response. Over 6 months, found no difference between the three conditions in rates of new abuse incidents |
| Dichter and Gelles (2012) | Cross-sectional study based on questionnaire | 164 female IPV victims | Assessed victims' perceptions of safety following police intervention related to IPV. Feeling unsafe was a function of partners having made death threats and use of sexual assault, but was not influenced by perpetrator having been arrested |
| Exum et al. (2014) | Group comparison between DV unit and standard patrol | 891 DV cases, of which 220 were DV unit cases | Evaluated the impact of a specialized police DV unit. Over 18–30-month follow-up recidivism prevalence was significantly lower amongst DV unit cases than in standard patrol cases (50% difference) involving arrest alone. There were insufficient data to explain the cause of the result |
| Friday et al. (2006) | Group comparison between DV unit (DVU) and routine patrol | 891 DV incidents analysed, 25% from the DV unit | Process evaluation of a specialized police DV unit. This showed the unit was selecting the most serious cases and that DVU suspects had lower offending prevalence after initial incidents than routine patrol cases (29% vs 37%). Victims showed no change in reporting rates for DV, but showed lower personal harm. DVU was less successful than routine patrol in securing prosecution at 2 years. Best predictor of DV prevalence was prior DV record |
| Goosey et al. (2017) | RCT of integrated IPV case management involving police + 10 agencies | 3 groups of 60 IPV dyads randomly allocated to treatments or control | *Domestic Abuse Service Coordination* intervention had three elements: victim support, perpetrator counselling with motivational techniques and follow-up home visits. Analysis over 24 months, interpretation hampered by presence of outliers. There was a significant drop in harm index in both groups but larger in treatment than control group, but no change in the frequency of repeat IPV incidents |
| Hatcher et al. (2020) | Mixed-methods process evaluation of a community mobilization intervention | Interviews with 114 participants + participant observation of programme delivery | Part of evaluation of the *CHANGE* intervention. A trial of this (not yet published) failed to find reductions in men's and discoveries from the process evaluation showed that poor implementation may have been a factor in this. Some aspects of the community mobilization process were weak due to insufficient institutional support and lack of staff training |

(continued)

**Table 4.4** (continued)

| Study | Methodology | Samples/data sources | Intervention and outcomes |
|---|---|---|---|
| Hester et al. (2019) | Multisite RCT | At the outset, 530 in experiment and 2085 control conditions. At 12 months: Site 1: 169 in each group Site 2: 184 in each group | Evaluation of *Drive*, a community-based, multi-agency initiative combining individual work with perpetrators, indirect work between agencies, information sharing, risk management, victim support and safeguarding. Intervention lasted 10 months. While both *Drive* and control group members showed reductions in domestic violence rates, the former sustained this and at follow-up showed a 10% incident rate as against 24% for controls |
| HMIC (2015) | Review report on focused inspection | HM inspectorate review of progress in responding to DA across all forces | Numerous findings, including improved standard of investigations and better supervision of frontline staff, but inconsistencies in use of DV Protection Orders and risk assessment practices. Found marked variations in charge rates (16% to 51%) and in rates of victims not supporting police action (1% to 46%). Made 11 recommendations |
| Messing et al. (2016) | Study of factors influencing programme participation | Interviews with 648 women IPV victims at high risk, comparing those who used a hotline with those who did not | Evaluates the *Lethality Assessment Program*, a joint police-social service intervention, to examine factors affecting levels of use of an advocacy hotline. Extent and form of violence in prior incidents, women's prior use of safety planning, increased likelihood of use, while increased PTSD symptoms reduced it |
| Millbank et al. (2000) | Monitoring study of early stage of large-scale project | 427 interventions following first police attendance | Evaluated partnerships between 500 specially trained police and local DV support providers in a project entailing increased support for victims and attention to perpetrators. Over 4 months, interim findings showed a 400% increase in recording of DV incidents but a low number of repeat call-outs |
| Muftić and Bouffard (2007) | Quasi-experimental design | Court-assessed individuals: 131 males 70 females | Evaluated a coordinated community response (CCR) involving police contact and victim advocacy. Compared differences in how males and females were processed and in outcomes. Found large differences on all variables examined. But the CCR approach failed to produce any impact on DV re-offending |
| Post et al. (2009) | Group comparison design with telephone survey | 12,039 telephone calls in 10 CCR test and 10 matched control sites | Tested the impact of CCR projects on general population knowledge of IPV, attitudes towards it, use of related services and its prevalence. CCRs were designed to increase community awareness of IPV. However, no differences were found on any variable between CCR and comparison sites |
| Salazar et al. (2007) | Interrupted time-series design | Arrests and court dispositions at 75 data points over 6 years | Evaluated the impact of a CCR comparing two counties implementing it (one urban, one rural) with areas not doing so. Found that CCRs were associated with significant increases in arrests and prosecutions of males, but also in arrests of females |

(continued)

**Table 4.4** (continued)

| Study | Methodology | Samples/data sources | Intervention and outcomes |
|---|---|---|---|
| Scott et al. (2015) | Quasi-experimental design | Male IPV offenders: 40 treatment 40 control | Evaluated a second responder programme. Follow-up rates for new DV charges were significantly lower for the experimental than the control group: 29.3% vs 65.9% at 1 year and 12.2% vs 41.5% at 2 years. Provides information on police time commitment to the intervention |
| Slaght and Hamilton (2005) | Qualitative study: interviews + content analysis | Number of respondents not given | Interviews were conducted with a range of professionals in two Family Violence Coordinating Councils in Illinois. Dominant emergent theme was that of a unified "judicial philosophy" across all levels of an agency that "integrated law enforcement and treatment responses" (p.58) |
| Stover (2012) | Interview-based survey | 52 DV victims from Stover et al. (2010) study | Evaluated partnerships between police and other agencies in responding to DA/IPV, including home visit and second responder programmes. Respondents reported high levels of satisfaction with the Domestic Violence Home Visit Intervention (DVHVI) in terms of their own and their children's safety and their confidence in police. No evaluation reported of rates of IPV incidents |
| Stover et al. (2008) | Group comparison + correlational study | 301 DV cases over an 18-month period, 204 with DVHVI contact | Examined factors influencing engagement with a conjoint Police-Advocacy home visit service as a method of preventing DV. Describes the DVHVI service in detail. The factors which best predicted engagement were victim-advocate ethnic match, number of children in the family and more weakly, severity of DV charges |
| Stover et al. (2009b) | Group comparison and monitoring study | 512 DV cases in 4 groups tracked for 12 months | Evaluated the impact of the DVHVI on police-reported incidents of repeat violence at follow-up. Divided groups according to dosage or level of contact: high, low, no contact and comparison condition in a non-DVHVI area. Survival analysis found no differences between DVHVI groups and no-contact groups. Higher levels of engagement were associated with increased calls to the police and substance use with decreased calls |
| Stover et al. (2010) | Quasi-experimental design | Women victims: 52 DVHVI group 55 control group | Evaluated the efficacy of the DVHVI involving joint visits to victims by a police officer and advocate team. Over 12 months DVHVI women reported more positive interaction with police, felt more respected and called the police significantly more often, with a trend towards more minor incidents (breach of peace, no physical injury) |

(continued)

**Table 4.4** (continued)

| Study | Methodology | Samples/data sources | Intervention and outcomes |
|---|---|---|---|
| Strang et al. (2017) | RCT of *Cautioning and Relationship Abuse* police-based experimental intervention | 293 males arrested for and admitting low-level IPV; random assignment to *Cautioning and Relationship Abuse* or no-treatment control | Evaluation of *Cautioning and Relationship Abuse* involving 2-day workshops run by a charitable trust for Hampshire Police. Over 1 year, members of *Cautioning and Relationship Abuse* groups had a 27% lower harm score than controls, a re-arrest rate 21% lower and prevalence rate 35% lower. Effect size for IPV recidivism was 0.299 |
| Tutty and Babins-Wagner (2019) | Before-and-after study of introduction of a specialized DV court | 382 males mandated to attend a group counselling programme | Evaluated specially designed 30-hour, 14-week, narrative therapy courses, *Responsible Choices for Men* (RCM) provided by Calgary Counselling Centre. There was a large drop in recidivism (41.2% to 8.2%) after the DV court was implemented, mandating attendance at the RCM courses |
| Tutty et al. (2020) | Differential impact court mandate on DV perpetrator participation | 964 males, who attended a group programme; 78% court-mandated, 22% not; 694 (72%) completed | Compared the effect of being court-mandated to attend RCM (see previous entry) with non-mandated attendance; also evaluated the effect on a set of mental health measures. The latter improved significantly across both groups, i.e. regardless of mandated/non-mandated status |
| Whetstone (2001) | Quasi-experiment in two districts, experimental and control | 18,044 IPV calls, 4004 incidents, 979 arrests | Studied the efficacy of a DVU comparing responses to calls 1 year before and 18 months after it was introduced. Results showed several more positive changes in the experimental DVU district in terms of total arrests and proportion of calls for service and IPV incidents, and in prosecutions, convictions and medical care for victims |

close attention needs to be paid to establishing a core set of expectations about their goals (Slaght & Hamilton, 2005).

It is difficult to draw conclusions regarding other types of intervention. Findings on the effects of CCRs are contradictory, with one study finding some positive outcomes, but also some unanticipated adverse effects (Salazar et al., 2007) and another finding no effect (Post et al., 2009). It is clearly a major challenge to generate greater public awareness of a problem that until not long ago was largely hidden or denied. Unfortunately, the early report by Millbank et al. (2000) on the project in Adelaide does not appear to have been followed by other reports of its progress or of final outcomes. A supplementary search was conducted to locate any other documents on this work but none could be found.

Also, in common with research on arrest, the designs used in these evaluations are for the most part not strong. Some were process evaluations only, and amongst the outcome studies just one employed random allocation. While other studies were fairly well designed given the constraints they operated under, differences between groups detracted from the chances of being able to draw firm conclusions. The statistical models developed in these studies however accounted for only rather small proportions of the variance. In other words, there are probably many other factors influencing the results that the studies have not measured. While this can only be speculated, the most likely explanation of such a pattern is that a large number of factors each explain a small amount of the variation in results.

Bates and Douglas (2020) provide an overview of the range of services available for victims of domestic violence in the UK and the USA, showing the extensive variety of types of provision, but simultaneously the gaps that remain in the support networks and in their connectivity. They make a series of recommendations for improving the position with reference to legislation, levels of resources and training, amongst other areas. The involvement of police in multi-agency responses to IPV continues to show wide variation from one location to another.

### *4.6.3 Women's Police Stations and Justice Centres*

The next set of studies, listed in Table 4.5, reported on the effects of a change that has perhaps offered potentially some of the most promising results to have appeared to date. This is the establishment of police stations staffed entirely or almost entirely by women officers – Women's Police Stations. While this may sound like a novel idea of recent origin, such stations have existed in India and in some parts of Latin America for several decades. Different documents date the opening of the first such stations to Kerala, India, in 1973; São Paulo in 1985; La Plata, Argentina, in 1988; and Tamil Nadu, India, in 1992. The services are known in Brazil as *Delegacias Especializadas de Atendimento das Mulheres* (Police Stations Specialized in Serving Women). By 2010 there were over 500 such stations in Brazil, and the model had been adopted in 14 other countries, almost all in the low- or middle-income range in global economic terms (Perova & Reynolds, 2017). In Argentina the stations have a multidisciplinary staff team, including social workers, lawyers and psychologists working alongside police.

Services of this nature are based on a model of empowering female victims of male violence, challenging patriarchal norms and facilitating women's access to justice, and creating a career pathway for more women in law enforcement. Implemented in this manner, they thus reach much farther across the spectrum of variables set out in the ecological model shown in Fig. 4.1. As the findings summarized in Table 4.5 show, this development has led to predominantly positive outcomes. These studies use large-scale official crime statistics rather than experimental trial designs. There have been reported reductions at statistically significant levels in rates of violence against women in Argentina, Brazil and Peru, in each of which women police stations provide access to a range of services relevant to responding to IPV. Carrington et al. (2020c) have proposed that there are valuable lessons to be learnt from this, and recommended that these services be adopted in Australia, one of several practices that Carrington (2021) suggests could be adapted from the global south.

We can view this innovation against a background in which to date, the influence of women officers on policing has been fairly limited. Prenzler and Sinclair (2013)

**Table 4.5** Studies of women's police stations (6 studies)

| Study | Methodology | Samples/data sources | Intervention and outcomes |
|---|---|---|---|
| Amaral et al. (2019) | Multivariate regression analysis of city-level trends in crimes against women including IPV | Data from the National Crime Records Bureau for 73 Indian cities over different years in the period 2005–2013 | Evaluated effects of *All-Women Police Units* as they were expanded across cities and states of India. Overall found a significant increase of 22% in the rate of crimes against women reported to the police. However, the recorded rates of crime showed no change in levels of violence |
| Carrington et al. (2020a, b) | Interview-based + observational study of patterns of work in women's police services in Buenos Aires province | 100 staff (81 police officers + social workers, psychologists and lawyers) from 10 women's police stations | Found a high level of collaboration between police and other professions, and evidence of an intensive victim-centred orientation, with accompanying emphasis on work with perpetrators and involvement in community crime prevention activities via links to 11 other named agencies. However, there were also major problems of under-resourcing. Court data showed Buenos Aires had one of the lowest rates of femicide in Latin America in 2018 |
| Jassal (2020) | Multivariate analysis of police data to compare states with all-women police stations at different times | Data from the Criminal Tracking and Network System for three Indian states in the period 2015–2017 | Compared data for Haryana with Bihar and Uttar Pradesh states. Found no evidence that all-women police stations provided greater access to justice than standard police stations and some evidence of negative effects. Staff in the former more often blamed victims and tried harder to persuade women to stay in abusive partnerships, and women officers expressed more dissatisfaction with their roles |
| Kavanaugh et al. (2017) | Multivariate analysis of three datasets (individuals, households and schools) | Data testing the effects of introducing 226 women's justice centres in Peru over the period 1999–2014 | Evaluation of the impact of the rollout of women's justice centres staffed by police, prosecutors, counsellors and others. The presence of a women's justice centre was associated with significantly lower rates of reported physical IPV, of assaults of women resulting in hospitalizations and in femicides. Also found that the presence of a women's justice centre was linked to increased levels of children's school enrolment and attendance |

(continued)

**Table 4.5** (continued)

| Study | Methodology | Samples/data sources | Intervention and outcomes |
|---|---|---|---|
| Natarajan (2005) | Retrospective single-cohort analysis of case reports and outcomes of dispute resolution processes | Analysis of a 25% random sample of 474 case records and interviews with 60 victims in Tamil Nadu, India, in 1999–2001 | Description of the working and impact of *All-Women Police Units* set up to deal with violence against women, especially when associated with dowry disputes. Reported mainly positive outcomes of police contact and positive perceptions of women police, but reports no comparative or pre-post analysis. Noted needs for more training in counselling and dispute resolution |
| Perova and Reynolds (2017) | Multivariate statistical analysis of rates of femicide using official data sources and using femicide as an index of severe IPV | Data on murders (rate per 100,000 population) of women aged 15–49 from 2074 municipalities in Brazil in the period 2004–2009 | Compared municipalities with and without women's police services. Controlled for other variables usually associated with homicide (e.g. population density, % females in district, GDP per capita). Did not find a significant overall effect, but in metropolitan districts there was a reduction of 17% in the average femicide rate and a 50% reduction amongst women aged 15–24. There were no effects in smaller towns or rural areas and no effect on rates of male homicide |

collected data on the proportions of female officers in police services from English language websites in 14 countries for 10 years up to July 2012. Some services provided no data on this. Where data were available, there was a considerable range from the highest figure of women officers of 28.8% in Tasmania to the lowest at 5.1% in India. But there was also evidence of a historical plateau effect, with further increases appearing less likely over recent years. In that context however, there is evidence that the involvement of women police has had a discernible effect in improving some aspects of the quality of policing, at least where such a comparison was done. Miller and Segal (2019) analysed several aspects of policing in the USA over the period from the late 1970s till the early 1990s as the proportions of women officers in the police workforce steadily grew, from 3.4% to 10.1%. They found that increases in the female officer share of the workforce were associated with increasing rates of reporting of domestic violence to police and more effective responses by police to reports of sexual assault. There was no association with the proportions of women employed by the police in civilian roles.

However, investigating the effects of Women's Police Stations in the Indian state of Haryana, Jassal (2020) sounded some cautionary notes. It is important for such stations not to develop into enclaves offering an exclusive service, as this results in deflection of workloads from one station to another, and negative perceptions of women officers. The extent to which this departure can yield benefits may also depend on the model of services that is adopted. Moreover, as with many other aspects of effective policing, it is vital for initiatives to take account of context and to consider potential unintended consequences as part of risk analysis prior to major strategy decisions.

### 4.6.4 Intervention Programmes for DA/IPV

This section summarizes findings from a total of 69 separate intervention/outcome evaluation studies. Several different approaches have been used in developing interventions designed to reduce DA/IPV. Though showing variety in many aspects of their methods and content, these are often collectively known as *Batterer Intervention Programmes* (BIPs), a generic name for structured treatment programmes for those convicted of these offences. Findings of the studies located in this review are presented in Table 4.6.

Over a lengthy period, the most widely used method of working with individuals who had committed domestic abuse was based on the *Duluth model*, an inter-agency approach devised by the *Duluth Domestic Abuse Intervention Project* in Minnesota in the 1980s. The main strand in this is the application of pro-feminist concepts of patriarchy/male dominance to the analysis of power, coercion and control in close relationships (Bowen, 2011b; Cluss & Bodea, 2011). Another widely used approach draws on more broadly based models of offender rehabilitation employing cognitive-behavioural methods focusing (for example) on development of self-control, problem-solving and social interaction skills. There are many variants and hybrids of both approaches, as well as other models of more recent origin.

The studies listed in Table 4.6 cover a very wide spectrum of interventions for the prevention of DA/IPV recidivism. The main features they have in common are that they presuppose that there are individual, dispositional, psychological factors associated with a preparedness or propensity to act violently towards a partner, within an underlying social context where there are ambivalent attitudes towards gender relations. These and other risk factors can putatively be addressed and altered through psychologically based treatments that combine elements of educational, therapeutic and skills-training approaches to personal change. The result is a plethora of treatment models, with a small number that have become well established and which are the most frequently used and evaluated, with a larger number of novel approaches represented by only a single evaluation each.

The majority of the retained studies measured a range of variables, and many details of the information collected and of the analyses conducted are not included here. Many used a well-established instrument, the *Conflict Tactics Scale*, which was designed for the assessment of controlling behaviours in couple relationships. Others used numerous different scales for measuring attitudes, personality traits, anger, impulsivity and in some studies symptom inventories for assessment of

**Table 4.6** Evaluations of DA/IPV treatment/intervention (69 studies)

| Study | Methodology | Samples/data sources | Intervention and outcomes |
|---|---|---|---|
| Alexander et al. (2010) | RCT | 528 male DV offenders | Compared offenders assigned to a stages-of-change motivational interviewing treatment with a CBT-based approach. No differences were found in self-reports of violence but significantly fewer partners of men in the stages-of-change motivational interviewing condition reported having been victimized at 12-month telephone follow-up |
| Ashburn et al. (2017) | Quasi-experimental design to compare those exposed or not exposed to the programme | 435 fathers aged 16–25 married or cohabiting, with children aged 1–3 in Northern Uganda: 256 exposed 179 unexposed | Post-test and follow-up evaluation of *REAL Fathers Initiative*, a 12-session mentoring programme + community posters, designed to reduce violence against partners and children. Outcome data were measures of attitudes to and perpetration of IPV and punishing children. *REAL* attenders had significantly greater odds (OR 2.4) of showing positive interactions with partners and lower odds of justifying IPV (0.63 at post-test and 0.50 at follow-up) |
| Bennett et al. (2007) | Large-scale follow-up of cohort of BIP offenders analysed using regression | 890 males attending one of 30 programmes | Followed up participants for 2.4 years to test relationship between programme completion and recidivism. Re-arrest rates were 14.3% and 34.7% for completers and non-completers, respectively. Reduced odds of re-arrest ranged from 39% to 61% |
| Bloomfield and Dixon (2015) | Quasi-experimental design | 6695 referrals to two programmes: 3349 completers 1188 dropouts 2158 controls | Evaluated two probation programmes (IDAP and CDVP)[a] over a 2-year follow-up. Found statistically significant reductions of 13.2% and 10.9% in any re-offending and in DV re-offending, respectively |
| Boira et al. (2013) | Two studies, one descriptive, one qualitative | 27 males in groups for IPV perpetrators | Process study of relationships between factors operating in treatment. Found significant correlations between markers of therapeutic alliance and rated usefulness; aspects of the former promoted treatment adherence |
| Bowen (2010) | Correlational study | 77 DV offenders 31 probation staff | Investigated the relationship between offender and tutor perceptions of cohesion of a treatment group; these were closely correlated, but neither had any association with re-offending outcomes |
| Bowen et al. (2005) | Before-and-after quasi-experiment | 86 DV offenders | Compared treatment completers and dropouts from the probation-based DVPP[b] at 11-month follow-up; 15% of the former and 33% of the later had allegedly committed a new offence. Only 1 of 13 psychological variables differentiated the groups; there were more marked differences in criminal histories |
| Bowen et al. (2008) | Before-and-after quasi-experiment | 52 DV offenders 32 non-offenders | Examined intermediate changes over 11-month follow-up of offenders mandated to attend treatment programme. Only 17% of offenders showed reliable change on mediating factors, but none showed association with re-offending |

(continued)

**Table 4.6** (continued)

| Study | Methodology | Samples/data sources | Intervention and outcomes |
|---|---|---|---|
| Braithwaite and Fincham (2014) | RCT | 52 married couples randomly assigned to treatment versus placebo control | Evaluated the impact of a computer-based preventive intervention "*ePREP*" on rates of IPV. Obtained self-report and other reports at three time points over 1 year. There was a 90% reduction in physical aggression and a more modest reduction in psychological aggression. Note that couples were not offenders and only 18% acknowledge IPV at baseline |
| Buttell (2002) | Quasi-experimental design | 91 women court-mandated to attend treatment | Examined the relationship between IPV and moral reasoning and any changes during treatment groups. Offenders (mean age 30) had moral reasoning scores similar to youths in early high school. The programme had no impact on moral reasoning scores at post-test or 2-year follow-up |
| Buttell and Carney (2004) | Single-cohort before-and-after study | 76 court-referred male DV offenders | Analysed a wide range of data to test for the extent of change following treatment and at 12-month follow-up. There were no differences in any test scores pre- to post-treatment. Only one participant had been re-arrested at follow-up. Comparisons between African-American and Caucasian offenders showed no differences |
| Carney and Buttell (2004) | Secondary analysis with one-group pre-test/ post-test | 26 female DV offenders | Evaluated a 16-week BIP + 12-week psycho-educational programme using several measures. At 12-month follow-up only one person was re-arrested. There were significant changes on scales of passive/aggressive responding but not in assertiveness |
| Cissner and Puffett (2006) | Comparison study of two BIPs | 291 defendants charged with DV | Evaluated two court-mandated BIPs in Brooklyn, compared on completion and recidivism rates. Completion rates were 66% and 77% and BIPs had similar rates of re-arrest at 1 year. The best predictor of re-arrest was criminal record |
| Connors et al. (2012) | Single-cohort before-and-after study with some sub-group analyses | 298 male Canadian federal prisoners convicted of IPV | Evaluation of MIFVPP[c] in prison or after release with pre-, mid- and post-test measures. Results showed significant improvements on all measures associated with IPV risk. Measures of motivation (readiness to change) were highly correlated with the extent of change |
| Connors et al. (2013) | Single-cohort before-and-after study with some sub-group analyses | 159 male Canadian federal prisoners convicted of IPV | Evaluation of changes linked to participation in the HIFVPP[d] in high-risk prisoners. Significant changes were found in most measures through pre-, mid- and post-programme assessments. Motivation to change was associated with changes in performance measures |
| Coulter and VandeWeerd (2009) | Pre-post study across series of programmes | 17,999 IPV offenders treated from 1995 to 2004 | Evaluation of a three-level programme system in successive groups over 10 years at six centres. Mean completion rate was 70%. IPV recidivism rate for completers was 8.4% compared to 21.2% for non-completers. Discusses changes in referral and success rates over time |

(continued)

**Table 4.6** (continued)

| Study | Methodology | Samples/data sources | Intervention and outcomes |
|---|---|---|---|
| Crane and Eckhardt (2013) | RCT | 82 males IPV perpetrators on probation | Evaluated the effect of a brief single-session motivational enhancement intervention on re-arrest at 6 months. There was evidence that the brief single-session motivational enhancement session increased programme compliance. Treatment versus control recidivism rates (25% vs 39%) not statistically significant |
| Crockett et al. (2015) | Single-cohort before-and-after study | 149 DV offenders (35 female) | Examined the effects of a form of BIP called RCIP[e] on several risk factors for IPV. There were significant gains in terms of accountability, anger management, stress levels and motives but not in controlling behaviours and in self-reported physical and psychological violence |
| Cunha and Goncalves (2015) | Quasi-experimental design | Male offenders:<br>26 treatment group<br>19 control group<br>Portugal | Evaluated psycho-educational BIP. Significant changes found in attitudes to DV, use of techniques of minimization and legitimation, maintained at 6-month follow-up. No re-offence in treatment group, 22% in control group |
| Dalton (2007) | Survey-based study | 150 directors of 2131 BIPs in 35 states (USA) | Distributed a 44-item questionnaire including questions on evaluation. Found overall mean BIP completion rate of 62%. Only 24.7% reported follow-ups but 51.3% collected data on recidivism, giving a mean rate of 16% for men and 10% for women |
| Day et al. (2010) | Single-cohort before-and-after study | 38 IPV males Australia | Evaluation of GCDVIR[f] programme. Graphs show reductions over time in facilitator ratings of minimization, denial, blame and manipulation and positive but non-significant trends in psychometric scales. At 12-month follow-up 7/20 completers and 16/18 non-completers had further charges against them |
| Dunford (2000) | RCT | 861 couples<br>US navy personnel | Servicemen who had assaulted their wives were randomly assigned to four groups: men's, conjoint, rigorous monitoring and controls. Data collected from victims and perpetrators at 6- and 12-month follow-up. No significant differences were found between any of the conditions on husband or wife reports or in rates of arrest |
| Easton et al. (2000) | Quasi-experimental design | 41 DV offenders<br>67% substance abuse problems | Focused on relation of substance abuse to IPV. Compared two anger management groups with or without motivational enhancement session. Those given session showed significant increase in motivation but data could not be calculated for controls |
| Easton et al. (2007) | RCT | 78 IPV offenders with substance use problems:<br>40: Substance Abuse DV Treatment<br>38: TSF | Compared persons seeking treatment at a substance abuse treatment unit, who had also been arrested for DV, using Substance Abuse DV Treatment and 12-step therapy (TSF). At 6-month follow-up, there were no group differences in alcohol use, but for Substance Abuse DV Treatment 1 episode of violence per month and for TSF: 2.4 episodes of violence per month |

(continued)

**Table 4.6** (continued)

| Study | Methodology | Samples/data sources | Intervention and outcomes |
|---|---|---|---|
| Echauri et al. (2013) | Quasi-experimental design | IPV males<br>300 immigrants<br>300 citizens<br>Spain | Tested whether a BIP (20 × 1 hour) used with citizens would also work with immigrants at post-test and 12-month follow-up. Found 34.6% success (= absence of abuse episodes and return to normal functioning) and 51.3% improvement (= absence of abuse episodes) in both groups, with similar results at follow-up |
| Echeburúa et al. (2006) | Single-cohort before-and-after study | 52 IPV convicted prisoners<br>Spain | Evaluation of a BIP with males convicted of serious IPV. Found 92% completion rate and significant reduction in irrational and pro-violence beliefs and in hostility |
| Eckhardt et al. (2008) | Quasi-experimental design | 190 male IPV perpetrators | Investigated role of anger in IPV and possible effect on BIP outcomes at 12-month follow-up. Placed participants in three anger clusters, though these were not related to prior arrest history. Low-anger men were more likely to complete BIP and had significantly lower rate of re-arrest |
| Feder and Dugan (2002); Feder and Forde (2000) | RCT<br>The Broward experiment | 404 male IPV defendants | Experimental group received probation and mandatory 26-week BIP, control group given probation only. No differences were found in attitudes, beliefs, behaviours or rates of re-arrest at 12-month follow-up. Men with a low "stake in conformity" were less compliant and more likely to re-offend |
| Fernández-Montalvo et al. (2015) | Single-cohort before-and-after study | 235 IPV males on suspended sentences, Spain | Study overlaps with Echauri et al. (2013) and used the same outcome criteria. Percentages counted as success, improvement and failure were at post-treatment, 37.4, 48.1 and 14.5, and at 12-month follow-up, 39.6, 47.6 and 12.8 |
| Gondolf (2000) | Quasi-experimental, longitudinal design | 618 IPV males + data from female partners (67%) in 4 US cities | Reports long-term outcomes of 4 BIPs over 30 months. 41% of men re-assaulted partners during that period. Re-assault rate for men attending a BIP for >3 months was significantly lower than for dropouts (36% vs 51%) |
| Gondolf (2007a) | RCT | 501 IPV males + data from 60% to 70% of partners | Compared impact of BIPs in relation to ethnicity when delivered in three formats, culturally focused, African-American only and racially mixed. Over 12-month follow-up no differences emerged between groups on reported re-assault or on women's perceptions of safety, but re-arrest rate for DV was higher for culturally focused than for racially mixed groups with African-American intermediate |
| Gondolf and Jones (2001) | Quasi-experimental design | 640 IPV males court-mandated to BIPs | Overlaps with Gondolf (2000). Multisite study in three cities with 15-month follow-up. Men had been abusing partners for a mean of 3½ years. Found that programme completion had a "significant and substantial" (p.699) effect on re-assault reducing its probability by 44–64% |

(continued)

**Table 4.6** (continued)

| Study | Methodology | Samples/data sources | Intervention and outcomes |
|---|---|---|---|
| Gordon and Moriarty (2003) | Quasi-experimental design | 248 male DV offenders<br>132 treatment<br>116 control | Evaluation of probation-based BIPs. Treatment had no significant effect in straight group comparison. But there was a significant association between the number of treatment sessions completed and rates of re-arrest and reconviction |
| Hendricks et al. (2006) | Single-cohort before-and-after study | 200 male DA offenders | Compares two interventions: one a BIP called SAFE[g], the other a general offender treatment programme R&R[h]. Tracking at 6, 12 and 18 months. 10.6% of SAFE completers failed, as compared with 38.8% non-completers, but non-completion offenders had lower risk scores |
| Herman et al. (2014) | Single-cohort before-and-after study | 156 male IPV perpetrators, court-mandated | Evaluation of Duluth model programme using three measures and recidivism data after long-term follow-up of 9 years. Completion rate of 66%. Completers showed short-term change in measures at post-test. However, there was no difference between completers and non-completers in re-offending rates at follow-up |
| Jones and Gondolf (2002) | Quasi-experimental design | 640 male DV perpetrators, some mandated, some voluntary | Evaluated effects of three programmes using an instrumental variable analysis, designed to counter possible selection bias. Mean completion rate 54.1%. Taking other variables into account, completion was associated with a reduction in re-assault of 40 percentage points |
| Kistenmacher and Weiss (2008) | RCT | 33 DV offenders court-mandated | Compared motivational interviewing versus control condition. There was a larger change in motivation and readiness to change in the motivational interviewing than control group, and a greater shift away from blaming others |
| Labriola et al. (2005) | RCT with 2 × 2 factorial design | 420 male IPV misdemeanour offenders | Random assignment to one of four conditions: BIP + judicial monitoring, BIP + graduated monitoring, monthly monitoring only and graduated monitoring only. Neither BIP nor any form of monitoring obtained any reduction in re-arrest rate at 12-month follow-up |
| Labriola et al. (2010) | Survey | 260 courts, BIPs and victim support agencies | Investigated court responses to BIP non-compliance. Found only 58% had monitoring data, 83% referred offenders to non-BIPs, only 40% imposed sanctions for dropout and only 27% of courts and 16% of BIPs used jail as sanction |
| Lawson (2010) | Quasi-experimental design | 18 CBT<br>27 integrated | Compared two types of therapy for partner violence, CBT alone versus CBT integrated with psychodynamic therapy. CBT group functioned at lower level at pre-test. Both groups showed improvement but on different variables. Partner reports showed recidivism of 50% (CBT) and 22.2% (integrated) at follow-up (time unclear) |

(continued)

**Table 4.6** (continued)

| Study | Methodology | Samples/data sources | Intervention and outcomes |
|---|---|---|---|
| Lee et al. (2004) | Single-cohort pre-post-test design | 90 DV offenders 77 men, 13 women | Evaluated solution-focused therapy (8 × 1-hour sessions) over 14 groups. Found a completion rate of 92.8% and recidivism rate of 16.7% over a 6-month follow-up |
| Levesque et al. (2012) | RCT | 492 male DV offenders | Compared Usual Care which included a BIP with Usual Care + "Journey to Change" and three computer-assisted sessions based on the trans-theoretical model. BIP completion rate 68% for both groups. At 12-month follow-up partners of Usual Care + Journey group showed lower reports of violence (31.6% vs 60%) but there was no difference in police arrest records |
| Lila et al. (2013) | Single-cohort pre-post-test design | 212 convicted IPV offenders on suspended sentences | Evaluated *Contexto*, a BIP used in Spain. Used a large number of measures to ascertain risk of IPV re-offending, which was associated with lower alcohol consumption, lower impulsivity and higher life satisfaction |
| Lin et al. (2009) | Quasi-experimental, case-control design | DV offenders in Taiwan:<br>70 treated<br>231 control | Compared a higher-risk group mandated to BIP under protective orders with a lower-risk group on protective orders only. At 9-month follow-up the treated group had a significantly higher rate of DV: 58.65% vs 45% but no difference in overall criminal recidivism |
| Lyon (2005) | Quasi-experimental design | Male DV offenders<br>420 treated<br>124 control | Compared EVOLVE, a new 52-session BIP, with an older 26-session BIP. Found similar completion rates (63.5% and 65.2%) and lower rates of recidivism amongst completers. At 6-month follow-up 83.4% of EVOLVE and 75.9% of control group completers were arrest-free |
| MacLeod et al. (2010) | Quasi-experimental design | 1303 male DV offenders in 5 districts of California | Reviews BIP systems across five jurisdictions. Found modest differences in re-arrest rates at 12 months averaging 19%, range 15–25% for DV and 40%, range 32–48% for any offence |
| Maxwell et al. (2010) | Secondary analysis of RCT data from Taylor et al. (2001) | 376 male DV offenders | Evaluated a Duluth model BIP *Alternatives to Violence*. Re-analysed data obtained in an earlier study. Found a small reduction in new DV incidents during treatment but no evidence of maintained change at 15-month follow-up. Highlighted the importance of court control of offenders combined with readiness to change |
| Mennicke et al. (2015) | Single-group design + quasi-experimental design | Male prisoners convicted of DV:<br>176 pre-post only<br>253 treated<br>253 controls | Evaluated a prison-based 20-week BIP (*STOP and Change Direction*). Obtained data on 5- and 7-year reconvictions after release. Found significant pre-post changes in study 1. No significant differences in re-incarceration rates |
| Miller et al. (2013b) | Follow-up study of RCT of dating violence prevention programme | 1513 male athletes from grades 9 to 11 in 16 high schools in California | Evaluated 12-month effectiveness of *Coaching Boys into Men*, a programme for reducing violence against women. There were reductions in behaviour supportive of violence in both treatment and control groups, but they were larger for the intervention group with a mean effect size of −0.41; that group also reported a lower rate of abuse perpetration than controls, with a lower effect size of −0.15 |

(continued)

**Table 4.6** (continued)

| Study | Methodology | Samples/data sources | Intervention and outcomes |
|---|---|---|---|
| Mills et al. (2013) | RCT | 152 DV offenders | Compared BIP with restorative justice (RJ) programme, *Circles of Peace*. Respective completion rates of 40% and 51%. Found differences in favour of RJ in general re-offending rates, but differences in DV recidivism were non-significant |
| Morrel et al. (2003) | Quasi-experimental design | 86 males seeking treatment for partner abuse | Compared CBT and supportive therapy (ST) programmes for IPV. Across treatment there were significant reductions in physical and psychological aggression, maintained at 6-month follow-up. There were no between-group differences in numbers of police visits or in new charges at 3-year follow-up |
| Muñoz-Fernández et al. (2019)<br>See also Chap. 5 | RCT of *Date-e Adolescence* dating violence prevention programme | 1423 teenagers aged 11–19 from 7 schools in Seville or Córdoba, Spain | The programme contained 7 × 1-hour sessions, based on the analysis of risk factors for conflict in romantic dyads. Data collected at pre-, post-test and 6-month follow-up. Treated group showed a significantly reduced rate of growth in moderate and severe dating and sexual violence compared to controls. However, some schools did not take part at the follow-up stage |
| Musser et al. (2008) | Quasi-experimental design | 108 male IPV offenders:<br>55 treatment (MI)<br>53 control | Evaluated a two-session pre-group motivational interviewing input. Reported impact on homework compliance and valuation of group and marginal effect on physical assault but not injury or psychological aggression at 6 months |
| Niolon et al. (2016, 2019). For results on bullying, see Vivolo-Kantor et al. (2020), in Chap. 5 | Cluster RCT of *Dating Matters* teen violence prevention programme | Female and male students from 46 schools in 4 American states;<br>1157 treatment<br>1192 controls | Developed and evaluated a multi-component programme for youth and parents, to reduce teen dating violence; provided in treatment group schools for 2 years, compared with standard care. Found significant changes in reported dating violence perpetration, reported victimization and negative conflict resolution, but not in positive relationship skills |
| Novo et al. (2012) | Single-cohort pre-post-test design | 130 male IPV offenders | Evaluated the extent of change in a series of psychological and offence risk variables following participation in the Galician Experimental Re-education Programme for IPV. Found significant pre-post changes but does not report re-arrest or re-offence data |
| O'Farrell et al. (2004) | Quasi-experiment, well-matched comparison group | 303 couples + 303 males and 303 females in comparison sample | Evaluation of *Behavioral Couples Therapy*. Found a reduction in violence amongst those with alcohol problems from 60% to 24% (though still higher than comparison sample). Used intent-to-treat (ITT) analysis; 84% sample involved at 2-year follow-up |
| Pascual-Leone et al. (2011) | Quasi-experimental design | Prisoners with histories of IPV<br>66 treated<br>184 controls | Reported evaluation of emotion-focused therapy programme, *Relating Without Violence*, 12 weeks, in Canadian prisons. Found a reduction in recidivism, significant at 1-year post-release but smaller and non-significant at years 2 and 3 |

(continued)

**Table 4.6** (continued)

| Study | Methodology | Samples/data sources | Intervention and outcomes |
|---|---|---|---|
| Pitts et al. (2009) | Quasi-experimental design | Male DV offenders<br>100 treated<br>100 controls | Evaluated a DV repeat offender programme. Treated group was significantly less likely to have new charges for DV or other offences at 29-month follow-up point, 6% versus 45% for DV, 15% versus 58% for any type of offence |
| Rosenbaum et al. (2001) | Quasi-experimental design | 326 IPV males:<br>82 self-referred<br>244 court-mandated | Evaluated a psycho-educational group treatment comparing court-referred and self-referred offenders and different programme lengths. The former had a higher completion rate 79.5% versus 58.5% and a lower recidivism rate 4.9% versus 13.4% for DV. Recidivism reduced with increasing programme length |
| Scott and Easton (2010) | Quasi-experimental group comparison | 75 IPV males:<br>39 Caucasian<br>36 African-American | Study of a population court-mandated to attend substance abuse and domestic violence treatment following arrest for an offence involving both. Found significant reductions in alcohol use ($p = .001$) but not drug use and in physical violence ($p < .001$) for both groups |
| Sharps et al. (2016) | Multisite RCT of enhanced perinatal visits in DV risk cases | 239 low-income women who reported perinatal IPV, randomized<br>124 intervention<br>115 usual care | Evaluated *Domestic Violence Enhanced Home Visitation Program* comprising abuse assessment + six additional home visit sessions. Found significant reductions in Conflicts Tactics Scale (CTS-2) IPV scores including reported violence at 6 time points up to 24 months after childbirth, with significantly larger changes in the *Domestic Violence Enhanced Home Visitation Program* intervention group than in usual care |
| Stewart et al. (2014) | Evaluation of RNR-based interventions | 572 male prisoners, 246 followed post-release | Collated evaluation data from Correctional Services Canada of high- and moderate-intensity programmes based on the risk-need-responsivity model located at several sites. Pre-post data showed significant positive changes on all measures. Following release untreated offenders were 3.76 times more likely to commit new offences of spousal abuse |
| Stith et al. (2004) | RCT | 89 couples, but at follow-up:<br>11 individual couples<br>8 multiple couples<br>4 control groups | Evaluation of multi-couples versus individual couples therapy and no treatment for DV offenders. At 6-month follow-up of female partners, reported rates of violence as multi-couple groups 25%, individual couples 43% and untreated 67%. At 2 years, only one woman reported violence but the rate was 50% in controls |
| Taylor et al. (2001) | RCT | 376 male DV offenders | Evaluated the impact of a 40-hour BIP as compared with 40 hours of community service. At 12-month follow-up found 93% of treated as compared to 86% of controls group has no new offences. Results were interpreted as encouraging but a later re-analysis altered this conclusion (Maxwell et al., 2010) |

(continued)

**Table 4.6** (continued)

| Study | Methodology | Samples/data sources | Intervention and outcomes |
|---|---|---|---|
| Taylor and Maxwell (2009) | RCT | 629 male arrestees held in local jail: 317 treatment 312 control | Evaluated a short, early-intervention BIP provided to prisoners in a local jail. there was evidence that the programme had an effect in reducing controlling behaviours within couples, but no significant effect on physical assault. However, 6-month follow-up data were only available on 20% of the sample |
| Tollefson and Gross (2006) | Single-cohort design + follow-up of predictive variables | 197 DV offenders 85% males | Evaluated a multi-modal 20-session BIP. Police records indicated that only 21% of the study sample re-offended during the 25-month follow-up. Key aim was to identify factors associated with recidivism; analysis showed four key variables: substance abuse, psychopathology, psychiatric history and child abuse history |
| Trebow et al. (2015) | Longitudinal, naturalistic, mixed-methods evaluation | 150 males convicted of DV and placed on probation | Evaluated a 52-session BIP and compared those whose first language was English or Spanish, respectively ($N = 75$ each). Re-offending rates were low: at 6 months 8% had a new DV conviction, but 39% had violated probation |
| Wray et al. (2013) | Longitudinal, single-cohort design | 121 couples referred by court, 92 mandated to programme | A pilot evaluation only of a three-phase group treatment for couples in violent conflict. Having a child was a prerequisite of inclusion. At 1-year follow-up there was a 33% reduction in recidivism amongst completers based on both self-report and partner report. From 92 couples, 62 men and 70 women completed the programme |
| Yorke et al. (2012) | Single-cohort pre-post-test design | 24 prisoners in 2 groups | Evaluated a 52-week BIP in a prison setting, using psychometric data and qualitative information. Tested the hypothesis that the intervention would enable participants to recognize their behaviour as abusive. Results supported the hypothesis with evidence of significant change. No offence data |

[a]IDAP = Integrated Domestic Abuse Programme, 27 group and 13 individual sessions; CDVP = Community Domestic Violence Programme, 25 group and 9 individual sessions; Both programmes were accredited by the NOMS Correctional Services Advisory and Accreditation Panel.
[b]DVPP = Domestic Violence Perpetrator Programme developed by the West Midlands Probation Service
[c]MIFVPP = Moderate Intensity Family Violence Prevention Program: 29 × 3-hour group + 3 individual sessions
[d]HIFVPP = High Intensity Violence Prevention Program: 75 × 5- or 3-hour group + 10 individual sessions
[e]RCIP = Resolution Counseling Intervention Program, a psycho-educational treatment group, 21 or 30 weeks
[f]GCDVIR = Gold Coast Domestic Violence Integrated Response, 24-week group-based BIP
[g]SAFE = Stop Abuse For Everyone, 1 × 1½-hour session and 15 × 2-hour sessions
[h]R&R = Reasoning and Rehabilitation, 26 × 2-hour sessions (the full version is 38 sessions)

mental health problems. Some devised specially made measures for use in a single study which have not been validated elsewhere.

The contents of Table 4.6 represent only a snapshot of the principal findings of each study. The overall pattern of results presents a slightly more positive overall picture than the one that has emerged from previous reviews, and there are some very encouraging findings. However, some reservations still need to be expressed regarding the work done in this field.

First, while there are some exceptions, results obtained from RCT designs are generally poorer, implying that some of the positive results in other studies could be a product of selection factors rather than a genuine treatment effect. There have been many calls for improved research methods and changes of focus in this area (e.g. Eckhardt et al., 2006; Saunders, 2008; Stuart et al., 2007), but it appears to take some time before such messages are properly heeded and acted upon. Second, there are often very tenuous links between scores on intermediate measures (of mediating variables, such as cognitions, attitudes) and the outcome variable of re-offending (whether IPV, other violence or offending in general). This may be a measurement problem given the challenges of assessing some of the variables that are operating, but it also raises questions about theories and explanations.

An exception to both of these is the evaluation of the *Drive* programme reported by Hester et al. (2019), which is the largest study of its kind to have been undertaken in the UK, and has several strengths, including its focus on high-risk, high-harm IPV perpetrators and the use of an RCT design. Participants were identified through Multi-Agency Risk Assessment Conferences. These include police, probation, health, child protection, housing practitioners, Independent Domestic Violence Advisors and other specialists from the statutory and voluntary sectors. They prepare a coordinated response to ensure the safety of those at risk of harm. Between intake and case closure, amongst *Drive* participants there was a statistically significant reduction in scores on the Domestic Abuse, Stalking and Honour-Based Violence risk assessment employed by Multi-Agency Risk Assessment Conferences. As seen earlier in Table 4.4, the *Drive* intervention had positive outcomes and similar patterns were observed at both sites. For individuals identified as serial IPV perpetrators, the mean number of police-recorded incidents amongst *Drive* participants at 12-month follow-up was 1.5, whereas for the control group the corresponding figure was 7.5. An approach that was thought to offer the prospect of saving lives (Orr, 2016) appears as if it may well have done so.

A third reservation is that some programmes are relatively brief in duration and it seems unlikely that significant change can be induced in some of the risk factors for DA/IPV after a comparatively limited short-term intervention. This was found, for example, in the meta-analysis by Arce et al. (2020) included earlier in Table 4.2. In some studies, this may explain why apparently good findings at post-test are not borne out by changed behaviour at follow-up.

Fourth, there are often high rates of attrition (dropout) and programme non-completion is associated with higher risk. There are several possible reasons for this. It could be a result of self-selection, where the more problematic individuals are resistant or even hostile to treatment, and deliberately absent themselves, but there could also be a proportion who are ambivalent about participation and who with some persuasion could still benefit from it. Methods of increasing engagement and of sustaining attendance become very important. Motivational enhancement sessions have produced some encouraging results and could be added to existing programmes, but compliance could also be strengthened by closer court or police monitoring of mandated programme attendance.

But it may also be that the limited power of these programmes is due in part to the fact that intervention needs to take place on multiple levels, for example, addressing beliefs and attitudes that remain widely influential, operating at the *society* level of the model shown earlier in Fig. 4.1. Some of the frameworks recommended by the WHO for reducing violence against women in low- and middle-income countries are attempts to go in that direction and have been at least partially successful (Bourey et al., 2015, included in Table 4.2). However, while police would be involved alongside other agencies if those interventions were implemented, they are not available as services that can be delivered by or commissioned through policing as they are likely to require major policy decisions probably at governmental level.

The results of some of the studies included here (Johnson & Goodlin-Fahncke, 2015; Piquero et al., 2005) and of others discussed in the review (Herrero et al., 2016; Huss & Ralston, 2008; Stare & Fernando, 2014) suggest there are sub-groups within those who perpetrate DA/IPV offences. There has been extensive work on heterogeneity and on typologies or sub-groups amongst DA/IPV offenders (Boxall et al., 2015; Cantos & O'Leary, 2014; Dixon & Browne, 2003). Offenders vary by risk level, but also by typology in terms of the type of violence in which they engage in close relationships. In extreme cases the ability to assess this could potentially be useful in estimating risk of femicide (Dixon et al., 2008; Dobash et al., 2007). It could also be used to gauge risk of officers themselves being assaulted (Johnson, 2011). These findings potentially highlight a differentiated approach to offender management, allocation to intervention programmes and required level of contact and monitoring. There is preliminary evidence of the potential usefulness of this from a study on the use of the *Spousal Assault Risk Assessment* by police officers in Sweden (Belfrage et al., 2012), although a related measure, *Brief Spousal Assault Form for the Evaluation of Risk*, produced somewhat better results (Storey et al., 2013).

### *4.6.5 Other Developments*

As noted earlier, the most frequently used approach since its inception has been the Duluth programme model. For example, in a survey of 116 probation departments in the state of Ohio, Ventura and Davis (2006) found that 80% of all the programmes in use were based on that model. Given the inconsistent evidence in support of it, there have been disputes over its continued use (Dutton & Corvo, 2006, 2007; Gondolf, 2007b). Interventions drawing on cognitive-behavioural methods are probably the second most widely used, and there have been several multi-modal formats developed that combine the two approaches. Many of those used in England and Wales, such as the Integrated Domestic Abuse Programme, Community

Domestic Violence Programme and Domestic Violence Perpetrator Programme (Bloomfield & Dixon, 2015; Bowen et al., 2005), adopted that approach.

Several other approaches have been attempted but to date were each represented in the present review by just one study or a very small number of studies in the research that was located. Some have adopted an innovative approach in applying a treatment model not previously evaluated in work with perpetrators of DA/IPV. They include solution focused therapy (Lee et al., 2004), emotion-focused therapy (Pascual-Leone et al., 2011), mandatory couples therapy (Wray et al., 2013) and a non-punitive paradigm examined by Crockett et al. (2015).

The present review has been concerned almost exclusively with outcomes, with "what works" to reduce the likelihood of IPV. A different approach was adopted in *Project Mirabal*, a UK-based investigation of the working of domestic violence prevention programmes that sought to move on from the rudimentary question of their effectiveness, to the development of a deeper understanding of the processes that occurred within them (Kelly & Westmarland, 2015). For example, Wistow et al. (2017) and Downes et al. (2019) have reported interview-based studies of aspects of coercive control strategies used by some perpetrators. This work identified how the balance of influences towards or away from the use of coercive control reflects men's changing levels of adherence to gender norms.

## 4.7 Discussion

This review focused on gathering evidence to answer the question: what general approaches and specific methods can be applied in work with those who have committed domestic abuse to reduce the likelihood of the behaviour recurring? We hoped that the answers obtained would have particular relevance to policing and would point towards initiatives that police officers could take to address the problem of IPV.

### *4.7.1 Strengths of This Literature*

The research reviewed here has a number of strengths. It covers a very wide range of the issues that need to be considered in addressing DA/IPV and uses a variety of methodologies and different perspectives in seeking answers to core questions. Many studies contain large participant samples, and although others have smaller sample sizes, they are often designed solely as pilot studies for which lower numbers are more appropriate. It is crucial to keep in mind the challenges of researching this field. It is an area of personal conflicts where many times there may be a great deal at stake, and where there are considerable sensitivities and barriers, ever-present legal and ethical dilemmas and often contradictory attitudes and expectations (Groves & Thomas, 2014).

### 4.7.2 Limitations of the Literature

A principal weakness of research in this area lies in the fundamental design of studies which still leaves many sets of results open to the effect of various biases. It is usually considered that the best way to reduce such problems is to conduct a randomized controlled trial (RCT). For a number of reasons random allocation is very difficult to implement in psychosocial treatment settings. Amongst the studies located in this review, for those on arrest none was an RCT, though some reported new analyses of trials conducted in the 1990s; only one of the coordinated community initiatives was evaluated via an RCT; and even in the intervention studies, where more randomized designs might be expected, there were only 18/69 (26%). A further weakness arises in that, while the variety of issues addressed is in some senses advantageous, its drawback is a lack of consolidated findings on specific issues that could give more confidence to anyone planning a novel departure in this area.

There is a cogent argument, put forward by Day et al. (2009), that programmes for men who commit DV offences are poorly articulated at a conceptual level and could be strengthened by adapting more of the approaches used in addressing other kinds of violence. Some have argued that DA/IPV interventions would benefit from more extensive use of the risk-needs responsivity model used in other areas of offender rehabilitation (Stewart et al., 2013). As many abusive incidents occur when males or both partners are intoxicated, there is also a sound rationale for closer links between DV interventions and work in the treatment of alcohol and other substance abuse (McMurran & Gilchrist, 2008), and some studies in the present review illustrate the value of this (e.g. Easton et al., 2007).

While an attempt has been made to make the present review as wide-ranging as possible, there are other areas of concern on which there is also a substantial amount of research not covered by it. They include work on vulnerable adults, who may be at risk in a range of settings not only in family relationships but in other contexts such as institutional care (Kalaga & Kingston, 2007). Oram et al. (2013) reviewed 42 studies on rates of domestic violence amongst psychiatric patients. Lifetime prevalence for in-patients ranged from 16% to 94% amongst women and 18–48% amongst men; the median prevalence for women was 33%. Beyond this, there are also problems, such as honour-related killings and coercion of women inside some cultural groups, which due to the controversies they raise remain under-researched. Focusing on these areas could identify other courses of action in which police involvement could potentially make a substantial difference to effectiveness. Alongside this however, it is also important to note that a review of seven studies by Mennicke and Ropes (2016) found that a proportion of law enforcement officers themselves admit to perpetrating violence against their partners, the rate across studies ranging from 4.8% to 40%. As shown in Table 4.3, Oehme et al. (2016) evaluated a training package specifically designed for preparing officers for responding to the problem of officer-involved domestic violence (OIDV) perpetrated by colleagues.

### 4.7.3 Principal Conclusions

Against the background of a highly influential research project, the MDVE, numerous other studies were conducted to evaluate the possible impact of arrest in reducing DA/IPV. Some of these did show beneficial results. However, research carried out over the last 15 years suggests that other than in situations where officers judge it as necessary, there is little convincing evidence that arrest in itself is an effective action to employ as a routine practice in deterring DA/IPV. Results of research on its effects are mixed. Arrest of both partners in a domestic dispute (dual arrest) is ineffective, and, given the preponderance of male perpetrators, it has resulted in inappropriate detention of many women. A study of police forces in North East England found that women were arrested to a disproportionate degree given the smaller number of incidents in which they were perpetrators (Hester, 2013). Some authors have questioned in general whether deterrence policies are likely to have much success with this problem (Sloan et al., 2013). On the other hand, there is tentative evidence that victims reporting to police may be effective, and that processes which increase actual or potential victims' confidence in police and empower them in making contacts may also increase their willingness to report assaults.

There is tentative evidence that arrest of some suspected IPV perpetrators may have an impact in reducing subsequent repeat offending, as a function of risk levels and previous patterns of DA and other types of offending. This raises the prospect of attempting to identify those factors and test the feasibility of such action. However, this may not be applicable to new calls for assistance, only to second and subsequent calls.

The strongest evidence regarding other initiatives first supports the use of specialized police DVUs that include a mixture of personnel. Although the total volume of work on this remains limited, the findings suggest they are perceived positively by victims and can have a significant impact in reducing repeat DA/IPV offending. The roles of the specialized DVUs that have been found to be effective include a combination of more intensive investigation, provision of victim support and preparation of case material to improve possibilities of successful prosecution. There are encouraging results from a recently published evaluation of a second responder intervention in which officers or advocates make return visits to couples within a pre-arranged time period, and this can be incorporated in the work of DVUs.

Second, mainly positive outcomes are associated with the establishment of police stations staffed largely, if not completely, by women officers. Based on the findings summarized in Table 4.5, this is associated with some very encouraging outcomes concerning IPV and other violence towards women. There are different models of implementing this with the most favourable being one where other professional groups work alongside police.

Amongst the conclusions reached by Dowling et al. (2018) in their wide-ranging review of research on policing and IPV was one to the effect that "it is wrong to assume that mandating an increase in the use of a particular police response (e.g., pro-arrest and pro-charge policies) will inevitably have desirable flow-on effects on subsequent police and criminal justice activities" (p. 76). That is, almost any method the police can employ has varying effects dependent on different types of cases.

One another level, based on previous reviews, there is provisional evidence of the usefulness of long-term developmental prevention of DA/IPV through the introduction of awareness or training sessions for secondary school students, and involvement of police in such an initiative would lend weight and credibility to its inception. This work was carried out in North America and has not been evaluated in England and Wales, and a proper evaluation of it would require lengthy timescales. It is however a plausible prospect for innovation in multi-agency working.

Results from the review of treatment interventions present, overall, a more positive pattern of positive effects that has been suggested in previous research reviews. Further work is necessary to analyse some of the detailed patterns within this. Caution is still required given that some of the seemingly largest effects come from the least well-designed studies, and some apparent changes in the short term (e.g. at the end of programmes) do not endure at follow-up.

The results of several treatment evaluation studies suggest there are sub-groups or separate patterns or trajectories of offending amongst those who perpetrate DA/IPV offences. Individuals vary by risk level but also by typology in terms of the type of violence in which they engage in partner relationships, often reflecting other aspects of criminal histories such as their involvement in non-partner violence or in substance misuse. These findings potentially highlight the need for a differentiated approach to offender management, which in turn would influence allocation to intervention programmes and specified levels of contact and monitoring.

The findings reported here did play a part in further research that the relevant police forces subsequently commissioned and were certainly cited in a number of internal documents. In the period following, plans were formulated for conducting controlled experimental trials or quasi-experimental evaluations of police-led IPV interventions. On a much larger canvas, this has parallels in a number of other contexts, within countries with only limited traditions of conducing and reporting research of this kind. Examples of studies where protocols have been prepared and research is underway at the time of writing include projects based in Bangladesh (Mamun et al., 2018), Ethiopia (Semahegn et al., 2017), Ghana (Addo-Lartey et al., 2019), Nepal (Clark et al., 2017) and South Africa (Christofides et al., 2018).

## References

Abramsky, T., Watts, C. H., Garcia-Moreno, C., Devries, K., Kiss, L., Ellsberg, M., Henrica, A. F. M., & Heise, L. (2011). What factors are associated with recent intimate partner violence? Findings from the WHO multi-country study on women's health and domestic violence. *BMC Public Health, 11*, 109.

Addo-Lartey, A., Alangea, D. O., Sikweyiya, Y., Chirwa, E. D., Coker-Appiah, D., Jewkes, R., & Adanu, R. K. M. (2019). Rural response system to prevent violence against women: Methodology for a community randomised controlled trial in the central region of Ghana. *Global Health Action, 12*, 1612604. https://doi.org/10.1080/16549716.2019.1612604

Akoensi, T. D., Koehler, J. A., Lösel, F. A., & Humphreys, D. K. (2012). Domestic violence perpetrator programs in Europe, Part II: A systematic review of the state of evidence. *International Journal of Offender Therapy and Comparative Criminology, 57*, 1206–1225.

Aldarondo, E. (2010). Understanding the contribution of common interventions with men who batter to the reduction of re-assaults. *Juvenile and Family Court Journal, 61*, 87–101.

Alexander, P. C., Morris, E., Tracy, A., & Frye, A. (2010). Stages of change and the group treatment of batterers: A randomized clinical trial. *Violence and Victims, 25*, 571–587.

Alhabib, S., Nur, U., & Jones, R. (2010). Domestic violence against women: Systematic review of prevalence studies. *Journal of Family Violence, 25*, 369–382.

Ali, P. A., & Naylor, P. B. (2013a). Intimate partner violence: A narrative review of the biological and psychological explanations for its causation. *Aggression and Violent Behavior, 18*, 373–382.

Ali, P. A., & Naylor, P. B. (2013b). Intimate partner violence: A narrative review of the feminist, social and ecological explanations for its causation. *Aggression and Violent Behavior, 18*, 611–619.

Ali, P. A., Dhingra, K., & McGarry, J. (2016). A literature review of intimate partner violence and its classifications. *Aggression and Violent Behavior, 31*, 16–25.

Amaral, S., Bhalotra, S., & Prakash, N. (2019). *Gender, crime and punishment: Evidence from women police stations in India*. University of Essex: Research Report to the Economic and Social Research Council.

An, S., & Choi, Y. J. (2017). A review and assessment of intimate partner violence interventions and trainings for service providers and frontline staff. *Violence and Victims, 31*(3), 379–404.

Aos, S., Miller, M., & Drake, E. (2006). *Evidence-based adult corrections: What works and what does not*. Washington State Institute for Public Policy.

Arce, R., Arias, E., Novo, M., & Fariña, F. (2020). Are interventions with batterers effective? A meta-analytical review. *Psychosocial Intervention, 29*(3), 153–164.

Arias, E., Arce, R., & Vilariño, M. (2013). Batterer intervention programmes: A meta-analytic review of effectiveness. *Psychosocial Intervention, 22*, 153–160.

Armenti, N. A., & Babcock, J. C. (2016). Conjoint treatment for intimate partner violence: A systematic review and implications. *Couple and Family Psychology: Research and Practice, 5*(2), 109–123.

Ashburn, K., Kerner, B., Ojamuge, D., & Lundgren, R. (2017). Evaluation of the Responsible, Engaged, and Loving (REAL) fathers initiative on physical child punishment and intimate partner violence in Northern Uganda. *Prevention Science, 18*, 854–864.

Babcock, J. C., Green, C. E., & Robie, C. (2004). Does batterers' treatment work? A meta-analytic review of domestic violence treatment. *Clinical Psychology Review, 23*, 1023–1053.

Badenes-Ribera, L., Frias-Navarro, D., Bonilla-Campos, A., Pons-Salvador, G., & Monterde-i-Bort, H. (2015). Intimate partner violence in self-identified lesbians: A meta-analysis of its prevalence. *Sexuality Research and Social Policy, 12*, 47–59.

Barelds, D. P. H., & Dijkstra, P. (2005). Reactive, anxious and possessive forms of jealousy and their relation to relationship quality among heterosexuals and homosexuals. *Journal of Homosexuality, 51*, 183–198.

Barner, J. R., & Carney, M. M. (2011). Interventions for intimate partner violence: A historical review. *Journal of Family Violence, 26*, 235–244.

Bartholomew, K., Regan, K. V., Oran, D., & White, M. A. (2008). Correlates of partner abuse in male same-sex relationships. *Violence and Victims, 23*, 344–360.

Bates, E. A., & Douglas, E. M. (2020). Services for domestic violence victims in the United Kingdom and United States: Where are we today? *Partner Abuse, 11*(3), 350–382.

Beeble, M. L., Bybee, D., & Sullivan, C. M. (2007). Abusive men's use of children to control their partners and ex-partners. *European Psychologist, 12*, 54–61.

Belfrage, H., Strand, S., Storey, J. E., Gibas, A. L., Kropp, P. R., & Hart, S. D. (2012). Assessment and management of risk for intimate partner violence by police officers using the Spousal Assault Risk Assessment Guide. *Law and Human Behaviour, 36*, 60–67.

Bell, K. M., & Naugle, A. E. (2008). Intimate partner violence theoretical considerations: Moving towards a contextual framework. *Clinical Psychology Review, 28*, 1096–1107.

Bennett, L. W., Stoops, C., Call, C., & Flett, H. (2007). Program completion and re-arrest in a batterer intervention system. *Research on Social Work Practice, 17*, 42–54.

Beyer, K., Wallis, A. B., & Hamberger, L. K. (2015). Neighborhood environment and intimate partner violence: A systematic review. *Trauma, Violence, & Abuse, 16*, 16–47.

Birkley, E. L., & Eckhardt, C. I. (2015). Anger, hostility, internalizing negative emotions, and intimate partner violence perpetration: A meta-analytic review. *Clinical Psychology Review, 37*, 40–56.

Bloomfield, S., & Dixon, L. (2015). *An outcome evaluation of the Integrated Domestic Abuse Programme (IDAP) and Community Domestic Violence Programme (CDVP). Analytic summary*. London: National Offender Management Service.

Boira, S., del Castillo, M. F., Carbajosa, P., & Marcuello, C. (2013). Context of treatment and therapeutic alliance: Critical factors in court-mandated batterer intervention programs. *Spanish Journal of Psychology, 16*, 1–13.

Bourey, C., Willliams, W., Bernstein, E. E., & Stephenson, R. (2015). Systematic review of structural interventions for intimate partner violence in low- and middle-income countries: Organizing evidence for prevention. *BMC Public Health, 15*, 1165. https://doi.org/10.1186/s12889-015-2460-4

Bowen, E. (2010). Therapeutic environment in a U.K. domestic violence perpetrator program. *Small Group Research, 41*, 198–220.

Bowen, E. (2011a). An overview of partner violence risk assessment and the potential role of female victim risk appraisals. *Aggression and Violent Behavior, 16*, 214–226.

Bowen, E. (2011b). *The rehabilitation of partner violent men*. Wiley-Blackwell.

Bowen, E., Gilchrist, E., & Beech, A. R. (2005). An examination of the impact of community-based rehabilitation on the offending behaviour of male domestic violence offenders and the characteristics associated with recidivism. *Legal and Criminological Psychology, 10*, 189–209.

Bowen, E., Gilchrist, E., & Beech, A. R. (2008). Change in treatment has no relationship with subsequent re-offending in U.K. domestic violence sample. *International Journal of Offender Therapy and Comparative Criminology, 52*, 598–614.

Boxall, H., Rosevear, L., & Payne, J. (2015). Domestic violence typologies: What value to practice? *Trends and Issues*, No. 494. Canberra: Australian Institute of Criminology.

Braithwaite, S. R., & Fincham, F. D. (2014). Computer-based prevention of intimate partner violence in marriage. *Behaviour Research and Therapy, 54*, 12–21.

Broidy, L., Albright, D., & Denman, K. (2016). Deterring future incidents of intimate partner violence: Does type of formal intervention matter? *Violence Against Women, 22*(9), 1113–1133.

Buttell, F. P. (2002). Levels of moral reasoning among female domestic violence offenders: Evaluating the impact of treatment. *Research on Social Work Practice, 12*, 349–363.

Buttell, F. P., & Carney, M. M. (2004). A multidimensional assessment of a batterer treatment program: An alert to a problem? *Research on Social Work Practice, 14*, 93–101.

Cantos, A. L., & O'Leary, K. D. (2014). One size does not fit all in the treatment of intimate partner violence. *Partner Abuse, 5*, 204–236.

Capaldi, D. M., Knoble, N. B., Shortt, J. W., & Kim, H. K. (2012). A systematic review of risk factors for intimate partner violence. *Partner Abuse, 3*, 231–280.

Carney, M. M., & Buttell, F. P. (2004). A multidimensional evaluation of a treatment program for female batterers: A pilot study. *Research on Social Work Practice, 14*, 249–258.

Carrington, K. (2021). Women's police stations: Unique innovations from the Global South. In T. P. de Ávila, A. Yamamoto, C. E. de Faria, J. McCulloch, & K. Carrington (Eds.), *Reflections on Prevention policies for gender based violence against women and girls: Debates in Brazil and Australia* (pp. 109–116). United Nations Entity for Gender Equality and the Empowerment of Women (UN Women) & Public Prosecutor's Office of the Federal District of Brazil (MPDFT).

Carrington, K., Guala, N., Puyol, M. V., & Sozzo, M. (2020a). How women's police stations empower women, widen access to justice and prevent gender violence. *International Journal for Crime, Justice and Social Democracy, 9*(1), 42–67.

Carrington, K., Sozzo, M., Guala, N., & Puyol, M. V. (2020b). *How women's police stations prevent gender violence*. Queensland University of Technology, Centre for Justice Briefing Paper, Issue 2.

Carrington, K., Sozzo, M., & Ryan, V. (2020c). *What Australia can learn from women's police stations to prevent gender violence*. Queensland University of Technology, Centre for Justice Briefing Paper, Issue 6.

Cattaneo, L. B., & Goodman, L. A. (2005). Risk factors for reabuse in intimate partner violence: A cross-disciplinary critical review. *Trauma, Violence & Abuse, 6*, 141–175.

Cavanaugh, M. M., & Gelles, R. J. (2005). The utility of male domestic violence offender typologies: New directions for research, policy, and practice. *Journal of Interpersonal Violence, 20*, 155–166.

Cho, H., & Wilke, D. J. (2010). Gender differences in the nature of the intimate partner violence and effects of perpetrator arrest on revictimization. *Journal of Family Violence, 25*, 393–400.

Christofides, N. J., Hatcher, A. M., Pino, A., Rebombo, D., McBride, R. S., Anderson, A., & Peacock, D. (2018). A cluster randomised controlled trial to determine the effect of community mobilisation and advocacy on men's use of violence in Periurban South Africa: Study protocol. *BMJ Open, 8*, e017579.

Cissner, A. B., & Puffett, N. K. (2006). *Do batter program length or approach affect completion or re-arrest rates?* Center for Court Innovation.

Clark, C. J., Spencer, R. A., Shrestha, B., Ferguson, G., Oakes, J. M., & Gupta, J. (2017). Evaluating a multicomponent social behaviour change communication strategy to reduce intimate partner violence among married couples: Study protocol for a cluster randomized trial in Nepal. *BMC Public Health, 17*, 75. https://doi.org/10.1186/s12889-016-3909-9

Cluss, P., & Bodea, A. (2011). *The effectiveness of batterer intervention programs: A literature review & recommendations for next steps* (Abridged Version). Pittsburgh, PA: University of Pittsburgh and FISA Foundation.

Connors, A. D., Mills, J. F., & Gray, A. L. (2012). An evaluation of intimate partner violence intervention with incarcerated offenders. *Journal of Interpersonal Violence, 27*, 1176–1196.

Connors, A. D., Mills, J. F., & Gray, A. L. (2013). Intimate partner violence intervention for high-risk offenders. *Psychological Services, 10*, 12–23.

Corcoran, J., Stephenson, M., Perryman, D., & Allen, S. (2001). Perceptions and utilization of a police-social work crisis intervention approach to domestic violence. *Families in Society: The Journal of Contemporary Human Services, 82*, 393–398.

Corradi, C., & Stöckl, H. (2014). Intimate partner homicide in 10 European countries: Statistical data and policy development in a cross-national perspective. *European Journal of Criminology, 11*, 601–618.

Coulter, M., & VandeWeerd, C. (2009). Reducing domestic violence and other criminal recidivism: Effectiveness of a multilevel batterers intervention program. *Violence and Victims, 24*, 139–152.

Crane, C. A., & Eckhardt, C. I. (2013). Evaluation of a single-session brief motivational enhancement intervention for partner abusive men. *Journal of Counseling Psychology, 60*, 180–187.

Crockett, E. E., Keneski, E., Yeager, K., & Loving, T. J. (2015). Breaking the mold: Evaluating a non-punitive domestic violence intervention program. *Journal of Family Violence, 30*, 489–499.

Cunha, O. S., & Goncalves, R. A. (2015). Efficacy assessment of an intervention program with batterers. *Small Group Research, 46*, 455–482.

Dalton, B. (2007). What's going on out there? A survey of batterer intervention programs. *Journal of Aggression, Maltreatment & Trauma, 15*, 59–74.

Davis, R. C., Smith, B. E., & Rabbitt, C. R. (2001). Increasing convictions in domestic violence cases: A field test in Milwaukee. *Justice System Journal, 22*, 61–72.

Davis, R. C., Weisburd, D., & Hamilton, E. E. (2007). *Preventing repeat incidents of family violence: A randomized field test of a second responder program in Redlands, CA*. Document no. 219840. Washington, DC: National Institute of Justice.

Davis, R. C., Weisburd, D., & Taylor, B. (2008). Effects of second responder programs on repeat incidents of family abuse. *Campbell Systematic Reviews, 2008*, 15. https://doi.org/10.4073/csr.2008.15

Davis, R. C., Weisburd, D., & Hamilton, E. E. (2010). Preventing repeat incidents of family violence: A randomized field test of a second responder program. *Journal of Experimental Criminology, 6*, 397–418.

Day, A., Chung, D., O'Leary, P., & Carson, E. (2009). Programs for men who perpetrate domestic violence: An examination of the issues underlying the effectiveness of intervention programs. *Journal of Family Violence, 24*, 203–212.

Day, A., Chung, D., O'Leary, P., Justo, D., Moore, S., Carson, E., & Gerace, A. (2010). Integrated responses to domestic violence: Legally mandated intervention programs for male batterers. *Trends and Issues*, No. 404. Canberra: Australian Institute of Criminology.

De Koker, P., Mathews, C., Zuch, M., Bastien, S., & Mason-Jones, A. J. (2014). A systematic review of interventions for preventing adolescent intimate partner violence. *Journal of Adolescent Health, 54*, 3–13.

Devries, K., Watts, C., Yoshihama, M., Kiss, L., Schraiber, L. B., Deyessa, N., Heise, L., Durand, J., Mbwambo, J., Jansen, J., Berhane, Y., Ellsberg, M., Garcia-Moreno, C., & WHO Multi-Country Study Team. (2011). Violence against women is strongly associated with suicide attempts: Evidence from the WHO multi-country study on women's health and domestic violence against women. *Social Science and Medicine, 73*, 79–86.

Dichter, M. E., & Gelles, R. J. (2012). Women's perceptions of safety and risk following police intervention for intimate partner violence. *Violence Against Women, 18*, 44–63.

Dixon, L., & Browne, K. (2003). The heterogeneity of spouse abuse: A review. *Aggression and Violent Behavior, 8*, 107–130.

Dixon, L., & Graham-Kevan, N. (2011). Understanding the nature and etiology of intimate partner violence and implications for practice and policy. *Clinical Psychology Review, 31*, 1145–1155.

Dixon, L., Hamilton-Giachristis, C., & Browne, K. (2008). Classifying partner femicide. *Journal of Interpersonal Violence, 23*, 74–93.

Dobash, R. E., Dobash, R. P., Cavanagh, K., & Medina-Ariza, J. (2007). Lethal and nonlethal violence against an intimate female partner: Comparing male murderers to nonlethal abusers. *Violence Against Women, 13*, 329–353.

Dowling, C., Morgan, A., Boyd, C., & Voce, I. (2018). *Policing domestic violence: A review of the evidence*. AIC Research Report 13. Canberra: Australian Institute of Criminology.

Downes, J., Kelly, L., & Westmarland, N. (2019). "It's a work in progress": Men's accounts of gender and change in their use of coercive control. *Journal of Gender-Based Violence, 3*(3), 267–282.

Dunford, F. W. (2000). The San Diego navy experiment: An assessment of interventions for men who assault their wives. *Journal of Consulting and Clinical Psychology, 68*, 468–476.

Dutton, D. G., & Corvo, K. (2006). Transforming a flawed policy: A call to revive psychology and science in domestic violence research and practice. *Aggression and Violent Behavior, 11*, 457–483.

Dutton, D. G., & Corvo, K. (2007). The Duluth model: A data-impervious paradigm and a failed strategy. *Aggression and Violent Behavior, 12*, 658–667.

Easton, C., Swan, S., & Sinha, R. (2000). Motivation to change substance use among offenders of domestic violence. *Journal of Substance Abuse Treatment, 19*, 1–5.

Easton, C. J., Mandel, D. L., Hunkele, K. A., Nich, C., Rounsaville, B. J., & Carroll, K. M. (2007). A cognitive behavioral therapy for alcohol-dependent domestic violence offenders: An integrated substance abuse-domestic violence treatment approach (SADV). *American Journal on Addictions, 16*, 24–31.

Echauri, J. A., Fernández-Montalvo, J., Martínez, M., & Azkarate, J. M. (2013). Effectiveness of a treatment programme for immigrants who committed gender-based violence against their partners. *Psicothema, 25*, 49–54.

Echeburúa, E., Fernández-Montalvo, J., & Amor, P. J. (2006). Psychological treatment of men convicted of gender violence: A pilot study in Spanish prisons. *International Journal of Offender Therapy and Comparative Criminology, 50*, 57–70.

Eckhardt, C. I., Murphy, C. M., Black, D., & Suhr, L. (2006). Intervention programs for perpetrators of intimate partner violence: Conclusions from a clinical health perspective. *Public Health Reports, 121*, 369–381.

Eckhardt, C. I., Samper, R. E., & Murphy, C. M. (2008). Anger disturbances among perpetrators of intimate partner violence: Clinical characteristics and outcomes of court-mandated treatment. *Journal of Interpersonal Violence, 23*, 1600–1617.

Eckhardt, C. I., Murphy, C. M., Whitaker, D. J., Sprunger, J., Dykstra, R., & Woodward, K. (2013). The effectiveness of intervention programs for perpetrators and victims of intimate partner violence. *Partner Abuse, 4*, 196–231.

Esquivel-Santoveña, E. E., & Dixon, L. (2012). Investigating the true rate of physical intimate partner violence: A review of nationally representative surveys. *Aggression and Violent Behavior, 17*, 208–219.

Esquivel-Santoveña, E. E., Lambert, T. L., & Hamel, J. (2013). Partner abuse worldwide. *Partner Abuse, 4*, 6–75.

Exum, M. L., Hartman, J. L., Friday, P. C., & Lord, V. B. (2014). Policing domestic violence in the Post-SARP era: The impact of a Domestic Violence Police Unit. *Crime & Delinquency, 60*, 999–1032.

Feder, L., & Dugan, L. (2002). A test of the efficacy of court-mandated counselling for domestic violence offenders: The broward experiment. *Justice Quarterly, 19*, 343–375.

Feder, L., & Forde, D. R. (2000). *Test of the efficacy of court-mandated counselling for domestic violence offenders: The Broward experiment, Executive Summary*. Document No. 184631. Washington, DC: National Institute of Justice.

Feder, L., & Wilson, D. B. (2005). A meta-analytic review of court-mandated batterer intervention programs: Can courts affect abusers' behaviour? *Journal of Experimental Criminology, 1*, 239–262.

Feder, L., Wilson, D. B., & Austin. (2008). Court-mandated interventions for individuals convicted of domestic violence. *Campbell Systematic Reviews, 2008*, 12. https://doi.org/10.4073/csr.2008.12

Felson, R. B., & Lane, K. J. (2010). Does violence involving women and intimate partners have a special etiology? *Criminology, 48*, 321–338.

Felson, R. B., Ackerman, J. M., & Gallagher, C. A. (2005). Police intervention and the repeat of domestic assault. *Criminology, 43*, 563–588.

Fernández-Montalvo, J., Echuari, J. A., Azcarate, J. M., & Lopez-Goñi, J. J. (2015). Impact of a court-referred psychological treatment program for intimate partner batterer men with suspended sentences. *Violence and Victims, 30*, 3–15.

Foran, H. M., & O'Leary, K. D. (2008). Alcohol and intimate partner violence: A meta-analytic review. *Clinical Psychology Review, 28*, 1222–1234.

FRA (European Union Agency for Fundamental Rights). (2014). *Violence against women: An EU-wide survey: Main results*. Publications Office of the European Union.

Friday, P. C., Lord, V. B., Exul, M. L., & Hartman, J. L. (2006). *Evaluating the impact of a specialized Domestic Violence Police Unit*. Document No. 215916. Washington, DC: National Institute of Justice.

García-Moreno, C., Pallitto, C., Devries, K., Stöckl, H., Watts, C., & Abrahams, N. (2013). *Global and regional estimate of violence against women: Prevalence and health effects of intimate partner violence and non-partner sexual violence*. World Health Organization.

García-Moreno, C., Zimmerman, C., Morris-Gehring, A., Heise, L., Amin, A., Abrahams, N., Montoya, O., Bhate-Doesthali, P., Kilonzo, N., & Watts, C. (2015). Addressing violence against women: A call to action. *The Lancet, 385*, 1685–1695.

Garner, J. H., & Maxwell, C. D. (2000). What are the lessons of the police arrest studies? *Journal of Aggression, Maltreatment & Trauma, 4*, 83–114.

Garner, J. H., & Maxwell, C. D. (2011). *The crime control effects of criminal sanctions for intimate partner violence*. Document no. 236959. Washington DC: National Institute of Justice.

Garner, J., Fagan, J., & Maxwell, C. (1995). Published findings from the spouse assault replication program: A critical review. *Journal of Quantitative Criminology, 11*, 3–28.

Garside, R. (2006). Right for the wrong reasons: Making sense of criminal justice failure. In R. Garside & W. McMahon (Eds.), *Does criminal justice work? The 'right for the wrong reasons' debate* (pp. 9–39). Crime and Society Foundation.

Gerstenberger, C. B., & Williams, K. R. (2012). Gender and intimate partner violence: Does dual arrest reveal gender symmetry or asymmetry? *Journal of Interpersonal Violence, 20*, 1–18.

Gondolf, E. W. (2000). A 30-month follow-up of court-referred batterers in four cities. *International Journal of Offender Therapy and Comparative Criminology, 44*, 111–128.

Gondolf, E. W. (2007a). Culturally-focused batterer counselling for African-American men. *Criminology & Public Policy, 6*, 341–366.

Gondolf, E. W. (2007b). Theoretical and research support for the Duluth model: A reply to Dutton and Corvo. *Aggression and Violent Behaviour, 12*, 644–657.

Gondolf, E. W., & Jones, A. S. (2001). The program effect of batterer programs in three cities. *Violence and Victims, 16*, 693–704.

Goosey, J., Sherman, L., & Neyroud, P. (2017). Integrated case management of repeated intimate partner violence: A randomized, controlled trial. *Cambridge Journal of Evidence-Based Policing, 1*, 174–189.

Gordon, J. A., & Moriarty, L. J. (2003). The effects of domestic violence batterer treatment on domestic violence recidivism: The Chesterfield County experience. *Criminal Justice and Behavior, 30*, 118–134.

Gracia, E., Lila, M., & Santirso, F. A. (2020). Attitudes toward intimate partner violence against women in the European Union. *European Psychologist, 25*(2), 104–121.

Groves, N., & Thomas, T. (2014). *Domestic violence and criminal justice*. Routledge.

Hamilton, L., Koehler, J. A., & Lösel, F. A. (2012). Domestic violence perpetrator programs in Europe, Part I: A survey of current practice. *International Journal of Offender Therapy and Comparative Criminology, 57*, 1189–1205.

Hatcher, A. M., McBride, R.-S., Rebombo, D., Munshi, S., Khumalo, M., & Christofides, N. (2020). Process evaluation of a community mobilization intervention for preventing men's partner violence use in peri-urban South Africa. *Evaluation and Program Planning, 78*, 101727. https://doi.org/10.1016/j.evalprogplan.2019.101727

Heise, L. L. (1998). Violence against women: An integrated, ecological framework. *Violence Against Women, 4*, 262–290.

Hendricks, B., Werner, T., Shipway, L., & Turinetti, G. J. (2006). Recidivism among spousal abusers: Predictions and program evaluation. *Journal of Interpersonal Violence, 21*, 703–716.

Henwood, K. S., Chou, S., & Browne, K. D. (2015). A systematic review and meta-analysis on the effectiveness of CBT informed anger management. *Aggression and Violent Behavior, 25*, 280–292.

Her Majesty's Inspectorate of Constabulary. (2015). *Increasingly everyone's business: A progress report on the police response to domestic abuse*. HMIC.

Herman, K., Rotunda, R., Williamson, G., & Vodanovich, S. (2014). Outcomes from a Duluth Model batterer intervention program at completion and long term follow-up. *Journal of Offender Rehabilitation, 53*, 1–18.

Herrero, J., Torres, A., Fernández-Suárez, A., & Rodríguez-Díaz, F. J. (2016). Generalists versus specialists: Toward a typology of batterers in prison. *The European Journal of Psychology Applied to Legal Context, 8*, 19–26.

Hester, M. (2013). Who does what to whom? Gender and domestic violence perpetrators in English police records. *European Journal of Criminology, 10*, 623–637.

Hester, M., Eisenstadt, N., Ortega-Avila, A., Morgan, K., Walker, S., & Bell, J. (2019). *Evaluation of the drive project: A three-year pilot to address high-risk, high-harm perpetrators of domestic abuse*. Unpublished Report. University of Bristol.

Hilton, N. Z., & Harris, G. T. (2005). Predicting wife assault: A critical review and implications for policy and practice. *Trauma, Violence & Abuse, 6*, 3–23.
Hilton, N. Z., Harris, G. T., & Rice, M. E. (2007). The effect of arrest on wife assault recidivism: Controlling for pre-arrest risk. *Criminal Justice and Behavior, 34*, 1334–1344.
Hirschel, D. (2008). *Domestic violence cases: What research shows about arrest and dual arrest rates*. U.S. Dept. of Justice, Office of Justice Programs, National Institute of Justice.
Hungerford, A., Wait, S. K., Fritz, A. M., & Clements, C. M. (2012). Exposure to intimate partner violence and children's psychological adjustment, cognitive functioning, and social competence: A review. *Aggression and Violent Behavior, 17*, 373–382.
Huss, M. T., & Ralston, A. (2008). Do batterer subtypes actually matter? Treatment completion, treatment response, and recidivism across a batterer typology. *Criminal Justice and Behavior, 35*, 710–724.
Jassal, N. (2020). Gender, law enforcement, and access to justice: Evidence from all-women police stations in India. *American Political Science Review, 114*(4), 1035–1054.
Jewell, L. M., & Wormith, J. S. (2010). Variables associated with attrition from domestic violence treatment programs targeting male batterers: A meta-analysis. *Criminal Justice and Behavior, 37*, 1086–1113.
Johnson, M. P. (2008). *A typology of domestic violence: Intimate terrorism, violent resistance, and situational couple violence*. Northeastern University Press.
Johnson, R. R. (2011). Predicting officer physical assaults at domestic assault calls. *Journal of Family Violence, 26*, 163–169.
Johnson, R. R., & Goodlin-Fahncke, W. (2015). Exploring the effect of arrest across a domestic batterer typology. *Juvenile and Family Court Journal, 66*, 15–30.
Jolliffe, D., & Farrington, D. P. (2007). *A systematic review of the national and international evidence on the effectiveness of interventions with violent offenders*. Ministry of Justice Research Series 16/07. London: Ministry of Justice, Research Development Statistics.
Jones, A. S., & Gondolf, E. W. (2002). Assessing the effect of batterer program completion on reassault: An instrumental variables analysis. *Journal of Quantitative Criminology, 18*, 71–98.
Kalaga, H., & Kingston, P. (2007). *A review of literature on effective interventions that prevent and respond to harm against adults*. Scottish Government Social Research.
Kavanaugh, G. E., Sviatschi, M. M., & Trako, I. (2017). *Inter-generational benefits of improving access to justice for women: Evidence from Peru*. Working paper, SSRN Electronic Journal. http://conference.iza.org/conference_files/Gender_2018/sviatschi_m23512.pdf
Kelly, L., & Westmarland, N. (2015). *Domestic violence perpetrator programmes: Steps towards change. Project Mirabal final report*. London Metropolitan University and Durham University.
Kiss, L., Schraiber, L. B., Heise, L., Zimmerman, C., Gouveia, N., & Watts, C. (2012). Gender-based violence and socioeconomic inequalities: Does living in deprived neighbourhoods increase women's risk of intimate partner violence? *Social Science and Medicine, 74*, 1172–1179.
Kistenmacher, B. R., & Weiss, R. L. (2008). Motivational interviewing as a mechanism for change in men who batter: A randomized controlled trial. *Violence and Victims, 23*, 558–570.
Klein, A. R., & Tobin, T. (2008). A longitudinal study of arrested batterers, 1995–2005. *Violence Against Women, 14*, 136–157.
Labriola, M., Rempel, M., & Davis, R. C. (2005). *Testing the effectiveness of batterer programs and judicial monitoring: Results from a randomized trial at the Bronx Misdemeanor Domestic Violence Court*. Center for Court Innovation.
Labriola, M., Rempel, M., O'Sullivan, C. S., & Frank, P. B. (2010). *Court responses to batterer program noncompliance: A national perspective*. Center for Court Innovation.
Langenderfer, L. (2013). Alcohol use among partner violent adults: Reviewing recent literature to inform intervention. *Aggression and Violent Behavior, 18*, 152–158.
Langhinrichsen-Rohling, J., Misra, T. A., Selwyn, C., & Rohling, M. L. (2012). Rates of bidirectional versus unidirectional intimate partner violence across samples, sexual orientations, and race/ethnicities: A comprehensive review. *Partner Abuse, 3*, 199–230.

Larsen, S. E., & Hamberger, L. K. (2015). Men's and women's experience of IPV part II: A review of new developments in comparative studies of clinical populations. *Journal of Family Violence, 30*, 1007–1030.

Lawson, D. M. (2010). Comparing cognitive behavioural therapy and integrated cognitive behavioural therapy/psychodynamic therapy in group treatment for partner violent men. *Psychotherapy: Theory, Research, Practice, Training, 47*, 122–133.

Lee, M. Y., Uken, A., & Sebold, J. (2004). Accountability for change: Solution-focused treatment with domestic violence offenders. *Families in Society, 85*, 463–476.

Levesque, D. A., Ciavatta, M. M., Castle, P. H., Prochaska, J. M., & Prochaska, J. O. (2012). Evaluation of a stage-based, computer-tailored adjunct to usual care for domestic violence offenders. *Psychology of Violence, 2*, 368–384.

Lila, M., Oliver, A., Galiana, L., & Gracia, E. (2013). Predicting success indicators of an intervention programme for convicted intimate-partner violence offenders: The Contexto programme. *The European Journal of Psychology Applied to Legal Context, 5*, 73–95.

Lilley-Walker, S.-J., Hester, M., & Turner, W. (2018). Evaluation of European domestic violence perpetrator programmes: Toward a model for designing and reporting evaluations related to perpetrator treatment intervention. *International Journal of Offender Therapy and Comparative Criminology, 62*(4), 868–884.

Lin, S.-C., Su, C.-Y., Chou, F. H.-C., Chen, S.-P., Huang, J.-J., Wu, G. T.-E., Chao, S.-S., & Chen, C.-C. (2009). Domestic violence recidivism in high-risk Taiwanese offenders after the completion of violence treatment programs. *Journal of Forensic Psychiatry & Psychology, 20*, 458–472.

Lyon, E. (2005). *Impact evaluation of special session domestic violence: Enhanced advocacy and interventions (Final Report Summary)*. National Institute of Justice.

MacLeod, D., Pi, R., Smith, D., & Rose-Goodwin, L. (2010). *Batterer intervention systems in California: An evaluation*. Judicial Council of California.

MacMillan, H. L., & Wathen, C. N. with the Canadian Task Force on Preventive Health Care (2001). *Prevention and treatment of violence against women: Systematic review & recommendations*. CTFPHC Technical Report #01-4. London, ON: Canadian Task Force.

Mamun, M. A., Parvin, K., Yu, M., Wan, J., Willan, S., Gibbs, A., Jewkes, R., & Naved, R. T. (2018). The HERrespect intervention to address violence against female garment workers in Bangladesh: Study protocol for a quasi-experimental trial. *BMC Public Health, 18*, 512. https://doi.org/10.1186/s12889-018-5442-5

Maxwell, C. D., & Garner, J. H. (2012). The crime control effects of criminal sanctions for intimate partner violence. *Partner Abuse, 3*, 469–500.

Maxwell, C. D., Garner, J. H., & Fagan, J. A. (2002). The preventive effects of arrest on intimate partner violence: Research, policy and theory. *Criminology & Public Policy, 2*, 51–80.

Maxwell, C. D., Davis, R. C., & Taylor, B. G. (2010). The impact of length of domestic violence treatment on the patterns of subsequent intimate partner violence. *Journal of Experimental Criminology, 6*, 475–497.

McCollum, E. E., & Stith, S. M. (2008). Couples treatment for interpersonal violence: A review of outcome research literature and current clinical practices. *Violence and Victims, 23*, 187–201.

McGuire, J. (2008). A review of effective interventions for reducing aggression and violence. *Philosophical Transactions of the Royal Society B, 363*, 2577–2597.

McGuire, J., & Duff, S. (2018). *Forensic psychology: Routes through the system*. Palgrave Macmillan.

McMurran, M., & Gilchrist, E. (2008). Anger control and alcohol use: Appropriate interventions for domestic violence? *Psychology, Crime, and Law, 14*, 107–116.

Mears, D. P., Carlson, M. J., Holden, G. W., & Harris, S. D. (2001). Reducing domestic violence revictimization: The effects of individual and contextual factors and type of legal intervention. *Journal of Interpersonal Violence, 16*, 1260–1283.

Mennicke, A. M., & Ropes, K. (2016). Estimating the rate of domestic violence perpetrated by law enforcement officers: A review of methods and estimates. *Aggression and Violent Behavior, 31*, 157–164.

Mennicke, A. M., Tripodi, S. J., Veh, C. A., Wilke, D. J., & Kennedy, S. C. (2015). Assessing attitude and reincarceration outcomes associated with in-prison domestic violence treatment program completion. *Journal of Offender Rehabilitation, 54*, 465–485.

Messing, J. T., Campbell, J. C., Ward-Lasher, A., Brown, S., Patchell, B., & Wilson, J. S. (2016). The lethality assessment program: Which survivors of intimate partner violence are most likely to participate? *Policing: An International Journal of Police Strategies & Management, 39*(1), 64–77.

Millbank, S., Riches, M., & Prior, B. (2000). *Reducing repeat victimisation of domestic violence: The NDV Project*. Paper presented at the conference reducing "Criminality: Partnerships and Best Practice". Ministry of Justice, Western Australia.

Miller, J. (2003). An arresting experiment: Domestic violence victim experience and perceptions. *Journal of Interpersonal Violence, 18*, 695–716.

Miller, A. R., & Segal, C. (2019). Do female officers improve law enforcement quality? Effects on crime reporting and domestic violence. *Review of Economic Studies, 86*, 2220–2247.

Miller, M., Drake, E., & Nafziger, M. (2013a). *What works to reduce recidivism by domestic violence offenders?* (Document No. 13-01-1201). Olympia, WA: Washington State Institute for Public Policy.

Miller, E., Tancredi, D. J., McCauley, H. L., Decker, M. R., Virata, M. C. D., Anderson, H. A., O'Connor, B., & Silverman, J. G. (2013b). One-year follow-up of a coach-delivered dating violence prevention program: A cluster randomized controlled trial. *American Journal of Preventive Medicine, 45*(1), 108–112.

Mills, L. G., Barocas, B., & Ariel, B. (2013). The next generation of court-mandated domestic violence treatment: A comparison study of batterer intervention and restorative justice programs. *Journal of Experimental Criminology, 9*, 65–90.

Moore, T. M., Stuart, G. L., Meehan, J. C., Rhatigan, D. L., Hellmuth, J. C., & Keen, S. M. (2008). Drug abuse and aggression between intimate partners: A meta-analytic review. *Clinical Psychology Review, 28*, 247–274.

Morrel, T. M., Elliott, J. D., Murphy, C. M., & Taft, C. T. (2003). Cognitive behavioural and supportive group treatments for partner-violent men. *Behavior Therapy, 34*, 77–95.

Morrow, W. J., Katz, C. M., & Choate, D. E. (2016). Assessing the impact of police body-worn cameras on arresting, prosecuting, and convicting suspects of intimate partner violence. *Police Quarterly, 19*(3), 303–325.

Muftić, L. R., & Bouffard, J. A. (2007). An evaluation of gender differences in the implementation and impact of a comprehensive approach to domestic violence. *Violence Against Women, 13*, 46–69.

Muñoz-Fernández, N., Ortega-Rivera, J., Nocentini, A., Menesini, E., & Sánchez-Jiménez, V. (2019). The efficacy of the "Dat-e Adolescence" prevention program in the reduction of dating violence and bullying. *International Journal of Environmental Research and Public Health, 16*, 408. https://doi.org/10.3390/ijerph16030408

Musser, P. H., Semiatin, J. N., Taft, C. T., & Murphy, C. M. (2008). Motivational interviewing as a pregroup intervention for partner-violent men. *Violence and Victims, 23*, 539–557.

Natarajan, M. (2005). Women police stations as a dispute processing system: The Tamil Nadu experience in dealing with dowry-related domestic violence. *Women and Criminal Justice, 16*(1/2), 87–106.

Natarajan, M. (2016). Police response to domestic violence: A case study of TecSOS mobile phone use in the London Metropolitan Police Service. *Policing, 10*(4), 378–390.

Nesset, M. B., Lara-Cabrera, M. L., Dalsbø, T. K., Pederson, S. A., Bjørngaard, J. H., & Palmstiema, T. (2019). Cognitive behavioural group therapy for male perpetrators of intimate partner violence: A systematic review. *BMC Psychiatry, 19*(11). https://doi.org/10.1186/s12888-019-2020-1

Niolon, P. H., Taylor, B. G., Latzman, N. E., Vivolo-Kantor, A. M., Valle, L. A., & Tharp, A. T. (2016). Lessons learned in evaluating a multisite, comprehensive teen dating violence prevention strategy: Design and challenges of the evaluation of dating matters: Strategies to promote healthy teen relationships. *Psychology of Violence, 6*, 452. https://doi.org/10.1037/vio0000043

Niolon, P. H., Vivolo-Kantor, A. M., Tracy, A. J., Latzman, N. E., Little, T. D., DeGue, S., Lang, K. M., Estefan, L. F., Ghazarian, S. R., McIntosh, W. L. K., Taylor, B., Johnson, L. L., Kuoh, H., Burton, B., Fortson, B., Mumford, E. A., Nelson, S. C., Joseph, H., Valle, L. A., & Tharp, A. T. (2019). An RCT of dating matters: Effects on teen dating violence and relationship behaviors. *American Journal of Preventive Medicine, 57*(1), 13–23.

Norlander, B., & Eckhardt, C. (2005). Anger, hostility, and male perpetrators of intimate partner violence: A meta-analytic review. *Clinical Psychology Review, 25*, 119–152.

Novo, M., Fariña, F., Seijo, M. D., & Arce, R. (2012). Assessment of a community rehabilitation programme in convicted male intimate-partner violence offenders. *International Journal of Clinical and Health Psychology, 12*, 219–234.

O'Farrell, T. J., Murphy, C. M., Stephan, S. H., Fals-Stewart, W., & Murphy, M. (2004). Partner violence before and after couples-based alcoholism treatment for male alcoholic patients: The role of treatment involvement and abstinence. *Journal of Consulting and Clinical Psychology, 72*, 202–217.

Oehme, K., Prost, S. G., & Saunders, D. G. (2016). Police responses to cases of officer-involved domestic violence: The effects of a brief web-based training. *Policing, 10*(4), 391–407.

Office for National Statistics (ONS). (2016a). *Chapter 4 – Intimate personal violence and partner abuse*. Statistical Bulletin. London: Office for National Statistics.

Office for National Statistics (ONS). (2016b). *Experimental Statistics 2: Domestic abuse offences recorded by the police, April to September 2015*. Statistical Bulletin. London: Office for National Statistics.

Okeke-Ihejirika, P., Salami, B., & Amodu, O. (2019). Exploring intimate partner violence from the perspective of African men: A meta-synthesis. *Aggression and Violent Behavior, 36*, 98–108.

Oram, S., Trevillion, K., Feder, G., & Howard, L. M. (2013). Prevalence of experiences of domestic violence among psychiatric patients: Systematic review. *British Journal of Psychiatry, 202*, 94–99.

Orr, D. (2016). 'Challenging the mindset of potential domestic abusers could save lives'. *The Guardian*, 17th February.

Pascual-Leone, A., Bierman, R., Arnold, R., & Stasiak, E. (2011). Emotion-focused therapy for incarcerated offenders of intimate partner violence: A 3-year outcome using a new whole-sample matching method. *Psychotherapy Research, 21*, 331–347.

Peitzmeier, S. M., Malik, M., Kattari, S. K., Marrow, E., Stephenson, R., Agénor, M., & Reisner, S. L. (2020). Intimate partner violence in transgender populations: Systematic review and meta-analysis of prevalence and correlates. *American Journal of Public Health, 110*, e1–e14. https://doi.org/10.2105/AJPH.2020.305774

Perova, E., & Reynolds, S. A. (2017). Women's police stations and intimate partner violence: Evidence from Brazil. *Social Science & Medicine, 174*, 188–196.

Piquero, A. R., Brame, R. Fagan, J., & Moffitt, T. E. (2005). *Assessing the offending activity of criminal domestic violence suspects: Offense specialization, escalation, and de-escalation evidence from the Spousal Assault Replication Program*. Document No. 212298. Washington, DC: National Institute of Justice.

Piquero, A. R., Brame, R., Fagan, J. A., & Moffitt, T. E. (2006). Assessing the offending activity of criminal domestic violence suspects: Offense specialization, escalation, and de-escalation evidence from the Spouse Assault Replication Program. *Public Health Reports, 121*, 409–418.

Piquero, A. R., Jennings, W. G., & Farrington, D. P. (2009). *Effectiveness of programs designed to improve self-control*. Swedish National Council for Crime Prevention (Brå).

Pitts, W. J., Givens, E., & McNeeley, S. (2009). The need for a holistic approach to specialized domestic violence court programming: Evaluating offender rehabilitation needs and recidivism. *Juvenile and Family Court Journal, 60*, 1–21.

Post, L. A., Klevens, J., Maxwell, C. D., Shelley, G. A., & Ingram, E. (2009). An examination of whether coordinated community responses affect intimate partner violence. *Journal of Interpersonal Violence, 25*, 75–93.

Prenzler, T., & Sinclair, G. (2013). The status of women police officers: An international review. *International Journal of Law, Crime and Justice, 41*(2), 115–131. https://doi.org/10.1016/j.ijlcj.2012.12.001

Rivas, C., Ramsay, J., Sadowski, L., Davidson, L. L., Dunne, D., Eldridge, S., Hegarty, K., Taft, A., & Feder, G. (2016). Advocacy interventions to reduce or eliminate violence and promote the physical and psychosocial well-being of women who experience intimate partner abuse. *Campbell Systematic Reviews, 2016*, 2. https://doi.org/10.4073/csr.2016.2

Rosenbaum, A., Gearan, P. J., & Ondoci, C. (2001). Completion and recidivism among court- and self-referred batterers in a psychoeducational group treatment program. *Journal of Aggression, Maltreatment & Trauma, 5*, 199–220.

Salazar, L. F., Emshoff, J. G., Baker, C. K., & Crowley, T. (2007). Examining the behaviour of a system: An outcome evaluation of a coordinated community response to domestic violence. *Journal of Family Violence, 22*, 631–641.

Santirso, F. A., Gilchrist, G., Lila, M., & Gracia, E. (2020). Motivational strategies in interventions for intimate partner violence offenders: A systematic review and meta-analysis of randomized controlled trials. *Psychosocial Intervention, 29*(3), 175–190.

Sartin, R. M., Hansen, D. J., & Huss, M. T. (2006). Domestic violence treatment response and recidivism: A review and implications for the study of family violence. *Aggression and Violent Behavior, 11*, 425–440.

Saunders, D. G. (2008). Group interventions for men who batter: A summary of program descriptions and research. *Violence and Victims, 23*, 156–172.

Schucan-Bird, K., Vigurs, C., Gough, D., & Quy, K. (undated). *Criminal justice interventions with perpetrators or victims of domestic violence: A systematic map of the empirical literature*. What works: Crime reduction review series, no. 3. University of London, Institute of Education, Evidence for Policy and Practice, Information and Coordinating Centre.

Scott, M. C., & Easton, C. J. (2010). Racial differences in treatment effect among men in a substance abuse and domestic violence program. *American Journal of Drug and Alcohol Abuse, 36*, 357–362.

Scott, K., Heslop, L., Kelly, T., & Wiggins, K. (2015). Intervening to prevent repeat offending among moderate- to high-risk domestic violence offenders: A second-responder program for men. *International Journal of Offender Therapy and Comparative Criminology, 59*, 273–294.

Semahegn, A., Torpey, K., Manu, A., Assefa, N., & Ankomah, A. (2017). Community based intervention to prevent domestic violence against women in the reproductive age in Northwestern Ethiopia: A protocol for quasi-experimental study. *Reproductive Health, 14*, 155. https://doi.org/10.1186/s12978-017-0414-2

Semahegn, A., Torpey, K., Manu, A., Assefa, N., Tesfaye, G., & Ankomah, A. (2019). Are interventions focused on gender-norms effective in preventing domestic violence against women in low and lower-middle income countries? A systematic review and meta-analysis. *Reproductive Health, 16*, 93. https://doi.org/10.1186/s12978-019-0726-5

Sharps, P. W., Bullock, L. F., Campbell, J. C., Alhusenm, J. L., Ghazarian, S. R., Bhandari, S. S., & Schminkey, D. L. (2016). Domestic violence enhanced perinatal home visits: The DOVE randomized clinical trial. *Journal of Women's Health, 25*(11), 1129–1138.

Sheehan, K. A., Thakor, S., & Stewart, D. E. (2012). Turning points for perpetrators of intimate partner violence. *Trauma, Violence, & Abuse, 13*, 30–40.

Sherman, L. W., & Berk, R. A. (1984). The specific deterrent effects of arrest for domestic assault. *American Sociological Review, 49*, 261–272.

Sherman, L. W., & Harris, H. M. (2015). Increased death rates of domestic violence victims from arresting vs. warning suspects in the Milwaukee Domestic Violence Experiment (MilDVE). *Journal of Experimental Criminology, 11*, 1–20.

Siddique, Z. (2013). Partially identified treatment effects under imperfect compliance: The case of domestic violence. *Journal of the American Statistical Association, 108*, 504–513.

Slaght, E., & Hamilton, N. (2005). A coordinated response to intimate partner violence: Lessons from an exploratory study. *Journal of Community Practice, 13*, 45–59.

Sloan, F. A., Platt, A. C., Chepke, L. M., & Blevins, C. E. (2013). Deterring domestic violence: Do criminal sanctions reduce repeat offenses? *Journal of Risk and Uncertainty, 46*, 51–80.

Smedslund, G., Dalsbø, T. K., Steiro, A., Winsvold, A., & Clench-Aas, J. (2011). Cognitive behavioural therapy for men who physical abuse their female partner. *Cochrane Database of Systematic Reviews*, (2), CD006048. https://doi.org/10.1002/14651858.CD006048.pub2

Stare, B. G., & Fernando, D. M. (2014). Intimate partner violence typology and treatment: A brief literature review. *The Family Journal: Counseling and Therapy for Couples and Families, 22*, 298–303.

Stewart, L. A., Flight, J., & Slavin-Stewart, C. (2013). Applying effective corrections principles (RNR) to partner abuse interventions. *Partner Abuse, 4*, 494–534.

Stewart, L. A., Gabora, N., Kropp, P. R., & Lee, Z. (2014). Effectiveness of risks-needs-responsibility-based family violence programs with male offenders. *Journal of Family Violence, 29*, 151–164.

Stith, S. M., Rosen, K. H., & McCollum, E. E. (2003). Effectiveness of couples treatment for spouse abuse. *Journal of Marital and Family Therapy, 29*, 407–426.

Stith, S. M., Rosen, K. H., McCollum, E. E., & Thomsen, C. J. (2004). Treating intimate partner violence within intact couple relationships: Outcomes of multi-couple versus individual couple therapy. *Journal of Marital and Family Therapy, 30*, 305–318.

Stöckl, H., Devries, K., Rotstein, A., Abrahams, N., Campbell, J., Watts, C., & García-Moreno, C. (2013). The global prevalence of intimate partner homicide: A systematic review. *Lancet, 382*, 859–865.

Storey, J. E., Kropp, P. R., Hart, S. D., Belfrage, H., & Strand, S. (2013). Assessment and management of risk for intimate partner violence by police officers using the Brief Spousal Assault Form for the Evaluation of Risk. *Criminal Justice and Behavior, 41*, 256–271.

Stover, C. S. (2012). Police-advocacy partnerships in response to domestic violence. *Journal of Police Crisis Negotiations, 12*, 183–198.

Stover, C. S., Rainey, A. M., Berkman, M., & Marans, S. (2008). Factors associated with engagement in a police-advocacy home-visit intervention to prevent domestic violence. *Violence Against Women, 14*, 1430–1450.

Stover, C. S., Meadows, A. M., & Kaufman, J. (2009a). Interventions for intimate partner violence: Review and implications for evidence-based practice. *Professional Psychology: Research and Practice, 40*, 223–233.

Stover, C. S., Poole, G., & Marans, S. (2009b). The domestic violence home-visit intervention: Impact on police-reported incidents of repeat violence over 12 months. *Violence and Victims, 24*, 591–606.

Stover, C. S., Berkman, M., Desai, R., & Marans, S. (2010). The efficacy of police-advocacy intervention for victims of domestic violence: 12 month follow-up data. *Violence Against Women, 16*, 410–425.

Strang, H., Sherman, L., Ariel, B., Chilton, S., Braddock, R., Rowlinson, T., Cornelius, N., Jarman, R., & Weinborn, C. (2017). Reducing the harm of intimate partner violence: Randomized controlled trial of the Hampshire Constabulary CARA Experiment. *Cambridge Journal of Evidence-Based Policing, 1*, 160–173.

Straus, M. A. (2008). Dominance and symmetry in partner violence by male and female university students in 32 nations. *Children and Youth Services Review, 30*, 252–275.

Straus, M. A. (2010). Thirty years of denying the evidence on gender symmetry in partner violence: Implications for prevention and treatment. *Partner Abuse, 1*, 332–362.

Straus, M. A. (2014). Addressing violence by female partners is vital to prevent or stop violence against women: Evidence from the Multisite Batterer Intervention Programme. *Violence Against Women, 20*, 889–899.

Stuart, G. L., Temple, J. R., & Moore, T. M. (2007). Improving batterer intervention programs through theory-based research. *Journal of the American Medical Association, 298*, 560–562.

Subirana-Malaret, M., Gahagan, J., & Parker, R. (2019). Intersectionality and sex and gender-based analyses as promising approaches in addressing intimate partner violence treatment programs among LGBT couples: A scoping review. *Cogent Social Sciences, 5*, 1644982. https://doi.org/10.1080/23311886.2019.1644982

Sugarman, D. B., & Boney-McCoy, S. (2000). Research synthesis in family violence: The art of reviewing research. *Journal of Aggression, Maltreatment & Trauma, 4*, 55–82.

Svalin, K., & Levander, S. (2020). The predictive validity of intimate partner violence risk assessments conducted by practitioners in different settings—a review of the literature. *Journal of Police and Criminal Psychology, 35*, 115–130.

Taylor, B. G., & Maxwell, C. D. (2009). *The effects of a short-term batterer treatment program for detained arrestees: A randomized experiment in the Sacramento County, California jail.* Document No. 228275. Washington, DC: National Institute of Justice.

Taylor, B. G., Davis, R. C., & Maxwell, C. D. (2001). The effects of a group batterer treatment program: A randomized experiment in Brooklyn. *Justice Quarterly, 18*, 171–201.

Tollefson, D. R., & Gross, E. R. (2006). Predicting recidivism following participation in a treatment program for batterers. *Journal of Social Service Research, 32*, 39–62.

Trebow, E. A., Berkanovic, E., & Harada, P. U. (2015). The outcomes and process improvement project: Batterers' intervention program evaluation comparing English-language and Spanish-language offenders. *Partner Abuse, 6*, 273–297.

Tutty, L. M., & Babins-Wagner, R. (2019). Outcomes and recidivism in mandated batterer intervention before and after introducing a specialized domestic violence court. *Journal of Interpersonal Violence, 34*(5), 1039–1062.

Tutty, L. M., Babins-Wagner, R., & Rothery, M. A. (2020). The responsible choices for men IPV offender program: Outcomes and a comparison of court-mandated to non-court-mandated men. *Journal of Aggression, Maltreatment & Trauma, 29*(3), 292–313.

VanderEnde, K. E., Yount, K. M., Dynes, M. M., & Sibley, L. M. (2012). Community-level correlates of intimate partner violence against women globally: A systematic review. *Social Science and Medicine, 75*, 1143–1155.

Ventura, L. A., & Davis, G. (2006). *An exploratory study of court-referred batterer intervention programs in Ohio.* Office of Criminal Justice Services.

Vigurs, C., Schucan-Bird, K., Quy, K. & Gough, D. (undated). *The impact of domestic violence perpetrator programmes or victim and criminal justice outcomes.* What works: Crime reduction review series, no. 5. University College London, Institute of Education, Evidence for Policy and Practice, Information and Coordinating Centre.

Vivolo-Kantor, A. M., Niolon, P. H., Estefan, L. F., Le, V. D., Tracy, A. J., Latzman, N. E., Little, T. D., Lang, K. M., DeGue, S., & Tharp, A. T. (2020). Middle school effects of the Dating Matters® comprehensive teen dating violence prevention model on physical violence, bullying, and cyberbullying: A cluster-randomized controlled trial. *Prevention Science*. https://doi.org/10.1007/s11121-019-01071-9

Walker, K., Bowen, E., & Brown, S. (2013). Desistance from intimate partner violence: A critical review. *Aggression and Violent Behavior, 18*, 271–280.

Wathen, C. N., MacMillan, H. L., & with the Canadian Task Force on Preventive Health Care. (2003). Prevention of violence against women: Recommendation statement from the Canadian Task Force on Preventive Health Care. *Canadian Medical Association Journal, 169*, 582–584.

Whetstone, T. S. (2001). Measuring the impact of a domestic violence coordinated response team. *Policing: An International Journal of Police Strategies and Management, 24*, 371–398.

Whitaker, D. J., Murphy, C. M., Eckhardt, C. I., Hodges, A. E., & Cowart, M. (2013). Effectiveness of primary prevention efforts for intimate partner violence. *Partner Abuse, 4*, 175–195.

Whittington, R., & McGuire, J. (2020). *Violence rewired: Evidence and strategies for public health action.* Cambridge University Press.

Wilkinson, D. L., & Hamerschlag, S. J. (2005). Situational determinants in intimate partner violence. *Aggression and Violent Behavior, 10*, 333–361.

Wistow, R., Kelly, L., & Westmarland, N. (2017). "Time Out": A strategy for reducing men's violence against women in relationships? *Violence Against Women, 23*(6), 730–748.

World Health Organization (WHO). (2013). *Global and regional estimates of violence against women: Prevalence and health effects of intimate partner violence and non-partner sexual violence.* WHO.

Wray, A. M., Hoyt, T., & Gerstle, M. (2013). Preliminary examination of a mutual intimate partner violence intervention among treatment-mandated couples. *Journal of Family Psychology, 27*, 664–670.

Yakubovich, A. R., Stöckl, H., Murray, J., Melendex-Torres, G. J., Steinert, J. I., Glavin, C. E. Y., & Humphreys, D. K. (2018). Risk and protective factors for intimate partner violence against women: Systematic review and meta-analyses of prospective–longitudinal studies. *American Journal of Public Health, 108*, e1–e11.

Yodanis, C. L. (2004). Gender inequality, violence against women, and fear: A cross-national test of the feminist theory of violence against women. *Journal of Interpersonal Violence, 19*, 655–675.
Yorke, N. J., Friedman, B. D., & Hurt, P. (2012). Implementing a batterer's intervention program in a correctional setting: A tertiary prevention model. *Journal of Offender Rehabilitation, 49*, 456–478.
Zeoli, A. M., Malinski, R., & Turchan, B. (2016). Risks and targeted interventions: Firearms in intimate partner violence. *Epidemiologic Reviews, 38*, 125–139.

# Chapter 5
# What Works in School-Based Interventions? A Systematic Review of Evaluation Research

## 5.1 Question to Be Addressed and Overall Objective

Our central question here is: what general approaches and specific methods can be employed that will effectively reduce risk of criminal offending/delinquency and other antisocial behaviour in schools? The key objective therefore was to conduct a Rapid Evidence Review and prepare a report summarizing what is known about effective approaches and methods in reducing antisocial behaviour and other conduct problems in schools, especially where they may lead to involvement in illegal activity. A related objective is to identify appropriate methods for possible use by police forces.

Some of the material covered in this chapter overlaps with that on relationship violence included in the preceding one, particularly with relevance to reviews or studies of aggression in schools and in teenage dating relationships (Muñoz-Fernández et al., 2019). Several programmes have been devised for the purpose of addressing those difficulties, and evaluations sometimes include both these and other types of variables.

At the outset of the revew, as in other areas, the work was planned using the PICO approach. The resultant framework devised for the review and the terms generated for conducting literature searches are shown in Table 5.1.

## 5.2 Background

Given their position in society, schools have a key role in influencing part of children's development. They can do so both early in development and later when there are more immediate risks of participation in criminal conduct. Thus, in respect of both their internal functioning and their responsibilities within a wider context,



J. McGuire et al., *Evidence-Based Policing and Community Crime Prevention*, Advances in Preventing and Treating Violence and Aggression,
https://doi.org/10.1007/978-3-030-76363-3_5

**Table 5.1** PICO framework: school-based interventions

| | |
|---|---|
| Population/ participants | *Setting*:<br>School (primary/elementary/secondary), academy<br>*People*:<br>Children/adolescents/teenagers. Pupils/students.<br>School head. Teachers. Teaching assistants. Kitchen staff. Cleaners. Janitor. Parents. Child-minders. Other caregivers<br>*Offences/problem behaviours*:<br>Crime, offending, delinquency<br>Violence, fight(ing), bullying, gang, sexual assault, indecency, sexting, cyberbullying, grooming, revenge porn, sharing indecent images, family abuse, drug-taking, drug-dealing, gang activities, theft, possess weapons, vandalism, property damage |
| Intervention/ indicator | School (based) interventions.<br>Anti-bullying programmes (ABPs)<br>Anti-vandalism programmes<br>Drugs, education/counselling<br>Advice on e-safety<br>Neighbourhood/community interventions<br>Police |
| Comparison/ control | Compare schools or districts with each other<br>Before-and-after studies<br>Comparisons between outcomes of different interventions<br>Where possible, extracting information from randomized controlled trials or quasi-experimental trials of interventions<br>Local, regional or international comparisons in rates of school violence |
| Outcome(s) | Recorded or self-reported rates of incidents (violent, sexual, damage)<br>Playground/classroom<br>Aggression/bullying/gangs<br>Levels of truancy<br>Children excluded/arrest/prosecuted<br>Mobile phone aggression/cyberbullying/sexting/grooming<br>Partner reports, third-party reports where available<br>Assaults on teachers or other staff<br>Conflicts with or between parents |

schools have often adopted policies and practices that complement those of police services.

Since schools are places where young people are brought together in large groups, they are also a major formative element of their experiences as they grow up. Spending a large part of most days in similarly aged peer groups means that there is also a powerful process of socialization at work. While that is fundamental for their growth, it can also generate difficulties for a proportion of them. It is well established that the early and middle adolescent years in particular are the phase of life when the majority of criminal careers begin. Many such problems are recognized and effectively managed by school staff. However, schools are often held accountable in the public arena for problems and issues that are outside their control or which they can have only limited impact upon.

For understandable reasons, the foremost attention of school staff is often on those problems that cause the greatest disruption inside the school itself. Probably the most frequently addressed problems are those of classroom disruption and bullying. Like other aggression the latter can take a variety of forms (physical, verbal, emotional), which can cause marked problems for victims. These include problems such as anxiety, depression and low self-esteem, which when bullying is prolonged may be very severe and in very serious cases can lead to self-harm and even suicide. It can also have adverse effects on witnesses or bystanders and may be an indicator of problems amongst those who engage in it themselves.

Due et al. (2009) reported an international survey of 35 countries from Europe and North America on rates of school bullying, investigating the association between it and socio-economic factors. This was based on data collected for the *Health Behaviour in School-Aged Children* survey for the World Health Organization (WHO). It involved a total sample of 162,305 students from 5998 schools. The data were collected in the 2001–2002 school year. On average across these samples, 11.0% of boys and 10.9% of girls were exposed to bullying. Rates of bullying in a country were associated not with its overall level of economic development but with its extent of income inequality (measured by the Gini index) and disparities of affluence within schools. Using the same data resource but extending it over 117 samples with a total of 594,638 adolescents surveyed across 4 separate years (1994, 1998, 2002, 2006), Elgar et al. (2013) noted that these relationships were also associated with the rate of homicide in each country. They suggested that cross-national differences in bullying prevalence were related to a "social milieu of interpersonal violence" (p. 237) as a function of income inequalities.

Levels of criminal victimization in school are however a function of many factors, including individual characteristics of children (their academic achievement, engagement in avoidant behaviour and experience of victimization outside school) and of their family backgrounds (notably their household income) and features of schools (such as the presence of gangs and availability of drugs) (Wynne & Joo, 2011). Perhaps surprisingly, perceptions that school rules were strictly enforced and certainty of punishment for violating them were not significant predictors of bullying rates.

There is no consensus definition of bullying, but one proposed by Norwegian researcher Dan Olweus, widely credited with having catalyzed the systematic study of school bullying from the 1970s onwards, is widely quoted: "A student is being bullied or victimized when he or she is exposed, repeatedly and over time, to negative actions on the part of one or more other students" (Olweus, 1993. p. 9; and see Olweus & Limber, 2010). Yet while a great deal of attention has been focused on bullying, some researchers have emphasized to need to view it in the wider context of other forms of school aggression (Donoghue & Raia-Hawrylak, 2016).

As well as being a problem in itself, longitudinal research indicates that bullying perpetration at school is a significant predictor of violence up to 11 years later. That applies also, although to a lesser extent, to being victimized (Ttofi et al., 2012). It has been suggested that anti-bullying programmes (ABPs) can be considered as an early form of crime prevention (Ttofi et al., 2011).

Summarizing a wide range of research, a leading sourcebook in the area drew together some key findings on school-based aggression and violence (Jimerson et al., 2012). With regard to bullying, Frey et al. (2012) have summarized key patterns in research results. This work shows that chronic victimization at school is associated with a series of later risks of anxiety, depression, self-injury, alcohol misuse and other problems. Repeated involvement in bullying is also linked to later risks to personal wellbeing, including failures in relationships. Witnessing bullying incidents as a bystander can lead in some cases to imitating them or in others to moral disengagement. Both produce negative emotional reactions. Research suggests that bystanders are present in 80% or more of bullying incidents (O'Connell et al., 1999).

Several other patterns that emerge while children are at school have been found to be associated with later involvement in delinquency and/or adult criminality. Those that have been investigated most extensively include other kinds of aggression such as general fighting, gang involvement, and the carrying of weapons; relational and sexual aggression including dating or partner violence; and under-age consumption of alcohol or involvement in illicit substance use.

There are other aspects to this, according to a news story in the British press (Grierson & agencies, 2017). Based on information released under a Freedom of Information Act request, large numbers of weapons were recovered from children attending school in England and Wales. Data from 32 police forces showed that between April 2015 and the end of 2016, 2579 weapons had been seized, including knives, air guns, in one case a metal rod and in another a police baton. Amongst the children discovered with weapons, 47 were less than 10 years old.

When these or other kinds of problems arise, one way to address them is to focus attention on those who are involved as perpetrators or affected as victims or bystanders. An alternative approach is to attempt to prevent such problems by taking broader-ranging action: addressing the problem on several levels or even at a school-wide or *universal* level. Many theories have been formulated to inform the development of bullying prevention programmes (Hawley & Williford, 2015). An important distinction that runs through this entire area is with respect to the breadth of compass of the interventions provided. Thus, there are *focused* or *indicated*, *selective*, *multilevel* and *universal* interventions. These distinctions are clarified in a general overview of school violence prevention research by Gottfredson (2017). Examples of each can be found in the research we will describe.

## 5.3 Specific Objectives

The specific objectives of this evidence review were first, to locate studies of interventions provided in school settings, with the objective of reducing some behavioural or attitudinal problem which evidence suggests may be a risk factor for delinquency, and second, to analyse the studies so located, to identify which approaches if any have generated evidence of effectiveness in reducing the likelihood of school-based antisocial behaviour or wider delinquent involvement.

## 5.4 Method

Prior to commencing the review, preliminary scoping searches identified a number of sources of relevant evidence in this area. In addition, it was known that there have been several experimental anti-bullying programmes and evaluations carried out in the UK, the USA, Norway and other countries. Several reviews published before 2010 were therefore used as sources for possible search terms (Ferguson et al., 2007; Flannery et al., 2003; Greenberg et al., 2003; Hahn, 2007; Merrell et al., 2008; Park-Higgerson et al., 2008; Vreeman & Carroll, 2007; Wilson et al., 2001, 2003; Wilson & Lipsey, 2007).

### *5.4.1 Search Strategy*

Initial scoping searches conducted for the purpose of developing the PICO framework shown in Table 5.1 located several relevant reviews. These suggested that the amount of published research in this area is very large, and also that it has already been extensively reviewed. For strategic reasons, it was therefore decided to limit the current searches and the review to the period from January 2010 onwards. The exact period covered in the initial search was from 1 January 2010 to 9 February 2017 when searches were conducted. Even so, the quantity of studies located was substantial.

A set of search terms was developed from Table 5.1, drawing on previous reviews and on the preliminary scoping searches already carried out. The search strategy focused on the databases most likely to contain materials relevant to the review question. Eight electronic databases were searched: EMBASE, ERIC, MEDLINE, National Criminal Justice Reference Service (USA), PsycINFO, PubMed (excluding MEDLINE), Scopus and the Social Sciences Citation Index. Searches produced a total of 14,247 items, which after removal of duplicates resulted in a total of 6331 items retained for first-stage screening. These items were recorded in an Endnote data file. As in other chapters of the book, a more limited updating search was carried out to take the period covered up to November 2020.

### *5.4.2 Inclusion and Exclusion Criteria*

The overall objective of the review was to survey the nature and the outcomes of school-based interventions. Therefore, the types of studies that were sought for inclusion were evaluations of school-based programmes or related activities designed to address potential or actual problems of antisocial behaviour linked to delinquency. Other inclusion criteria were set in order to make the review feasible and practicable, given the volume of studies that could be considered relevant on a broad interpretation of the objectives. To be retained for review, a study had to meet the following criteria:

1. To have been published in the period from 1 January 2010 to 30 November 2020.
2. To be published in a peer-reviewed research journal or government report. Research dissertations and articles from non-peer-reviewed periodicals were excluded.
3. To be published in English. Resources were not available for carrying out translation.
4. To consist of empirical research, presenting either quantitative or qualitative data from either an outcome or process evaluation of a delivered intervention, or from analysis of relationships between features of the schools and levels of problems.
5. To be focused on young people as actual or potential perpetrators of antisocial or delinquent acts or who are assessed on the basis of other evidence as being at risk of becoming involved (manifesting risk factors for future involvement) in illegal acts.

Conversely, studies were excluded if they did not focus on an intervention provided wholly or partly in a school setting. Many studies of that kind were found, involving work with families or in youth or community centres; in primary care, hospital emergency or mental health settings; and in youth or teen courts, or youth justice agencies, either in the community or in institutions. A few studies were found that described an intervention that involved one of those settings and were retained if part of the work was also undertaken in a school. All such studies reported on work carried out in a combination of school and family settings. The only other exception made to this was the retention of studies carried out in truancy centres.

Similarly, studies were excluded if they consisted of basic research on the factors associated with children's problems, for example, investigating which variables might be associated with becoming a target for bullying. Studies of developmental risk factors, correlational studies and other types of research were excluded, as were articles that consisted of discussion, analysis, theoretical or policy statements unless they also contained original empirical data. Studies that evaluated the impact of interventions on teachers only but not on pupils were excluded (e.g. Leuschner et al., 2017). Finally, large numbers of studies have been conducted on the effects of victimization on school-age children. This includes research on the effects of physical or sexual abuse in the family, witnessing parental violence in the home or having been a victim of bullying. These issues are clearly important but are the subject of separate reviews, and in terms of both volume and clarity of objectives they could not be included in the present work.

At a later stage of the review process, given the volume of material accumulated, a decision was made to restrict the focus to studies of interventions undertaken in secondary or high school settings or with children within the age range likely to attend those schools in England and Wales (11–18). This was based on several considerations. First, the age of criminal responsibility in England and Wales is 10 (one of the lowest in Europe), but that does not map neatly on to ages of transition to different levels of schooling. In addition, while some countries or district or county education departments have two tiers of schools (primary and secondary), others have a third, middle school tier. Where that exists, the ages of entry to and departure from it vary, as does the age of beginning school attendance overall. Some middle schools cover the age range 7–11, while in others the age range is 9–13. Unfortunately, a sizeable number of the located studies reported the school grades of study participants, but not their ages. Thus, school grades are not reliable indicators of children's ages. There were also longer-term follow-up studies in which children were tracked over time, across the standard ages for transition between school levels.

Accordingly, the retained studies were divided into five categories as follows. They respectively included children who were in (a) primary school only (elementary school in the USA and some other countries), (b) middle school only, (c) secondary school only, (d) primary and secondary school and (e) middle and secondary school. The present report deals only with the third of these groups, research based in secondary or high school settings, or with middle school children known to be aged 11 or over. A flowchart representing this sequence of selection decisions is shown in Fig. 5.1.

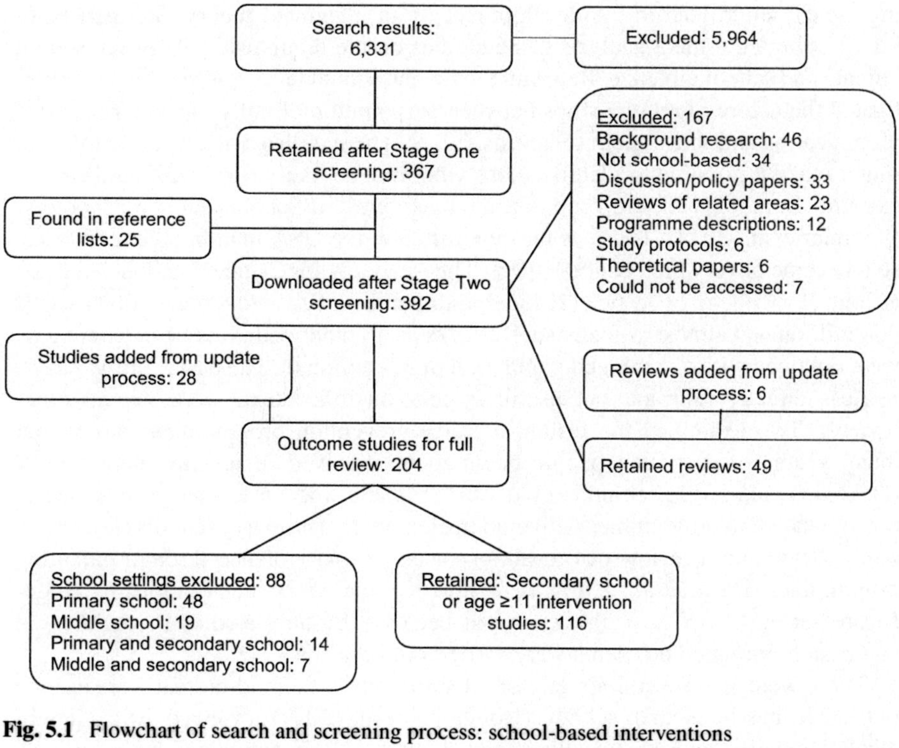


**Fig. 5.1** Flowchart of search and screening process: school-based interventions

## 5.5 Previous Reviews

Given the amount of research published in this area, there have also been numerous systematic reviews and meta-analyses of it. In combination, the electronic searches and checks in reference lists identified a total of 66 potentially relevant reviews. Several of them overlapped with each other in coverage, but many addressed separate aspects of the topic. Some reviews focused on background factors, including correlates of or risk factors for bullying or other problem behaviour. For example, Hong and Espelage (2012) examined evidence on a range of individual and ecological/system factors associated with bullying, as a framework for understanding how anti-bullying initiatives work in schools in South Korea (Hong et al., 2014). Other researchers have drawn together evidence on the classroom and other contextual variables that are associated with bullying (Saarento et al., 2015). Still others have conducted reviews to isolate individual factors or formulate combinations of them that might be used to predict bullying (Álvarez-García et al., 2015). Another review focused on the relationship between socio-economic status and antisocial behaviour in schools (Piotroswka et al., 2015).

In a very wide-ranging overview, Zych et al. (2015) integrated findings from 66 systematic reviews in an effort to distil key findings about bullying and cyberbullying, which could lead to the development of an integrated theory. Steffgen et al. (2013) reported a meta-analysis of 36 studies on the relationships between school climate and school violence. Returning to the individual level, another review investigated the nature of relationships between perpetration of bullying, experiences of victimization and self-esteem (Tsaousis, 2016). There is also a review of factors that might make it possible to identify those who may be likely to embark on the most extreme form of violence, committing massacres in schools (school shooters) (Sommer et al., 2014). These occur more often in the USA than in other countries, so it became of very high concern there. The Academy for Critical Incident Analysis at John Jay College of Justice (2017) found that the USA with a population then of 308 million had almost as many such attacks as 36 other countries from where data were obtained with a combined population of 3.8 billion (see also McCarthy, 2012).

Less directly relevant, but useful in relation to context, were several other reviews. Two examined the results of early prevention programmes, carried out many years before young people begin to be involved in juvenile delinquency (Deković et al., 2011; Schindler et al., 2015). There was a meta-analysis of mediators of change in programmes delivered in elementary (primary) schools (Dymnicki et al., 2011) and a review of prevention of childhood violence through parenting programmes (Desai et al., 2017). A review of social work interventions by Allen-Meares et al. (2013) was also excluded because the only studies that addressed aggression or related problems were carried out in primary schools.

There were also several reviews of interventions with children that were carried out in settings other than schools. Rongione et al. (2011) reviewed 20 studies of alcohol and drug abuse counselling carried out mainly in outpatient clinic settings. Results in relation to alcohol were inconsistent at therapy end-point but disappeared by follow-up, while results for other drugs were positive at termination but inconsistent by follow-up. Özabaci (2011) reviewed six studies of cognitive-behaviour therapy to reduce violence with an average modest effect size, but none was conducted in a school setting. Melendez-Torres et al. (2016a) reviewed three trials of community-based violence prevention. Fagan and Catalano (2012) reviewed 17 studies of youth violence prevention, but only 1 was undertaken in a secondary school and it was included in other reviews. A review by Farahmand et al. (2011) did report school-based interventions but almost entirely for mental health or *internalizing* problems. For the reasons given, each of these reviews was therefore excluded.

For present purposes the only reviews considered directly relevant were those that focused on studies involving evaluation of interventions carried out in secondary schools or in middle schools where age ranges upwards from 11 were given. Thus, a review by Kingston et al. (2016) of the implementation of Youth Violence Prevention Centre packages delivered at six sites in different American states was excluded from consideration as it contained no outcome data. Evans et al. (2014) reported a review of programmes evaluating a mixture of bullying and victimization effects but restricted it to primary and middle schools.

Another review of evidence of interventions to reduce alcohol and cannabis use amongst young people, by Smedslund et al. (2017), was also excluded. This was not based on work carried out in schools and included research with participants in the age range of 15–25, and therefore it did not meet inclusion criteria. A separate review published in the same year addressed the usefulness of Mindfulness-Based Interventions in school settings. However, this did not cover behaviours or attitudes associated with offending (Maynard et al., 2017), and therefore, it too was outside the scope of the present objectives.

After removing these and other reviews that did not include evaluative information, the number of relevant reports fell but was still substantial at 49. Some were unusual in consisting of reviews of reviews – instead of collecting primary studies they collated systematic reviews themselves, given the volume of work in this field. Three publications of this kind were found. Matjasko et al. (2012) collated results of 52 reviews of youth violence prevention published prior to 2010; five focused on studies carried out in schools. Another meta-review on preventing school violence was reported by Lester et al. (2017). Das et al. (2016) compared reviews of interventions designed to prevent adolescent substance abuse. These proved useful in supplementing the list of documents located in literature searches. They are not included in the series of reviews itemized in Tables 5.2, 5.3, 5.4, 5.5, and 5.6.

To facilitate the summary process, reviews were divided into five groups, each presented in one of the summary tables to follow. These were (1) reviews of anti-bullying interventions (12 studies); (2) interventions designed to address other forms of aggression or violence (15 studies); others with dating, sexual and relational violence (7 studies); (those concerned with alcohol or substance use (13 studies); and (5) those with after-school programmes (2 studies). Some publications reported different versions of the same study, in which case more than one source is listed in the left-hand column. A few reviews had multiple objectives, e.g.

**Table 5.2** Reviews of anti-bullying programmes and related interventions

| Review | Focus | Number of studies | Findings |
|---|---|---|---|
| Cantone et al. (2015) | Interventions to reduce bullying and cyberbullying | 17 | All included studies were RCTs. Most focused on primary schools: 1 on adolescents only and 4/17 mainly on them. Positive effects were short term with no evidence of long-term gains. Better effects were found for universal, whole-school interventions than for those with focused or multilevel components |
| Chalamandaris and Piette (2015) | Review of intervention evaluation methods | 62 | This report differs from others in not examining intervention outcomes but was retained as it focuses on analysing the relationship between intervention study designs and results that are obtained. This enables links to be made between questions asked, methodology and study designs, results and theories concerning the causes and remedies of bullying |
| Della Cioppa et al. (2015) | Evaluation of cyberbullying intervention programmes | 12 | Reviewed nine programmes to reduce cyberbullying and three focused on internet safety, mainly amongst 12–13-year-olds. Appraised on a 20-point scientific merit scale, most studies were found to be weak, lacking half of the criteria set. Programmes did not employ a whole-school approach. The authors suggested that more and better research is required before any conclusions can be drawn regarding effectiveness |
| Huang et al. (2019) | Meta-analysis of anti-bullying programmes with parent involvement | 22 | Reviews research based on the role that parents may have in the prevention of bullying amongst children up to 12th grade. Located prevention studies that included any of five types of parental component, from simply providing information to direct training. Mean effect sizes were small but statistically significant on both bullying perpetration ($d = 0.179$) and peer victimization ($d = 0.162$) |
| Jiminéz-Barbero et al. (2012) | Review of anti-bullying by evidence levels | 32: 5 reviews 12 RCTs 11 QEs 4 pre-post or cohort studies | Divided studies of ABPs into four groups according to the methodological quality of evaluation designs. In all four categories there was a similar pattern of beneficial effects. Studies covered the full school-age range. There were similar patterns of findings across all evidence levels in relation to changes in attitudes, beliefs and behaviours and in the frequency of violent behaviour |

(continued)

**Table 5.2** (continued)

| Review | Focus | Number of studies | Findings |
|---|---|---|---|
| Jiminéz-Barbero, Hernández, et al. (2016) | Efficacy of anti-bullying programmes (ABPs) | 14 RCTs 8 with children aged >10 | Examined the effect of ABPs on the frequency of bullying and victimization and on attitudes to bullying, in a total sample of 30,934 participants. Samples included children in the age range 7–16. Most interventions showed positive effects, but they were smaller for the age group >10: For bullying, −0.08, and for victimization, −0.07 |
| Lee et al. (2015) | Effects of school-based anti-bullying programmes | 13 | Across an aggregate sample size of 19,619, meta-analysis found a mean effect size favouring intervention of −0.15. No interventions had negative effects. Those focused on emotional control, peer counselling and establishing school-wide policies on bullying emerged with larger effect sizes than other approaches |
| Nocentini et al. (2015) | Use of information and communication technologies (ICTs) in ABPs | 13 | Covers 1 evaluation of each of 13 specially devised ABPs. Only four of the programmes were found to be effective. Two using ICTs only were effective and two containing both face-to-face and ICT elements were also effective; thus, the added value of ICT could not be established. Makes proposals for what should be included in ICT-mediated ABPs |
| Polanin et al. (2012) | Investigation of the effects of ABPs on bystanders | 12 (8 RCTs) | Synthesized ABP studies to test for their impact on the behaviour of bystanders and if they increase the likelihood of intervention in bullying situations. The mean effect size across studies was 0.20 and statistically significant: ABPs made bystanders more likely to intervene, and the effect was larger in secondary schools than lower tiers |
| Rivara and Le Menestrel (2016); see also Flannery et al. (2016) | Wide-ranging review of other reviews of preventive interventions | Na | A major initiative addressing several aspects of the bullying problem, including a review of prevention research covering universal, selective and indicated approaches. Summarizes findings of other review and provides descriptions of best-supported ABPs. Tabulates findings in terms of ecological context |

(continued)

**Table 5.2** (continued)

| Review | Focus | Number of studies | Findings |
|---|---|---|---|
| Ttofi and Farrington (2011) | School-based programmes to reduce bullying (across all tiers of schooling) | 44 | Meta-analysis of studies with a range of designs. Found an overall effect size (odds ratio) of 1.36 for bullying and 1.29 for victimization. This corresponds to an overall reduction of 17–23% in bullying events in experimental as compared to control samples. The review provides extensive detail on features of the more effective interventions |
| Yeager et al. (2015) | Investigation of whether ABP effects vary for different age groups | 19 | Review showed that the nature of bullying alters with age, with direct bullying (e.g. hitting) declining from sixth to 12th grade while indirect bullying (e.g. rumour, social exclusion) increased. Overall, there was evidence of a decline in the effectiveness of ABPs with increasing age, and some had negative effects for older teenage groups: From age 15 there were iatrogenic outcomes |

addressing both the issues of substance use and violence. They were placed in the category that reflected the strongest emphasis of the work reported.

Some reviews dealt only with randomized controlled trials (RCTs), while others included non-randomized, quasi-experimental evaluations (QEs). Those acronyms will be used throughout this chapter. Table 5.2 focuses on anti-bullying interventions.

The trend of results emerging from these reviews is fairly mixed but some conclusions can be drawn. First, the research is of variable quality and a disappointing portion of it involves weak designs from which it is difficult to identify clear results. Second, many studies report only short-term effects, sometimes at the end of interventions; therefore, it is uncertain whether reported gains remain over time. Third, there is little or no evidence to support the use of some strategies, such as information and communication technologies. Fourth, on balance whole-school or universal approaches emerge as more effective than selective or targeted interventions (e.g. focused on identified high-risk groups), a finding that runs counter to what is found in work with convicted offenders. Fifth, there are some indications that anti-bullying interventions are more effective with younger adolescents and their effects may decline for those aged 15 and beyond, and there may even be iatrogenic consequences. Finally, however, there is repeated evidence of positive outcomes from several of the reviews, notably those by Jiminéz-Barbero, Hernández, et al. (2016), Lee et al. (2015), Polanin et al. (2012) and Ttofi and Farrington (2011). Anti-bullying programme clearly can be effective, and that includes work with bystanders as well as with perpetrators of bullying.

Bullying involves repeated aggression (physical or psychological) towards one person as an exercise of power but as noted previously aggression and violence in school can take several other forms, such as fighting or aggression by one person

**Table 5.3** Prevention of other aggression and violence in schools

| Review | Focus | Number of studies | Findings |
|---|---|---|---|
| Alford and Derzon (2012) | School-based programmes with multiple targets for reducing violence | 24 | All 24 programmes showed some positive effect on reduction of violence or antisocial behaviour. Mean effect sizes were for physical aggression 0.26, antisocial behaviour 0.15, aggressive/disruptive behaviour 0.12 and delinquent behaviour 0.08. Amongst eight programmes measuring multiple outcomes however, only one showed more than one positive effect. But little evidence that programmes had multiple benefits |
| Atienzo et al. (2017) | Interventions to reduce youth violence | 9 | Focused on studies carried on in Latin American countries. Six were delivered in school settings and the majority of studies yielded positive results in terms of reductions in violence mostly over substantial follow-up periods; however, evaluation designs were often weak |
| Barnes et al. (2014) | Cognitive-behavioural interventions to reduce aggression | 25 | Meta-analysis: Mean effect size across all studies: −0.14. Mean weighted effect size, correcting for interdependence within studies: −0.23.<br>In 74% of studies, aggression was lower after treatment. File drawer number[a] = 224 |
| Blank et al. (2010) | Whole-school behavioural interventions to promote wellbeing | 37 (16 RCTs) | Narrative review of a series of interventions with a range of planned outcomes including reductions in bullying, conduct problems and violence. Found that conflict resolution training was effective in the short term with involvement of "peer mediators" yielding longer-term effects. The paper contains very little quantitative results and no tabulated comparisons |
| Bonell, Wells, et al. (2016) | Effect of altering school environments | 16 reports of 10 studies | Review focused on whether making changings in classroom or school environments influenced health-related behaviour. A few studies examined effects on aggression and violence. In two there were trends towards reductions based on improved teacher-student relations, but results were non-significant |
| Brännström et al. (2016) | Evaluation of Aggression Replacement Training | 16 | Aggression Replacement Training is a structured programme designed to reduce aggression and violence. Mixed review containing studies of adolescents and adults, only two in school settings, one showing some positive changes, the other a significant reduction in anger and increased levels of interaction skills |

(continued)

**Table 5.3** (continued)

| Review | Focus | Number of studies | Findings |
|---|---|---|---|
| Cox et al. (2016) | Violence prevention and intervention programmes in schools | 19 studies of 17 programmes | Review of Australian studies of violence prevention for age groups 12–18. Outcomes were mainly self-reports but four studies had other sources of information. Universal programmes obtained modest success levels; there were positive results for some alcohol programmes. Targeting high-risk youths was ineffective, while parent training produced better results |
| Durlak et al. (2011) | Effects of social and emotional learning | 213 | Extensive review and meta-analysis with a total of 270,034 participants; 27 studies undertaken in high schools. Interventions entailed social and emotional learning components. Effect sizes for a range of outcomes were positive and significant including prosocial behaviour (0.24) and conduct problems (0.22), but not disaggregated by age group |
| Gavine et al. (2016) | Effectiveness of universal school-based programmes | 21 of 16 programmes | Focused on violence prevention with outcomes from physical and non-physical aggression to attitudes to violence and use of prosocial skills. There were seven RCTs. Interventions were concerned either with *social development* through skills learning or with *social norms* through influencing school climates. Largest effects came from combining the two |
| Oliver et al. (2011) | Classroom management of disruptive behaviour | 12 (3 in high school grades) | The dependent variables were inappropriate and disruptive behaviour. Overall effect size at an average 12-month follow-up was large at 0.80 and statistically significant. However, it was not possible to analyse effects by age level so conclusions about ages ≥11 cannot be drawn |
| Price and Khubchandani (2019) | Practices and policies to reduce firearm offences in schools at primary, secondary and tertiary levels | 89 (including 6 media or website reports) | Narrative review of research on epidemiology but also covering prevention practices. Concludes that no school security measures, e.g. employing school resources officers, installing video cameras and metal detectors, random locker searches, etc., have been shown "to unequivocally reduce or eliminate school shootings" (p.162). Tertiary prevention assumes there is a shooter on campus and evidence on methods to respond to this is lacking and "unlikely to be forthcoming" (p. 163) |

(continued)

**Table 5.3** (continued)

| Review | Focus | Number of studies | Findings |
|---|---|---|---|
| Reingle Gonzalez et al. (2016) | School safety measures and school-related delinquency | 29 studies, 32 study samples | Analysed outcome studies of school violence prevention measures, e.g. metal detectors, surveillance cameras, controlled access, security guards and resource officers. Most outcomes were of perceived safety, only a few on actual safety (incidents, disciplinary actions, arrests). Results "almost uniformly suggest that the presence of more structural safety measures… results in a decline of student-perceived safety" (p. 450) |
| Sawyer et al. (2015) | Prevention or treatment of youth antisocial behaviour | 66 studies: 34 on prevention, 32 on therapy | Meta-analysis: Mean effect size of 0.31 over at least 1 year from the end of intervention. Almost half (29) of the studies were with age range ≥11 but it is not clear what proportion were carried out in schools (not analysed separately). Two identifiable studies with children aged ≥11 in schools had large effect sizes on antisocial behaviour |
| Sklad et al. (2012) | Effectiveness of social, emotional and behavioural programmes | 75 (48 in secondary schools) | Extensive review covering several sets of skills and wellbeing outcome variables but also including antisocial/aggressive behaviour and substance abuse. Focused on universal programmes. There was a moderately large and significant reduction in antisocial behaviour and a small reduction in substance use. The former gain was smaller in secondary schools (−0.25) but still notable, and had increased at follow-up. Similar trends were found in US and European studies |
| Tancred et al. (2018) | Qualitative/ thematic synthesis of process in reducing substance use and violence | 16 evaluations from 15 studies of factors influencing change processes | Reviewed studies that examined the process of change in implementing school-based interventions. Identified five overarching themes that affect the process of implementation, related to senior staff support, aspects of immediate working environment, attitudes to features of interventions of (a) teachers and (b) students, and parental support. Emphasized the importance of addressing these issues if useful interventions are to be properly delivered, and the relative neglect of them in many intervention efforts |

[a]In meta-analysis, the *file drawer number* (sometimes called the *fail-safe number*) is an estimate of how many unpublished studies with zero effect sizes would be necessary to reverse or overturn the observed effect size obtained from the published studies that have been located and reviewed

**Table 5.4** Dating, sexual and relationship violence in schools

| Review | Focus | Number of studies | Findings |
|---|---|---|---|
| DeGue et al. (2014) | Prevention of sexual violence | 140 (20 in secondary schools) | Extensive review of strategies for primary prevention of sexual violence. Of studies based in high schools, one produced short-term positive outcomes in attitudes at 1-year follow-up but effects on sexual violence were not measured. Another dating violence prevention programme (*Safe Dates*) evaluated in an RCT had significant effects on self-reported sexual violence (perpetration or victimization) at 4-year follow-up |
| De La Rue et al. (2014) | Interventions to reduce dating violence | 23 | Evaluated programmes based in middle or high schools to reduce or prevent dating/sexual violence or change attitudes to it. Studies found significant gains post-test in knowledge, attitude change and reduced acceptance of rape myths and four studies with follow-ups found a significant reduction in dating violence |
| De Koker et al. (2014) | Preventing adolescent IPV | 6 | Reviewed nine studies based on six RCTs from the USA, Canada and South Africa on prevention programmes for adolescents to reduce risks of IPV perpetration or victimization. Four of the programmes had significant beneficial effects over some long-term follow-up periods, and two shorter programmes did not |
| Fellmeth et al. (2013, 2015) | Preventing relationship violence | 38 | Review of studies of educational and skills-based interventions. Meta-analysis of 33 studies. Found no convincing evidence of effects on attitudes to violence or episodes of violence in relationships |
| Fryda and Hulme (2015) | Prevention of child sexual abuse | 31 studies of 23 programmes | Educational interventions to prevent children being sexually abused at home. Most studies were with primary schools; two studies focused on the aged range 11–14 or 11–15 and two others included ages 12–13. Studies found gains in knowledge and in self-protection skills. In one study disclosures increased |
| Prezensky et al. (2018) | Systematic review of prevention of gender-based school violence | 11 (Brazilian) 30 (worldwide) | Review of Brazilian and international databases. Found only 45% of the first but 83% of the latter were concerned with preventive actions. More of the former were in the curriculum, while the latter were more often extra-curricular. Found only six experiments. Only 34% of studies reported indicators of change in actions, 27% addressed gender awareness, and just 22% reported changes in occurrence of gender violence |
| Whitaker et al. (2013) | Primary prevention of partner violence | 19 | Reviewed studies of interventions designed to prevent intimate partner violence (IPV). Most studies (13) were conducted in schools; 15 were randomized studies and 4 quasi-experiments. Follow-up from 1–60 months but only six studies had follow-up >12 months. Outcomes were IPV-related behaviour. Several studies showed positive effects but others nil effects |

**Table 5.5** Drugs and alcohol in schools: previous reviews

| Review | Focus | Number of studies | Findings |
|---|---|---|---|
| Bonell, Dickson, et al. (2016); Bonell, Hinds, et al., (2016); Melendez-Torres et al. (2016b) | Positive youth development interventions | 10 studies (1 each on 10 different types of intervention) | A series of interconnected reviews on positive youth developments, which are focused on the promotion of positive assets of young people in preference to working on "risk reduction". Positive youth developments were delivered in the community outside school hours but were targeted towards school pupils. No evidence was found indicating that these interventions produced an effect "of statistical or public health significance" in reducing substance use or violence by young people |
| Espada et al. (2015) | School-based prevention of substance use | 21 | Meta-analysis of school-based substance use prevention programmes in Spain in the period 2002–2013. Found low-to-moderate effect sizes for changes in knowledge and attitudes, in many cases sustained at 12-month follow-up, but no firm effects on consumption. But study quality rated as low and it is suggested more rigorous evaluations are needed |
| Espada-Sánchez and Hernández-Serrano (2015) | School-based prevention of substance use | 8 studies of 1 programme | Narrative review of *Saluda*, a ten-session programme used in Spanish schools. Several controlled studies of different aspects of the programme. Results indicate positive effects on knowledge, attitudes and intentions, but results for drinking or other substance use behaviour are limited, with only one study showing a reduction in episodes of drunkenness |
| Faggiano et al. (2016) | Prevention of illicit drug use | 51 RCTs | Cochrane review of universal school-based programmes with a total of 127,146 participants. Compared outcomes for different programme models of three types: Social competence, social influence and combined approach. The first had supportive evidence for marijuana in short term and 12+ months but no effect on hard drug use. The second had no significant effects. Combined model: Significant effects for marijuana at 12+ months, but mixed findings for hard drug use |

(continued)

**Table 5.5** (continued)

| Review | Focus | Number of studies | Findings |
|---|---|---|---|
| Hennessy and Tanner-Smith (2015) | Brief alcohol interventions in schools | 17 | Part of a larger meta-analysis of interventions with adolescents and young adults across a variety of settings (Tanner-Smith & Lipsey, 2015; Tanner-Smith & Risser, 2016). Evaluated the impact of brief alcohol interventions ranging in duration from 17 to 240 minutes on alcohol consumption. Individual delivery was slightly superior to group delivery. Use of motivational enhancement was associated with larger effect sizes than other interventions. But these two features were usually combined |
| Hale et al. (2014) | Reduction of multiple health risks | 44 RCTs | Reviewed studies on reduction of alcohol and drug use alongside other outcomes (e.g. tobacco use, sexual risk). Effects sizes were small, but amongst the interventions, 18 showed a significant effect for 2 types of outcome and 9 affected alcohol, tobacco and illicit drug use. Effective programmes involved life skills training, problem-solving and stress management |
| Hodder et al. (2017) | Interventions to increase resilience in avoiding drug and alcohol use | 13 RCTs<br>6 others | Meta-analysis of programmes designed to strengthen resilience. Found positive and significant effects in relation to illicit substances (odds ratio 0.78, sustained after 1 year, odds ratio 0.84) but not for alcohol |
| Jackson et al. (2011) | Prevention of substance use and risky sexual behaviour | 18 | Based on studies with children aged ≥11 but also with young adults up to age 25. Of studies located, 13 were rated methodologically strong or moderate, 5 as weak. Findings were varied, but most programmes had some positive effect. But attrition was generally high. The largest effects were for interventions with multiple objectives. The authors stated intervention should start earlier, e.g. at ages 6–10 |
| MacArthur et al. (2015) | Peer-led methods for reducing substance use | 14 | Review of studies across 220 schools with 13,706 participants. Selected interventions that emphasized involvement of peers in delivering parts of sessions on alcohol (six studies) and cannabis use (three studies). Effects for alcohol showed a positive but limited trend; those for cannabis were stronger (odds ratio 0.71). Most studies found positive outcomes but in two, peer-led interventions had adverse effects |

(continued)

**Table 5.5** (continued)

| Review | Focus | Number of studies | Findings |
|---|---|---|---|
| Mason et al. (2015) | Impact of text messaging interventions on substance use | 14 RCTs | Evaluated the usefulness of text messaging as a method of influencing patterns of substance use. There were large differences between studies in sample sizes, numbers of texts sent and periods of delivery. There was a mean effect size of 0.25 but large variations across studies. Of 12 effect sizes computed, 10 were positive but only 5 statistically significant |
| Onrust et al. (2016) | Programmes to reduce substance use | 154 alcohol 110 drug use | Meta-analysis and meta-regression across a large number of studies to test for associations with target age groups, length of follow-up, programme type and methodological features. Compared effects when delivered on a universal basis with those provided to groups assessed as high risk. Methods of self-control and problem-solving training and cognitive-behaviour therapy were widely successful. Some methods (social influence, health education) had adverse effects in high-risk groups |
| Sancassiani et al. (2015) | Emotional and social skills training | 22 RCTs | Synthesis of evaluations of life skills and other similar training programmes applied at both universal and specific levels. Searches used one database only. Some studies were still ongoing. All programmes were effective in relation to at least one outcome variable (e.g. substance use, anger control, health-related behaviours) and most effective for several others |
| Sharma and Branscum (2013) | Prevention of drugs abuse | 18 (12 RCTs) on 12 interventions | Evaluation of a series of prevention programmes (with five studies of one). Most showed positive effects at post-test, but most found little or no effect at follow-up of 3 or more months. However, three studies found significant differences were maintained at 6-month follow-up. Most programmes were short |

towards several others. Table 5.3 summarizes reviews of interventions designed to address this.

The trend amongst this second set of reviews is more consistently positive than for those of bullying prevention programmes. In some cases, clear conclusions cannot be drawn about the secondary school-age group, as reviews included younger samples or studies conducted in other settings and did not analyse them separately.

**Table 5.6** Previous reviews of after-school programmes

| Review | Focus | Number of studies | Findings |
|---|---|---|---|
| Cid (2016) | After-school programmes in the Caribbean and Latin America | 6 | Reviewed studies of after-school programmes in Haiti, Jamaica, Peru, Uruguay and Venezuela. Only two were for age ≥10. Both had significant effects: One of violence prevention involving sports-reduced conflicts with authorities, the other involving an orchestra-improved behaviour and self-confidence |
| Taheri and Welsh (2015) | Results of after-school programmes for preventing delinquency | 12 | Reviewed three types of after-school interventions respectively with academic, recreational or skills-training focus, carried out in the USA, Canada and Sweden. Most were for secondary school children. Found large variations in effects; mean effect was small and non-significant. After allowing for other influences (moderators), the authors concluded that none of the interventions was shown to be effective |

The majority of the reviews however reported positive effects, sometimes with moderate-to-large effect sizes, and as some also considered other problem behaviour, they have addressed the kinds of multiple problems that are often found to have a link to risk of involvement in delinquency.

Several interventions have been developed to focus specifically on risks of violence in close relationships or of a sexual nature. Some are planned for their short-term effects on adolescent behaviour but with the longer-term objective of reducing risks of engaging in intimate partner violence (IPV) in adulthood. Several reviews were found of this area of research and are summarized in Table 5.4.

The latter findings, although not wholly consistent, are moderately encouraging: five out of seven studies reported positive results. Given the likely challenges of working on problems of this kind with adolescents, the outcomes suggest they can be overcome. On the other hand, the largest review included here (Fellmeth et al., 2013, 2015) found few positive outcomes, and studies often report effects on intermediate variables such as cognitions and attitudes but do not report whether these are associated with changes in behaviour. The findings of the Whitaker et al. (2013) review are perhaps the most encouraging amongst this group.

Table 5.5 summarizes key findings from reviews of interventions designed to reduce substance use by young people. This mainly focused on alcohol and illicit drugs, but in several reviews, it also included evaluations of efforts to reduce tobacco use. Given the objectives of the present review, that information has not been extracted for inclusion here.

In relation to the above set of reviews, it should be noted first that many of the studies which have a general objective of health promotion also focus on tobacco use but data concerning this have not been focused upon here. Second, it should be borne in mind that there is a general trend towards increasing use of alcohol and of other substances from earlier to later adolescence. Prevention or intervention programmes are therefore often evaluated in terms of the extent to which they can slow that process down, and if experimental (treated) groups have lower rates than comparison groups, even if they are still drinking alcohol or using drugs. Given patterns of behaviour that are widely understood to be difficult to alter, a mixture of results is a realistic expectation in this context. It is for that reason of course that early intervention is often seen as essential, and the authors of some reviews proposed that work of this kind needs to start even earlier, before the age of 10 (and many other studies have investigated such effects).

As with other sets of reviews there are recurrent problems of weak research designs and also in this case with the additional difficulty of sometimes high attrition (dropout) rates. Also, as with other areas, there is an over-reliance on self-report rather than being able to record actual behavioural change.

Nevertheless, there are also numerous positive findings in these reviews. There are fairly consistent effects in reducing levels of cannabis and other illicit substance use, though by contrast there is little evidence of any impact on reducing involvement in the use of hard drugs. The latter however is considerably less common in this age group. With regard to methods of working, the strongest support is for the use of social-learning-based or cognitive-behavioural interventions, which also have the clearest support within treatment of alcohol and drug problems amongst adults. There is also support for the use of social-emotional learning methods, and for motivational interventions, and these are sometimes combined within other types of programmes. There is tentative support for the innovative use of text messaging in supporting change.

Two reviews belong in a separate category as they specifically focused on activities provided in schools but outside normal school hours. Schools have many facilities of this kind but not usually focused on violence prevention. This has been tried in several countries, summarized in Table 5.6. Given the more limited availability of studies in this area, and the inconsistent findings reported, it is difficult to draw any firm conclusions from these reviews.

The overall pattern that emerges from the above collection of reviews is a very complex one. Given the volume of material, it is not straightforward to draw simple messages from it. Some findings emerge with reasonable consistency, but they are very often subject to the influence of various moderators and contextual factors.

Some conclusions can however be drawn regarding the factors associated with more successful outcomes, with the proviso that no programme exists that can guarantee success and there is always likely to be a proportion of any target group that is not responsive to an intervention. The features that are most regularly present when better results emerge include the use of a universal or school-wide approach (especially applicable to anti-bullying programmes); the use of active, participatory learning processes rather than didactic sessions; the use of methods that draw on generating cognitive, emotional and attitudinal change; and the acquisition of interpersonal and other behavioural skills. Results from some of the strongest reviews such as those by Cox et al. (2016), Durlak et al. (2011), Jiminéz-Barbero et al. (2012), Sawyer et al. (2015) and Ttofi and Farrington (2011) support these suggestions.

The interventions that have been applied in this area point towards possible opportunities for crime prevention. Some of the best outcomes have been obtained using universal or whole-school approaches, which are further strengthened when families, and in some cases other agencies, are also involved. Multi-agency collaboration involving police forces as partners could strengthen such interventions still further.

## 5.6 Results of the Present Review

This section presents details from the individual empirical studies located for the purposes of the present review. The 116 empirical studies that met all criteria for inclusion in the full review were divided into 5 categories according to the main focus of the intervention (the problem it was designed to address). These were first, interventions to reduce risks of alcohol or other drug abuse (37 studies, Table 5.7); second, anti-bullying programmes (26 studies, Table 5.8); third, interventions to reduce other kinds of aggression, violence or delinquency (26 studies, Table 5.9); fourth, studies of the effects of security, sanctions or disciplinary procedures (16 studies, Table 5.10); and fifth, programmes to reduce dating and other relational violence (11 studies, Table 5.11).

It is important to bear in mind when considering the results that appear in this section that many of the studies described will probably have been subsumed in one (and in some cases more than one) of the reviews listed above. This duplication is unavoidable given the scale of task that would be needed to check that the only studies considered here were the ones that had not appeared in any previous review.

Many different outcome targets or dependent variables are recorded in the studies summarized in the tables above and below. Measured outcomes differ markedly across studies, and most studies reported several kinds of data. They include self-reports, teacher reports or recorded frequencies of bullying and of victimization (which do not always coincide) or of other types of incident; responses on psychological measures of numerous variables including anger, anxiety, self-esteem, hostility, social interaction skills, sense of belonging, empathy, conflict resolution skills and attitudes; measures of school climate; and other indices of the environment or social ecosystem. In the summaries of studies presented in Tables 5.7, 5.8, 5.9, 5.10, and 5.11, space allows only a selection of the variables reported in each study to be described.

Where not specifically stated, studies were carried out in the USA. Full details are not given for each study but all included a mixture of male and female students, usually on a close to 50:50 basis. Most (especially in the USA) included participants from a range of ethnic backgrounds (often forming a majority of study samples).

Several sets of studies included in Table 5.7 are interconnected as they report an evaluation of the same programme with discrete groups or in a variety of settings. For example, there are seven evaluations of the European Drug Addiction Prevention Trial (EU-Dap, linked to the *Unplugged* programme) carried out in different

**Table 5.7** Interventions to reduce risk of alcohol or other substance misuse (37 studies)

| Study | Methodology | Samples/data sources | Intervention and outcomes |
|---|---|---|---|
| Belur et al. (2014) | QE pilot feasibility trial of programme to reduce substance use | 492 pupils in schools 492 in control sample in community | Evaluation of a motivational enhancement and cognitive-behavioural therapies programme (5–7 sessions). Self-report data collected in interviews + data on the nature of settings; control group was drawn from a larger sample but statistically matched with experimental group. At 6-month follow-up, no significant differences were found between groups |
| Bortes et al. (2016) | Single-cohort longitudinal study with subgroup analyses | 518 children aged 13–14 from 5 schools in Sweden | Evaluation of the Swedish government's SMART programme, a project in which children volunteer to enter into a contractual arrangement concerning their avoidance of substance abuse. Data were collected at baseline and 1-year and 2-year follow-ups. Those who had participated in the contracts for a longer period had lower rates of alcohol use, drunkenness and delinquency (theft and criminal damage) at the second (2-year) follow-up |
| Calder and Schulze (2015) | Single-cohort, qualitative case study of a psycho-educational programme | 26 students (grades 10–11) from schools in Pietermaritzburg, South Africa | Exploration of a structured programme *Above the Influence* to prevent substance abuse (seven sessions over 2 months). Based on social cognitive and self-efficacy theory and making extensive use of audio-visual material. The report consists mainly of interview-based analysis of participants' comments on changes in knowledge, self-esteem, family and peer relationships, assertiveness, communication skills and increased resistance to drugs |
| Caria et al. (2011) | Cluster RCT of a school-based substance use prevention programme | 7079 students aged 12–14 from 143 schools in 7 European countries (EU-Dap trial) | Evaluation of a 12-session standardized programme *Unplugged* based on a social influence model, with an 18-month follow-up. Data were self-reports of patterns of alcohol-related behaviour. Results were mixed with a moderate effect size of 0.78 for the primary outcome and alcohol-related problems, but no clear effects for others, notably overall frequency of alcohol consumption |
| Caria et al. (2013) | Secondary analysis of data on how classrooms affected results of Caria et al. (2011) | 3547 students aged 12–14 from 173 classes in 78 schools in 7 European countries (EU-Dap trial) | Secondary evaluation of *Unplugged* data (see previous entry), testing possible relationships between the extent of fidelity of application of the programme and target outcomes (here also including cannabis use). Implementation was affected by class sizes and by the prevalence of substance use at baseline |

(continued)

**Table 5.7** (continued)

| Study | Methodology | Samples/data sources | Intervention and outcomes |
|---|---|---|---|
| Conrod et al. (2013) | Cluster RCT of a programme to prevent alcohol misuse | 1202 high-risk and 1433 low-risk students in 21 London schools (mean age 13.7) | Evaluation of a school-based programme (2 × 90-minute sessions) to reduce alcohol use/misuse amongst youths assessed as at high risk. Risk defined in terms of survey-based personality variables. Reports 24-month outcomes. All groups drank more over time. As compared with high-risk group not given the intervention, participants drank less (−29%) had a lower frequency of binge drinking (−43%) and lower odds of problem drinking (−29%) |
| Dembo et al. (2014) | RCT of a brief intervention to reduce truancy | 180 youths (aged 11–17) referred to a Truancy Centre linked to a county Juvenile Assessment Centre | Evaluation of a brief intervention (BI) programme provided for young people with drug abuse problems truanting from school. Three conditions compared: BI (2 sessions), BI + session with parent and standard service which involved three home visits. Participants had prior arrest records. Follow-up at 3, 6 and 12 months. BI had a lower arrest rate but it fell just short of statistical significance ($p = 0.052$) |
| Espada et al. (2013) | Dismantling[a] QE of a drug use prevention programme | 341 students aged 12–15 from 2 schools in Spain | Evaluation of *Saluda* prevention programme (Espada-Sánchez et al., Table 5.5). Compared three different variants of Saluda with each other and with no-treatment condition. At 12 months' follow-up, the largest effect was in reduced alcohol use for the full version of the programme, but versions without social skills training or problem-solving training also did well. Rates of other substance use were low |
| Estefan et al. (2020) | Cluster RCT of multiple effects: Comprehensive prevention model | 3301 participants from 46 schools, sites assigned to treatment (1662) or control (1639) conditions. The latter was *Safe Dates* standard-of-care programme | Evaluated *Dating Matters* programme designed to promote healthy relationships in teenagers, measuring effects on weapon carrying, alcohol and drug use and delinquent involvement. Data collection twice yearly over 6–eighth grades. Found risk reductions for weapon carrying 9%, alcohol/drug use 9% and delinquency 8%. However, for one cohort of males, no difference emerged as the control condition was also associated with lower risk |
| Faggiano et al. (2013) | Cluster RCT of substance use prevention programme (EU-Dap trial) | Students aged 12–14 from 170 schools in 7 European countries; 7079 pre-test 6604 post-test 5812 at follow-up | Evaluation of the *Unplugged* programme at 18-month follow-up. All substance use increased across the study period but was lower amongst programme participants than amongst controls. Significant differences were found in episodes of drunkenness, frequent drunkenness and frequent cannabis use (respective PORs[b] of 0.80, 0.62 and 0.74) |

(continued)

**Table 5.7** (continued)

| Study | Methodology | Samples/data sources | Intervention and outcomes |
|---|---|---|---|
| Gabrhelik et al. (2012) | RCT of a substance abuse prevention programme | 914 experimental 339 control children from 74 schools in the Czech Republic (mean age 11.38) | Evaluation of the *Unplugged* programme (see Vigna-Taglianti et al.). Data collected at baseline and 1, 3, 12, 15 and 24 months. At wave 6 (24 months) there were no differences in the experimental group for "any drunkenness", but significant reductions for frequent drunkenness, any cannabis use, frequent cannabis use and any other drug use |
| Gianotta et al. (2014) | Cluster RCT of a school-based substance use prevention programme | 6370 students (mean age 13.25) from 143 schools in 7 European countries (EU-Dap trial) | Short-term evaluation of the *Unplugged* social influence programme (12 × 1-hour classroom sessions) after 3 months. Data collected on a range of mediating variables and analysed using multilevel statistics. Treatment group showed positive significant changes in beliefs, knowledge, attitudes and skills related to substance use. There were reported reductions in episodes of drunkenness and in cannabis use |
| Guo et al. (2015) | Cluster RCT of illicit drug use prevention programme | 2091 students (grade 7, mean age 13.4) from 24 schools in Taiwan | Reports pre- and post-test, 6- and 12-month follow-up of data on a multi-modal programme described by Huang et al. (below). Treatment group also received booster sessions. Found a significantly lower rate of illicit drug use as compared to controls at 6 + 12 months but no effect for alcohol consumption. There were significant group differences for all mediating variables (attitudes, intentions and life skills) |
| Guo et al. (2010) | RCT of skills programme to develop drugs resistance | 798 students (mean age 16.43) from 3 schools in Wuhan, China | Evaluation of a multi-modal programme CMER (cognition-motivation-emotional intelligence resistance skills, 6 × 40-minute sessions) designed to help prevent involvement in drug use. Intervention and control groups were well matched at baseline. At 3-month follow-up, there were significant differences in knowledge of drugs, understanding consequences of drug use, motivation to use drugs and skills for peer resistance. There was also a significant difference in reported illegal substance use, though the numbers of users were very small |
| Hall et al. (2013) | RCT of a drug prevention programme stratified by risk levels | 10,762 students (age range 11–12) from 40 schools in Florida | Evaluated the programme *Too Good for Drugs* (TGFD) comprising 10 × 50-minute sessions based on social learning theory and social-emotional learning. Collected data using the *Student Behavior and Risk and Protective Factor Survey*. At 6-month follow-up there was a significantly reduced level of alcohol, of binge drinking and of marijuana use, and there was evidence showing a particular effect in strengthening gains made and skills used by high-risk students within the sample |

(continued)

**Table 5.7** (continued)

| Study | Methodology | Samples/data sources | Intervention and outcomes |
|---|---|---|---|
| Hernández-Serrano et al. (2013) | Dismantling RCT of a drug use prevention programme | 480 students (aged 14–16) from 5 schools in Spain | Evaluation of *Saluda* prevention programme (Espada-Sánchez et al., Table 5.5) with or without different components. Four schools ran different variants of the programme, one acted as waiting-list control. At post-test, alcohol use was lowest for the full programme; the version without the health promotion module performed almost as well. At 6-month follow-up differences were no longer significant |
| Huang et al. (2012) | Pilot RCT of drug prevention programme | 441 adolescents (seventh grade, age 13.1–13.4) from 2 schools in Taiwan | Evaluated a multi-modal programme combining theory of planned behaviour and life skills exercises (10 × 45-minute sessions + homework). Compared this with conventional didactic teaching and control condition. At 24-week follow-up the intervention group showed significantly changed attitudes, subjective norms regarding drugs, planning strategies and life skills, all with medium effect sizes (0.35–0.62), compared to the controls |
| Kiewik et al. (2016) | Cluster RCT of e-learning substance use prevention programme | 210 students (mean age 13.6) from 5 schools in the Netherlands | Evaluation of the efficacy of *Prepared on Time* e-learning programme with a group identified as having mild or borderline intellectual difficulties. Alcohol-related knowledge increased in the intervention group but there was no evidence of behavioural change or in drinking intentions |
| Konishi et al. (2013) | Single-cohort survey sample analysed to evaluate role of school policies in preventing problem substance use | 29,315 pupils from 1760 classes in 461 schools in the British Columbia Adolescent Health Survey, Canada | Analysed whether lesbian/gay/bisexual and heterosexual students had differential outcomes with regard to substance abuse as a function of varying school policies in relation to homophobia, notably Gay-Straight Alliances. Results showed that Gay-Straight Alliances and anti-homophobic bullying policies were linked to lower odds of some (but not all) types of harm from alcohol or substance use amongst lesbian/gay/bisexual girls and also amongst heterosexual children. No such clear association emerged for boys |
| Li et al. (2011) | Longitudinal cohort study with survival analysis[c] | 6864 children from 4-H Study of Positive Youth Development, followed from age 10.97 for 7 years | Examined relationships between indicators of behavioural and emotional engagement in school, measured using a series of self-report items and later rates of substance abuse and delinquent involvement. With other variables controlled, higher levels of school engagement predicted significantly lower likelihood of using substances or committing delinquent acts |

(continued)

**Table 5.7** (continued)

| Study | Methodology | Samples/data sources | Intervention and outcomes |
|---|---|---|---|
| Lisha et al. (2012) | RCT of a drug abuse prevention programme | 1426 youths (age range 14–21, mean 16.8) from 24 schools | Evaluation of *Project Towards No Drug Abuse* programme, 12 × 45-minute sessions. Study with three conditions: TND only, TND + motivational interviewing follow-up and no treatment control. Results (post-test only) showed gains in knowledge, decrease in belief of drug use myths and intention to continue using alcohol, marijuana or hard drugs |
| Malmberg et al. (2014) | Cluster RCT of a substance use prevention programme | 3748 students (aged 11–15) from 21 schools in the Netherlands | Evaluated the *Healthy School and Drugs* programme, comparing e-learning educational component (three sessions per substance), integral version with parent and counselling involvement and no-treatment controls. Outcome targets were alcohol and marijuana use. At 32-month follow-up there were no differences between groups; it was concluded the programme was ineffective |
| Marsiglia et al. (2014) | RCT of alcohol use prevention programme | 432 adolescents (mean age 13) from 10 classrooms in 2 schools in Mexico | Short-term valuation of the *Keepin' It REAL* programme, translated from English but not culturally adapted. Comprises 10 weekly sessions + skills demonstration videos. At post-test, while the control group alcohol use rose significantly, the treatment group did not change. Regression analysis showed that the between-group difference was significant |
| McKay et al. (2014) | Secondary analysis of data from a QE of an alcohol education intervention | 2349 students (mean age 13.76) from 29 schools in Northern Ireland | Analysis of differential effects of the *School Health and Alcohol Harm Reduction Project*. Data collected at baseline, 12, 24 and 32 months. Using baseline data, children were divided into abstainer, supervised and unsupervised drinkers. Compared to controls, the unsupervised group, thought to be at highest risk, also made the largest gains in alcohol knowledge and attitudes |
| Medeiros et al. (2016) | Process evaluation, mixed qualitative methods | 1267 students from 62 classes in 8 schools in Brazil. Also 36 teachers, 11 administrators, 6 coaches, 16 stakeholders | The study was conducted to explore the suitability of the *Unplugged* programme (see Vigna-Taglianti et al.) for use in Brazilian schools. Collected data by questionnaires and focus groups, also recorded fidelity of delivery. It was concluded the programme was suitable for use but required some adaptation to reduce the numbers of activities in sessions |

(continued)

**Table 5.7** (continued)

| Study | Methodology | Samples/data sources | Intervention and outcomes |
|---|---|---|---|
| Midford et al. (2014) | Cluster RCT of school drug education/harm minimization programme | School students (ages 13–14)<br>1163 treatment<br>589 control group<br>In 21 schools in Victoria, Australia | Evaluation of *Drugs Education Victorian Schools*, a ten-lesson programme, focused mainly on alcohol, compared with the usual drug education curriculum which varied between schools. At 9-month follow-up, found a significantly greater increase in knowledge and in communication with parents and a smaller increase in alcohol consumption and in alcohol-related harms, than for the controls, and a decrease in harmful drinking, while for the control group this increased |
| Mogor-Wilson et al. (2017) | QE, pre-post evaluation of a brief substance use prevention programme | 1352 students from 12 schools (mean age 15) | Evaluation of *Refuse, Remove, Reasons,* a five-session programme designed to influence the acceptance of drinking or substance use. This had no effect on students' expectations of drinking alcohol, but did have on those of getting drunk, on the likelihood of using drugs and on acceptance of and perceived negative consequences of using drugs |
| Nieri et al. (2015)[d] | Longitudinal QE of substance use prevention programme | 259 treated 322 untreated students (mean age 11) from 30 schools in Phoenix, Arizona | Secondary analysis of data from a large RCT. Evaluation of the impact of the *Keepin' It REAL* programme on delinquent behaviours of stealing, fighting and weapon use. At post-test there were differences in the percentages of the three behaviours favouring the treatment group, but only one, for using or carrying a weapon, was statistically significant |
| Rohrbach, Gunning, et al. (2010), Rohrbach, Sun, & Sussman, 2010) | RCT of a drug abuse prevention programme | 2983 students (mean age 14.8) from 65 schools in 14 school districts<br>2538 at follow-up | Evaluation of the *Project Towards No Drug Abuse, a* 12 × 45-minute sessions, focused on motivation, skills and decision-making. Evaluation involved three conditions: Comprehensive programme, regular workshop or standard care. The two papers respectively report immediate outcomes and 1-year follow-up. For the former, there were significant improvements on 8/10 of the dependent variables, such as drops in intentions regarding marijuana and hard drug use and in acceptance of pro-drug myths. For the latter, there were no statistically significant effects for most variables. The authors concluded that the effects may be attenuated when a programme is disseminated too widely to diverse groups |

(continued)

**Table 5.7** (continued)

| Study | Methodology | Samples/data sources | Intervention and outcomes |
|---|---|---|---|
| Sanchez, Sanudo, et al. (2016) | QE of a substance abuse prevention programme in Brazil | 2185 students (ages 11–12 and 13–15) from 16 schools in 3 cities in Brazil | Efficacy evaluation of *Unplugged* programme (see Medeiros et al.). Follow-up at 4 months. There was a significant effect in holding back binge drinking amongst 13–15-year-olds and a marginal effect on marijuana use, but no differences amongst 11–12-year-olds |
| Sanchez, Valente, et al. (2016) | RCT of a substance use prevention programme in Brazil, intent-to-treat analysis | Children aged 11–15 from 72 schools: 2030 treatment 2183 control | Second evaluation of the 12-session *Tamojunto* (unplugged) programme to prevent first use of substances. At 9-month follow-up, there was a 30% higher rate of initiation of alcohol use but a 22% lower rate of initiation of inhalant use; no differences were found for tobacco, marijuana or cocaine experimentation. Expressed concerns over the possibility the programme stimulated curiosity about alcohol use |
| Serafini et al. (2016) | Single-cohort, before-and-after trial | 264 adolescents (mean age 16.1, range 14–18) from 7 schools, who had used alcohol or drugs in the last 3 months | Investigated the effect of 8-week, 16-session motivational enhancement intervention based on the trans-theoretical model of change. Outcome data were alcohol and marijuana use and negative consequences. Data collected at pre-test, mid-treatment, post-treatment and 12- and 16-week follow-up. There were large reductions in alcohol use and negative consequences of substance use and a smaller reduction in marijuana use |
| Stewart et al. (2016) | RCT of a motivational interviewing intervention | 244 students (mean age 16.30 but wide range) in high schools in north-West USA | Evaluation of *READY First* project comparing participants with waiting-list control groups who then received the intervention (4 weeks sessions + 4 weeks of check-ins + 2 follow-up appointments, total 16 weeks). Intervention led to larger reductions in marijuana use but both groups reduced alcohol use almost equally, i.e. there was no treatment effect on alcohol |
| Sussman et al. (2012) | Cluster RCT of a drug abuse prevention programme | 1186 youths (age range 14–21, mean 16.8) from 24 schools | Reports further evaluation of *Project Towards No Drug Abuse* programme (see Lisha et al. above). Results at 1-year follow-up showed *Project Towards No Drug Abuse* with or without the motivational component was associated with a significant lowering of proportions of abusers of alcohol and hard drugs, but not marijuana. Results did not generalize to risky sexual behaviours |
| Turham et al. (2016) | QE of modified healthy school and drug intervention | 363 special education students (mean age 13.9) from 13 schools in the Netherlands | Examined whether a pre-existing programme (*Healthy School and Drugs*, 4 x 50-minute sessions) could be adapted for use with students with a variety of types of special needs. Compared those attending the programme with those in usual curriculum. At 5-month follow-up, there was no difference found on any of the measured variables |

(continued)

**Table 5.7** (continued)

| Study | Methodology | Samples/data sources | Intervention and outcomes |
|---|---|---|---|
| Véronneau et al. (2016) | RCT of family check-up model: a "family intervention embedded in schools" | 998 students from 3 schools baseline age 12.2 follow-up age 22 | Long-term evaluations of progress of study participants relative to controls in terms of substance use. The intervention entailed contact with families in supporting children's development, with additional family check-up sessions for high-risk youth with motivational interviewing[e]. the intervention was associated with lower growth of marijuana use than amongst controls. Those who engaged with family check-ups had lower rates of alcohol use or dependence (69.9% vs 94.7%) and of marijuana use or dependence (59.3% vs 84.4%) by age 22 |
| Williams et al. (2014) | QE of a substance abuse programme | 65 pupils in 2 school districts (ages 14–15) | Evaluation of *One-Life* mentoring programme, delivered over a 4-month period in rural schools, based on a social ecology model and involving small groups. The intervention group showed significant reductions in alcohol and inhalant but not marijuana use over a 30-day period, and significantly increased interest in pursuing education |

[a]A type of research in which the objective is to evaluate the relative contribution of each component of a multi-component intervention to its overall effect, sometimes called *component analysis*
[b]POR = prevalence odds ratio, a measure of effect size where 1.00 = no effect
[c]In this analysis, survival means the probability of not becoming involved in substance abuse or delinquency over the ages 11–17; on average this gradually diminishes over time
[d]Although this study focuses on outcomes other than substance misuse, it was included in this table as the intervention was a drug use prevention programme
[e]This was based on the model of the *Drinker's Check-Up* developed by Miller and Rollnick (2002)

countries. Vigna-Taglianti et al. (2014) provide an overview of this programme which was jointly developed by researchers and practitioners in Austria, Belgium, Germany, Greece, Italy, Spain and Sweden. They report reductions at a 15-month follow-up for several types of outcome: any episode of drunkenness −20%, frequent drunkenness −38%, any cannabis use −17% and frequent cannabis use −26%. There were some differential effects by gender. Effects on drunkenness were stronger in schools with lower socio-economic status (SES). Overall, this programme has generated more studies than any other within the timespan of the current review, yielding mainly positive results, but there are also several inconsistent findings, for example, showing impact on some dependent variables but not on others. These evaluations have almost all involved randomized controlled trials.

Other examples include the four studies of the *Towards No Drug Abuse* programme, which has also led to favourable results, and *Saluda*, which has produced some positive but also some inconsistent results, reviewed by Espada-Sánchez and Hernández-Serrano (2015; see Table 5.5). However, findings for the *Keepin' it REAL* intervention are contradictory, and more research would be needed to draw

**Table 5.8** Anti-bullying programmes (26 studies)

| Study | Methodology | Samples/data sources | Intervention and outcomes |
|---|---|---|---|
| Albayrak et al. (2016) | QE of a bullying prevention programme (BPP) | 367 pupils aged 12–15 (grades 6–8) in 2 schools in Istanbul | Evaluation of a programme designed applying behavioural ecology and system models: 1 hour per week for 5 weeks + work with parents and staff. 5-month follow-up. Used self-report scales of bullying and victimization. Found significant reductions in assaults, threats and intimidating behaviour, teasing, attacks on personal belongings and relational aggression in the BPP groups as compared to controls |
| Allen (2010) | Parallel surveys 2 years apart: Non-matched samples | Independent samples at 2 time points: Self-reported victimization N = 874, 817 Self-reported bullying N = 870, 818 | Evaluated a whole-school anti-bullying intervention influenced by ecological-system theory. Reports data on both victimization and bullying. After 2 years, there was no overall change in the reported level of victimization: Some indicators rose but others fell. However, males reported more incidents. Self-reported bullying decreased by 50% or more on all indicators. There was an increase in level of empathy for victims |
| Beckman and Svensson (2015) | Cost-effectiveness evaluation of the Olweus Bullying Prevention Programme | Hypothetical model of a secondary school in Sweden with 300 pupils | Economic evaluation of the Olweus BPP, a whole-school multilevel intervention. Uses Swedish survey data to apply a baseline rate for bullying, then compares costs of providing the programme with savings made when bullying is prevented. Concluded that OBPP is cost-effective, saving €450 per pupil over a 3-year period (grades 7 to 9) |
| Bonell et al. (2015) | Pilot of cluster RCT of method to reduce bullying + other aggression | 1144 students (ages 12–13) 387 teachers from 8 schools in England | Pilot study to examine the feasibility of the *INCLUSIVE* anti-bullying whole-school initiative entailing action groups, using external facilitators to plan and monitor school-level actions, social and emotional skills curriculum |
| Bradshaw et al. (2015) | Preliminary work towards an RCT of a whole-school anti-bullying project | 31 schools in Maryland, planned as the treatment arm of an RCT (total students enrolled: 41,280) | An implementation rather than evaluation of an anti-bullying programme *Positive Behavioral Interventions and Supports*, a systemic approach to promoting a positive school environment which was already evaluated and widely disseminated (22,000 US schools) but not evaluated in a high school. Noted that fidelity of programme delivery was higher in schools with higher levels of bullying |
| Choi et al. (2016) | Qualitative evaluation of views of the capable guardian role in addressing bullying | Semi-structured interviews with 18 school-based police officers reached through snowball sampling | Considers the placement of law enforcement (schools resources) officers as fulfilling the role of "capable guardians" in routine activities theory. Officers interpreted their roles in those terms and perceived their principal task as one of building trust within the school rather than solely use of their authority |

(continued)

**Table 5.8** (continued)

| Study | Methodology | Samples/data sources | Intervention and outcomes |
|---|---|---|---|
| Fekkes et al. (2015) | Cluster RCT of health promotion programme | 1394 students (ages 13–16) from 27 schools in the Netherlands<br>511 at follow-up | Evaluated effect of *Skills for Life* programme on bullying alongside health-related behaviours, including focus on social and emotional learning. Some of original 38 schools dropped out. At 20-month follow-up: Found a positive effect in reducing alcohol consumption, a reduction in reported bullying in the experimental schools, but increase in sexual coercion (though total numbers low) |
| Gradinger et al. (2015) | RCT of programme for prevention of bullying and cyberbullying | 2042 students (mean age 11.7)<br>1377 programme<br>665 control from 18 schools in Vienna | Evaluation of the ViSC social competence programme which contains multiple elements. Data collection on 78 variables. Over 1-year cyberbullying increased in controls but not in the experimental group, cyber-victimization was stable in controls but decreased in the experimental group, and the between-group difference was significant at post-test. Effect sizes were larger than for most other ABPs |
| Kärnä et al. (2011) | Cohort longitudinal study of an anti-bullying programme | 75,984 students (grades 7–9) of Finnish schools | Reports the findings of wide dissemination on the KiVa ABP across grades 1–9 of Finnish schools. KiVa involves analysis of roles involved in bullying, linked to a social learning model. Using lagged time comparisons, the study analysed differences after 1 year with those just commencing the programme. There were significant and positive effects for grades 1–5, but for the upper grades differences between experimental and control groups fell slightly short of significance |
| Kärnä et al. (2013) | Cluster RCT of anti-bullying programme with multilevel regression analysis | 16,503 students (grades 7–9, age range 13–15) from 1000 classes in 73 schools in Finland | Evaluation of the KiVa programme in two age cohorts including secondary school sample. At 12-month follow-up, results were less uniform for grades 7–9 than for primary school groups. However, there were statistically significant results for 5/7 dependent variables, but they were moderated by age and gender. Positive effects found for bullying, victimization, assisting and reinforcing, but not for peer-reported outcomes |
| Masho et al. (2019) | Multiple-baseline design evaluation of external effects of the Olweus Bullying Prevention Programme | 2859 police-recorded incidents of violence involving youths aged 10–18 over a 6-year period in Richmond, VA | Investigated external effects of Olweus Bullying Prevention Programme on rates of violence in low-income neighbourhoods. The programme entails school-level and family intervention components. Analysed relative risk of violence as the Olweus Bullying Prevention Programme was introduced to two schools in sequence with a third acting as control. There were larger decreases in relative risk for the intervention communities than in the control area, with changes linked to the phased arrival of Olweus Bullying Prevention Programme |

(continued)

**Table 5.8** (continued)

| Study | Methodology | Samples/data sources | Intervention and outcomes |
|---|---|---|---|
| Perkins et al. (2011) | Case study experiment involving two anonymous online surveys | 2 surveys: Baseline: 2589 Post-test: 3024 Students (grades 6–8, ages 11–14) from 5 schools in New Jersey | Reports two consecutive surveys of school bullying (perpetration and victimization) and attitudes towards bullying. Results of first survey were fed back to the school to test whether knowledge of the school norms regarding bullying had an impact on reported levels of it in the second survey. 4/5 schools changed in predicted directions in terms of responses to the norms – That is, feedback on their own attitudinal norms influenced their perceptions of the school. However, there were differences between schools in the extent of this |
| Persson et al. (2018) | Cost-effectiveness evaluation of *Kiva* ABP in Sweden | Three classes (est. 75 children) in an elementary school covering ages up to 15/16 | Economic evaluation with outcome variables (a) number of victim-free years of bullying and (b) quality-adjusted life years (QALYs). Assumed a base prevalence of 4% based on national survey data within a 9-year timeframe. Analysis showed that investment in KiVa is cost-effective, but only when applied over more grades of schooling, for 6 or 9 rather than just 3 years |
| Raskauskas (2007) | Quasi-experimental evaluation of the *Kia Kaha* ABP designed by New Zealand police | 3155 students and 67 teachers from 49 schools: 31 experimental, (1572 students) 22 comparison (1583 students) | The *Kia Kaha* whole-school programme was delivered by teachers and police education officers. After 3 years of delivery, Kia Kaha schools reported significantly lower bullying victim rates than comparison (52% vs 62%), and significantly lower self-reported bullying. There were also positive effects on reported school climate + student self-esteem |
| Renshaw and Jimerson (2012) | Pilot QE of a brief universal-level bullying prevention curriculum | 636 students (grades 7 and 8) 320 intervention 316 control From 1 school in California | Pilot evaluation of the *P3R* curriculum, a psycho-educational programme involving film-based resources, with other classroom and community-oriented activities. At post-test there was a significant group main effect indicating improved perceptions of the school's anti-bullying supports and altered and more prosocial attitudes |
| Scheithauer et al. (2012)[a] | Pilot and QE studies (× 3) of an anti-bullying programme | 562 intervention 116 control (ages 11–21) in several schools in Germany | Describes ingredients of the *fairplayer. manual* programme model, designed to raise awareness of bullying, influence attitudes and provide skills training, then summarizes four studies of its effects. Reported results are positive with noticeable declines in reported bullying and victimization and significant increases in prosocial behaviour. But patterns of results varied across classes |

(continued)

**Table 5.8** (continued)

| Study | Methodology | Samples/data sources | Intervention and outcomes |
|---|---|---|---|
| Shriberg et al. (2017) | Qualitative study, action research with interview data | 10 students (seventh grade, 5 m 5f) from 1 school | Exploration of the potential role of developing student leadership in addressing bullying issues, using a sequential model over 10 x 45-minute sessions. The main objective was "the development of student-initiated ideas to address bullying in their school". Ideas included production of videos of role-play scenes of how to deal with bullying, pursuit of fairer discipline practices, representation on school boards, intercom announcements with messages about bullying, online anonymous forum, peer mediation and several others |
| Solomontos-Kountouri et al. (2016) | Longitudinal QE evaluation of an anti-bullying programme | 1752 students (mean age 12.6, grades 7 and 8) from 6 schools in Cyprus | Evaluation of the ViSC programme (see Gradinger), 6 × 90-minute sessions +2-hour parent session, with 3 experimental and 3 control schools. Data collection in three waves. At post-test and follow-up found mixed results: After declines in physical aggression and victimization in grade 7, there were changes of direction for different variables in grade 8 |
| Timmons-Mitchell et al. (2016) | Pilot, single-cohort, before-and-after study of a bullying prevention programme | 113 students (grades 9–12) 88 completers From one high school in mid-western USA | Pilot study of *StandUp*, an online three-session, interactive, skills-training programme, based on the trans-theoretical model of change. For those who completed all sessions, there was evidence of reported increased use of social skills and reduced likelihood of passivity towards bullying, with odds ratios 0.29–0.42. Other results were close to significance, but there was no clear effect for physical bullying perpetration but its prevalence was low |
| Trip et al. (2015) | QE of a bullying prevention programme | 970 students (grade 6) in 35 classes from 11 schools in Romania | Comparison of the *REBE-ViSC* programme, applying rational-emotive behavioural education, with reverse order of presentation (*ViSC-REBE*) and no treatment. At post-test intervention groups showed a larger decrease in low frustration tolerance than the control group, and one group a stronger decrease in expressing anger in aggression. Other differences non-significant |
| Usó et al. (2016) | QE of a peer mediation programme | 323 children (ages 12–14) and 17 teachers from 1 experimental and 1 control school in Spain | Evaluated the effects of peer mediation on bullying, based on an integrated model of conflict resolution. Involves some work in small groups + school-wide awareness. Data collection using questionnaires focused on perceptions of school climate and pro-victim attitudes, at baseline and 6 months later. At post-test the school with mediation showed significantly more pro-victim attitudes and more evidence of a harmonious climate. But missing data make results difficult to interpret |

(continued)

**Table 5.8** (continued)

| Study | Methodology | Samples/data sources | Intervention and outcomes |
|---|---|---|---|
| Vivolo-Kantor et al. (2020) For results on dating violence, see Niolon et al. (2019) in Chap. 4 | Cluster RCT of *Dating Matters* violence prevention programme | Female and male students from 46 schools with elevated risk of violent crime in 4 US states: 1662 treatment 1639 standard *Safe Dates* programme | Developed and evaluated a multi-component programme for youth and parents, to reduce adolescent violence; provided in treatment group schools for 2 years, compared with standard care. Found 11% reduction in reports of bullying perpetration, 9% in physical violence and 5% in both perpetration and victimization via cyberbullying amongst females, but zero effect for bullying and physical violence victimization |
| Williford et al. (2013) | RCT of a multilevel anti-bullying programme | 3351 treatment 4980 control Students (eighth and ninth grades) from 78 schools in Finland | Evaluation of the ABP KiVa (two components of *universal* and *indicated* actions) in its effect on cyberbullying. Study included primary and secondary school cohorts, and results are not reported for separate age groups, but age was used as a correlate in analysing results. KiVa was less effective for older groups in reducing cyberbullying; cyber-victimization decreased as age increased |
| Wong et al. (2011) | QE of whole-school anti-bullying programme | 1480 students (grades 7–9) from 4 schools in Hong Kong | Evaluation of the *Restorative Whole-School Approach*. Compared schools that implemented it fully with those that did so only partially or not at all. Measured physical, verbal, exclusion and extortion bullying. At 2-year follow-up, overall bullying and most types dropped significantly in the *Restorative Whole-School Approach* and partial *Restorative Whole-School Approach* schools, but worsened at other sites, with more mixed changes in other variables |
| Wurf (2012) | QE comparison of anti-bullying interventions | 545 students (grade 7) from 21 classes in 4 international schools in Hong Kong | Evaluation study with 4 conditions: (a) whole-school intervention, (b) curriculum + *Method of Shared Concern*, (c) *Method of Shared Concern* alone and (d) control school. *Method of Shared Concern* provides a model of mediation and conflict resolution. At 7-month follow-up conditions (a) and (b) showed significantly reduced bullying, but (c) and (d) showed small increases; (a) had best effects |
| Yaakub et al. (2010) | QE of Olweus bullying prevention programme | 3816 students from 6 secondary schools in Kuala Lumpur | Evaluated efficacy of the Olweus programme. Results showed a mixed pattern: In 1 of 3 experimental schools, bullying decreased while in the two others it increased; a similar pattern was found in control schools. Effects were moderated by gender. Reported victimization declined in girl's schools but the reverse occurred in co-educational schools. There is no information on trends or effect sizes as no quantitative data are reported |

[a]In part this is a review article, as one of its objectives is to summarize findings of several other studies. However, it was included in this table because (a) all the studies are of one programme, (b) the programme itself and those articles were written by the same group of authors and (c) the article does not employ any of the standard procedures of research review

**Table 5.9** Interventions to reduce other aggression in school (26 studies)

| Study | Methodology | Samples/data sources | Intervention and outcomes |
|---|---|---|---|
| Castillo et al. (2013) | QE study of a structured programme | 590 adolescents from 8 schools in 3 cities in Spain, mean age 13.73 | Evaluation of an intervention *INTEMO* based on an Emotional Intelligence (EI) model: 12 × 1-hour sessions spread over 6 months in each of 2 years +6-month follow-up. EI group showed significant reductions in anger and hostility, and EI group girls showed increases in perspective taking. Only one improvement in controls, other changes nil or negative |
| Cardwell et al. (2019) See also Chap. 6 | RCT of truancy and violence prevention programme, partnership between police and schools | 102 young people with school attendance problems and their parents: 51 experimental 51 control | Evaluation of the *Ability School Engagement Program* designed to reduce truancy and crime in disadvantaged settings, using family group conferences (FGCs). Data collected at 5 points up to 2 years. Created a model of individual and social risk factors to predict progress and outcomes. Results supported the expectation that risk factors for truancy and violence would decrease in the *Ability School Engagement Program* but not the control groups over 2 years |
| Castro-Olivo et al. (2013) | Comparison of two violence prevention programmes | Secondary analysis of data from the California Healthy Kids Survey: 667,610 cases in grades 7, 9 and 11 | Evaluated two programmes from promoting resilience and reducing violence; analysed measures used to collect data in a state-wide school survey. Statistical modelling showed that a comprehensive ecological model was associated with more effective prevention of several types of maladaptive behaviour in children |
| Coker et al. (2017) | Cluster RCT of a bystander programme to reduce sexual violence in high schools | 26 high schools in Kentucky; data collection 5 years 13 experimental 13 control | Evaluated *Green Dot* bystander intervention, a 4-day programme designed to engage those observing an aggressive act to recognize and take actions to prevent it. Outcomes were self-reported perpetration and victimization over 12 months. Intervention was associated with significant reductions in all outcomes except reported victimization in year 4 |
| Crooks et al. (2011) | Secondary analysis of data from a cluster RCT of a violence prevention programme | 1722 students (grade 9) from 20 schools in Ontario, Canada 1520 at follow-up | Tested effectiveness of *Fourth R* programme for children with histories of maltreatment: 21 × 75-minute sessions. At 2-year follow-up there was a significant interaction between condition and number of types of maltreatment in affecting delinquency: The risk of delinquency for those subject to greater maltreatment was lower in the intervention than control condition |
| Dymnicki et al. (2013) | Analysis of moderator effects in an RCT of a violence prevention project | 5256 students (sixth grade) from 37 schools from 4 cities | Analysed one aspect of the results from the multisite violence research project with 1-year follow-up. Measured school climate with a set of 7 scales covering indicators of levels of support and cooperation. It was discovered that the programme's effects were moderated to some extent by the baseline climate in a school, meaning the quality of relationships between principals, staff and students. These influenced support for non-violent norms |

(continued)

**Table 5.9** (continued)

| Study | Methodology | Samples/data sources | Intervention and outcomes |
|---|---|---|---|
| Edwards et al. (2019) | RCT of a bystander programme to reduce several types of school violence | 2403 students, mean age 15.8, 25 high schools in New England: High attrition to 1172 at time 4 | Evaluation of a 7-session classroom-based programme, *Bringing in the Bystander* testing at baseline, post-test, T3 at 98 days and T4 at 424 days on average. Recorded violence, victimization and perpetration, measures of bystander behaviour and readiness, victim empathy and other variables. Results were mixed with only short-lived changes in key outcomes but some marginally significant T4 effects on sexual harassment and stalking |
| Espelage et al. (2013); Espelage, Low, Polanin, and Brown (2015); Espelage, Low, Van Ryzin, and Polanin (2015) | Cluster RCT of *Second Step* programme to reduce aggression | 3658 children aged 11–13 in 36 schools in two American states | Two evaluations of a structured, multi-component social and emotional learning programme of 15 + 13 sessions. At 1-year follow-up found significant reduction in physical aggression only. At 2-year follow-up, found significant intervention effects on only 2/7 outcomes: Homophobic name-calling (56% drop) and sexual violence perpetration (39% drop). No significant effects on bullying or physical aggression variables. At 3-year follow-up no direct effects of intervention were detectable, but there were significant indirect effects on bullying, cyberbullying and homophobic name-calling (but not in sexual harassment) mediated by reductions in delinquency in year 2 |
| Espelage, Rose, and Polanin (2015) | Cluster RCT of *Second Step* programme to reduce aggression | 123 students (aged 11–12) with disability from the larger study sample above) | Separate study to analyse effects of the *Second Step* programme on students with disabilities. Over the 3-year follow-up there was a significant reduction in reported bullying perpetration amongst this group, although not in reported victimization or other aggression |
| Fingar and Jolls (2014) | QE of a media literacy curriculum to prevent violence | 1580 students (6–eighth grades) from 20 schools in California 426 second post-test | Evaluation of *Beyond Blame*, a specially devised curriculum of 10 × 50-minute lessons. Compared three groups, (a) where staff were trained to deliver the curriculum, (b) delivered without training and (c) no-treatment controls. At post-test there were significant changes in beliefs about the impact of media violence and some evidence of effect of reported aggression at second post-test, but involving only a small portion of the initial sample |
| Franco et al. (2016) | RCT of a mindfulness programme (waiting-list control group) | 27 adolescents (mean age 15.85) referred with disruptive classroom behaviour | Evaluation of the usefulness of a mindfulness-based intervention (10 weekly sessions + practice). Results based on psychometric assessments only. Found a significant reduction in impulsivity and in aggressiveness (with large effect sizes) for the experimental group; no significant changes in controls |

(continued)

**Table 5.9** (continued)

| Study | Methodology | Samples/data sources | Intervention and outcomes |
|---|---|---|---|
| Garaigordobil and Martinez-Valderrey (2016) | QE study of a violence prevention programme | 176 adolescents aged 13–15 in a Spanish school | Evaluation of a *Cyberprogram* designed to reduce cyberbullying: 19 x 1-hour sessions. As compared to controls, the programme was associated with a decrease in (a) several types of school violence and (b) premeditated and impulsive aggression, with a medium effect size of 0.57 and a small effect size of 0.37, respectively |
| Goossens et al. (2016) | Cluster RCT of a personality-focused problem prevention programme | 699 students assessed as high risk (mean age 14) from 15 schools in the Netherlands | Reports results of the *Dutch Preventure Trial*, focused mainly on mental health but also including delinquency as an outcome. Entailed 2 × 90-minute workshops but of 4 different types according to personality profiles. Follow-up at 2, 6 and 12 months. Of 24 variables tested, no effects were found for 22. Rate of delinquency very low at baseline. Called into question the knowledge transfer in applying methods developed elsewhere (Canada) |
| Jiminéz-Barbero, Ruiz-Hernández et al. (2016) | RCT of a programme to change attitudes supporting violence | 252 students aged 12–15 (mean age 13.54) from 10 Spanish schools. 180 at post-test | Evaluated the effects of *Count on Me*, a cognitive restructuring programme (5 × 1-hour sessions) designed to reduce attitudes supportive of violence. Most changes were non-significant, but effects on variables *Rejecting* and *Perceived playground violence* were significant, and *Violence perceived as legitimate* fell just short of significance |
| Kliewer et al. (2011) | RCT with three writing conditions: Non-emotional, standard and enhanced | 258 adolescents from 17 classes in 3 schools in a high-violence neighbourhood | Compared the effects of two expressive writing interventions with a control condition with 2- and 6-month follow-up. There were indicators of short-term benefit, including larger effects amongst children with greater exposure to violence, but no significant evidence of change at 6 months |
| Lo et al. (2011) | Multilevel statistical modelling of links between school climate and delinquency | Analysis of data from the Alabama student survey: 92,128 students in grades 6–12 from 577 schools (214 secondary) | Not an intervention study but an investigation of school environmental factors that may be associated with delinquency (carrying a gun, selling drugs, stealing vehicle, assault, being drunk in school). Found that secondary schools had a weaker prosocial climate than other types, and features of schools including physical structure, level of student participation in decisions and the extent to which environments were tailored to age-related needs had associations with delinquency |
| Miller et al. (2015) | Cluster RCT to evaluate a school health centre | 1011 students, ages 14–19, from 11 school health centres (SHCs) | Evaluation of the effects of attending school health centres in reducing abusive relationships amongst adolescents. Results were mixed with no significant impact on recognition of abuse or intentions to intervene, but there were effects of more intensive intervention on self-efficacy and a reduction in reported abuse amongst those who had reported it at baseline |

(continued)

**Table 5.9** (continued)

| Study | Methodology | Samples/data sources | Intervention and outcomes |
|---|---|---|---|
| Multisite Violence Research Project (2013) | Cluster RCT of project to reduce school aggression | 1241 high-risk students from 37 schools in 4 areas + families | Evaluation study with four conditions: Universal classroom-based, selective family-based, both combined or no intervention. Only the second condition produced significant reductions in aggression. Other results were fairly mixed |
| Pfetsch et al. (2011) | QE of an intervention training programme for bystanders | 187: Seventh grade<br>73: Eighth grade pupils from 15 school classes in Luxembourg | Evaluated the impact of a training intervention on the behaviour of witnesses/bystanders in incidents of school aggression. Total of 16–18 hours provided in primary and secondary schools. Measured bystander intentions and levels of victimization reported by pupils and by teachers to 3-month follow-up. Assessed quality of implementation: High levels were associated with significant reductions in pupil-reported victimization |
| Piotrowski (2014) | Cluster RCT of a violence prevention programme | 419 treatment<br>1407 control (11–12-year-olds) from 14 schools in Indiana | Only abstract available. Positive youth development curriculum intervention: 5 × 50-minute sessions +1 assembly session, participatory format. At 12-month follow-up there was a positive impact on violent behaviour, a significant reduction in treatment as compared to the control group ($p < 0.039$) |
| Seçer and Ogelman (2011) | QE of programme to reduce aggression | 30 children aged 14–15 in one school in Turkey | Evaluation of a nine-session social problem-solving programme. Groups were matched on test scores at pre-test. At post-test there was a significant reduction in scores on physical aggression, hostility and indirect aggression. However, there are inconsistencies in the tables in the paper and it is difficult to interpret the results |
| Sevigny and Zhang (2018) | Regression analysis of survey data on school barriers to use of situational crime prevention methods | *School Survey on Crime and Safety* 2008 data from the US Department of Education:<br>996 high schools where violence is classed as a salient threat | The dependent variable was the number of violent incidents occurring in a school in 2007–2008, including rape, attempted rape, robbery actual or threatened attack. Recorded variables on situational crime prevention policies + practice. Found a complex interaction between situational crime prevention policies and outcome variables moderated by "limiting factors": Some situational crime prevention practices (e.g. target hardening) were not diluted by external influences, but others (e.g. controlling access to grounds) were and thus had varied effects |
| Shetgiri et al. (2011) | RCT of a programme to reduce violence and substance use | 55 intervention<br>53 control<br>At-risk students (ninth grade) in 1 high school | Evaluation of a 28 × 45-minute sessions programme (1 per week) with students meeting in groups of 6–9 + facilitator. At-risk students had high absenteeism, discipline problems and evidence of family dysfunction. Data were collected at 4- and 8-month follow-up. No differences were found between intervention and control groups in fighting, drug or alcohol use from baseline to follow-up |

(continued)

**Table 5.9** (continued)

| Study | Methodology | Samples/data sources | Intervention and outcomes |
|---|---|---|---|
| Smokowski et al. (2016) | Investigation of programme dosage effects using statistical modelling | 5894 students in grades 6–8 (mean baseline age 12.78) from 13 schools | Focused on the *Positive Action Program*, designed to decrease problem behaviour and increase positive behaviour in schools; to determine the effects of different dosage levels (time attended). Previous research supports the programme's efficacy. However, there was no consistent or significant association between dosage level and aggression scores |
| Thompkins et al. (2014) | Multisite quasi-experimental design | 1112 children from 13 schools followed over 4 years | Evaluation of the *Violence Prevention Project* (12 × 45-minute sessions) in New York City. Programme participants showed improved academic self-concept, lower reported verbal aggression and antisocial or avoidant conflict resolution strategies, as compared with control participants |
| Webb and Martin (2012) | QE of a media literacy-based violence prevention programme | 2209 students (6–eighth grade) from 21 schools in California 1693 at post-test | Evaluation of *Beyond Blame*, a specially devised curriculum of 10 × 50-minute lessons. Compared three groups, (a) where staff were trained to deliver the curriculum, (b) delivered without training (c) no treatment controls. Groups (a) + (c) increased knowledge of the effects of media violence at post-test, largest for group (a) |

any conclusions with confidence. By contrast the two studies of the *Healthy School and Drugs* intervention did not find any significant benefits, and it may be that this programme is too brief to secure a meaningful impact. There are other single studies of programmes showing positive outcomes, for example, the results of the *Too Good for Drugs* trial by Hall et al. (2013), which also have strong effects in boosting protective factors amongst students assessed as high risk.

A recurrent difficulty is that several studies demonstrate short-term effects with mediating variables such as knowledge of substances, reported attitudes to them or rejection of drug myths, but provide little or no information on actual drug use. In addition, there are few studies with sufficiently long follow-ups to draw conclusions about the durability of changes, especially given evidence that most forms of substance use become gradually more frequent as the teenage years progress. In summary however, there is enough encouraging information here to suggest that provision of suitable interventions in schools can be shown to have effects in reducing alcohol and other substance abuse.

Tables 5.8 and 5.9 focus on studies of interventions designed to reduce aggression, first in its particular manifestation as school bullying and then in more varied forms. Regarding the former, studies such as that of Doğan et al. (2017), an evaluation of the Viennese Social Competence (ViSC) programme, the first evidence-based ABP to be provided in Turkey, involving 26 classes from 6 schools, were excluded as the participating children were aged 10; and ViSC was initially developed for use within the younger age ranges. Similarly a study by Lam et al. (2018)

of the *Be Safe* programme in Sri Lanka was excluded from Table 5.9 as children were aged 5–9 years.

For similar reasons (restriction to elementary school) a study by Salimi et al. (2020) was excluded. This contained a key salutary lesson. The authors reported a mixed-methods evaluation of *Iranian Health Promoting Schools* (IHPS) framework, devised to address the problem of bullying. This was an ambitious study with a cross-sectional component involving 900 students, 104 staff and 563 parents and a qualitative component with 24 policy makers. However, there were major problems of implementation of the IHPS policy, with weak coordination between stakeholder agencies, insufficient training for staff and poor levels of support for the delivery process. No differences were found in bullying between IHPS and non-IHPS schools, drawing attention to the difficulties that arise when seemingly sound ideas are not supported in practice.

Considering the trends found in the review studies summarized earlier (Table 5.2), where despite some inconsistencies there were several positive sets of findings, we would expect to see that pattern consolidated. This is difficult to discern to some extent because several of the reports included here are pilot studies only, and others are implementation trials, to test if a programme is usable and deliverable rather than to investigate its impact. Some of the studies in Table 5.8 do report very positive findings, but, overall, there was a mixed pattern of results and relatively fewer RCTs than were found in the drugs and alcohol research. There were three evaluations of the *ViSC* programme which produced some positive but also some less consistent results. More promising studies were found of the already widely used *KiVa* programme, developed in Finland but employed in several other countries. To date, this had been evaluated mainly with primary school samples, but the review located some studies done with secondary school groups, with mainly positive results, but moderated by other variables including gender. Finding smaller effects for teenage as compared to middle-childhood samples is not uncommon in bullying research.

One of the most striking results is that reported by Masho et al. (2019) of the OBPP using a relatively uncommon type of experimental design. "Our findings provide support for the premise that a school-based prevention program has the potential to reduce community-level rates of serious incidents of youth violence in the attendance zone served by the school" (p. 527). These patterns are sometimes known as *spillover* effects.

Studies in adjacent areas show it is possible to reduce the likelihood of both violence and alcohol misuse amongst adolescents. This has an obvious bearing on whether young people may act aggressively in school. For example, an RCT by Walton et al. (2010) reported a reduction of violence and alcohol misuse amongst young people aged 14–18 after only a quite brief intervention. However, as the work was undertaken in a clinical setting (a hospital emergency department), in accordance with inclusion and exclusion criteria, this study was not retained for review. However, 26 studies were located of evaluations of interventions to reduce various forms of school aggression (some with other objectives in addition). They are summarized in Table 5.9.

Amongst intervention studies, a sizeable number found positive effects of programmes of several types. There were a few where no positive outcomes were observed, and results with minimal effects or ones that were complex due to the number of moderator variables operating. However, the studies by Castro-Olivo et al. (2013), Crooks et al. (2011), Franco et al. (2016), Garaigordobil and Martinez-Valderrey (2016), Pfetsch et al. (2011), Piotrowski (2014), Thompkins et al. (2014) and Webb and Martin (2012) have all reported predominantly favourable outcomes.

The next set of studies to be discussed centres on other kinds of organizational strategies schools might employ in efforts to reduce problem behaviour. They focus more on the atmosphere of strictness or permissiveness that prevails in a school or on the nature of security, discipline or other measures taken to ensure student and staff safety. In some cases, these have involved direct involvement of police.

Moving forward, several of the studies described in Table 5.10 are not direct tests of planned interventions. Instead, they were designed to test hypotheses about the relationships between various aspects of school environments or climates and rates of aggression. That is, they analyse the relationships between independent variables at different levels and test the relationships between them and an outcome or dependent variable, usually levels of violence or other antisocial behaviour within a school. A few use a form of statistical analysis, multilevel modelling which makes it possible to compare the relative power of variables such as features of pupils/students, of teachers and of the school itself in predicting the dependent variable. With large samples, it is also possible to estimate the effect of each variable separately from the others or of different variables in combination.

That applies to studies of *School Resources Officers* (SROs), sworn police officers placed inside schools, a role that came to prominence from the 1990s onwards in the USA but has since been adopted in other countries. Prior to that period this had been uncommon, but reported increases in disorder, and the horror of shooting massacres led to a far greater emphasis on preserving safety (Brown, 2006). By the year 2000 it was estimated there were over 17,000 sworn police officers in such roles, and school authorities directly employed more than 3200 (Brown, 2006). These are distinct from the post of Schools Liaison Officer in the UK, which has more of a social welfare than law enforcement function.

Fisher and Hennessey (2015) reported a meta-analysis of ten effects from seven reports of the association between the presence of SROs on school campuses and the use of school exclusion as a disciplinary measure. Their review was not directly concerned with impacts on school violence but was an attempt to test competing expectations of the effects of the officers on other aspects of a school's operation. One view is that SROs function as guardians in reducing crime opportunities. Another is that they have a criminalizing effect by mirroring the wider law-and-order environment. The main analysis yielded more support for the latter view, but it was difficult to exclude the possible roles of other, moderator variables in this. Concerns have been expressed that the presence of SROs might contribute to a process whereby disruptive teenagers would be labelled in a first stage of their entry into a life of crime, in figurative terms forming a "school-to-prison pipeline".

The number of relevant studies here is more modest; therefore, conclusions are necessarily more tentative than was possible in areas discussed earlier. While there are some exceptions, the general trend of the results of studies reviewed in Table 5.10 is towards the near absence of intended effects of formal controls, punitive sanctions and enhanced security measures in reducing rates of aggression or other forms of misconduct in school. The presence of police staff in school security roles often appears to have an almost counter-productive effect. That may be a result of the additional scrutiny identifying larger numbers of rule violations, or potentially of heightened tensions amongst a proportion of youth who resent the proximity of authority. In some locations such as Greater Manchester there has been resistance to the placement of police officers, called safety officers, in schools (Connelly et al., 2020).

In several respects, the studies included in Table 5.10 have the closest relevance to policing as it has traditionally been practised, given that such posts are usually held by qualified police officers. There are differences however in the responsibilities involved, for example, between School Liaison Officers in the UK (Trotman & Thomas, 2016) and SROs in the USA (Bolger et al., 2019; Devlin & Gottfredson, 2018) or in Korea (Han & Connell, 2020). However, the specifications of the role may vary considerably (Lamont et al., 2011); the demands and function reportedly differ according to the level of social and educational disadvantage in schools (Lynch et al., 2016); and the work may require specialized training provision (Martinez-Prather et al., 2016).

Apart from bullying which has received considerable attention and was one of the first forms of interpersonal aggression or coercion to be investigated in schools, the other category of antisocial behaviour that has been a specific focus of research is relational aggression including harassment and dating violence. Eleven studies testing interventions to address this were located and are summarized in Table 5.11.

**Table 5.10** Effects of sanctions, school climate and security measures (16 studies)

| Study | Methodology | Samples/data sources | Intervention and outcomes |
|---|---|---|---|
| Bolger et al. (2019) | Survey on the influence of training on school police officer decisions | 179 school police officers, recorded responses to three hypothetical vignettes of student misbehaviour | Compared the effects of different training levels and models on police officers' use of discretion in school disciplinary decisions. The dependent variable was officers' decisions on how to respond to each of three scenarios. Results were at odds with the formal training advice given, with no difference related to trained/untrained status. The findings called the value of training for the role into question |
| Crawford and Burns (2015, 2016) | Regression analysis of survey data on associations of school security measures with violence levels | *School Survey on Crime and Safety* 2006 data from the US Department of Education: 2724 responses: 758 high schools | Examined different forms of security including controlled doors, cameras, metal detectors, specially trained teachers, school resources officers and incident policies. Dependent variables were reports of different forms of serious violence and were linked to some school variables. In high schools, the presence of security guards was associated with increased numbers of weapon attacks and cases of gun possession. Results counter to expectations |

(continued)

**Table 5.10** (continued)

| Study | Methodology | Samples/data sources | Intervention and outcomes |
|---|---|---|---|
| Devlin and Gottfredson (2018) | Comparison of schools with and without resource officers and with different SRO roles | *School Survey on Crime and Safety* (SSOCS) 2006 data from the US Department of education: Years 2003–2008, 480 schools | Tested hypotheses about whether the presence of Schools Resources Officers (SROs)[a] and whether they had teaching roles influenced the recording and reporting of school-based crimes of different types. SRO presence was associated with more reporting of all categories of crime |
| Gerlinger and Wo (2016) | Survey data analysed by statistical modelling (logistic regression) | Data from US national school survey: $n = 23{,}974$ in four cohorts 2005, 2007, 2009, 2011 | Compared the relative effects of deterrence (security measures) and of authoritative[b] school climate on rates of bullying victimization amongst 12–18-year-olds. Analysis showed that while security measures were associated with lower victimization rates, there were larger effects for authoritative approaches |
| Han and Connell (2020) | Effects of introducing Korean School Police Officers on school violence | Regression analysis of data from the 2014 *Korean Youth Victimization Survey* | Investigated associations between the presence of Korean School Police Officers (independent variable) and in-school violence, reported victimization and fear of school crime (dependent variables). Rates of all crimes were reported as low. The Korean school police officers' presence had no association with a lower fear of crime overall, but a higher rate of reporting delinquent property acts. It had no association with any type of victimization. Other school factors (e.g. level of disorder, attachment to teachers) had larger associations with several outcome variables |
| Hemphill et al. (2013) | Longitudinal study, two time points, logistic regression | 3677 students, grades 7 and 9 from 60 schools, USA and Australia | Investigated whether school suspension affects self-reported non-violent antisocial behaviour. No association was found between suspension and non-violent antisocial behaviour separately from other risk factors. Earlier work by the same authors had found suspension increased the likelihood of violence and non-violent antisocial behaviour |
| Jennings et al. (2011) | Regression analysis of survey data on associations of school security measures to violence levels | *School Survey on Crime and Safety* (SSOCS) 2006 data from the US Department of education: 954 high schools | Independent variables in five groups: Security enforcement, school security measures, level of coordination with external agencies, school characteristics and school demographics. Dependent variables were reported rates of violence and serious violence. There were higher levels of violence in schools where security guards were armed, but lower levels where they wore uniform. Numbers of guards were positively linked to higher levels of serious violence, but the number of SROs were linked to lower levels |

(continued)

**Table 5.10** (continued)

| Study | Methodology | Samples/data sources | Intervention and outcomes |
|---|---|---|---|
| Maimon et al. (2012) | Survey data and multivariate statistical modelling | $N = 7660$ in 119 schools data from the US National Longitudinal Study of Adolescent Health survey | Investigated the role of school sanctions in preventing school misconduct and adolescent violent offending. Tested the relationship between the school sanctioning climate, pupil engagement in "thoughtfully relevant decision-making" and violent behaviour. School sanctions were of five types: Verbal warning, minor action, school suspension, home suspension and expulsion. Most schools were found to use sanctions "at the harsher end" of the continuum. Thoughtfully relevant decision-making was more likely to operate in schools with less harsh sanctions: Stricter regimes "disarmed" the process of cognitive reflection. Harsher sanctions had no effect in reducing violence. Activating thoughtfully relevant decision-making had a significant effect |
| Martinez-Prather et al. (2016) | Qualitative evaluation of training for school-based law enforcement officers | Semi-structured interviews with a convenience sample of 26 school-based law enforcements from 11 Texas police departments | Investigated a dilemma between the role of SBLEs as preserving safety on school campuses and the risk of criminalizing pupil misconduct. 62% stated they needed specialized training for the role. 39% had no training, and 15% did on-the-job training. Roles were varied and often not clearly defined. School-based law enforcement used counselling (58%), legal intervention (54%) and referral for disciplinary procedures (27%) in response to incidents. Lower training level was associated with likelier use of legal intervention |
| McDevitt and Panniello (2005) | Analysis of survey data on perceptions of SROs and influence on crime reporting | 907 students from schools in 4 districts in different parts of the USA | Investigated which factors were associated with students' level of comfort in reporting crimes to the SRO. The main influences were positive perceptions of the SRO and general feelings of safety in school, which were influenced by victimization and crime rates in the neighbourhood. Suggested SROs should find ways to promote a positive image |
| Na and Gottfredson (2013) | Correlational and longitudinal analysis of large-scale survey data | Data from >3000 schools (all tiers), in the School Survey on Crime and Safety, USA | Examined the effect of SROs on the levels of crime in schools. Found no evidence that SROs contributed to school safety and their presence did not lead to reductions in crime; on the contrary reported rates of non-serious crimes rose |
| Swartz et al. (2016) | Regression modelling with large dataset | Data from 1699 schools (all tiers), in the School Survey on Crime and Safety, USA | Examined the effect of SROs on the numbers of serious violent acts in schools. Used statistical correction (propensity score matching) to take account of other variables. The presence of SROs was associated with an increase in the rate of reporting of serious violent acts. The effect held with other key variables controlled |

(continued)

**Table 5.10** (continued)

| Study | Methodology | Samples/data sources | Intervention and outcomes |
|---|---|---|---|
| Theriot and Orme (2016) | Analysis of survey data on perceptions of SROs and feelings of safety | Interviews with 1126 middle and 830 high school students from 12 schools in one district | Statistical analysis led to the identification of two student groups, one (61%) predominantly feeling safe, the other (39%) unsafe (in relative terms). Those in the former were less likely to have experienced violence at school, had more feelings of connectedness with school and were less likely to be African-American. The amount of interaction with the SRO was not predictive of students' feelings of safety |
| Tillyer et al. (2011) | Large single-cohort study with multilevel modelling, hierarchical logistic regression | 2644 pupils aged 12–13 in 58 Kentucky schools | Tested the effects on violent victimization and fear of violence of reducing crime opportunities in schools, using measures such as police involvement, metal detectors, locker checks and banning backpacks. While some individual-level variables were associated with the target outcomes, prevention practices did not significantly reduce the likelihood of violent victimization, perceptions of risk or fear |
| Trotman and Thomas (2016) | Qualitative study of pilot training for school Liaison officers | Focus group and interview study in secondary schools in West Midlands, UK | Evaluation of joint police-school project after induction process involving 2-day training in liaison roles, mentoring and coaching processes and a small-scale research project. Illustrates the possibility of altering negative concerns about surveillance, by building trust and incorporating a police liaison role into the standard working of schools |
| Waddell (2012) | Large single-cohort study analysed using instrumental variables | Data from Add Health: 80 high schools, 12,642 participants | Tested the effect of school sanctions on self-reported marijuana use amongst 9–12th grade students. Found that a policy of expulsion for second-time offenders was associated with lower reported use |

[a]These are specially created roles with a responsibility for maintaining security and keeping order in a school. Some SROs are police officers who may also have other duties. Others, usually employed by local police authorities, have powers of arrest but are not fully qualified police officers
[b]Defined as an ethos combining two features, *structure*, the consistent and fair enforcement of rules, and *support*, the provision of care and attention by adults (Gregory et al., 2010)

**Table 5.11** Interventions to reduce gender, dating and other relationship violence (11 studies)

| Study | Methodology | Samples/data sources | Intervention and outcomes |
|---|---|---|---|
| Bowen et al. (2014) | Qualitative study of a programme implementation | 13 children aged 13–15 in 3 focus groups in UK schools | Evaluation of how an online game-based programme (*Green Acres High*) specially devised for working with adolescents on dating violence was received by potential participants. Identified themes included emphasis on the importance of experiential learning as contrasted with traditional teaching and the acceptability of using a structured game format as a method of approaching sensitive issues |

(continued)

**Table 5.11** (continued)

| Study | Methodology | Samples/data sources | Intervention and outcomes |
|---|---|---|---|
| Coker et al. (2017) | Cluster RCT of a bystander programme to reduce sexual violence in high schools | 26 high schools in Kentucky:<br>13 experimental<br>13 control<br>Data collection over 5 years | Evaluated *Green Dot* bystander intervention, a 4-day programme designed to engage those observing an aggressive act to recognize and take actions to prevent it. Outcomes were self-reported perpetration and victimization over 4 × 12 months. Intervention was associated with significant reductions in all outcomes except reported victimization in year 4 |
| Gonzalez-Guarda et al. (2015) | RCT of a dating violence prevention programme, *JOVEN* | 82 student-parent dyads; students aged 13–16, female and male, from one school in Florida | Evaluated a programme designed for Cuban-American adolescents: Six groups for children, two for parents and two for school staff. Psycho-education and skill-building exercises. Employed intent-to-treat[a] analysis. Found medium effect sizes on partner victimization and perpetration in both groups for females, but a medium size treatment effect for the programme group only for males. At 12-month follow-up gains were maintained amongst males only |
| Kearney et al. (2016) | Multi-method evaluation of a whole-school violence prevention project | 1587 students (grades 8 and 9)<br>740 staff from 19 schools in Victoria, Australia | Evaluation of the delivery of *Respectful Relationships Education*, a curriculum designed to prevent gender-based violence. Staff and student surveys were complemented with focus groups and audit information. The main objective of this study was to illustrate the integral role of evaluation in project implementation |
| Meiksin et al. (2019, 2020) | Pilot cluster- RCT and process evaluation of *Project Respect* programme | 6 secondary schools:<br>4 intervention<br>2 control | Envisaged as an evaluation of a whole-school relationships and sex education programme. The process aspect focused on fidelity of implementation. However, following process evaluation it was concluded that the research should not proceed to the next phase. It was found that the delivery of the programme as planned was not feasible as part of the school curriculum, without a longer preparatory phase and more commitment from senior staff. The findings underline the importance of allotting sufficient time to process and delivery issues |
| Muñoz-Fernández et al. (2019) See also Chap. 4 | RCT of *Dat-e Adolescence* violence prevention programme | 1423 teenagers aged 11–19 from 7 schools in Seville or Córdoba, Spain | Evaluation of efficacy of a school-based dating aggression intervention programme. Collected pre- and post-test +6-month follow-up data. Bullying perpetration and victimization were assessed using the European Bullying Intervention Project Questionnaire. No effect was found for reported aggression, but for bullying victimization there was a significant decrease in the treatment group's growth trajectory, compared with the controls, with a large effect size ($d = 0.98$) |

(continued)

**Table 5.11** (continued)

| Study | Methodology | Samples/data sources | Intervention and outcomes |
|---|---|---|---|
| Sinclair et al. (2014) | Single-cohort before-and-after study | 1250 boys from 5 slum areas of Kenya, 1086 at post-test and 889 at follow-up | Only abstract available. Evaluated the impact of a curriculum (6 × 2-hour sessions) to raise awareness of gender-based violence. Measures used at the start and end of programme and after 6 months. There was a significant improvement in attitudes to gender violence and at post-test sustained at follow-up and a reduction in negative sexual stereotypes |
| Sosa-Rubi et al. (2016) | Pilot quasi-experimental trial of a school-based programme | Children (age range 15–16) from 2 low-income schools in Mexico City: 381 classroom + climate elements 540 climate elements only | Short-term evaluation of *True Love*, designed to reduce relational aggression, with 16-week individual/classroom-based and school climate components, evaluated separately and in combination. Found significant reduction in perpetrated (58%) and experienced (58%) violence amongst males in the combined programme condition, and smaller but still significant reductions in attitudes and beliefs concerning violence |
| Splett et al. (2015) | RCT of a programme to reduce relational aggression | 30 females aged 12–15 | Evaluation of growing interpersonal relationships through learning and systemic supports, a 10-week group school counselling programme, linked to parent training and support. Intervention group showed a significantly reduced rate of relational aggression at post-test; no change in control group. Data were based on counsellor and teacher reports but observations were not blinded |
| Taylor et al. (2011) | RCT of a programme to reduce gender-based violence | 764 students in 16 schools in KwaZulu-Natal, South Africa | Only abstract available. Provision of the programme was linked to avoidance of HIV in a high-risk infection area. 16 modules, 8-month follow-up. Intervention groups were three times less likely to be forced to have sex |
| Taylor et al. (2015) | RCT of dating violence prevention programme | 2655 students in 117 classes in 6–seventh grades from 30 schools in new York City | Evaluation of *Shifting Boundaries* teen dating programme for reducing violence/harassment. Measures pre- and post-test and at 6 months. Significant reductions were found in frequency of sexual harassment perpetration and victimization, and of dating violence, reported by both boys and girls |

[a]In ITT analysis data are analysed for all participants regardless of whether they completed treatment, or dropped out, or moved between study conditions, as compared to a *treatment received* or *per protocol* analysis, in which data are analysed only for those who remained in assigned groups

Table 5.11 shows a smaller number of studies than that available for other areas considered in the review; therefore, interpretations are necessarily more tentative. Three of the studies summarized are accounts of implementation rather than evaluations as such. Of the remaining eight, all found some positive results of interventions. Clearly that is an encouraging trend, but as has been found in other areas, the outcome variables are sometimes attitudinal or perceptual or are reliant on participants' self-reports. Given that six of those studies were based on randomized designs, this is still a demonstration of a valuable effect, and in some studies this is confirmed by reports of actual behaviour or of events.

## 5.7 Discussion

The problems discussed in this report are ubiquitous in their occurrence. School bullying, relational aggression and involvement to varying degrees in under-age drinking or other substance abuse may be examples of short-lived or *adolescence time-limited* rule-breaking, but in a proportion of cases may be precursors of adult, *life-course-persistent* criminality. The terms come from the work of Moffitt (1993, 2003) who introduced and researched these distinctions. Similar patterns appear in many societies, and the research assembled here attests to this. The studies summarized in Tables 5.7, 5.8, 5.9, 5.10, and 5.11 originated from 23 countries. The largest single group comes from the USA but there are also reports of research carried out in Australia, Austria, Brazil, Canada, China, Cyprus, Czech Republic, Finland, Germany, Hong Kong, Kenya, Luxembourg, Malaysia, Mexico, the Netherlands, Romania, South Africa, Spain, Sweden, Taiwan, Turkey and the UK.

### *5.7.1 Strengths and Limitations of the Research*

The volume of research in this field is substantial relative to the wider study of social problems and the rate of publication is fairly high. That may explain the quite large number of reviews found even in the period of a few years covered here – and there were many more prior to 2010. The quantity in itself is a strength as it means there is a larger body of evidence available to test propositions and judge the viability of different approaches to addressing the target problems.

A second strength is that many studies have very large sample sizes, often in the hundreds and sometimes in the tens of thousands. Occasionally, entire school systems have been involved in the evaluation of a method forwarded to prevent bullying or reduce adolescent substance use. While there are smaller-scale studies and also some case reports, alongside qualitative studies of process these also play a part in developing a clearer picture of what is most likely to work in different contexts, and why. There is unlikely to be a single solution in the form of a general prevention programme that will be equally effective wherever it is used, as studies here already show poorer results when an initiative is transferred from its original location to one that differs from it in some crucial respects.

A third advantage is the extensive use of experimental or quasi-experimental designs. Amongst the 43 relevant review articles collated in Tables 5.2, 5.3, 5.4, 5.5, and 5.6, many located a high proportion of RCTs, and some focused exclusively on them. Of the 94 studies retained in the review itself in Tables 5.7, 5.8, 5.9, 5.10, and 5.11, 42 were RCTs, including some that were cluster RCTs in which schools, not students, were randomly assigned to either experimental or control conditions (or other comparators). A further 23 were QEs or were based on secondary analysis of data from them. Nine of the reports reviewed were not intervention/outcome studies, instead using survey data or statistical modelling to test relationships between school variables and rates of problem behaviour, and four were qualitative process or implementation studies. Overall, within intervention studies therefore, 80% had reasonably sound designs with equivalent or non-equivalent comparison samples.

However, the reviewed studies inevitably also show some limitations. As found when addressing related questions in adjoining fields, even where the total number of available studies is large, there are often discrepancies in the number of studies on any specific question. Hence, there are issues, such as prevention of relational violence, that have received less attention and far more research is required before we can be confident about any patterns that seem to be emerging.

Notwithstanding the previous comments about research design, the use of randomization in school-based studies also contains internal weaknesses. Research in human service settings cannot be conducted blind as usually done in medical trials as the activity itself makes it obvious to which group an individual or school has been assigned. That in turn can create what are known as *demand characteristics* through which participants are inadvertently influenced by their interpretations of what researchers are looking for. These and other factors can introduce biases in research, making results especially difficult to comprehend when (as is often the case) they produce complex patterns of interactions.

### 5.7.2 Limitations of This Review

It is important to note some features of the present review itself. Although a large number of prior reviews and empirical studies have been summarized within it, it also has some internal limitations.

First, all the decisions made with regard to screening and selection, assigning studies to categories and extracting information to be presented in tables, were made by one author and it would be preferable if at least a proportion of those decisions could be subject to ratification by a second researcher and any resultant discrepancies resolved.

Second, due to time limitations given the volume of material located, the retained studies have not been subject to a quality appraisal process as regards their methodological quality or scientific robustness. There are several methods of achieving this and ideally that work too should also be validated by a second rater. The basic types of research design employed in each study have been recorded, but that information alone is not always sufficient to judge the quality of a piece of research and whether it is potentially subject to biases.

Third, more details of each study could be extracted for insertion in Tables 5.7, 5.8, 5.9, 5.10, and 5.11. It is recognized that amassing very large amounts of information can also make material difficult to access; therefore, all the studies reviewed are available in pdf form and can be transferred in files for the use of readers of this document who require more details of any specific study.

Fourth, also as a result of the numbers of studies located, only research focusing on children aged 11 and upwards was retained for full review. Some designers and evaluators of school-based prevention suggest that work of this kind ideally should begin before that age, in primary school. As shown earlier in Fig. 5.1, numerous studies were found that focus on research in those settings, which therefore needs to be reviewed separately. Also, given the (relatively) speedy pace of publication in this field, even within 1 year there will be numerous additional studies to review.

Finally, as a further step in integrating the findings of the studies examined, it would be advantageous to employ meta-analysis for each of the separate sets of studies reviewed. This might clarify some of the issues on which findings are not wholly consistent. The strength of different factors influencing the success or failure of different interventions could be quantified using meta-regression.

## 5.8 Conclusions

Drawing together the findings of this review, there are several conclusions that can be drawn with reasonable confidence. The key conclusion is that there is ample, indeed abundant, evidence that it is possible to reduce rates of bullying perpetration and victimization amongst school students. There is also evidence that other kinds of aggression and violence can be reduced, including relational and dating violence which may be a forerunner of intimate partner violence in longer-term relationships. In addition, it is possible to reduce young people's involvement in alcohol and other substance abuse, or at the very least to slow down the speed with which they might otherwise take them up, in the face of their own urges and the powerful influences on them to become involved in this.

A second major conclusion is that before embarking on any project in this area, it is crucial to take into account the findings of research review and use them as a template for assessing ready-made intervention packages, many of which are branded within a commercial marketplace. That is not a criticism of them, as some have track records of success, but rather a recommendation that any decision to work in a particular way should be informed by relevant findings of research.

### *5.8.1 Summary of the Best-Supported Interventions*

A third conclusion concerns what can be said about the interventions most likely to accomplish their planned objectives in this area. As already noted, there are several examples of programme that appear to have worked well in the context in which they were originally devised, but which are less successful when transported to another setting. This is a salutary lesson when making decisions on whether or not to adopt a programme that has been piloted or tested elsewhere: detailed thought needs to be given to how it could and should be adapted to local contexts.

It was not considered useful and it would have required additional time for this report to include a comparative list of the advantages and disadvantages of all the anti-bullying or drug abuse prevention programmes that have been tested in research. Only a few have been evaluated in two or more studies. But if features of programmes can be compared, it should be possible to identify the most likely combination of ingredients that can maximize the chances of success. Programmes such as *Unplugged* and *KiVa* are probably the ones best supported by several pieces of research, but there are also some inconsistent findings for them so it is difficult simply to endorse them as treatments of choice to the exclusion of other possible options.

Rather than selecting an intervention from the range currently available, another direction to take is to draw up a list of criteria for effective interventions. Which types of intervention are best supported in terms of the size of the effects they produce and in the consistency with which they do so? Regrettably there is no clear-cut answer to this given the complexity and sometimes contradictory nature of the results that emerge. However, for prevention of bullying, for example, the conclusions drawn by Ttofi and Farrington (2011, p. 41) are a useful summary that is also applicable to the studies reviewed here: "The most important program elements that were associated with a decrease in bullying were parent training/meetings, improved playground supervision, disciplinary methods, classroom management, teacher training, classroom rules, a whole school anti-bullying policy, school conferences, information for parents, and cooperative group work. In addition, the total number of elements and the duration and intensity of the program for teachers and children were significantly associated with a decrease in bullying". Similar features were found in relation to victimization.

In terms of methods of change, the likelihood of success appears to increase when the following three principles are applied. One is the use of a social influence perspective. In relation to bullying this is likely to be based on recognizing the pressures operating on the roles of bully, victim and bystander. A similar approach can be applied to other conflict resolution and to relational aggression. The second is emphasizing social norms both of the school and the wider community and reinforcing them in a consistent way. While it is crucial that schools promote awareness of rules and norms and have disciplinary responses to violations of them, that is best done within a positive and supportive school climate. The third is employing methods of teaching or training that enhance competence, develop self-management and strengthen interpersonal skills.

For interventions designed to reduce alcohol or other substance use, several quality criteria were identified some time ago by Cuijpers (2002) for drug use prevention programmes, and most of them are sustained by the current findings. The more successful interventions are the ones which employ an interactive delivery method, make use of social influence processes, focus on social norms and are connected to broader community interventions, including links to families. Effective interventions include exercises for development of life skills in structured sessions or programmes. Most of these interventions can be delivered on a group basis, within the wider context of a whole-school approach, but motivational enhancement interventions work better when provided on an individual basis.

If any work along such lines is to be undertaken, and intervention projects are formulated and embarked on, it is important that they should be evaluated, incorporating baseline, monitoring, before-and-after and follow-up methods.

### 5.8.2 Practical Implications

The research reviewed here has implications for police services seeking to establish or strengthen liaison with schools for the twin purposes of helping them to manage current challenging behaviour and to engage in preventive work with at-risk young people. For the police forces which commissioned this research, the findings were used as part of their internal review of Police Community Support Officer deployment in schools, and of their overall pattern of working with schools. Thus, a principal result of the review was a remodelling of their approach including redeployment of resources.

First, there is no evidence supporting the use or the benefits of having police officers or other personnel placed in schools, even on a time-limited or rota basis. On the basis of the small number of studies pertaining to this, it does not appear to be an appropriate use of police resources.

Second, there is a wide array of evidence showing it is possible to reduce levels of several types of aggression, violence and involvement in alcohol and drug abuse amongst children attending school. With a review of information on this, police can be equipped to advise or to engage in multi-agency initiatives with the objective of addressing these problems. One strength of the police role in this context is the specific issue of highlighting the links between problems that are exhibited in schools that may later evolve into delinquent and criminal activity.

Third, drawing on the research reviewed, it should be possible either to identify existing programmes that could be used in school-based prevention, and make a selection as to which ones to implement, or to establish a set of criteria for developing new interventions or programmes for use in local areas.

## References

Academy for Critical Incident Analysis, John Jay College of Justice. (2017). New York. *Shooting incidents in educational settings*. Accessible at: http://aciajj.org/archive/cgi-bin/hsda?harcsda+Shootings_Database

Albayrak, S., Yildiz, A., & Erol, S. (2016). Assessing the effect of school bullying prevention programs on reducing bullying. *Children and Youth Services Review, 63*, 1–9. https://doi.org/10.1016/jchildyouth.201602.005

Alford, A. A., & Derzon, J. (2012). Meta-analysis and systematic review of the effectiveness of school-based programs to reduce multiple violent and antisocial behavioral outcomes. In S. R. Jimerson, A. Nickerson, M. J. Mayer, & M. J. Furlong (Eds.), *Handbook of school violence and school safety: International research and practice* (2nd ed., pp. 593–606). Routledge.

Allen, K. P. (2010). A bullying intervention system in high school: A two-year school-wide follow-up. *Studies in Educational Evaluation, 36*, 83–92.

Allen-Meares, P., Montgomery, K. L., & Kim, J. S. (2013). School-based social work interventions: A cross-national systematic review. *Social Work, 58*, 253–262.

Álvarez-García, D., Garcia, T., & Núñez, J. C. (2015). Predictors of school bullying perpetration in adolescence: A systematic review. *Aggression and Violent Behavior, 23*, 126–136.

Atienzo, E. E., Baxter, S. K., & Kaltenhaaler, E. (2017). Interventions to prevent youth violence in Latin America: A systematic review. *International Journal of Public Health, 62*, 15–29.

Barnes, T. N., Smith, S. W., & Miller, M. D. (2014). School-based cognitive-behavioral interventions in the treatment of aggression in the United States: A meta-analysis. *Aggression and Violent Behavior, 19*, 311–321.

Beckman, L., & Svensson, M. (2015). The cost-effectiveness of the Olweus bullying prevention program: Results from a modelling study. *Journal of Adolescence, 45*, 127–137.

Belur, V., Dennis, M. L., Ives, M. L., Vincent, R., & Muck, R. (2014). Feasibility and impact of implementing motivational enhancement therapy–cognitive behavioral therapy as a substance use treatment intervention in school-based settings. *Advances in School Mental Health Promotion, 7*, 88–104.

Blank, L., Baxter, S., Goyder, E., Naylor, P. B., Guillaume, L., Wilkinson, A., Hummel, S., & Chilcott, J. (2010). Promoting well-being by changing behaviour: A systematic review and narrative synthesis of the effectiveness of whole secondary school behavioural interventions. *Mental Health Review Journal, 15*, 43–53.

Bolger, P. C., Kremser, J., & Walker, H. (2019). Detention or diversion? The influence of training and education on school police officer discretion. *Policing: An International Journal, 42*(2), 255–269.

Bonell, C., Dickson, K., Hinds, K., Melendez-Torres, G. J., Stansfield, C., Fletcher, A., et al. (2016). The effects of Positive Youth Development interventions on substance use, violence and inequalities: Systematic review of theories of change, processes and outcomes. *Public Health Research, 4*(5). https://doi.org/10.3310/phr04050.

Bonell, C., Fletcher, A., Fitzgerald-Yau, N., Hale, D., Allen, E., Elbourne, D., Jones, R., Bond, L., Wiggins, M., Miners, A., Legood, R., Scott, S., Christie, D., & Viner, R. (2015). Initiating change locally in bullying and aggression through the school environment (INCLUSIVE): A pilot randomised controlled trial. *Health Technology Assessment, 19*(53).

Bonell, C., Hinds, K., Dickson, K., Thomas, J., Fletcher, A., Murphy, S., Melendez-Torres, G. J., Bonell, C., & Campbell, R. (2016). What is positive youth development and how might it reduce substance use and violence? A systematic review and synthesis of theoretical literature. *BMC Public Health, 16*, 135. https://doi.org/10.1186/s12889-016-2817-3

Bonell, C., Wells, H., Harden, A., Jamal, F., Thomas, J., Campbell, R., Petticrew, M., Whitehead, M., Murphy, S., & Moore, L. (2016). The effects on student health of interventions modifying the school environment: Systematic review. *Journal of Epidemiology and Community Health, 67*, 677–681.

Bortes, C., Geidne, S., & Eriksson, C. (2016). Evaluating the effectiveness of the SMART contract-signing strategy in reducing the growth of Swedish adolescents' substance use and problem behaviors. *BMC Public Health, 16*. https://doi.org/10.1186/s12889-016-3131-9

Bowen, E., Walker, K., Mawer, M., Holdsworth, E., Sorbring, E., Helsing, B., Bolin, A., Leen, E., Held, P., Awouters, V., & Jans, S. (2014). "It's like you're actually playing as yourself": Development and preliminary evaluation of 'Green Acres High', a serious game-based primary intervention to combat adolescent dating violence. *Psychosocial Intervention, 23*, 43–55.

Bradshaw, C. P., Pas, E. T., Debnam, K. J., & Johnson, S. L. (2015). A focus on implementation of Positive Behavioral Interventions and Supports (PBIS) in high schools: Associations with bullying and other indicators of school disorder. *School Psychology Review, 44*, 480–498.

Brännström, L., Kaunitz, C., Andershed, A.-K., South, S., & Smedslund, G. (2016). Aggression replacement training (ART) for reducing antisocial behaviour in adolescents and adults: A systematic review. *Aggression and Violent Behavior, 27*, 30–41.

Brown, B. (2006). Understanding and assessing school police officers: A conceptual and methodological comment. *Journal of Criminal Justice, 34*, 591–604.

Calder, B. D., & Schulze, S. (2015). A psycho-educational programme using audio-visual media to prevent adolescent substance abuse. *Education as Change, 19*, 36–53.

Cantone, E., Piras, A. P., Vellante, M., Preti, A., Daníelsdóttir, S., D'Aloja, E., Lesinkiene, S., Angermeyer, M. C., Carta, M. G., & Bhugra, D. (2015). Interventions on bullying and cyberbullying in schools: A systematic review. *Clinical Practice & Epidemiology in Mental Health, 11*(Suppl 1: M4), 58–76.

Cardwell, S. M., Mazerolle, L., & Piquero, A. R. (2019). Truancy intervention and violent offending: Evidence from a randomized controlled trial. *Aggression and Violent Behavior, 49*. https://doi.org/10.1016/j.avb.2019.07.003

Caria, M. P., Faggiano, F., Bellocco, R., Galanti, M. R. & EU-Dap Study Group. (2013). Classroom characteristics and implementation of a substance use prevention curriculum in European countries. *European Journal of Public Health, 23*, 1088–1093.

Caria, M. P., Faggiano, F., Bellocco, R., Ganalti, M. R., & EU-Dap Study Group. (2011). Effects of a school-based prevention program on European adolescents' patterns of alcohol use. *Journal of Adolescent Health, 48*, 182–188.

Castillo, R., Salguero, J. M., Fernández-Berrocal, P., & Balluerka, N. (2013). Effects of an emotional intelligence intervention on aggression and empathy among adolescents. *Journal of Adolescence, 36*, 883–892.

Castro-Olivo, S. M., Tran, O. K., Begum, G. F., Arellano, E. M., Garcia, N. M., & Tung, C. Y. (2013). A comprehensive model for promoting resiliency and preventing violence in schools. *Contemporary School Psychology, 17*, 23–34.

Chalamandaris, A.-G., & Piette, D. (2015). School-based anti-bullying interventions: Systematic review of the methodology to assess their effectiveness. *Aggression and Violent Behavior, 24*, 131–174.

Choi, K.-S., Cronin, S., & Correia, H. (2016). The assessment of capable guardianship measures against bullying victimization in the school environment. *Police Practice and Research: An International Journal, 17*(2), 149–159.

Cid, A. (2016). Interventions using regular activities to engage high-risk school-age youth: A review of after-school programs in Latin America and the Caribbean. *Prevention Science, 18*, 879–886.

Coker, A. L., Bush, H. M., Cook-Craig, P. G., DeGuem, S. A., Clear, E. R., Brancato, C. J., Fisher, B. S., & Recktenwald, E. A. (2017). RCT testing bystander effectiveness to reduce violence. *American Journal of Preventive Medicine, 52*(5), 566–578.

Connelly, L., Legane, R., & Joseph-Slisbury, R. (2020). *Decriminalise the Classroom: A Community Response to Police in Greater Manchester's Schools*. Kids of Colour and Northern Police Monitoring Project.

Conrod, P. J., O'Leary-Barnett, M., Newton, N., Topper, L., Castellanos-Ryan, N., Mackie, C., & Girard, A. (2013). Effectiveness of a selective, personality-targeted prevention program for adolescent alcohol use and misuse: A cluster randomized controlled trial. *JAMA Psychiatry, 70*, 334–342.

Cox, E., Leung, R., Baksheev, G., Day, A., Toumbourou, J. W., Miller, P., Kremer, P., & Walker, A. (2016). Violence prevention and intervention programmes for adolescents in Australia: A systematic review. *Australian Psychologist, 51*, 206–222.

Crawford, C., & Burns, R. (2015). Preventing school violence: Assessing armed guardians, school policy, and context. *Policing: An International Journal of Police Strategies & Management, 38*(4), 631–647.

Crawford, C., & Burns, R. (2016). Reducing school violence: Considering school characteristics and the impact of law enforcement, school security, and environmental factors. *Policing: An International Journal of Police Strategies & Management, 39*(3), 455–477.

Crooks, C. V., Scott, K., Ellism, W., & Wolfe, D. A. (2011). Impact of a universal school-based violence prevention program on violent delinquency: Distinctive benefits for youth with maltreatment histories. *Child Abuse & Neglect, 35*, 393–400.

Cuijpers, P. (2002). Effective ingredients of school-based drug prevention programs: A systematic review. *Addictive Behaviors, 27*, 1009–1023.

Das, J. K., Salam, R. A., Arshad, A., Finkelstein, Y., & Bhutta, Z. A. (2016). Interventions for adolescent substance abuse: An overview of systematic reviews. *Journal of Adolescent Health, 59*, 561–575.

De Koker, P., Mathews, C., Zuch, M., Bastien, S., & Mason-Jones, A. J. (2014). A systematic review of interventions for preventing adolescent intimate partner violence. *Journal of Adolescent Health, 54*, 3–13.

De La Rue, L., Polanin, J. R., Espelage, D. L., & Pigott, T. D. (2014). School-based interventions to reduce dating and sexual violence: A systematic review. *Campbell Systematic Reviews, 2014*, 7. https://doi.org/10.4073/csr.2014.7

DeGue, S., Valle, L. A., Holt, M. K., Massetti, G. M., Matjasko, J. L., & Tharp, A. T. (2014). A systematic review of primary prevention strategies for sexual violence perpetration. *Aggression and Violent Behavior, 19*, 346–342.

Deković, M., Slagt, M. I., Asscher, J. J., & Boendermaker, L. (2011). Effects of early prevention programs on adult criminal offending: A meta-analysis. *Clinical Psychology Review, 31*, 532–544.

Della Cioppa, V., O'Neil, A., & Craig, W. (2015). Learning from traditional bullying interventions: A review of research on cyberbullying and best practice. *Aggression and Violent Behavior, 23*, 61–68.

Dembo, R., Briones-Robinson, R., Wareham, J., Schmeidler, J., Winters, K. C., Barrett, K., Ungaro, R., Karas, L. M., & Belenko, S. (2014). Impact of brief intervention services on drug-using, truant youth arrest charges over time. *Journal of Child & Adolescent Substance Abuse, 23*, 375–388.

Desai, C. C., Reece, J.-A., & Shakespeare-Pellington, S. (2017). The prevention of violence in childhood through parenting programmes: A global review. *Psychology, Health & Medicine, 22*, 166–186.

Devlin, D. N., & Gottfredson, D. C. (2018). The roles of police officers in schools: Effects on the recording and reporting of crime. *Youth Violence and Juvenile Justice, 16*(2), 208–223.

Doğan, A., Keser, E., Şen, Z., Yanagida, T., Gradinger, P., & Strohmeier, D. (2017). Evidence based bullying prevention in Turkey: Implementation of the ViSC social competence program. *International Journal of Development Science, 11*, 93–108.

Donoghue, C., & Raia-Hawrylak, A. (2016). Moving beyond the emphasis on bullying: A generalized approach to peer aggression in high school. *Children & Schools, 38*, 30–39. https://doi.org/10.1093/cs/cdv042

Due, P., Merlo, J., Harel-Fisch, Y., Damsgaard, M. T., Holstein, B. E., Hetland, J., & Lynch, J. (2009). Socioeconomic inequality in exposure to bullying during adolescence: A comparative, cross-sectional, multilevel study in 35 countries. *American Journal of Public Health, 99*, 907–914.

Durlak, J. A., Weissberg, R. P., Dymnicki, A. B., Taylor, R. D., & Schellinger, K. B. (2011). The impact of enhancing students' social and emotional learning: A meta-analysis of school-based universal interventions. *Child Development, 82*, 405–432.

Dymnicki, A. B., & Multisite Violence Prevention Project. (2013). Moderating effects of school climate on outcomes for the multisite violence prevention project universal program. *Journal of Research on Adolescence, 24*, 383–398.

Dymnicki, A. B., Weissberg, R. P., & Henry, D. B. (2011). Understanding how programs work to prevent overt aggressive behaviors: A meta-analysis of mediators of elementary school–based programs. *Journal of School Violence, 10*, 315–337.

Edwards, K. M., Banyard, V. L., Sessarego, S. N., Waterman, E. A., Mitchell, K. J., & Chang, H. (2019). Evaluation of a bystander-focused interpersonal violence prevention program with high school students. *Prevention Science, 20*, 488–498.

Elgar, F. J., Pickett, K. E., Pickett, W., Craig, W., Molcho, M., Hurrelmann, K., & Lenzi, M. (2013). School bullying, homicide and income inequality: A cross-national pooled time series analysis. *International Journal of Public Health, 58*, 237–245.

Espada, J. P., Gonzálvez, M. T., Orgilés, M., Lloret, D., & Guillén-Riquelme, A. (2015). Meta-analysis of the effectiveness of school substance abuse prevention programs in Spain. *Psicothema, 27*, 5–12.

Espada, J. P., Griffin, K. W., Pereira, J. R., Orgilés, M., & García-Fernández, J. M. (2013). Component analysis of a school-based substance use prevention program in Spain: Contributions of problem solving and social skills training content. *Prevention Science, 13*, 86–95.

Espada-Sánchez, J. P., & Hernández-Serrano, O. (2015). Effects of the Saluda prevention program: A review of controlled evaluation studies. *Electronic Journal of Research in Educational Psychology, 35*. https://doi.org/10.14204/ejrep.35.14052

Espelage, D. L., Low, S., Polanin, J. R., & Brown, E. C. (2013). The impact of a middle school program to reduce aggression, victimization, and sexual violence. *Journal of Adolescent Health, 53*, 180–186.

Espelage, D. L., Low, S., Polanin, J. R., & Brown, E. C. (2015). Clinical trial of Second Step© middle-school program: Impact on aggression & victimization. *Journal of Applied Developmental Psychology, 37*, 52–63.

Espelage, D. L., Low, S., Van Ryzin, M. J., & Polanin, J. R. (2015). Clinical trial of Second Step middle-school program: Impact on bullying, cyberbullying, homophobic teasing, and sexual harassment perpetration. *School Psychology Review, 44*, 464–479.

Espelage, D. L., Rose, C. A., & Polanin, J. R. (2015). Social-emotional learning program to reduce bullying, fighting, and victimization among middle school students with disabilities. *Remedial and Special Education, 36*, 299–231.

Estefan, L. F., Vivolo-Kantor, A. M., Niolon, P. H., Le, V. D., Tracy, A. J., Little, T. D., DeGue, S., Latzman, N. E., Tharp, A., Lang, K. M., & McIntosh, W. L. (2020). Effects of the Dating Matters® comprehensive prevention model on health- and delinquency-related risk behaviors in middle school youth: A cluster-randomized controlled trial. *Prevention Science*. https://doi.org/10.1007/s11121-020-01114-6

Evans, C. B. R., Fraser, M. W., & Cotter, K. L. (2014). The effectiveness of school-based bullying prevention programs: A systematic review. *Aggression and Violent Behavior, 19*, 532–544.

Fagan, A. A., & Catalano, R. F. (2012). What works in youth violence prevention: A review of the literature. *Research on Social Work Practice, 23*, 141–156.

Faggiano, F., Minozzi, S., Verso, E., & Buscemi, D. (2016). Universal school-based prevention for illicit drug use (review). *Cochrane Database of Systematic Reviews, 2014*, 12. https://doi.org/10.1002/14651858.CD003020.pub3

Faggiano, F., Vigna-Taglianti, F., Burkhart, G., Bohrn, K., Cuomo, L., Gregori, D., Panella, M., Scatigna, M., Siliquini, R., Varona, L., van der Kreeft, P., Vassara, M., Wiborg, G., Galanti, M. R., & EU-Dap Study Group. (2013). The effectiveness of a school-based substance abuse prevention program: 18-month follow-up of the EU-Dap cluster randomized controlled trial. *Drug and Alcohol Dependence, 108*, 56–64.

Farahmand, F. K., Grant, K. E., Polo, A. J., Duffy, S. N., & DuBois, D. L. (2011). School-based mental health and behavioral programs for low-income, urban youth: A systematic and meta-analytic review. *Clinical Psychology: Science and Practice, 18*, 372–390.

Fekkes, M., can de Sande, M. C. E., Gravesteijn, J. C., Pannebakker, F. D., Buijs, G. J., Diekstra, R. F. W., & Kocken, P. L. (2015). Effects of the Dutch Skills for Life program on the health behavior, bullying, and suicidal ideation of secondary school students. *Health Education, 116*, 2–15. https://doi.org/10.1108/HE-05-2014-0068

Fellmeth, G. L. T., Heffernan, C., Nurse, J., Habubula, S., & Sethi, D. (2013). Educational and skills-based interventions for preventing relationship and dating violence in adolescents and young adults. *Campbell Systematic Reviews, 2013*, 14. https://doi.org/10.4073/csr.2013.14

Fellmeth, G. L. T., Heffernan, C., Nurse, J., Habubula, S., & Sethi, D. (2015). Educational and skills-based interventions for preventing relationship violence in young people. *Research on Social Work Practice, 25*, 90–102.

Ferguson, C. J., Miguel, C. S., Kilburn, J. C., & Sanchez, P. (2007). The effectiveness of school-based anti-bullying programs: A meta-analytic review. *Criminal Justice Review, 32*, 401–414.

Fingar, K. R., & Jolls, T. (2014). Evaluation of a school-based violence prevention media literacy curriculum. *Injury Prevention, 20*, 183–190.

Fisher, B. W., & Hennessey, E. A. (2015). School resource officers and exclusionary discipline in US high schools: A systematic review and meta-analysis. *Adolescent Research Review, 1*, 217–233.

Flannery, D. J., Todres, J., Bradshaw, C. P., Amar, A. F., Graham, S., Hatzenbuehler, M., Masiello, M., Moreno, M., Sullivan, T., Le Menestrel, S. M., & Rivara, F. (2016). Bullying prevention: A summary of the report of the National Academies of Sciences, Engineering, and Medicine. *Prevention Science, 17*, 1044–1053.

Flannery, D. J., Vazsonyi, A. T., Liau, A. K., Guo, S., Powell, K. E., Atha, H., Vesterdal, W., & Embry, D. (2003). Initial behavior outcomes for the peacebuilders universal school-based violence prevention program. *Developmental Psychology, 39*, 292–308.

Franco, C., Amutio, A., López-González, L., Oriol, X., & Martinez-Taboada, C. (2016). Effect of a mindfulness training program on the impulsivity and aggression levels of adolescents with behavioural problems in the classroom. *Frontiers in Psychology, 7*, 1385. https://doi.org/10.3389/fpsyg.2016.01385

Frey, K. S., Newman, J. B., Nolen, S. B., & Hirschstein, M. K. (2012). Reducing bullying and contributing peer behaviors. In S. R. Jimerson, A. B. Nickerson, M. J. Mayer, & M. J. Furlong (Eds.), *Handbook of school violence and school safety: International research and practice* (2nd ed., pp. 383–395). Routledge.

Fryda, C. M., & Hulme, P. A. (2015). School-based childhood sexual abuse prevention programs: An integrative review. *Journal of School Nursing, 31*, 167–182.

Gabrhelik, R., Duncan, A., Miovsky, M., Furr-Holden, C. D. M., Stastna, L., & Jurystova, L. (2012). "Unplugged": A school-based randomized control trial to prevent and reduce adolescent substance use in the Czech Republic. *Drug and Alcohol Dependence, 124*, 79–87.

Garaigordobil, M., & Martinez-Valderrey, V. (2016). Impact of Cyberprogram 2.0 on different types of school violence and aggressiveness. *Frontiers in Psychology, 7*, 428. https://doi.org/10.3389/fpsyg.2016.00428

Gavine, A. J., Donnelly, P. D., & Williams, D. J. (2016). Effectiveness of universal school-based programs for prevention of violence in adolescents. *Psychology of Violence, 6*, 390–399.

Gerlinger, J., & Wo, J. C. (2016). Preventing school bullying: Should schools prioritize an authoritative school discipline approach over security measures? *Journal of School Violence, 15*, 133–157.

Gianotta, F., Vigna-Taglianti, F., Galanti, M. R., Scatigna, M., & Faggiano, F. (2014). Short-term mediating factors of a school-based intervention to prevent youth substance use in Europe. *Journal of Adolescent Health, 54*, 565–573.

Gonzalez-Guarda, R. M., Guerra, J. E., Cummings, A. A., Pino, K., & Becerra, M. M. (2015). Examining the preliminary efficacy of a dating violence prevention program for Hispanic adolescents. *Journal of School Nursing, 31*, 411–421.

Goossens, F. X., Lammers, J., Onrust, S. A., Conrodm, P. J., de Castro, B. O., & Monshouwer, K. (2016). Effectiveness of a brief school-based intervention on depression, anxiety, hyperactivity, and delinquency: A cluster randomized controlled trial. *European Child and Adolescent Psychiatry, 25*, 639–648.

Gottfredson, D. C. (2017). Prevention research in schools: Past, present, and future. *Criminology & Public Policy, 16*(1), 7–27.

Gradinger, P., Yanagida, T., Strohmeier, D., & Spiel, C. (2015). Prevention of cyberbullying and cybervictimization: Evaluation of the ViSC social competence program. *Journal of School Violence, 14*, 87–110.

Greenberg, M. T., Weissburg, R. P., O'Brien, M. U., Zins, J. E., Fredericks, L., Resnik, H., & Elias, M. J. (2003). Enhancing school-based prevention and youth development through coordinated social, emotional, and academic learning. *American Psychologist, 58*, 466–474.

Gregory, A., Cornell, D., Fan, X., Sheras, P., Shih, T.-H., & Huang, F. (2010). Authoritative school discipline: High school practices associated with lower bullying and victimization. *Journal of Educational Psychology, 102*, 483–496. https://doi.org/10.1037/a0018562

Grierson, J., & Agencies. (2017). Hundreds of knives seized in 18 months at UK schools, figures show. *The Guardian*, 12th May. https://www.google.co.uk/search?hl=en&q=Hundreds+of+knives+seized+in+18+months+at+UK+schools,+figures+show&meta=&gws_rd=ssl

Guo, J.-L., Lee, T.-C., Liao, J.-Y., & Huang, C.-M. (2015). Prevention of illicit drug use through a school-based program: Results of a longitudinal, cluster-randomized controlled trial. *Journal of Adolescent Health, 56*, 314–322.

Guo, R., He, Q., Shi, J., Gong, J., Wang, H., & Wang, Z. (2010). Short-term impact of cognition-motivation-emotional intelligence-resistance skills program on drug use prevention for school students in Wuhan, China. *Journal of Huazhong University of Science and Technology [Medical Science], 30*, 720–725. https://doi.org/10.1007/s11596-010-0647-6

Hahn, R. (2007). Effectiveness of universal school-based programs to prevent violent and aggressive behaviour: A systematic review. *American Journal of Preventive Medicine, 33*, S114–S129.

Hale, D. R., Fitzgerald-Yau, N., & Viner, R. M. (2014). A systematic review of effective interventions for reducing multiple health risk behaviors in adolescence. *American Journal of Public Health, 104*, e19–e41.

Hall, B. W., Bacon, T. P., & Ferron, J. M. (2013). Randomized controlled evaluation of the *Too Good for Drugs* prevention program: Impact on adolescents at different risk levels for drug use. *Journal of Drugs Education, 43*, 277–300.

Han, S., & Connell, N. M. (2020). The effects of school police officers on victimization, delinquency, and fear of crime: Focusing on Korean youth. *International Journal of Offender Therapy and Comparative Criminology*, 1–17. https://doi.org/10.1177/0306624X20946933.

Hawley, P. H., & Williford, A. (2015). Articulating the theory of bullying prevention programmes: Views from, social psychology, social work, and organizational science. *Journal of Applied Developmental Psychology, 37*, 3–15.

Hemphill, S. A., Kotevski, A., Herrenkohl, T. I., Toumbourou, J. W., & Catalano, R. F. (2013). Does school suspension affect subsequent youth non-violent antisocial behaviour? A longitudinal study of students in Victoria, Australia and Washington State, United States. *Australian Journal of Psychology, 65*, 236–249.

Hennessy, E. A., & Tanner-Smith, E. E. (2015). Effectiveness of brief school-based interventions for adolescents: A meta-analysis of alcohol use prevention programs. *Prevention Science, 16*, 463–474.

Hernández-Serrano, O., Griffin, K. W., García-Fernández, J. M., Orgilés, M., & Espada, J. P. (2013). Public commitment, resistance to advertising, and leisure promotion in a school-based drug abuse prevention program: A component dismantling study. *Journal of Drugs Education, 43*, 331–351.

Hodder, R. K., Freund, M., Wolfenden, L., Bowman, J., Nepal, S., Dray, J., Kingsland, M., Yoong, S. L., & Wiggers, J. (2017). Systematic review of universal school-based 'resilience' interventions targeting adolescent tobacco, alcohol or illicit substance use: A meta-analysis. *Preventive Medicine*. https://doi.org/10.1016/j.ypmed.2017.04.003

Hong, J. S., & Espelage, D. L. (2012). A review of research on bullying and peer victimization in school: An ecological system analysis. *Aggression and Violent Behavior, 17*, 311–322.

Hong, J. S., Lee, C.-H., Lee, J., Lee, N. Y., & Garbarino, J. (2014). A review of bullying prevention and intervention in South Korean schools: An application of the social–ecological framework. *Child Psychiatry and Human Development, 45*, 433–442.

Huang, C.-M., Chien, L.-Y., Cheng, C.-F., & Guo, J.-L. (2012). Integrating life skills into a theory-based drug-use prevention program: Effectiveness among junior high students in Taiwan. *Journal of School Health, 82*, 328–335.

Huang, Y., Espelage, D. L., Polanin, J. R., & Hong, J. S. (2019). A meta-analytic review of school-based anti-bullying programs with a parent component. *International Journal of Bullying Prevention, 1*, 32–44.

Jackson, C., Geddes, R., Haw, S., & Frank, J. (2011). Interventions to prevent substance use and risky sexual behaviour in young people: A systematic review. *Addiction, 107*, 733–747.

Jennings, W. C., Khey, D. N., Maskaly, J., & Donner, C. M. (2011). Evaluating the relationship between law enforcement and school security measures and violent crime in schools. *Journal of Police Crisis Negotiations, 11*(2), 173–192.

Jimerson, S. R., Nickerson, A. B., Mayer, M. J., & Furlong, M. J. (Eds.). (2012). *Handbook of school violence and school safety: International research and practice* (2nd ed.). Routledge.

Jiminéz-Barbero, J. A., Hernández, J. A., Esteban, B. L., & García, M. P. (2012). Effectiveness of antibullying school programmes: A systematic review by evidence levels. *Children and Youth Services Review, 34*, 1646–1658.

Jiminéz-Barbero, J. A., Hernández, J. A. R., Llor-Zaragoza, L., García, M. P., & Llor-Esteban, B. (2016). Effectiveness of anti-bullying programs: A meta-analysis. *Children and Youth Services Review, 61*, 165–175.

Jiminéz-Barbero, J. A., Ruiz-Hernández, J. A., Llor-Esteban, B., Llor-Zaragoza, L., & García, M. P. (2016). Efficacy of a brief intervention on attitudes to reduce school violence: A randomized clinical trial. *Children and Youth Services Review, 35*, 1313–1318.

Kärnä, A., Voeten, M., Little, T. D., Alanen, E., Poskiparta, E., & Salmivalli, C. (2013). Effectiveness of the KiVa antibullying program: Grades 1–3 and 7–9. *Journal of Educational Psychology, 105*, 535–551.

Kärnä, A., Voeten, M., Little, T. D., Poskiparta, E., Alanen, E., & Salmivalli, C. (2011). Going to scale: A nonrandomized nationwide trial of the KiVa antibullying program for grades 1–9. *Journal of Consulting and Clinical Psychology, 79*, 796–805.

Kearney, S., Leung, L., Joyce, A., Ollis, D., & Green, C. (2016). Applying systems theory to the evaluation of a whole school approach to violence prevention. *Health Promotion Journal of Australia, 27*, 230–235.

Kiewik, M., VenDerNagel, J. E. L., Kemna, L. E. M., Engels, R. C. M. E., & DeJong, C. A. J. (2016). Substance use prevention program for adolescents with intellectual disabilities on special education schools: A cluster randomised control trial. *Journal of Intellectual Disability Research, 60*, 191–200.

Kingston, B., Bacallao, M., Smokowski, P., Sullivan, T., & Sutherland, K. (2016). Constructing "packages" of evidence-based programs to prevent youth violence: Processes and illustrative examples from the CDC's youth violence prevention centers. *Journal of Primary Prevention, 37*, 141–163.

Kliewer, W., Lepore, S. J., Farrell, A. D., Allison, K. W., Meyer, A. L., Sullivan, T. N., & Greene, A. Y. (2011). A school-based expressive writing intervention for at-risk urban adolescents' aggressive behavior and emotional lability. *Journal of Clinical Child & Adolescent Psychology, 40*, 693–705.

Konishi, C., Saewyc, E., Homma, Y., & Poon, C. (2013). Population-level evaluation of school-based interventions to prevent problem substance use among gay, lesbian and bisexual adolescents in Canada. *Preventive Medicine, 57*, 929–933.

Lam, S., Zwart, C., Chahal, I., Lane, D., & Cummings, H. (2018). Preventing violence against children in schools: Contributions from the be safe program in Sri Lanka. *Child Abuse & Neglect, 76*, 728–737.

Lamont, E., Macleod, S., & Wilkin, A. (2011). *Police officers in schools: A scoping study*. National Foundation for Educational Research.

Lee, L., Kim, C.-J., & Kim, D. H. (2015). A meta-analysis of the effect of school-based anti-bullying programs. *Journal of Child Health Care, 19*, 136–153.

Lester, S., Lawrence, C., & Ward, C. L. (2017). What do we know about preventing school violence? A systematic review of systematic reviews. *Psychology, Health & Medicine, 22*, 187–223.

Leuschner, V., Fielder, N., Schultze, M., Ahlig, N., Göbel, K., Sommer, F., Scholl, J., Cornell, D., & Scheithauer, H. (2017). Prevention of targeted school violence by responding to students' psychosocial crises: The NETWASS program. *Child Development, 88*, 68–82.

Li, Y., Zhang, W., Liu, J., Arbeit, M. R., Schwartz, S. J., Bowers, E. P., & Lerner, R. M. (2011). The role of school engagement in preventing adolescent delinquency and substance use: A survival analysis. *Journal of Adolescence, 34*, 1181–1192.

Lisha, N. E., Sun, P., Rohrbach, L. A., Spruijt-Metz, D., Unger, J. B., & Sussman, S. (2012). An evaluation of immediate outcomes and fidelity of a drug abuse prevention program in continuation high schools: Project towards no drug abuse (TND). *Journal of Drug Education, 42*, 33–57.

Lo, C. C., Kim, Y. S., Allen, T. M., Allen, A. N., Minugh, P. A., & Lumoto, N. (2011). The impact of school environment and grade level on student delinquency: A multilevel modeling approach. *Crime & Delinquency, 57*, 622–657.

Lynch, C. G., Gainey, R. R., & Chappell, A. T. (2016). The effects of social and educational disadvantage on the roles and functions of schools resources officers. *Policing: An International Journal of Police Strategies & Management, 39*(3), 521–535.

MacArthur, G. J., Harrison, S., Caldwell, D. M., Hickman, M., & Campbell, R. (2015). Peer-led interventions to prevent tobacco, alcohol and/or drug use among young people aged 11–21 years: A systematic review and meta-analysis. *Addiction, 111*, 391–407.

Maimon, D., Antonaccio, O., & French, M. T. (2012). Severe sanctions, easy choice? Investigating the role of school sanctions in preventing adolescent violent offending. *Criminology, 50*, 495–524.

Malmberg, M., Kleinjan, M., Overbeek, G., Vermulst, A., Monshouwer, K., Lammers, J., Vollebergh, W. A. M., & Engels. (2014). Effectiveness of the 'Healthy School and Drugs' prevention programme on adolescents' substance use: A randomized clustered trial. *Addiction, 109*, 1031–1040.

Marsiglia, F. F., Booth, J. M., Ayers, S. L., Nuño-Guiterrez, B. L., Kulis, S., & Hoffman, S. (2014). Short-term effects on substance use of the Keepin' it REAL pilot prevention program: Linguistically adapted for youth in Jalisco, Mexico. *Prevention Science, 15*, 694–704.

Martinez-Prather, K. E., McKenna, J. M., & Bowman, S. W. (2016). The impact of training on discipline outcomes in school-based policing. *Policing: An International Journal of Police Strategies & Management, 39*(3), 478–490.

Masho, S. W., Zirkle, K. W., Wheeler, D. C., Sullivan, T., & Farrell, A. D. (2019). Spatial analysis of the impact of a school-level youth violence prevention program on violent crime incidents in the community. *Prevention Science, 20*, 521–531.

Mason, M., Ola, B., Zaharakis, N., & Zhang, J. (2015). Text messaging interventions for adolescent and young adult substance use: A meta-analysis. *Prevention Science, 16*, 181–188.

Matjasko, J. L., Vivolo-Kantor, A. M., Massetti, G. M., Holland, K. M., Holt, M. K., & Dela Cruz, J. (2012). A systematic meta-review of evaluations of youth violence prevention programs: Common and divergent findings from 25 years of meta-analyses and systematic reviews. *Aggression and Violent Behavior, 17*, 540–553.

Maynard, B. R., Solis, M. R., Miller, V. L., & Brendel, K. E. (2017). Mindfulness-based interventions for improving cognition, academic achievement, behavior, and socioemotional functioning of primary and secondary school students. *Campbell Systematic Reviews, 2017*, 5. https://doi.org/10.4073/csr.2017.5

McCarthy, D. (2012). How can the Sandy Hook atrocity happen? A statistical look at the perpetrators of school violence. *The Media Transformation*. http://www.themediatransformation.com/2012/12/16/how-can-the-sandy-hook-atrocity-happen-a-statistical-look-at-the-perpetrators-of-school-violence/

McDevitt, J., & Panniello, J. (2005). *National Assessment of School Resource Officer Programs: Survey of Students in Three Large New SRO Programs*. Unpublished report. Washington, DC: National Institute of Justice.

McKay, M., Sumnall, H., McBride, N., & Harvey, S. (2014). The differential impact of a classroom-based, alcohol harm reduction intervention, on adolescents with different alcohol use experiences: A multi-level growth modelling analysis. *Journal of Adolescence, 37*, 1057–1067.

Medeiros, P. F. P., Cruz, J. I., Schneider, D. R., Sanudo, A., & Sanchez, Z. M. (2016). Process evaluation of the implementation of the *Unplugged* program for drug use prevention in Brazilian schools. *Substance Abuse Treatment, Prevention and Policy, 11*, 2. https://doi.org/10.1186/s13011-015-0047-9

Meiksin, R., Allen, A., Crichton, J., Morgan, G. S., Barter, C., Elbourne, D., Hunt, K., Melendez-Torres, G. J., Morris, S., McNaughton Reyes, H. L., Sturgess, J., Taylor, B., Young, H., Campbell, R., & Bonell, C. (2019). Protocol for pilot cluster RCT of project respect: A school-based intervention to prevent dating and relationship violence and address health inequalities among young people. *BMC Pilot and Feasibility Studies, 5*, 13. https://doi.org/10.1186/s40814-019-0391-z

Meiksin, R., Campbell, R., Crichton, J., Morgan, G. S., Williams, P., Willmott, M., Tilouche, N., Ponsford, R., Barter, C. A., Sweeting, H., Taylor, B., Young, H., Melendez-Torres, G. J., McNaughton, H. L., & Bonell, C. (2020). Implementing a whole-school relationships and sex education intervention to prevent dating and relationship violence: Evidence from a pilot trial in English secondary schools. *Sex Education, 20*(6), 658–674. https://doi.org/10.1080/14681811.2020.1729718

Melendez-Torres, G. J., Dickson, K., Fletcher, A., Thomas, J., Hinds, K., Campbell, R., Murphy, S., & Bonell, C. (2016a). Systematic review and meta-analysis of effects of community-delivered positive youth development interventions on violence outcomes. *Journal of Epidemiology and Community Health, 70*, 1171–1177.

Melendez-Torres, G. J., Dickson, K., Fletcher, A., Thomas, J., Hinds, K., Campbell, R., Murphy, S., & Bonell, C. (2016b). Positive youth development programmes to reduce substance use in young people: Systematic review. *International Journal of Drug Policy, 36*, 95–103.

Merrell, K. W., Gueldner, B. A., Ross, S. W., & Isava, D. M. (2008). How effective are school bullying intervention programs? A meta-analysis of intervention research. *School Psychology Quarterly, 23*, 26–42.

Midford, R., Mitchelll, J., Lester, L., Cahill, H., Foxcroft, D., Ramsden, R., Venning, L., & Pose, M. (2014). Preventing alcohol harm: Early results from a cluster randomised, controlled trial in Victoria, Australia of comprehensive harm minimisation school drug education. *International Journal of Drug Policy, 25*, 142–150.

Miller, E., Goldstein, S., McCauley, H. L., Jones, K. A., Dick, R. N., Jetton, J., Silverman, J. G., Blackburn, S., Monasterio, E., James, L., & Tancredi, D. J. (2015). A school health center intervention for abusive adolescent relationships: A cluster RCT. *Pediatrics, 135*, 76–85.

Miller, W. R., & Rollnick, S. (2002). *Motivational interviewing: Preparing people for change* (2nd ed.). Guilford Press.

Moffitt, T. E. (1993). Adolescence-limited and life-course-persistent antisocial behavior: A developmental taxonomy. *Psychological Review, 100*, 674–701.

Moffitt, T. E. (2003). Life-course-persistent and adolescence-limited antisocial behaviour: A 10-year research review and a research agenda. In B. B. Lahey, T. E. Moffitt, & A. Caspi (Eds.), *Causes of conduct disorder and delinquency* (pp. 49–75). Guilford Press.

Mogor-Wilson, C., Allen, E., & Cavallucci, C. (2017). Short-term mediating factors of a school-based intervention to prevent youth substance use in Europe. *Social Work Research, 41*, 53–62.

Multisite Violence Research Project. (2013). Targeting high-risk, socially influential middle school students to reduce aggression: Universal versus selective preventive intervention effects. *Journal of Research on Adolescence, 24*, 364–382.

Muñoz-Fernández, N., Ortega-Rivera, J., Nocentini, A., Menesini, E., & Sánchez-Jiménez, V. (2019). The efficacy of the "Dat-e adolescence" prevention program in the reduction of dating violence and bullying. *International Journal of Environmental Research and Public Health, 16*, 408. https://doi.org/10.3390/ijerph16030408

Na, C., & Gottfredson, D. C. (2013). Police officers in schools: Effects on school crime and the processing of offending behaviors. *Justice Quarterly, 30*, 619–650.

Nieri, T., Apkarian, J., Kulis, S., & Marsiglia, F. F. (2015). Effects of a youth substance use prevention program on stealing, fighting, and weapon use. *Journal of Primary Prevention, 36*, 41–49.

Niolon, P. H., Vivolo-Kantor, A. M., Tracy, A. J., Latzman, N. E., Little, T. D., DeGue, S., Lang, K. M., Estefan, L. F., Ghazarian, S. R., McIntosh, W. L. K., Taylor, B., Johnson, L. L., Kuoh, H., Burton, B., Fortson, B., Mumford, E. A., Nelson, S. C., Joseph, H., Valle, L. A., & Tharp, A. T. (2019). An RCT of dating matters: Effects on teen dating violence and relationship behaviors. *American Journal of Preventive Medicine, 57*(1), 13–23.

Nocentini, A., Zambuto, V., & Menesini, E. (2015). Anti-bullying programs and Information and Communication Technologies (ICTs): A systematic review. *Aggression and Violent Behavior, 23*, 52–60.

O'Connell, P., Pepler, D., & Craig, W. (1999). Peer involvement in bullying: Insights and challenges for intervention. *Journal of Adolescence, 22*, 437–452.

Oliver, R. M., Wehby, J. H., & Reschly, D. J. (2011). Teacher classroom management practices: Effects on disruptive or aggressive student behaviour. *Campbell Systematic Reviews, 2011*, 4. https://doi.org/10.4073/csr.2011.4

Olweus, D. (1993). *Bullying at school: What we know and what we can do*. Blackwell.

Olweus, D., & Limber, S. P. (2010). Bullying in school: Evaluation and dissemination of the Olweus Bullying Prevention Program. *American Journal of Orthopsychiatry, 80*, 124–134.

Onrust, S. A., Otten, R., Lammers, J., & Smit, F. (2016). School-based programmes to reduce and prevent substance use in different age groups: What works for whom? Systematic review and meta-regression analysis. *Clinical Psychology Review, 44*, 45–59.

Özabaci, N. (2011). Cognitive behavioural therapy for violent behaviour in children and adolescents: A meta-analysis. *Children and Youth Services Review, 33*, 1989–1993.

Park-Higgerson, H.-K., Perumean-Chaney, S. E., Bartoluca, A. A., Grimley, D. M., & Singh, K. P. (2008). The evaluation of school-based violence prevention programs: A meta-analysis. *Journal of School Health, 78*, 465–479.

Perkins, H. W., Craig, Q. W., & Perkins, J. M. (2011). Using social norms to reduce bullying: A research intervention among adolescents in five middle schools. *Group Processes & Intergroup Relations, 14*, 703–722.

Persson, M., Wennberg, L., Beckman, L., Salmivalli, C., & Svensson, M. (2018). The cost-effectiveness of the KiVa antibullying program: Results from a decision-analytic model. *Prevention Science, 19*, 1044–1053.

Pfetsch, J., Steffgen, G., Gollwitzer, M., & Ittel, A. (2011). Prevention of aggression in schools through a bystander intervention training. *International Journal of Developmental Science, 5*, 139–149.

Piotroswka, P. J., Stride, C. B., Croft, S. E., & Rowe, R. (2015). Socioeconomic status and antisocial behaviour among children and adolescents: A systematic review and meta-analysis. *Clinical Psychology Review, 35*, 47–55.

Piotrowski, H. (2014). Evidence of reduction of aggression and violent behaviors after the positive youth potential curriculum intervention in the sixth grade: A 12-month follow-up in a rural Indiana middle school cluster randomized controlled trial. *Journal of Adolescent Health, 54*, S26.

Polanin, J. R., Espelage, D. L., & Pigott, T. D. (2012). A meta-analysis of school-based bullying prevention programs' effects on bystander intervention behavior. *School Psychology Review, 41*, 47–65.

Prezensky, B. C., Galli, E. F., Bachega, D., & de Mello, R. R. (2018). School actions to prevent gender-based violence: A (quasi-)systematic review of the Brazilian and the international scientific literature. *Frontiers in Education, 3*, 89. https://doi.org/10.3389/feduc.2018.00089

Price, J. H., & Khubchandani, J. (2019). School firearm violence prevention practices and policies: Functional or folly? *Violence and Gender, 6*(3), 154–167.

Raskauskas, J. (2007). *Evaluation of the Kia Kaha Anti-Bullying Programme for Students in Years 5–8*. Report for New Zealand Police. Wellington: New Zealand Police. https://www.police.govt.nz/about-us/publication/evaluation-kia-kaha-anti-bullying-programme-students-years-5-8

Reingle Gonzalez, J. M., Jetelina, K. K., & Jennings, W. G. (2016). Structural school safety measures, SROs, and school related delinquent behavior and perceptions of safety: A state-of-the-art review. *Policing: An International Journal of Police Strategies & Management, 39*(3), 438–454.

Renshaw, T. L., & Jimerson, S. R. (2012). Enhancing student attitudes via a brief, universal-level bullying prevention curriculum. *School Mental Health, 4*, 115–128.

Rivara, F. P., & Le Menestrel, S. M. (Eds.). (2016). *Preventing bullying through science, policy and practice*. The National Academies Press. https://doi.org/10.17226/23482

Rohrbach, L. A., Gunning, M., Sun, P., & Sussman, S. (2010). The Project Towards No Drug Abuse (TND) dissemination trial: Implementation fidelity and immediate outcomes. *Prevention Science, 11*, 77–88.

Rohrbach, L. A., Sun, P., & Sussman, S. (2010). One-year follow-up evaluation of the Project Towards No Drug Abuse (TND) dissemination trial. *Preventive Medicine, 51*, 313–319. https://doi.org/10.1016/j.ypmed.2010.07.016

Rongione, D., Erfordm, B. T., & Broglie, C. (2011). Alcohol and other drug abuse counseling outcomes for school-aged youth: A meta-analysis of studies from 1990 to 2009. *Counseling Outcome Research and Evaluation, 2*, 8–24.

Saarento, S., Garandeau, C. F., & Salmivalli, C. (2015). Classroom- and school-level contributions to bullying and victimization: A review. *Journal of Community and Applied Social Psychology, 25*, 104–218.

Salimi, N., Karimi-Shahanjarin, A., Rezapur-Shahkolai, F., Hamzeh, B., & Roshanaei, & Babamiri, M. (2020). Use of a mixed-methods approach to evaluate the implementation of violence and bullying prevention programs in schools. *Education and Urban Society*, 1–22. https://doi.org/10.1177/0013124520972090

Sancassiani, F., Pintus, E., Holte, A., Paulus, P., Moro, M. F., Cossu, G., Angermeyer, M. C., Carta, M. G., & Lindert, J. (2015). Enhancing the emotional and social skills of the youth to promote their wellbeing and positive development: A systematic review of universal school-based randomized controlled trials. *Clinical Practice & Epidemiology in Mental Health, 11*(Suppl 1: M2), 21–40.

Sanchez, Z. M., Sanudo, A., Andreoni, A., Schneider, D., Pereira, P. D., & Faggiano, D. (2016). Efficacy evaluation of the school program *Unplugged* for drug use prevention among Brazilian adolescents. *BMC Public Health, 16*, 1206. https://doi.org/10.1186/s12889-016-3877-0

Sanchez, Z. M., Valente, J. Y., Sanudo, A., Pereira, A. P. D., Cruz, J. I., Schneider, D., & Andreoni, S. (2016). The #Tamojunto drug prevention program in Brazilian schools: A randomized controlled trial. *Prevention Science, 18*, 772–782.

Sawyer, A. M., Borduin, C. M., & Dopp, A. R. (2015). Long-term effects of prevention and treatment on youth antisocial behavior: A meta-analysis. *Clinical Psychology Review, 42*, 130–144.

Scheithauer, H., Hess, M., Schultze-Krumbholtz, A., & Bull, H. D. (2012). School-based prevention of bullying and relational aggression in adolescence: The fairplayer.manual. *New Directions for Youth Development, 133*, 55–70. https://doi.org/10.1002/yd.20007

Schindler, H. S., Kholoptseva, J., Oh, S. S., Yoshikawa, H., Duncan, G. J., Magnusson, K. A., & Shonkoff, J. P. (2015). Maximizing the potential of early childhood education to prevent externalizing behavior problems: A meta-analysis. *Journal of School Psychology, 53*, 243–263.

Seçer, Z., & Ogelman, H. G. (2011). Analysis of the effect of a social problem-solving program on the aggression of children. *Australian Journal of Guidance and Counselling, 21*, 142–153.

Serafini, K., Shipley, L., & Stewart, D. G. (2016). Motivation and substance use outcomes among adolescents in a school-based intervention. *Addictive Behaviors, 53*, 74–79.

Sevigny, E. L., & Zhang, G. (2018). Do barriers to crime prevention moderate the effects of situational crime prevention policies on violent crime in high schools? *Journal of School Violence, 17*(2), 164–179.

Sharma, M., & Branscum, P. (2013). School-based drug abuse prevention programs in high school students. *Journal of Alcohol & Drug Education, 57*, 51–65.

Shetgiri, R., Kataoka, S., Lin, H., & Flores, G. (2011). A randomized, controlled trial of a school-based intervention to reduce violence and substance use in predominantly Latino high school students. *Journal of the National Medical Association, 103*, 932–940.

Shriberg, D., Brooks, K., Jenkins, K., Immen, J., Sutter, C., & Cronin, K. (2017). Using student voice to respond to middle school bullying: A student leadership approach. *School Psychology Forum: Research in Practice, 11*, 20–33.

Sinclair, J., Githua, O. W., Omond, B., Kapphahn, C. J., Sinclair, L., Mulinge, M. M., & Golden, N. H. (2014). The impact of a six-week school curriculum on boys' attitudes and behaviors related to gender based violence (GBV) in Kenya. *Journal of Adolescent Health, 54*, S6. https://doi.org/10.1016/jadohealth.2013.10.028

Sklad, M., Diekstra, R., De Ritter, M., & Ben, J. (2012). Effectiveness of school-based universal social, emotional, and behavioral programs: Do they enhance students' development in the area of skill, behavior, and adjustment? *Psychology in the Schools, 49*, 892–909.

Smedslund, G., Wollscheid, S., Fang, L., Nilsen, W., Steiro, A., & Larun, L. (2017). Effects of early, computerized brief interventions on risky alcohol use and risky cannabis use among young people. *Campbell Systematic Reviews, 2017*, 6. https://doi.org/10.4073/csr.2017.6

Smokowski, P. R., Guo, S., Wu, Q., Evans, C. B. R., Cotterm, K. L., & Bacallao, M. (2016). Evaluating dosage effects for the positive action program: How implementation impacts internalizing symptoms, aggression, school hassles, and self-esteem. *American Journal of Orthopsychiatry, 86*, 310–322.

Solomontos-Kountouri, O., Gradinger, P., Yanagida, T., & Strohmeier, D. (2016). The implementation and evaluation of the ViSC program in Cyprus: Challenges of cross-national dissemination and evaluation results. *European Journal of Developmental Psychology, 13*, 737–755.

Sommer, F., Leuschner, V., & Scheithauer, H. (2014). Bullying, romantic rejection, and conflicts with teachers: The crucial role of social dynamics in the development of school shootings – A systematic review. *International Journal of Developmental Science, 8*, 3–24.

Sosa-Rubi, S. G., Saavedra-Avendano, B., Piras, C., Can Buren, S. J., & Bautista-Arredondo, S. (2016). True love: Effectiveness of a school-based program to reduce dating violence among adolescents in Mexico City. *Prevention Science, 18*, 804–817.

Splett, J. D., Maras, M. A., & Brooks, C. M. (2015). GIRLSS: A randomized, pilot study of a multisystemic, school-based intervention to reduce relational aggression. *Journal of Child and Family Studies, 24*, 2250–2261.

Steffgen, G., Recchia, S., & Viechtbauer, W. (2013). The link between school climate and violence in school: A meta-analytic review. *Aggression and Violent Behavior, 18*, 30–309.

Stewart, D. G., Siebert, E. C., Arlt, V. K., Moise-Campbell, C., & Lehinger, E. (2016). READY or not: Findings from a school-based MI intervention for adolescent substance use. *Journal of Substance Abuse Treatment, 71*, 23–29.

Sussman, S., Sun, P., Rohrbach, L. A., & Spruijt-Metz, D. (2012). One-year outcomes of a drug abuse prevention program for older teens and emerging adults: Evaluating a motivational interviewing booster component. *Health Psychology, 31*, 476–485.

Swartz, K., Osborne, D. L., Dawson-Edwards, C., & Higgins, G. E. (2016). Policing schools: Examining the impact of place management activities on school violence. *American Journal of Criminal Justice, 41*, 465–483.

Taheri, S. A., & Welsh, B. C. (2015). After-school programs for delinquency prevention: A systematic review and meta-analysis. *Youth Violence and Juvenile Justice, 14*, 272–290.

Tancred, T., Paparini, S., Melendex-Torres, G. J., Fetcher, A., Thomas, J., Campbell, R., & Bonell, C. (2018). Interventions integrating health and academic interventions to prevent substance use and violence: A systematic review and synthesis of process evaluations. *Systematic Reviews, 7*, 227. https://doi.org/10.1186/s13643-018-0886-3

Tanner-Smith, E. E., & Lipsey, M. W. (2015). Brief alcohol interventions for adolescents and young adults: A systematic review and meta-analysis. *Journal of Substance Abuse Treatment, 51*, 1–18. https://doi.org/10.1016/j.jsat.2014.09.001

Tanner-Smith, E. E., & Risser, M. D. (2016). A meta-analysis of brief alcohol interventions for adolescents and young adults: Variability in effects across alcohol measures. *American Journal of Drug and Alcohol Abuse, 42*, 140–151.

Taylor, B. G., Mumford, E. A., & Stein, N. D. (2015). Effectiveness of “shifting boundaries” teen dating violence prevention program for subgroups of middle school students. *Journal of Adolescent Health, 56*, S20–S26.

Taylor, M., Jinabhai, C., Diamini, S., Sathiparsad, R., Meyer-Wetiz, A., Eggers, M., & de Vries, H. (2011). Examining a school-based RCT to reduce gender based violence among high school students in Kwazulu-Natal, South Africa. Poster abstract. *Journal of Epidemiology and Community Health, 65*, A354. https://doi.org/10.1136/jech.2011.142976m.9

Theriot, M. T., & Orme, J. G. (2016). School resource officers and students’ feelings of safety at school. *Youth Violence and Juvenile Justice, 14*(2), 130–146.

Thompkins, A. C., Chauveron, L. M., Harel, O., & Perkins, D. F. (2014). Optimizing violence prevention programs: An examination of program effectiveness among urban high school students. *Journal of School Health, 84*, 435–443.

Tillyer, M. S., Fisher, B. S., & Wilcox, P. (2011). The effects of school crime prevention on students’ violent victimization, risk perception, and fear of crime: A multilevel opportunity perspective. *Justice Quarterly, 28*, 249–277.

Timmons-Mitchell, J., Levesque, D. A., Harris, L. A., III, Flannery, D. J., & Falcome, T. (2016). Pilot test of StandUp, an online school-based bullying prevention program. *Children & Schools, 38*, 71–79.

Trip, S., Bora, C., Sipos-Gug, S., Tocai, I., Gradinger, P., Yanagida, T., & Strohmeier, D. (2015). Bullying prevention in schools by targeting cognitions, emotions, and behavior: Evaluating the effectiveness of the REBE-ViSC program. *Journal of Counseling Psychology, 62*, 732–740.

Trotman, D., & Thomas, L. (2016). Police community support officers in schools: Findings from an evaluation of a pilot training programme for school liaison officers. *Policing, 10*(3), 288–299.

Tsaousis, I. (2016). The relationship of self-esteem to bullying perpetration and peer victimization among schoolchildren and adolescents: A meta-analytic review. *Aggression and Violent Behavior, 31*, 186–199.

Ttofi, M. M., & Farrington, D. P. (2011). Effectiveness of school-based programs to reduce bullying: A systematic and meta-analytic review. *Journal of Experimental Criminology, 7*, 27–56.

Ttofi, M. M., Farrington, D. P., & Lösel, F. (2012). School bullying as a predictor of violence later in life: A systematic review and meta-analysis of prospective longitudinal studies. *Aggression and Violent Behavior, 17*, 405–418.

Ttofi, M. M., Farrington, D. P., Lösel, F., & Loeber, R. (2011). The predictive efficiency of school bullying versus later offending: A systematic/meta-analytic review of longitudinal studies. *Criminal Behaviour and Mental Health, 21*, 80–89.

Turham, A., Onrust, S. A., ten Klooster, P. M., & Pieterse, M. E. (2016). A school-based programme for tobacco and alcohol prevention in special education: Effectiveness of the modified ‘healthy school and drugs’ intervention and moderation by school subtype. *Addiction, 112*, 533–543.

Usó, I., Villanueva, L., & Adrián, J. E. (2016). Impact of peer mediation programmes to prevent bullying behaviours in secondary schools. *Infancia y Aprendizaje, Journal for the Study of Education and Development, 39*, 499–527.

Véronneau, M.-H., Dishion, T. J., Connell, A. M., & Kavanagh, K. (2016). A randomized, controlled trial of the family check-up model in public secondary schools: Examining links between parent engagement and substance use progressions from early adolescence to adulthood. *Journal of Consulting and Clinical Psychology, 84*, 526–543.

Vigna-Taglianti, F. D., Galanti, M. R., Burkhart, G., Caria, M. P., Vadrucci, S., Faggiano, F., & for the EU-Dap Study Group. (2014). “Unplugged”: A European school-based program for substance use prevention among adolescents: Overview of results from the EU-Dap trial. *New Directions for Youth Development, 141*, 67–82. https://doi.org/10.1002/yd.20087

Vivolo-Kantor, A. M., Niolon, P. H., Estefan, L. F., Le, V. D., Tracy, A. J., Latzman, N. E., Little, T. D., Lang, K. M., DeGue, S., & Tharp, A. T. (2020). Middle school effects of the Dating Matters® comprehensive teen dating violence prevention model on physical violence, bullying, and cyberbullying: A cluster-randomized controlled trial. *Prevention Science*. https://doi.org/10.1007/s11121-019-01071-9

Vreeman, R. C., & Carroll, A. E. (2007). A systematic review of school-based interventions to prevent bullying. *Archives of Pediatrics and Adolescent Medicine, 161*, 78–88.

Waddell, G. R. (2012). Adolescent drug use and the deterrent effect of school-imposed penalties. *Economics of Education Review, 31*, 961–969.

Walton, M. A., Chermack, S. T., Shope, J. T., Bingham, C. R., Zimmerman, M. A., Blow, F. C., & Cunningham, R. M. (2010). Effects of a brief intervention for reducing violence and alcohol misuse among adolescents: A randomized controlled trial. *Journal of the American Medical Association, 304*, 527–535.

Webb, T., & Martin, K. (2012). Evaluation of a US school-based media literacy violence prevention curriculum on changes in knowledge and critical thinking among adolescents. *Journal of Children and Media, 6*, 430–449.

Whitaker, D. J., Murphy, C. M., Eckhardt, C. I., Hodges, A. E., & Cowart, M. (2013). Effectiveness of primary prevention efforts for intimate partner violence. *Partner Abuse, 4*, 175–195.

Williams, R. D., Barnes, J. T., Holman, T., & Hunt, B. P. (2014). Substance use prevention among at-risk rural youth: Piloting the social ecological *One Life* program. *Journal of At-Risk Issues, 18*, 19–26.

Williford, A., Elledge, L. C., Boiulton, A. J., DePaolis, K. J., Little, T. D., & Salmivalli, C. (2013). Effects of the KiVa antibullying programme on cyberbullying and cybervictimisation frequency among Finnish youth. *Journal of Clinical Child & Adolescent Psychology, 42*, 820–833.

Wilson, D. B., Gottfredson, D. C., & Najaka, S. S. (2001). School-based prevention of problem behaviors: A meta-analysis. *Journal of Quantitative Criminology, 17*, 247–272.

Wilson, S. J., & Lipsey, M. W. (2007). School-based interventions for aggressive and disruptive behaviour: Update of a meta-analysis. *American Journal of Preventive Medicine, 33*, S130–S143.

Wilson, S. J., Lipsey, M. W., & Derzon, J. H. (2003). The effects of school-based intervention programs on aggressive behaviour: A meta-analysis. *Journal of Consulting and Clinical Psychology, 71*, 136–149.

Wong, D. S. W., Cheng, C. H. K., Ngan, R. M. H., & Ma, S. K. (2011). Program effectiveness of a restorative whole-school approach for tackling school bullying in Hong Kong. *International Journal of Offender Therapy and Comparative Criminology, 55*, 846–862.

Wurf, G. (2012). High School Anti-Bullying Interventions: An evaluation of curriculum approaches and the method of shared concern in four Hong Kong international schools. *Australian Journal of Guidance and Counselling, 22*, 139–149.

Wynne, S. L., & Joo, H. J. (2011). Predictors of school victimization: Individual, familial, and school factors. *Crime & Delinquency, 57*, 458–488. https://doi.org/10.1177/0011128710389586

Yaakub, N. F., Huron, F., & Leong, G. C. (2010). Examining the efficacy of the Olweus prevention programme in reducing bullying: The Malaysian experience. *Procedia Social and Behavioral Sciences, 5*, 595–598.

Yeager, D. S., Fong, C. J., Lee, H. Y., & Espelage, D. L. (2015). Declines in efficacy of anti-bullying programs among older adolescents: Theory and a three-level meta-analysis. *Journal of Applied Developmental Psychology, 37*, 36–51.

Zych, I., Ortega-Ruiz, R., & Del Rey, R. (2015). Systematic review of theoretical studies on bullying and cyberbullying: Facts, knowledge, prevention, and intervention. *Aggression and Violent Behavior, 23*, 1–21.

# Chapter 6
# Preventing Young People from Involvement in Violence, Gangs and Organized Crime

## 6.1 Overall Objective

The objective of this evidence review as it was initially conceived was to provide an overview of the available research on the effectiveness of methods for preventing young people from committing violent offences or becoming involved in gangs or organized crime. However, that goal was modified after preliminary searches located a number of reviews of the designated areas. It was agreed that a new review would have been largely a duplication of those efforts. The first part of the chapter therefore presents a summary of the other reviews and discussion of some key points arising from them.

## 6.2 Background

Police already engage in a large variety of crime prevention activities, and there has been a steadily growing emphasis on the importance of that work as a component of policing, particularly through actions that can be taken in the community in conjunction with other agencies. Alongside this development, as we saw in Chap. 1, progressively more extensive use is being made of research evidence as a basis for informing operational policy and practice. This chapter addresses the question of whether young people can be prevented from becoming involved in crimes of violence, or of entering a cycle of violence, and more specifically where doing so results from participation in gangs, and whether young people can be diverted from possible involvement in organized crime. As a starting point, it is useful to examine the meanings of the terms being used, as follows.



J. McGuire et al., *Evidence-Based Policing and Community Crime Prevention*, Advances in Preventing and Treating Violence and Aggression,
https://doi.org/10.1007/978-3-030-76363-3_6

***Violence*** While this can be defined in numerous ways, for immediate practical purposes, the most readily applicable definition is in terms of criminal law and what is codified in the relevant legal statutes.

***Gangs*** We might expect that this too is straightforward, but studies have found that it is not always easy to say precisely what a gang consists of and there is no consensus on how to define a gang (Sierra-Arévalo & Papachristos, 2017). Esbensen et al. (2001) surveyed a large sample ($N = 5935$) of young people aged 13–15 from 42 high schools in 11 American cities. Using a loose definition of gang participation – whether someone had ever been in a gang, which respondents could construe in any way they wished – 16.8% of the sample reported that they had. When a stricter definition was used, entailing current core membership of an active delinquent gang, only 2.3% described themselves as members. Thus, sometimes what appear to be gangs are very loosely organized groups with unclear boundaries; and offences they commit may more often be spontaneous than planned. Only a small proportion of those groups appear to have shared aims, named leaders, sets of rules, entry procedures or penalties for leaving.

***Organized crime*** This is also difficult to define, and while it is sometimes carried out by gangs, it is usually considered to have distinct characteristics of its own. Clearly, many crimes involve planned and coordinated effort by two or more people, but this is not usually classified as organized crime, which involves more continuity over time as in recognized and self-proclaimed criminal fraternities. The variety of criminal activities that are organized at this level is very wide: from illegal vehicle trafficking, cigarette smuggling, racketeering, professional white collar crime or cybercrime to the operation of illicit drug markets or human including sexual trafficking. Several criminologists have illustrated the difficulties of pinning down what these different patterns have in common (Albanese, 2000; Finckenauer, 2005). Adolescents or young adults are unlikely to be involved in many crimes of this type: to the extent that they enter into organized criminality, it is most likely to be at the lower levels of drug distribution networks. Recent research by the Police Foundation suggests young people are more likely to be victims of organized crime than perpetrators of it, for example, through sexual exploitation (Crocker et al., 2017).

That appears to apply also in the expansion of so-called *county lines* networks, in which organized gangs based in urban centres recruit vulnerable young people and sometimes adults to act as distributors or couriers of illicit drugs in smaller towns or rural areas (Children's Commissioner for England, 2019). With reference to the individuals drawn into this, the issue seems to be primarily one of safeguarding, and at the time of writing, there was not as yet any research available that evaluated mechanisms whereby this particular form of exploitation, which is reportedly often blatantly coercive, could be prevented.

There are several kinds of overlap between the three areas listed, to an extent that it is probably impossible to keep them entirely separate, especially the first two. Solitary individuals obviously do commit violent crimes, but the majority of violence occurs in the context of interaction, in small group settings or between couples. A proportion of more serious violent crime is gang-related, and within the groups that are known as gangs, there may be individuals who would also be likely to offend on their own, but others who are brought into acting violently through a setting that promotes the use of violence. Organized crime is a relatively less common pattern and as noted is mainly committed by adults. However, some young people may be "groomed" as potential new entrants and prepared for induction into adult criminal networks. It would be invaluable to be able to identify any attributes of individuals that make this more likely or to have a clearer understanding of the process by which it occurs.

### *6.2.1 From Definitions to Policy Developments*

Debates over the definition of a gang became a central issue in public policy formation in England and Wales in the period from 2004 to 2005 onwards. One relatively broad formulation was set out in a Home Office publication by Sharp et al. (2006). This conceptualized a "delinquent youth group" as consisting of three or more young people, who spend a lot of time in public places, where the group has existed for 3 months or more, where members have engaged in delinquent or criminal behaviour together in the last 12 months and where the group has at least one structural feature – either a name, an area, a leader or rules. In their research, Sharp et al. (p.vi) found that 63% of those belonging to such groups had committed "at least one 'core offence' in the last year", as compared to 26% for non-members. The most common feature of a delinquent youth group was the "possession of an area or place the group 'called its own'" (p. viii).

A slightly stricter definition was devised by the Centre for Social Justice (2009, p. 21), which defined a gang as:

> A relatively durable, predominantly street-based group of young people who (1) see themselves (and are seen by others) as a discernible group, (2) engage in a range of criminal activity and violence, (3) identify with or lay claim over territory, (4) have some form of identifying structural feature, and (5) are in conflict with other, similar, gangs.

Almost simultaneously, the *Eurogang* project, a collaboration between American and European researchers, offered a more succinct definition (Weerman et al., 2009, p. 20):

> A street gang (or troublesome youth group corresponding to a street gang elsewhere) is any durable, street-oriented youth group whose involvement in illegal activity is part of its group identity.

Nevertheless, a joint thematic inspection report by the HM Chief Inspectors of Prisons, Probation and Constabulary (2010, p. 22) concluded that there was "no single accepted definition of what constituted a 'gang' or indeed what should be the focus of local problem-solving efforts". Following the episodes of unrest in a number of urban centres in the UK in 2011, the government launched an *Ending Gang and Youth Violence* initiative (HM Government, 2011), adopting the Centre for Social Justice (2009) definition. Critics later commented that the overall policy framework potentially criminalized fairly large numbers of young people and that the focus on gangs was a distraction from the underlying causes of youth crime and violence (Cottrell-Boyce, 2013; Smithson & Ralphs, 2016). As a result of an independent review (HM Government, n.d.), this policy was redesigned with modified aims (HM Government, 2016). Simultaneously the National Crime Agency (2016) published its own research highlighting patterns of activity in which gangs from urban centres committed offences in smaller towns adjoining those areas, mostly related to sale of drugs.

Apart from ambiguities of definition, another core difficulty in research on gang involvement is whether it is possible to discern the direction of influence between individual variables and group interaction processes. Do young people with certain features join gangs because of an unmet need to belong, a quest for status, for opportunity to engage in new kinds of crime or more serious crime – or for other reasons, such as being unable to find friends anywhere else? Are gangs therefore composed of individuals who are in some ways similar or like-minded – sometimes called the "birds of a feather" or "selection" hypothesis? Or do gangs influence their members – a well-attested effect of group interaction – in such a way that they will do things they would not otherwise have done, sometimes called the "socialization" or "facilitation" hypothesis? There is no clear answer to this. Research suggests that both sets of variables, individual and group influence, play a part, so the process is described as *bidirectional* (Matsueda & Anderson, 1998; Melde & Esbensen, 2013; Winfree et al., 1994; Wright et al., 2001). However, some have concluded that the facilitation process is the more influential of the two (Decker et al., 2013). Another possibility however is that there are different processes occurring for "adolescence-limited" as compared to "life-course-persistent" offenders and that research studies to date have conflated the two (Wong et al., 2013).

## 6.3 Method

This report as initially planned was to employ the methodology of a rapid evidence review, which applies some elements of the methods used in systematic review but with elements of the procedure simplified and certain kinds of material excluded such as unpublished research dissertations. A preliminary search of the Scopus database was conducted in August 2017, using the search string:

> young *AND* people *OR* youth *OR* adolescent *OR* juvenile *AND* crime *OR* delinquency *OR* offending *AND* prevention *OR* intervention

This retrieved 2133 documents. Scrutiny of those documents, together with a number of supplementary searches suggested by some of the documents, resulted in location of a number of recently published reviews of the area designated for the planned review. Subsequently, five other databases were searched: PsycINFO, Web of Science, the Cochrane and Campbell libraries and the National Criminal Justice Reference Service. This resulted in discovery of some other recent reviews.

Given that several of the reviews that were found were comparatively new and that the results of some had already been incorporated into guideline documents issued by official bodies in the UK, including justice and social welfare agencies, it appeared an unnecessary duplication to review the field again. We considered it more useful simply to provide what researchers call a review of reviews in this area. To be included, a review had to have the objective of collating a number of studies on a given relevant issue and to contain results that reflected that aim in the form of a narrative or systematic review, rapid evidence assessment or meta-analysis. The first part of this chapter is therefore a summary of the main points from the previous recent reviews. The second part of the chapter reviews studies in this area, involving collaborative work between police and other agencies, published in the period 2017–2020.

## 6.4 Previous Reviews

There is already a very large research literature on youth violence and on criminal gangs. The largest proportion of both has been carried out within criminology, a smaller but still substantial volume in psychology and recently a small but growing proportion in the field of public health. By comparison, the study of organized crime is much less well developed. There are many case studies of it, but given its usually hidden nature, systematic knowledge is limited. For the same reason, as far as could be established, there are no research evaluations of preventive methods designed to reduce its emergence or occurrence.

There have also been numerous research studies of interventions to reduce youth violence, and a sizeable body of research has accumulated on how to address the gang problem and to reduce gang violence. Given evidence that the presence of gangs is associated with higher rates of serious offending, numerous efforts have been made to carry out direct work with young people in the context of the gangs themselves. Proposals regarding how to do this have taken a variety of forms, and some practical applications were developed on the basis of them, and evaluation research showed some modest degrees of success (Goldstein & Huff, 1992).

The present review was however intended to examine research on the process of *entry* into violence, gangs or organized crime and how it could be prevented. Given the multiple and overlapping areas within this, some of the reviews that were found covered more than one area of interest. However, none of them addressed the precise question asked or the area delineated for the present review, i.e. to reduce the likelihood of young people's initial involvement or entry into participation in gang violence or organized crime. Only one review was found on the effects of interventions to reduce organized crime, but that was based on criminal justice procedures rather than on preventive work.

A bibliography of government and academic research studies and related reports and documents was compiled by researchers at the House of Commons Library (Lalic & Holland, 2016). Four of the documents found were interconnected reports prepared for the Home Office by the Early Intervention Foundation, consisting of a review of risk and protective factors, a review of prevention programmes, a short summary of those two reviews and a document distilling key advice for commissioners of programmes (Cordis Bright Consulting, 2015; O'Connor & Waddell, 2015a, 2015b; Waddell, 2015). Other reviews were reported in more standard academic format of articles in research journals. The 16 reviews that were found are summarized in Table 6.1; only two of these (Hodgkinson et al., 2009, not located previously; Roth & Pierce, 2019) came from the updating process. Another that has been added was an update of previous reviews on the *pulling levers* strategy first reviewed by Braga and Weisburd (2012a, 2012b). Five of the included articles are narrative reviews only; given the less formalized processes applied in such reviews, in four of them there was no statement of the number of studies included, and it was not possible to make a meaningful count of that number: some studies were discussed in detail, but others only cursorily. In the remaining reviews, a more formal methodology of systematic review or rapid evidence assessment was used, and two employed meta-analysis. All of these gave an exact number of located studies.

## 6.5 Findings

The types of research carried out in this area and summarized in the retained reviews can be divided into three main categories (though one review fitted two of them) with a few remaining that were unique in their coverage. The largest group involves the study of individual gang members and of the risk and protective factors associated with joining or remaining in a gang (Cordis Bright Consulting, 2015; Decker et al., 2013; O'Brien et al., 2013; Petrosino et al., 2015; Raby & Jones, 2016). A second group consists of the study of law-enforcement-based interventions known as *pulling levers* (Braga & Weisburd, 2012a, 2012b, 2015; Petrosino et al., 2015). The third is a collection of reviews focused on evaluations of community interventions (Abt & Winship, 2016; Higginson et al., 2015; Hodgkinson et al., 2009; O'Connor & Waddell, 2015a). Finally, however, there are several reviews each with separate stand-alone aims and content, dealing with social network analysis of gangs (Sierra-Arévalo & Papachristos, 2017), with law enforcement in drug markets (Werb et al., 2011) and with the role of social media in coordinating gang violence (Patton et al., 2014). Two other reviews that were focused on interventions of specific types, carried out to Cochrane Collaboration standards, found no studies that satisfactorily met the criteria that were set for methodological rigour (Fisher, Gardner, & Montgomery, 2008; Fisher, Montgomery, & Gardner, 2008).

**Table 6.1** Previous reviews of related areas

| Review | Focus | No. of studies | Findings |
|---|---|---|---|
| Abt and Winship (2016) | Systematic meta-review of previous review studies of interventions to reduce community violence. Tabulates findings but does not report a quantitative synthesis | 43 reviews with a total of 1435 studies | Large-scale and wide-ranging overview of existing reviews, including a quality assessment that found the methodology of most reviews to be good. The report is supplemented by field site visits in the USA and in parts of the Northern Triangle of El Salvador, Guatemala and Honduras, an area with extremely high rates of violence. Found that the forms of intervention with the firmest support were those classed as *pulling levers* and *cognitive-behavioural therapies*. The report however combines reviews of offender rehabilitation research with those on prevention, making it more difficult to isolate whether there are any distinctive markers of projects or methods that will work for prevention of youth violence or of entry into gangs before offences are committed |

(continued)

**Table 6.1** (continued)

| Review | Focus | No. of studies | Findings |
|---|---|---|---|
| Braga and Weisburd (2012a, 2012b, 2015); Braga et al. (2018) | Meta-analysis of *pulling levers*: focused deterrence strategies designed to reduce gang violence. Strategies entailed: selecting a specific crime problem, convening an inter-agency working group, designing a set of sanctions, providing services to targeted offenders and directly communicating plans to offender groups | 24 (QE designs) 12 with matched controls | Review of interventions to reduce gang violence by young people, following on an initial study in Boston (*Operation Ceasefire*, a problem-oriented policing initiative) concerning gang-related gun homicides amongst youth (<24 years). The operation meant communicating with gangs about the enforcement consequences of retaliating to actions by other gangs and carrying out a coordinated criminal justice response to the gang's other activities, including stiffer plea bargains and sentences, but also offering other multi-agency community services. This approach was subsequently tested in several US cities. The first review reported a meta-analysis of 10 studies, finding a medium-to-large mean effect size of 0.604 across studies, representing a significant drop in key target outcomes including homicide rates. The later review (2018) found a mean effect size of 0.383 across a range of outcomes from gun violence to general crime, though with a large range of effects from one marginally negative outcome to an effect size of 1.186. Effect sizes were lower in matched-design evaluations. Overall, there were statistically significant crime reduction effects on a targeted crime problem in 19 of the 24 studies |
| Cordis Bright Consulting (2015) | Research review based on analysis of risk and protective factors identified in 8 longitudinal studies of delinquent development and 15 other quantitative studies | 23 | Focused separately on risk and protective factors for youth violence and for gang involvement. Risk and protective factors were divided into 5 domains (individual, family, school, peer group and community), and a total of 16 factors were identified as *strong* for youth violence and 8 factors identified as *strong* for gang involvement. Factors were also sorted by a series of six age bands (0–2, 3–6, 7–9, 10–12, 13–15 and 16–25) |

(continued)

**Table 6.1** (continued)

| Review | Focus | No. of studies | Findings |
|---|---|---|---|
| Decker et al. (2013) | Narrative review of research on gang membership and of theories and models of the processes involved | n/a | Categorizes research studies according to level of focus: individual (studies of gang members, including risk factors), micro (group processes in gangs) and macro (explanation of the uneven distribution of gangs across geographic areas, e.g. neighbourhoods). Also reviews theoretical statements on how gangs emerge and persist |
| Fisher, Gardner, and Montgomery (2008) | Cognitive-behavioural intervention to prevent gang involvement in children and youths aged 7–16 | 0 | Review using standard search strategies located an initial 2284 records. After inspection, all were excluded as there were no RCTs or QEs, or the studies did not address the target problem. This is cited as it was located as part of the relevant literature, but does not contain any findings that add to knowledge in the area. Authors emphasized the need for more rigorous research |
| Fisher, Montgomery, and Gardner (2008) | Review of the effects of opportunities provision for preventing youth gang involvement for children and young people | 0 | The review focused on the effects of providing youths at risk of involvement in gangs with opportunities for education, employment or training. Review using standard search strategies located an initial 2696 records. After applying inclusion and exclusion criteria, only two studies (both US-based) were found that were partially relevant to the issue of opportunity provision, but due to methodological flaws, they too were excluded. No RCTs or QEs were located, and the authors concluded that in the absence of more rigorous research, there were no conclusions that could be drawn and more research is urgently needed |

(continued)

**Table 6.1** (continued)

| Review | Focus | No. of studies | Findings |
|---|---|---|---|
| Higginson et al. (2015) | Review of evidence on the effectiveness of interventions to prevent youth involvement in gangs and gang crime in low- and middle-income countries and identify reasons for success or failure using thematic analysis | 4 | Searches conducted in 7 languages of a total of 17 databases, 8 individual journals and 8 repositories of "grey literature". No studies were found that used an experimental design (RCT or QE) which were inclusion criteria for evaluating effectiveness. Therefore, no conclusions could be drawn about effectiveness. Four studies were retained for thematic analysis of whether or not implementation was successful. On this basis four factors emerged as important in intervention design and delivery: including components that appeal to youth, active engagement, offering continuity of social ties outside the gang and focusing on "demobilization" and "reconciliation" |
| Hodgkinson et al. (2009) | Systematic review and meta-analysis of interventions designed to reduce gang-related crime | 17 | From an initial large number of potentially relevant records (20,672) found in literature search, after screening 208 were retained, narrowed further to 17 that focused on comprehensive interventions, i.e. those involving multi-agency partnerships and targeted several dimensions of gang activity. Meta-analysis of 12 studies found a positive but not statistically significant impact in reducing crime. When two studies were removed due to suspected invalid calculations, the mean effect size was 0.12 and marginally significant |

(continued)

**Table 6.1** (continued)

| Review | Focus | No. of studies | Findings |
|---|---|---|---|
| O'Brien et al. (2013) | Narrative review of research on motivational, risk and protective factors related to youth gang affiliation and its relationship to violence | Approx. 200 | Review focused on the factors and psychological processes associated with young people joining and leaving gangs (engagement and desistance), risk and protective factors for gang membership and the relationship of gang affiliation to violent and other types of crime. Searched 3 databases, >3 relevant websites and Google. From 672 tests located, "approximately 200" were reviewed. Risk factors for gang involvement and youth violence were allocated under five headings: individual, peer, family, school and community. Many overlapped, but there were fewer factors for gang involvement than for youth violence more generally. Their focus on protective factors was more limited. Desistance from gangs showed two patterns, abrupt or more gradual; both were driven mainly by maturation |
| O'Connor and Waddell (2015a) | Report using rapid evidence assessment conducted as part of HO *Ending Gang and Youth Violence* programme | 67 | Review of intervention programme evaluations. All the located studies were carried out in the USA. 54/67 studies reported positive outcomes and were divided into 2 main groups. *Well-evidenced interventions* included skills-based or skill-building methods and group and family counselling, home visiting, parent training and family therapy. *Promising approaches* included mentoring, community-based programmes and hospital-based programmes. The remaining 13 studies were of ineffective and even harmful approaches including deterrence and discipline. Note that the positive outcomes were primarily measured in terms of reductions in behaviour problems or delinquency in general and results are not specific to violence or involvement in gangs |

(continued)

**Table 6.1** (continued)

| Review | Focus | No. of studies | Findings |
|---|---|---|---|
| Patton et al. (2014) | Narrative review of the uses of social media in relation to youth violence | 56 | Extensive review of research on several forms of interpersonal violence conducted through social media, including cyberbullying and victimization, electronic dating aggression and cyber-stalking, gang violence and use of social media in support of it. Found 10 QEs, 18 surveys and a variety of other studies. Found that there is evidence of increasing use of violence in online space, but research was insufficiently rigorous to allow conclusions to be drawn regarding its role as almost all research was descriptive only, and there are no agreed definitions or standards for measurement or recording of online violence |
| Petrosino et al. (2015) | Rapid evidence assessment of studies on interventions to reduce firearms violence by urban youth | 11 | Collated findings from studies published in the period 1996–2013. Amongst the studies, three involved targeting high-risk individuals, and eight were broader and tested strategies involving neighbourhoods. The latter overlapped with those reviewed by Braga and Weisburd (see above). Overall, 10/11 studies reported large decreases in violence outcomes including homicides and nonfatal shootings. The single study without positive effects, which had potentially harmful results, showed a number of key weaknesses in implementation |
| Raby and Jones (2016) | Systematic review of research on risk factors for gang affiliation | 102 | Review carried out as a component of the "Ending Serious Group Violence" work at the HO. Searched 6 databases locating 244 studies of which 102 met inclusion criteria; 8 were carried out in the UK. Applied quality appraisal procedure to studies. Classified risk variables under seven major headings: family, school, individual (which included antisocial behaviour history, drug use and ethnicity), poverty, psychological difficulties, peers and community. Proposed a "cumulative developmental risk" model or "meta-narrative" as a means to understanding key risk parameters |

(continued)

**Table 6.1** (continued)

| Review | Focus | No. of studies | Findings |
|---|---|---|---|
| Roth and Pierce (2019) | Narrative review of initiatives to reduce burglary by youthful offenders | n/a | A wide-ranging review that considers different approaches to working with young people who have been convicted of burglary. Summarizes the methods involved in several initiatives and offers an overall evaluation of issues and challenges arising from each. They include mentoring programmes, drug and alcohol treatment, transfer of juveniles to adult courts, multi-modal education/ employment interventions and victim involvement (including mediation and restorative justice) |
| Sierra-Arévalo and Papachristos (2017) | Narrative review of research on the role of social networks in attempts to reduce gang violence | n/a | Historically based narrative review examining the concepts used in *network analysis*, an approach to understanding the formation and activities of gangs by mapping the connections between individuals in a gang and between gangs in the same or adjoining areas. The maps produced are then used to guide which groups to target in focused deterrence. The review explains the theoretical basis of this and illustrates the use of methods from previous and ongoing research |
| Werb et al. (2011) | Systematic review of the effects of law enforcement on drug market violence | 15 | Focused on organized crime in drug markets. The located research included 11 longitudinal studies with follow-up periods extending to 6 years, 2 studies employing mathematical models and 2 qualitative studies. 14/15 studies and 91% of the outcomes analysed found that law enforcement had an adverse impact on levels of violence; there was evidence that drug prohibition was associated with increased violence |

Abbreviations used in the table are as follows: *HO* Home Office, *RCT* randomized controlled trial, *QE* quasi-experimental (non-randomized) design

### 6.5.1 Risk and Protective Factors

The objective of many research projects in this field has been to gain an understanding of the factors and processes that draw young people into gang membership. This is part of the larger field of research on risk factors for offending in general, and this information has been used to inform the design of interventions with adjudicated young offenders in criminal justice settings. The reviews considered here address the related question of whether there are any separate or additional factors, or combination of factors, that specifically predict involvement in violent crime or in gangs.

Table 6.2 lists the factors found by Corbis Bright Consulting to overlap in being associated with both youth violence and gang involvement. The importance of each of these varied by age band, reflecting developmental changes and processes at each stage. O'Brien et al. (2013) arrived at a longer list of risk factors and also noted a high degree of overlap for those connected to youth violence and gang membership, respectively. There was a high level of agreement between the sets of risk factors identified in the two reviews. For individuals whose gang membership results in committing serious offences that led to custodial sentences, an additional factor may be at work. *Social dominance theory* emphasizes the part played in criminal offending by a search for status and an individual's perceived position in a social hierarchy. In a recent UK-based study with 188 prisoners aged 16–18 in a Young Offender Institution, Alleyne et al. (2016) found that prisoners who were gang members while in custody had previously committed more aggressive and violent crimes. They also showed more evidence of being influenced by a social dominance orientation and were also more likely to endorse hypermasculine values, anti-authority attitudes and moral disengagement than non-gang offenders.

It is important to realize however that in many cases, the risk factors that are associated with violence, or with involvement in gangs, are not distinct from those that are well established for involvement in delinquency more generally. This presents an obstacle to the identification of those individuals who may be susceptible to gang participation and also lends support to the socialization concept of gang formation and continuation. However, Hennigan et al. (2015) have devised and provide preliminary validation data on a risk assessment measure concerned exclusively with gang involvement.

**Table 6.2** Overlapping factors associated with both youth violence and gang involvement (from Cordis Bright Consulting, 2015)

| Domain | Factor |
|---|---|
| Individual | Hyperactivity<br>Lack of guilt and empathy<br>Physical violence/aggression<br>Positive attitude towards delinquency<br>Previous criminal activity |
| Family | Family poverty<br>Family violence and abuse<br>Broken home/change in the primary carer<br>Antisocial parents |
| School | Low academic performance<br>Low commitment to school<br>Frequent truancy |
| Peers | Delinquent peers<br>Commitment to delinquent peers<br>Peer rejection |
| Community | Neighbourhood disorganization<br>Exposure to drugs |

An understanding of the development of risk and its links to the processes through which young people join gangs can be gained from the type of theory developed by Howell and Egley Jr. (2005) which combines the risk factors approach with evidence from longitudinal studies of development. The associations between variables as depicted in their integrated model are shown in Fig. 6.1. This shows key sets of variables applying at different phases of the life span. Some are *distal*, having their origins in early family experiences, but their relative influence progressively alters over time. Others are *proximal*, that is, they are more recent and closer to the process through which a youth joins a gang. A clearer grasp of this could be very useful if planning preventive work with youths of different ages, when selecting which risk factors to focus on with separate cohorts.

### 6.5.2 Best-Supported Interventions

On the basis of the research reviewed here and having the advantage of several reviews conducted in the area, it is possible to identify a number of interventions that have received fairly good and, in some cases, comparatively strong support from research findings. They include the following.

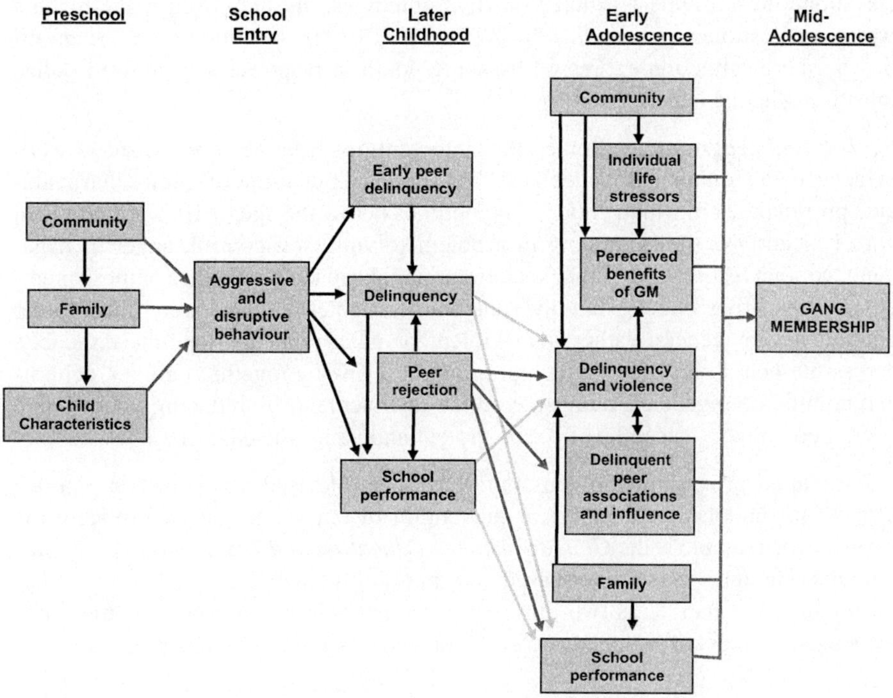


**Fig. 6.1** A developmental model of gang involvement. (From Howell and Egley Jr. (2005))

***Pulling levers*** This refers to an intervention that entails a variety of components that act in a complementary way. The original evaluation of a study of this kind was reported by Braga et al. (2001) in Boston (*Operation Ceasefire*), but similar approaches were developed in other American cities and were reviewed by Braga and Weisburd (2012a, 2012b, 2015) and Braga et al. (2018) in the reviews listed in Table 6.1. These had significant and in some instances large effects, with outcome variables ranging from gun homicide to other kinds of violence. The projects involved a combination of law enforcement with provision of services to gang members, implemented through direct communication with gangs in efforts to avoid immediate resort to striking back when a gang member was victimized by a member of another gang.

***Working with high-risk cases*** Petrosino et al. (2015) found three studies with individuals aged 15–24 who were assessed as showing high risk for violence and were targeted for intervention. This included community notification, making social and community services available, street worker support, supervision to reduce crime opportunities and aggressive law enforcement. Reductions in violence were reported in all three studies.

Both of these approaches are notable in the mixture of direct use of law enforcement with making available other kinds of provision for gang members, recognizing the circumstances in which many live. Deterrence-based or control-oriented policies alone do not appear to have positive outcomes and may even make matters worse, as illustrated in the review by Werb et al. (2011). Such effects may be amplified by the disaffection expressed by some youth in response to perceived police injustice (Zapolski et al., 2018).

***Skills-based programmes*** Some other interventions have been described as well-evidenced. O'Connor and Waddell (2015a) surveyed outcomes of studies that evaluated programmes in which children, sometimes below the age of 10, were provided with education or skills training in problem-solving, self-control, anger management, conflict resolution or other social-emotional capacities. Studies of these methods had positive effects, but the outcome variables studied were most often delinquency in general rather than violent or gang-related offending. Arguably, across-the-board provision of such programmes, linking together families, schools and community agencies, alongside police involvement, by reducing youth crime overall could have a specific effect on violent and gang-related crime.

Structured programmes of this kind have been devised for delivery by police officers in schools, specifically for prevention of entry into gangs. Probably the best-known example is the *Gang Resistance Education and Training* (GREAT) programme. Though this is school-based, it did not fulfil the inclusion criteria for studies retained in Chap. 5, as two-thirds of participants in the largest evaluation of it were aged 11 years or younger, and evaluation analysis does not report outcomes for separate age groups. The primary objectives of *Gang Resistance Education and Training* are described as being, first, to teach youth to avoid gang membership; second, to prevent violence and criminal activity; and, third, to assist youth in developing positive relationships with law enforcement.

While initial piloting of this programme produced some positive and promising outcomes, in an early longitudinal follow-up study, results were less encouraging (Esbensen & Osgood, 1999). The programme content was subsequently redesigned, and a fuller multisite RCT evaluation was conducted (Esbensen et al., 2011, 2013). Participants in this study were 3820 students from 195 classrooms in 31 schools in 7 US cities. Researchers measured a total of 33 outcome variables, including gang membership, delinquency and violent offending. Over the period of the project, with six waves of data collection, the retention rate at the 4-year follow-up point was 71.9%. However, results at a 4-year follow-up were again mixed. Approximately one-third of outcome measures showed significant improvements, but the effect sizes were uniformly small. The single most impressive findings were a reduction in the odds of belonging to a gang which at the 4-year follow-up point were 24% lower for programme participants than for controls and that participants showed significantly more positive attitudes to police, although the effect size for this was fairly small. The principal limitation of this programme is probably one of dosage, in that it consists of just 13 sessions each lasting 40 minutes. In addition, it relies on school-based delivery only, with no parental dimension or other community involvement.

A further set of interventions have been described as promising. They include *mentoring* (O'Connor & Waddell, 2015a). This refers to a process in which an adult is appointed who can provide both individual support and liaison with practical services for each young offender. In a meta-analysis of 39 studies, this has been shown to have positive outcomes with young offenders (Tolan et al., 2008). One of the outcomes focused on, and for which positive outcomes were obtained, was aggressive behaviour. However, that review did not address the issue of gang involvement. Another possibility is that of community-based interventions that incorporate a wide range of service provision, where young people, families, communities and public services are coordinated to identify both individuals and features of communities that are associated with increased risk (O'Connor & Waddell, 2015a). This also includes sports-based programmes. However, findings from some reviews of this area found only rather weak effects on criminal recidivism variables (e.g. Hodgkinson et al., 2009).

On organized crime unfortunately, given the substantial challenges presented by trying to do research in this area, conclusions are more or less impossible to draw. Tackling organized crime is often the responsibility of specialized police agencies that work across regional or county boundaries, and as Mackenzie and Hamilton-Smith (2011) note, the difficulty in defining organized crime has been an impediment to measuring police impact on this problem. The process by which individuals are inducted into organized criminal networks appears to be one in which there is little or no reliable information available.

## 6.6 Implications of Review Findings

There are compelling reasons for the level of research interest in the areas covered in this review summary. First, as can be seen immediately in the familiar *age-crime curve*, the middle and late adolescent years are the peak age for participation in delinquency and are also a highly influential and formative period for those who will continue in criminal activity into adulthood. Given the additional concern arising from the prospect of involvement in gangs or in organized crime, the need to address this appears even more urgent. Second, it is widely recognized that the earlier those prevention efforts can be undertaken, the more likely they are to succeed. That may be partly because of the opportune moment in the maturation process, but also because of the possibility of harnessing support from other sources (families and schools) and potentially averting the risk that individuals will become entrenched in what is called a criminal lifestyle.

On the basis of some of the reviews listed in Table 6.1, sets of guidelines have been issued by criminal justice departments, law enforcement agencies or associated research bodies in several jurisdictions, including England and Wales (College of Policing, 2014; Factor et al., 2015; Home Office, 2015), the USA (Esbensen, 2000; Howell, 2010; National Gang Center, 2017; Simon et al., 2013) and Canada (Public Safety Canada, 2007).

### *6.6.1 Strengths and Limitations of the Reviews*

It was expected that the volume of research found potentially relevant to this review question would be large. Despite a sizeable volume of research with an indirect bearing on the issues however, there was far less that can be described as clearly and explicitly addressing the core objective of the review, which was concerned with evaluation of interventions to reduce youth violence and participation in gangs or in organized crime.

The reviews summarized in Table 6.1 are very diverse in the ground they cover and in their methodology. This makes it difficult to discern a trend across the set of reviews as a whole. Nevertheless, there is sufficient uniformity in the findings of some studies to make it possible to arrive at clear conclusions on the effects of some interventions.

As in many other areas of research on crime, North American studies are far more numerous amongst both the primary studies and the reviews. Given evidence that gangs in Europe including the UK are both fewer in number and less violent than in the USA, it seems important not to extrapolate findings from that context to application elsewhere without careful consideration of the differences in crime patterns, neighbourhood environments and the criminal justice context (Pyrooz & Sweeten, 2015; Klein et al., 2006). However, there have been studies of factors that influence gang involvement in the UK (e.g. Medina Ariza et al., 2014), and some researchers have suggested that gangs in the USA and the UK have enough in common to make it a useful process to apply the findings of US-based research (Alleyne & Wood, 2010).

There are large challenges in conducting research in this area. The processes through which individuals join gangs are not likely to be directly observable. Unless individuals are already known to the police as a result of prior delinquency, they cannot be assessed, and the likelihood of joining gangs cannot be estimated. For those whose first conviction arises from an offence committed in a gang, it is difficult to be sure whether individual characteristics or social facilitation processes were the main influences on their offending.

### *6.6.2 Primary and Tertiary Prevention*

This is of less immediate relevance to our present objectives. But if efforts at primary prevention fail and young people do commit offences of violence, there is well-established evidence concerning the possibility of reducing rates of criminal reoffending amongst them at the *tertiary prevention* or criminal justice intervention stage.

Lipsey and Wilson (1998) reviewed 200 studies, and Garrido and Morales (2007) a further 30 studies, concerned with young people between the ages of 12 and 21 who had committed serious violent or sexual offences. Both reviews found clear evidence of positive outcomes from several types of intervention. However, a later study suggests that gang membership can reduce the effectiveness of evidence-based interventions (Boxer et al., 2015). This places further stress on the need for giving priority emphasis to prevention and intervention efforts that can reduce levels of participation in gangs at earlier stages of involvement and, if possible, to avert it entirely.

In as far as it is possible to achieve it, prevention is a preferable strategy in dealing with these problems as with so many others. Moreover, as Decker (2013, p. 61) notes, "it is difficult to imagine a successful gang-membership prevention program without police involvement". Even so, police usually form partnerships with other agencies including schools, youth justice, health services and community agencies including local government and voluntary sector groups, to stand the best chance of providing effective approaches. Some recent research findings have illustrated the potential of such a combined approach.

## 6.7 Review of Recent Evaluations

In the remaining part of this chapter, we report a review of research studies published in the period 2017 to 2020 (with one exception of a 2016 study that was not detected in earlier searches). As with the pattern of updating used elsewhere in the book, this is based on a more limited form of search than that employed in the initial reviews. Three databases were searched: Scopus, PsycINFO and the National Criminal Justice Reference Service, using the following search string:

> offenders OR juvenile delinquents OR juvenile offenders AND gang involvement AND police AND interventions OR strategies OR best practices AND effect* AND gangs OR organized crime AND polic* AND (effectiveness or efficacy or effective)

This yielded only 67 relevant studies, the low number probably reflecting the inclusion of polic* as a search term (though that often locates items concerned with policy rather than policing or police). After downloading and screening, eight of these studies were retained for review. A report by Gahunia et al. (2019) of a police initiative to reduce restaurant-based violence in Vancouver was considered but excluded as it was not primarily designed to reduce youth involvement in the gangs.

The quality of research design in each study was rated using the Maryland *Scientific Methods Scale* (SMS). Many different forms of research can be used for the purpose of evaluating interventions, and examples of several of them are found throughout this book. Designs vary in their robustness, and approaches have been devised for appraising the quality of studies and comparing them with each other. The Maryland Scale is one method widely used for this purpose in criminal justice research (Farrington et al., 2002; Sherman et al., 1998) which allocates a score to studies on a scale from 1 to 5 according to their design. Higher scores denote more robust types of design as set out in Table 6.3.

Adopting this framework, the key details of the eight studies retained, including their scores on the Maryland Scale, are presented in Table 6.4.

Some of the studies summarized in Table 6.4 were derivatives of, or further applications of, models of intervention first tested elsewhere. The *Growing Against Gangs and Violence* intervention evaluated by Densley et al. (2016) was inspired by and in many respects evolved from the GREAT programme described earlier (Esbensen et al., 2013). However as noted in Table 6.4, implementation problems made it difficult to draw any clear conclusions about its effectiveness.

*Project Safe Neighborhoods* (Jeffries et al., 2019) was one of a series of applications of the *pulling levers* initiative which involved direct communication between police and members of violent gangs in a form of problem-oriented policing. This had its origins in the earlier *Project Ceasefire* begun in Boston in the 1990s, an attempt to reduce gun-related homicides and other violence by youth gangs (Braga et al., 2001), as described earlier. The *pulling levers* strategy was later conceptualized as a form of *focused deterrence* because at its core, as a method of behaviour change, it centres on seeking "to enhance offender perceptions of the certainty, swiftness, and severity of punishment, while providing social service opportunities and potential rewards for law-abiding behavior" (Jeffries et al., 2019, p. 328). Thus, while it does include what would be defined in behavioural terms as a form of punishment of undesired behaviour, it also includes a form of positive reinforcement of desired behaviour.

Some other interventions here, such as those by Bennett et al. (2018) and Mazerolle et al. (2017, 2019), are conceptualized as forms or variations of

**Table 6.3** The Maryland Scientific Methods Scale

| Score and level | Type of study |
|---|---|
| 1: Correlational study | Correlation between a crime prevention measure or intervention programme and a measure of crime, or with risk factors at a given point in time |
| 2: Pre-post comparison with no equivalent comparator | Before-and-after measurement with an experimental cohort, with no untreated comparison group available, or the presence of a comparison group without demonstrated comparability to the treatment group |
| 3: Group comparison or case-control design | A comparison between two or more comparable groups or units of analysis, one with and one without the intervention, or between two or more types of intervention |
| 4: Quasi-experimental design with statistical or other controls | Comparison between multiple equivalent groups or units, one with and one without the treatment programme, statistically controlling for confounding factors, or using comparison samples that evidence only minor differences |
| 5: Randomized controlled trial (RCT) | Fully random assignment of comparable units to intervention/ experimental and comparison groups and analysis of data at end-point and/or follow-up |

*third-party policing* (Mazerolle & Ransley, 2005). This is based on the fundamental precept that "the role of the police is arguably most important in conveying sanction certainty" (Mazerolle et al., 2020, p. 896). Thus other, non-police personnel whose roles involve contact with at-risk youth can cooperate with police in seeking to reduce difficulties before they escalate to a more serious level. With reference to truancy, for example, it is well established as having a link to delinquency. Therefore, if it can be reduced, the risk of criminal involvement will also decrease as a result. As Mazerolle et al. (2020, p. 887) suggest, "Through the Third Party Policing approach, police strive to influence a young person's antisocial behavior by working with schools and parents to better communicate the nature of education legislation and the consequences of noncompliance".

Another study in this series by Mazerolle et al. (2020) was not strictly an evaluation study, but an analysis of data from 86 children, together with their parents, from the participant group in the studies by Mazerolle et al. (2017, 2019). The objective was to test for factors correlated with outcome variables. The study was embedded within the *Ability School Engagement Program* (ASEP) experimental trial described in Table 6.4, examining the relationship between youth self-reported antisocial behaviour and their parents' knowledge of their legal responsibilities, perceptions of the likelihood of prosecution and risk choices. Results showed that the experimental condition was associated with a reduction in the link between children's willingness to attend school and their level of self-reported antisocial behaviour.

**Table 6.4** Recent evaluation studies of interventions (eight studies)

| Study: author(s), (date), country | Design and Maryland Scientific Methods Scale (SMS) quality of evidence | Samples/data sources | Interventions and outcomes |
|---|---|---|---|
| Aalsma et al. (2018) USA | Pilot study using a pre-post single-cohort design to evaluate a training event SMS = 2 | 232 participants in a training event: 148 law enforcement (police) officers 84 probation and other correctional staff | Evaluated *Policing the Teen Brain*, a two-day training programme which explains aspects of the neurological and behavioural features of adolescent development, designed to reduce conflict and misunderstanding between police officers and young people. Participants provided demographic information and completed a set of knowledge and attitudes scales before and after attending the event, concerning beliefs about adolescents and wider beliefs concerning punitiveness. Results showed positive and significant change on almost all scales employed, concerning perceptions of adolescents and beliefs about punishment |
| Bennett et al. (2018) Australia | RCT SMS = 5 | Study group as in Mazerolle et al. (2017) | One of a series of studies to evaluate *Ability School Engagement Program (*ASEP) (see Mazerolle et al., 2017, below). The present study reports findings on levels of delinquency from official police records before and after the programme. At pre-test there were no significant differences between the experimental and control groups in prior numbers of crime incidents. At 1-year post-test, there was a significant time *x* condition interaction. Control participants showed a significant increase in rate of offending. Experimental participants showed a non-significant decline. Authors concluded this demonstrated that "a truancy reduction program slowed the progression of increased offending, relative to a control group who evinced significantly higher crime incidents" (p. 323) |

(continued)

**Table 6.4** (continued)

| Study: author(s), (date), country | Design and Maryland Scientific Methods Scale (SMS) quality of evidence | Samples/data sources | Interventions and outcomes |
|---|---|---|---|
| Densley et al. (2016) UK | RCT outcome evaluation and qualitative process evaluation SMS =5 | 391 school students aged 12–14 at 4 school sites:<br>198 intervention<br>193 control<br>92.3 retention at post-test but only 64% at follow-up | Evaluated the efficacy of *Growing Against Gangs and Violence*, a primary prevention partnership programme between the Metropolitan Police and other agencies, delivered by police officers in schools in London. *Growing Against Gangs and Violence* consists of six lessons and involves skills training in combination with other elements. Process evaluation findings were mixed regarding mode of delivery and adherence to the model. Outcome evaluation showed a small but non-significant reduction in gang involvement in the intervention compared to the control groups. At 1-year follow-up, there were small but again non-significant reductions in general and violent offending, improvements in youth-police relationships and reductions in adherence to "street code". Other problematic aspects of delivery detracted from the evaluator's ability to draw clear conclusions |
| De Vries et al. (2018) Netherlands | RCT with long-term follow-up SMS = 5 | Two groups of at-risk youth aged 12–19:<br>47 intervention<br>45 care-as-usual<br>47% arrested at least once before | Evaluated *New Perspectives* a prevention programme designed to reduce offending behaviour in a group assessed as being at risk of involvement in it (secondary intervention). NP involves an intensive 3-month programme followed by 3 months' aftercare and targets a number of identified criminogenic risk variables: poor relationships, cognitive distortions and poor parenting. Recidivism was measured at 12 and 18 months and at a mean of 2.4 years using both self-report and official information sources. However, no between-group differences were found on any outcome measure. Care as usual was as effective as the NP programme. The authors suggested the New Perspectives programme lacked theoretical focus and that treatment integrity was compromised in that treatment adherence was unacceptably low during the aftercare phase |

(continued)

**Table 6.4** (continued)

| Study: author(s), (date), country | Design and Maryland Scientific Methods Scale (SMS) quality of evidence | Samples/data sources | Interventions and outcomes |
|---|---|---|---|
| Hobson et al. (2018) UK | Process and outcome evaluation, using a quasi-experimental waiting-list design SMS = 4 | 97 at-risk youth aged 9–17 in 3 locations: 69 active cases 28 in waiting-list control group | Evaluated the *Aston Project*, a police-led initiative to reduce crime and harm by young people through increasing engagement in constructive community-focused activities, entailing extensive use of volunteer workers. Reports a process evaluation based on interviews with a wide range of stakeholders in the project, highlighting a number of difficulties in delivery. Outcome evaluation does not however clarify the data sources or specify precise measures of effectiveness, reporting only that of 69 young people involved, over 11 months of activity, only 4 offended. The estimated £8000 per capita savings from this is used as part of a cost-benefit evaluation. Based on projected figures, authors suggest that the project would lead to significant savings, returning 170% of the sums invested by Police and Crime Commissioners |
| Jeffries et al. (2019) USA | Quasi-experimental design SMS = 4 | 133 young people aged 13–19 either involved in serious crimes or assessed as at risk of becoming involved | Evaluated *Project Safe Neighborhoods* in Connecticut, part of the pulling levers initiative. This combined individual assessment, a school-based programme, support in career planning and a media outreach campaign, in working with identified at-risk young people, who completed a number of job-related certificates. The project reached fewer youths than initially planned. There was a significant drop (48% to 33.8%) in extent of justice involvement across the project as a whole and at both participating sites. Rates of re-adjudication (return to court, 31.3% at 12 months) were however "less encouraging" (p. 341) and indicated a need for longer-term support services for participating youth |

(continued)

**Table 6.4** (continued)

| Study: author(s), (date), country | Design and Maryland Scientific Methods Scale (SMS) quality of evidence | Samples/data sources | Interventions and outcomes |
|---|---|---|---|
| Mazerolle et al. (2017) Australia | Process evaluation and RCT SMS = 5 | 102 young people (age range 10–16) from 11 schools, involved in truanting: 51 assigned to ASEP 51 business-as-usual controls | Evaluation of the ASEP, a police-schools partnership designed to reduce levels of truancy. To be eligible, participants had to have missed ≥15% of school days with no legitimate reason. Police worked with school facilitators in a series of family group conferences with children and parents over a period of 6 months. Objectives were to increase parent's awareness of truancy laws, and halt likely increases in truancy. Control children were seen by School Resource Officers. There was a significant effect over time in perceptions of the likelihood of prosecution for ASEP but not control participants. Children whose parents believed prosecution was likely made significantly more efforts to go to school, as compared to control participants where children's efforts to attend school reduced |
| Mazerolle et al. (2019) Australia | RCT SMS = 5 | Study group as in Mazerolle et al. (2017) | Reports a 2-year follow-up evaluation of the ASEP project described in the preceding entry. Also collected data on self-reported antisocial behaviour. There was a reduction in ASB for the ASEP but not the control group at 1- and 2-year follow-up, and the differences were statistically significant (effect size −0.27 at 2 years). There was a significant association between lower antisocial behaviour and greater willingness to attend school at 1- but not 2-year follow-up. This was considered to be a short-term effect, drawing attention to the need for sustained work to maintain gains over time |

### 6.7.1 Possible Future Directions

For the two police forces that commissioned the review reported here, the findings played a part in the gradual changes that they each implemented in addressing this area. Particularly in one county, the results influenced initiatives taken in 2019, focused on county lines drug distribution networks, alongside programmes to develop key skills of young people to challenge offending behaviour and learn how to manage conflict safely as part of a new initiative designed to prevent them from falling into crime.

While the following suggestions have not been sufficiently well researched to be the basis for translation into practice, they highlight some additional directions in which research on methods of prevention of youth violence and gang involvement might proceed in the next few years.

First, Hennigan et al. (2015) developed a risk assessment measure for gang involvement and reported a validation study. Having an accessible tool for this purpose could be very advantageous for implementing some of the risk-focused strategies that have to date produced positive results and for disseminating them more widely.

Another departure that may grow in extent of use is the adoption of a *public health perspective* which involves coordinating support from a wide range of services including health. Such an approach has been piloted by Strathclyde Police, and Williams et al. (2014) have reported positive outcomes of an intervention based on these principles for reducing gang-related violence in Glasgow. However, Gebo (2016) advises caution in applying this to all levels of violence prevention and sees its main role at the primary prevention stage of work. This would however correspond well to the objectives of police and allied agencies working with at-risk adolescents.

In examining the role of police in preventing gang membership, Decker et al. (2013) consider the Scanning, Analysis, Response and Assessment (SARA) model which grew out of problem-oriented policing, as a strategy for crime prevention concerned with gang-related activity. This could potentially be employed as an organizing framework in formulating plans for a coordinated approach to community-based initiatives in violence and gang prevention. Subsequently, Abt (2017), drawing on the review summarized earlier in Table 6.1, proposed a possible framework for organizing community prevention that combines public health with criminal justice perspectives.

It may be possible to gain a clearer understanding of why young people become gang members by examining what happens at the eventual end of the process, when they leave gangs and desist from crime. Dong and Krohn (2016) have reported results that suggest this could be a fruitful area of further work. As with criminal offending more generally, this change is often associated with the development of other supportive relationships, including those with close partners, and parenthood. This also draws attention to the need for more in-depth qualitative research involving interviews with gang members (e.g. Peterson, 2017).

## References

Aalsma, M. C., Schwartz, K., & Tu, W. (2018). Improving police officer and justice personnel attitudes and de-escalation skills: A pilot study of policing the teen brain. *Journal of Offender Rehabilitation, 57*(7), 415–430.

Abt, T. P. (2017). Towards a framework for preventing community violence among youth. *Psychology, Health & Medicine, 22*, 266–285.

Abt, T. P., & Winship, C. (2016). *"What works" in reducing community violence: A meta-review and field study for the northern triangle*. United States Agency for International Development (USAID).

Albanese, J. S. (2000). The causes of organized crime: Do criminals organise around opportunities for crime or do criminal opportunities create new offenders? *Journal of Contemporary Criminal Justice, 16*, 409–423.

Alleyne, E., & Wood, J. L. (2010). Gang involvement: Psychological and behavioral characteristics of gang members, peripheral youth and non-gang youth. *Aggressive Behavior, 36*, 423–436.

Alleyne, E., Wood, J. L., Mozova, K., & James, M. (2016). Psychological and behavioural characteristics that distinguish street gang members in custody. *Legal and Criminological Psychology, 21*, 266–285.

Bennett, S., Mazerolle, L., Antrobus, E., Eggins, E., & Piquero, A. R. (2018). Truancy intervention reduces crime: Results from a randomized field trial. *Justice Quarterly, 35*(2), 309–329.

Boxer, P., Kubic, J., Ostermann, M., & Veysey, B. (2015). Gang involvement moderates the effectiveness of evidence-based intervention for justice-involved youth. *Children and Youth Services Review, 52*, 26–33.

Braga, A. A., Kennedy, D. M., Waring, E. J., & Piehl, A. M. (2001). Problem-oriented policing, deterrence, and youth violence: An evaluation of Boston's operation ceasefire. *Journal of Research in Crime and Delinquency, 38*, 195–225.

Braga, A. A., & Weisburd, D. L. (2012a). The effects of 'pulling levers' focused deterrence strategies on crime. *Campbell Systematic Reviews, 8*(1), 1–10. https://doi.org/10.4073/csr.2012.6

Braga, A. A., & Weisburd, D. L. (2012b). The effects of focused deterrence strategies on crime: A systematic review and meta-analysis of the empirical evidence. *Journal of Research in Crime and Delinquency, 49*, 323–358.

Braga, A. A., & Weisburd, D. L. (2015). Focused deterrence and the prevention of violent gun injuries: Practice, theoretical principles, and scientific evidence. *Annual Review of Public Health, 36*, 55–68.

Braga, A. A., Weisburd, D., & Turchan, B. (2018). Focused deterrence strategies and crime control: An updated systematic review and meta-analysis of the empirical evidence. *Criminology and Public Policy, 17*(1), 205–250.

Centre for Social Justice. (2009). *Dying to belong: An in-depth review of street gangs in Britain*. The Centre for Social Justice.

Children's Commissioner for England. (2019). *Keeping kids safe: Improving safeguarding responses to gang violence and criminal exploitation*. Children's Commissioner for England.

College of Policing. (2014). Preventing youth gang involvement for children and young people (7–16) using opportunities provision. In *What works briefing*. CoP.

Cordis Bright Consulting. (2015). *Preventing gang and youth violence: A review of risk and protective factors. Early Intervention Foundation report*. Home Office.

Cottrell-Boyce, J. (2013). Ending gang and youth violence: A critique. *Youth Justice, 13*, 193–206.

Crocker, R., Webb, S., Garner, S., & Skidmore, M. (2017). *The impact of organized crime in local communities*. The Police Foundation.

Decker, S. H. (2013). What is the role of police in preventing gang membership? In T. R. Simon, N. M. Ritter, & R. R. Mahendra (Eds.), *Changing course: Preventing gang membership* (pp. 50–61). US Department of Justice and Centers for Disease Control and Prevention, US Department of Health and Human Services.

Decker, S. H., Melde, C., & Pyrooz, D. C. (2013). What do we know about gangs and gang members and where do we go from here? *Justice Quarterly, 30*, 369–402.

Densley, J. A., Adler, J. R., Zhu, L., & Lambine, M. (2016). Growing against gangs and violence: Findings from a process and outcome evaluation. *Psychology of Violence, 7*(2), 242–252.

De Vries, S. L. A., Hoeve, M., Asscher, J. J., & Stams, G. J. J. M. (2018). The long-term effects of the youth crime prevention program "New Perspectives" on delinquency and recidivism. *International Journal of Offender Therapy and Comparative Criminology, 62*(12), 3639–3661.

Dong, B., & Krohn, M. D. (2016). Escape from violence: What reduces the enduring consequences of adolescent gang affiliation? *Journal of Criminal Justice, 47*, 41–50.

Esbensen, F.-A. (2000). *Preventing Adolescent Gang Involvement*. Office of Juvenile Justice and Delinquency Prevention, US Department of Justice.

Esbensen, F.-A., & Osgood, D. W. (1999). Gang Resistance Education and Training (GREAT): Results from the national evaluation. *Journal of Research in Crime and Delinquency, 36*(2), 194–225.

Esbensen, F.-A., Osgood, D. W., Peterson, D., Taylor, T., & Carson, D. (2013). Short- and long-term outcome results from a multisite evaluation of the G. R. E. A. T. program. *Criminology & Public Policy, 12*, 375–411.

Esbensen, F.-A., Peterson, D., Taylor, T. J., Freng, A., Osgood, D. W., Carson, D. C., & Matsuda, K. N. (2011). Evaluation and evolution of the Gang Resistance Education and Training (G.R.E.A.T.) program. *Journal of School Violence, 10*, 53–70.

Esbensen, F.-A., Winfree, L. T., He, N., & Taylor, T. J. (2001). Youth gangs and definitional issues: When is a gang a gang, and why does it matter? *Crime and Delinquency, 47*, 105–130.

Factor, F., Pitts, J., & Bateman, T. (2015). *Gang-involved young people: Custody and beyond.* Beyond Youth Custody Partnership.

Farrington, D. P., Gottfredson, D. C., Sherman, L. W., & Welsh, B. C. (2002). The Maryland scientific methods scale. In L. W. Sherman, D. P. Farrington, B. C. Welsh, & D. L. MacKenzie (Eds.), *Evidence-based crime prevention* (pp. 13–21). Routledge.

Finckenauer, J. O. (2005). Problems of definition: What is organized crime? *Trends in Organized Crime, 8*, 63–83.

Fisher, H., Gardner, F., & Montgomery, P. (2008). Cognitive-behavioural interventions for preventing youth gang involvement for children and young people (7–16*). Cochrane Database of Systematic Reviews*, (2), CD007008. https://doi.org/10.1002/14651858.CD007008.pub2

Fisher, H., Montgomery, P., & Gardner, F. (2008). Opportunities provision for preventing youth gang involvement for children and young people (7–16). *Cochrane Database of Systematic Reviews*, (2), CD007002. https://doi.org/10.1002/14651858.CD007002.pub2

Gahunia, S., McConnel, K., & Bain, A. (2019). The positive perception of reduced gang violence through a public safety initiative. *Police Journal, 92*(2), 167–188.

Garrido, V., & Morales, L. A. (2007). *Serious (violent and chronic) juvenile offenders: a systematic review of treatment effectiveness in secure corrections*. Campbell Collaboration Reviews of Intervention and Policy Evaluations (C2-RIPE). Available at: www.campbellcollaboration.org/doc-pdf/Garrido_seriousjuv_review.pdf

Gebo, E. (2016). An integrated public health and criminal justice approach to gangs: What can research tell us? *Preventive Medicine Reports, 4*, 376–380.

Goldstein, A. P., & Huff, C. R. (Eds.). (1992). *The gang intervention handbook.* Research Press.

Hennigan, K. M., Kolnick, K. A., Vindel, F., & Maxson, C. L. (2015). Targeting youth at risk for gang involvement: Validation of a gang risk assessment to support individualized secondary prevention. *Children and Youth Services Review, 56*, 86–96.

Higginson, A., Benier, K., Shenderovich, Y., Bedford, L., Mazerolle, L., & Murray, J. (2015). Preventive interventions to reduce youth involvement in gangs and gang crime in low- and middle-income countries: A systematic review. *Campbell Systematic Reviews, 2015*, 28. https://doi.org/10.4073/csr.2015.18

Hobson, J., Lynch, K., Payne, B., & Ellis, L. (2018). Are police-led social crime prevention initiatives effective? A process and outcome evaluation of a UK youth intervention. *International Criminal Justice Review, 2018, 1*, –22. https://doi.org/10.1177/1057567718814891

Hodgkinson, J., Marshall, S., Berry, G., Newman, M., Reynolds, P., Burton, E., Dickson, K., & Anderson, J. (2009). *Reducing gang related crime: A systematic review of 'comprehensive' interventions*. Technical report. In *Research evidence in education library*. EPPI-Centre, Social Science Research Unit, Institute of Education, University of London.

Home Office. (2015). *Preventing youth violence and gang involvement: Practical advice for schools and colleges*. Home Office.

HM Government. (2011). *Ending gang and youth violence. A cross-government report.* Cm 8211. Crown copyright.

HM Government. (2016). *Ending gang violence and exploitation*. HM Government.

HM Government. (n.d.). *Ending gang and youth violence programme 2012–15: Assessment.* https://www.gov.uk/government/uploads/system/uploads/attachment_data/file/570476/egyv-assessment-programme-2012-15-full-report.pdf

HM Chief Inspector of Prisons, HM Chief Inspector of Probation, HM Chief Inspector of Constabulary (2010). *The management of gang issues among children and young people in prison custody and the community: A joint thematic review*. Crown copyright.

Howell, J. C. (2010). *Gang prevention: An overview of research and programs*. Office of Juvenile Justice and Delinquency Prevention, US Department of Justice.

Howell, J. C., & Egley, A., Jr. (2005). Moving risk factors into developmental theories of gang membership. *Youth Violence and Juvenile Justice, 3*, 334–354.

Jeffries, S. A., Myers, D., Kringen, J. A., & Schack, R. (2019). Evaluating project safe neighborhoods in Connecticut: A youth opportunity initiative. *Crime Prevention and Community Safety, 21*, 325–345.

Klein, M. W., Weerman, F. M., & Thornberry, T. P. (2006). Street gang violence in Europe. *European Journal of Criminology, 3*, 413–437.

Lalic, M., & Holland, S. (2016). *Gangs: A select bibliography*. House of Commons Library.

Lipsey, M. W., & Wilson, D. B. (1998). Effective intervention for serious juvenile offenders: A synthesis of research. In R. Loeber & D. P. Farrington (Eds.), *Serious and violent juvenile offenders: Risk factors and successful interventions* (pp. 313–345). Sage Publications.

Mackenzie, S., & Hamilton-Smith, N. (2011). Measuring police impact on organized crime: Performance management and harm reduction. *Policing: An International Journal of Police Strategies and Management, 34*, 7–30.

Matsueda, R. L., & Anderson, K. (1998). The dynamics of delinquent peers and delinquent behavior. *Criminology, 36*, 269–308.

Mazerolle, L., Bennett, S., Antrobus, E., Cardwell, S. M., Eggins, E., & Piquero, A. R. (2019). Disrupting the pathway from truancy to delinquency: A randomized field trial test of the longitudinal impact of a school engagement program. *Journal of Quantitative Criminology, 35*, 663–689.

Mazerolle, L., Bennett, S., Antrobus, E., & Eggins, E. (2017). The coproduction of truancy control: Results from a randomized trial of a police–schools partnership program. *Journal of Research in Crime and Delinquency, 54*(6), 791–823.

Mazerolle, L., Cardwell, S. M., Antrobus, E., & Piquero, A. R. (2020). Policing partnerships to address youth antisocial behavior: How parental risk-taking shapes child outcomes. *Criminology & Public Policy, 19*, 883–904.

Mazerolle, L., & Ransley, J. (2005). *Third party policing*. Cambridge University Press.

Medina Ariza, J. J., Cebulla, A., Aldridge, J., Shute, J., & Ross, A. (2014). Proximal adolescent outcomes of gang membership in England and Wales. *Journal of Research in Crime and Delinquency, 51*, 168–199.

Melde, C., & Esbensen, F.-A. (2013). Gangs and violence: Disentangling the impact of gang membership on the level and nature of offending. *Journal of Quantitative Criminology, 29*, 143–166.

National Crime Agency. (2016). *County lines gang violence, exploitation & drug supply 2016. 0346-CAD National Briefing Report*. National Crime Agency.

National Gang Center. (2017). *A law enforcement official's guide to the OJJDP comprehensive gang model*. Office of Juvenile Justice and Delinquency Prevention, US Department of Justice.

O'Brien, K., Daffern, M., Chu, C. M., & Thomas, S. D. M. (2013). Youth gang affiliation, violence, and criminal activities: A review of motivational, risk, and protective factors. *Aggression and Violent Behavior, 18*, 417–425.

O'Connor, R. M., & Waddell, S. (2015a). *What works to prevent gang involvement, youth violence and crime: A rapid review of interventions delivered in the UK and abroad. Early Intervention Foundation report*. Home Office.

O'Connor, R. M., & Waddell, S. (2015b). *Preventing Gang Involvement and Youth Violence: Advice for those Commissioning Mentoring Programmes. Early Intervention Foundation report*. Home Office.

Patton, D. U., Hong, J. S., Ranney, M., Patel, S., Kelley, C., Eschamm, R., & Washington, T. (2014). Social media as a vector for youth violence: A review of the literature. *Computers in Human Behavior, 35*, 548–553.

Peterson, K. E. (2017). Voices from a gang – A study of young gang members and stories as told by themselves about upbringing, school and gang life – Gang research in a Danish context. *Journal of Gang Research, 24*, 35–52.

Petrosino, A., Campie, P., Pace, J., Fronius, T., Guckenburg, S., Wiatrowski, M., & Rivera, L. (2015). Cross-sector, multi-agency interventions to address urban youth firearms violence: A rapid evidence assessment. *Aggression and Violent Behavior, 22*, 87–96.

Public Safety Canada. (2007). *Youth gang involvement: What are the risk factors?* National Crime Prevention Centre, Public Safety Canada/Sécurité publique Canada.

Pyrooz, D. C., & Sweeten, G. (2015). Gang membership between ages 5 and 17 years in the United States. *Journal of Adolescent Health, 56*, 414–419.

Raby, C., & Jones, F. (2016). Identifying risks for male street gang affiliation: A systematic review and narrative synthesis. *Journal of Forensic Psychiatry and Psychology, 27*, 601–644.

Roth, J. J., & Pierce, M. B. (2019). Improving responses to juvenile burglary offenders. *Safer Communities, 18*(3/4), 94–106.

Sharp, C., Aldridge, J., & Medina, J. (2006). *Delinquent youth groups and offending behaviour: findings from the 2004 Offending, Crime and Justice Survey. Home Office Online Report 14/06*. Home Office.

Sherman, L. W., Gottfredson, D. C., MacKenzie, D. L., Eck, J., Reuter, P., & Bushway, S. D. (1998). *Preventing crime: What works, what doesn't, what's promising*. National Institute of Justice.

Sierra-Arévalo, M., & Papachristos, A. V. (2017). Social networks and gang violence reduction. *Annual Review of Law and Social Science, 13*, 373–393.

Simon, T. R., Ritter, N. M., & Mahendra, R. R. (Eds.). (2013). *Changing course: Preventing gang membership*. Office of Justice Programs, US Department of Justice and Centers for Disease Control and Prevention, US Department of Health and Human Services.

Smithson, H., & Ralphs, R. (2016). Youth in the UK: 99 problems but the gang ain't one? *Safer Communities, 15*, 11–23.

Tolan, P., Henry, D., Schoeny, M., & Bass, A. (2008). Mentoring interventions to affect juvenile delinquency and associated problems. *Campbell Systematic Reviews, 2008*, 16. https://doi.org/10.4073/csr.2008.16

Waddell, S. (2015). *Preventing Gang and Youth Violence: Spotting Signals of Risk and Supporting Children and Young People: An Overview. Early Intervention Foundation report*. Home Office.

Weerman, F. M., Maxson, C. L., Esbensen, F.-A., Aldridge, J., Medina, J., & van Gemert, F. (2009). *Eurogang program manual: Background, development, and use of the Eurogang instruments in multi-site, multi-method comparative research*. Available at: http://www.umsl.edu/ccj/Eurogang/EurogangManual.pdf

Werb, D., Rowell, G., Guyatt, G., Kerr, T., Montaner, J., & Wood, E. (2011). Effect of drug law enforcement on drug market violence: A systematic review. *International Journal of Drug Policy, 22*, 87–94.

Williams, D. J., Currie, D., Linden, W., & Donnelly, P. D. (2014). Addressing gang-related violence in Glasgow: A preliminary pragmatic quasi-experimental evaluation of the Community Initiative to Reduce Violence (CIRV). *Aggression and Violent Behavior, 19*, 686–691.

Winfree, L. T., Bäckström, T. V., & Mays, G. L. (1994). Social learning theory, self-reported delinquency, and youth gangs: A new twist on a general theory of crime and delinquency. *Youth & Society, 26*, 147–177.

Wright, B. R. E., Caspi, A., Moffitt, T. E., & Silva, P. A. (2001). The effects of social ties on crime vary by criminal propensity: A life-course model of interdependence. *Criminology, 39*, 321–351.

Wong, I. W., Toh, D. P., Hung, P. P. L., & Ang, R. P. (2013). Delinquency in gangs – Selection or socialization? *Aggression and Violent Behavior, 18*, 784–791.

Zapolski, T. C. B., Banks, D. E., Lau, K. S. L., & Aalsma, M. C. (2018). Perceived police injustice, moral disengagement, and aggression among juvenile offenders: Utilizing the general strain theory model. *Child Psychiatry and Human Development, 49*, 290–297.

# Chapter 7
# Multi-agency Safeguarding for Vulnerable and At-Risk Adults

## 7.1 Overall Objective

The objective of this evidence review is to provide an overall descriptive account of the available research on the effectiveness of methods of safeguarding or protecting vulnerable adults through multi-agency services in the community.

## 7.2 Background

Amongst the broad range of tasks performed by the police, there are several that are associated with the community-based protection of vulnerable individuals, carried out in collaboration with other agencies. The present chapter focuses on one part of that, concerned with protection or safeguarding of vulnerable adults. Large amounts of research have been carried out in the adjoining field of child protection, which is a highly developed area that has generated a very large body of research literature informing both practice and policy. By contrast work on adult protection has received considerably less attention. The chapter is therefore focused on that area and issues arising within it. A decision to focus the review in this way was also taken in order to ensure the task of reviewing was manageable within the allocated time.

Used in this context, the term *community-based* refers to the work of large network of agencies that provide services to vulnerable or at-risk adults, other than those that involve direct hospital-based care as an in-patient or hospital detention under the Mental Health Act. Thus, it includes those with statutory responsibilities for health and social care, such as NHS trusts and local authority social services departments, but it also encompasses a range of voluntary, charitable or "third sector" providers. While some of these are coordinated nationally, the patterning of others varies considerably according to local needs. But as used in the research that



J. McGuire et al., *Evidence-Based Policing and Community Crime Prevention*, Advances in Preventing and Treating Violence and Aggression,
https://doi.org/10.1007/978-3-030-76363-3_7

was located here, the term also denotes some kinds of residential care provision, which, despite in one sense taking service users out of their communities, also rely on the maintenance of strong links with families and with agencies providing home-based services.

As a result of several different developmental factors, there is a proportion of adults who are unable to protect themselves and are partially or entirely dependent on others. Individuals with one or more types of disability (or in some cases multiple disabilities) may have difficulty in protecting themselves from several kinds of risk, and in older adulthood a significant proportion of the population come to rely on others for regular help. The phrase *vulnerable adult* is widely used as a general term when referring to individuals in these positions. They may have long-term difficulties such as some form of disability, or they may become incapacitated as a result of the onset of problems or adverse circumstances. They may then be at risk of being abused, neglected, exploited or victimized in some other way.

In the UK the General Medical Council considers that family doctors (general practitioners [GPs]) have a pivotal role to play in protecting patients and in ensuring their safety is not compromised. Based on the Department of Health's (2000) *No Secrets* guidance, Boland et al. (2013) listed the types of abuse to which vulnerable adults are sometimes subjected. Abuse was divided into six categories, *physical*, *sexual*, *psychological*, *financial*, *neglect* (acts of omission) and *discriminatory*. However, that list was significantly augmented following the implementation of the Care Act 2014 which placed safeguarding on a statutory basis. Gibson et al. (2016) subsequently published a paper offering more extensive guidance to GPs on making safeguarding referrals. They provide a fuller list of the different forms of abuse, now divided into ten categories as follows:

1. *Physical*. Assault, physical coercion or inappropriate restraint, including misuse of medication
2. *Domestic*. Psychological, physical, sexual, financial, emotional and including honour-based abusiveness
3. *Sexual*. Rape, indecent assault or exposure, sexual harassment or involvement in unwanted touching or sexual acts, including witnessing without consent
4. *Psychological*. Emotional abuse, threats of harm or abandonment, deprivation of contact or support, intimidation or other forms of control, verbal or cyberbullying
5. *Financial or material*. Theft or fraud; coercion over financial affairs; misuse of property, possessions or benefits; interference with wills or other transactions
6. *Modern slavery*. Forced labour, human trafficking, domestic servitude and other forms of exploitation or inhumane treatment
7. *Discriminatory*. Harassment, slurs, humiliation or maltreatment based on gender, race, age, gender identity, sexual orientation, disability or religion
8. *Organizational*. Neglect or inadequate care within an institution or other care setting, including someone's own home, resulting from poor professional practice

9. *Neglect and acts of omission*. Ignoring medical, physical or emotional care needs, failing to provide access to health or other care or withholding necessities of life
10. *Self-neglect*. Including a range of behaviour such as neglect of personal hygiene, health or surroundings

One of the objectives of Boland et al.'s (2013) earlier paper was to offer advice to GPs regarding when to refer someone for safeguarding support. They summarized six principles of good safeguarding practice as follows: *(1) empowerment*, proceed on a person-led basis that involves informed consent; *(2) protection*, support and represent those in greatest need; *(3) prevention*, where possible act before harm occurs; *(4) proportionality*, select the least intrusive action appropriate to the risk; *(5) partnership*, search for solutions first through local community-based services; and *(6) accountability*, provide transparent grounds for the safeguarding actions taken. Adding to this Gibson et al. (2016) incorporated a decision-making flowchart as a format for guiding a family doctor who becomes aware of a possible need for safeguarding, indicating a sequence of steps to be taken to arrive at a referral decision.

## 7.2.1 Extent of Need for Safeguarding

Thus, there are numerous reasons why adults may be vulnerable, but those who are most frequently seen as requiring protection or safeguarding are often considered under one of three major categories: people with intellectual disabilities, those with severe and enduring mental health problems and older adults. However, there are many other specific causes of vulnerability including sensory and physical impairments, and some people experience multiple levels of difficulty. Victimization or other mistreatment of people who are vulnerable for these or other reasons is, sadly, far from uncommon. Surveys of the prevalence of such abuse or neglect often tend to focus on each of these broad areas separately, but a proportion have reviewed evidence concerning disadvantage and vulnerability of various kinds. One area that has been quite extensively researched is that of violent victimization.

### 7.2.1.1 Overview

Hughes et al. (2012) carried out an integrative overview of research on violence towards people with disabilities of one kind or more. They noted World Health Organisation (2015) data showing that globally, 15% of people have a disability. They located 26 studies from 7 countries with a cumulative participant sample of 21,557. They examined reported levels of physical, sexual and intimate partner violence. Studies were found in the areas of mental illness (17 studies), intellectual impairment (5 studies), physical disability (3 studies), sensory impairments (3 studies) and non-specific impairments (9 studies). Overall, they found that "…violence is a major problem in adults with disabilities, who are at an increased risk of violence compared with non-disabled adults" (p. 6). The prevalence of this problem was highest amongst those with mental illnesses and lowest for those with non-specific impairments. Other studies of prevalence have tended to focus on specific types of vulnerability.

#### 7.2.1.2 Intellectual Disabilities

Horner-Johnson and Drum (2006) reviewed a set of 5 studies, and later Fisher et al. (2016) reviewed a series of 23 studies, finding that people with intellectual disabilities are far more often victims of crime or abuse than those without such disabilities. An illustration of what this may mean at a local level can be seen in the work of Beadle-Brown et al. (2010). These authors reported a survey of referrals for adult protection during 1 year in a single local authority in England and found that one-third (1926 of 6148) were for individuals with intellectual disabilities. This group experienced a higher rate of physical and sexual abuse in various care settings than adults without an intellectual disability.

#### 7.2.1.3 Severe and Enduring Mental Health Problems

In a systematic review locating 34 studies, Latalova et al. (2014) found that people with severe mental illness were considerably more likely to suffer violent victimization than other members of the community. There is evidence that this applies not only to those experiencing severe mental illnesses but also to those experiencing what are called common mental health disorders (Meijward et al., 2015). On the basis of an analysis of 41 studies, Trevillion et al. (2012) found that for this group there is also a higher risk of being a victim of domestic violence across all diagnostic categories. The trend is particularly pronounced amongst women with depressive, anxiety or post-traumatic stress disorders.

#### 7.2.1.4 Older Adults

Biggs et al. (2009) reported findings of the *First National Prevalence Study of Elder Mistreatment* in the UK. In a sample of 2111 respondents, over a 12-month period, 2.6% reported mistreatment by a family member, friend or care worker. Extrapolated to the UK as a whole, this would imply an annual figure of 227,000 adults aged 65 or older who were subjected to mistreatment. The most frequently reported type of mistreatment was neglect, followed by financial, psychological, physical and sexual abuse. De Donder et al. (2011) reviewed findings from the *Abuse and Violence against Older Wome*n study, conducted across five European countries, but were able to access data from a total of ten countries. On average across countries, psychological abuse had the highest prevalence rates, and sexual abuse the lowest, but on some issues such as violation of personal rights, there was very little research. The first systematic review of this area by Cooper et al. (2008) found 49 studies of the prevalence of elder abuse based on victim reports and family or caregiver reports or recorded using objective measures (e.g. screening measures administered by third parties). Overall, they found that 6% of older adults, a quarter of vulnerable adults and a third of family carers "…report being involved in significant abuse, but only a small proportion of this is currently known to protective services" (p. 159). More recently Yon et al. (2017) found a total of 234 studies of the prevalence of elder abuse and meta-analysed results from 52 studies of 12-month neglect or abuse of adults aged 60 years or over from 28 countries. As suggested by the World Health Organisation (see Hughes et al., 2012), the average prevalence rate across studies was 15.7%, i.e. approaching one in six of older adults worldwide, but there were large national variations in abuse rates.

Slightly more is known about the abuse of older adults in situations where this can be monitored and recorded, such as residential care homes, although even here, as some recent notorious cases illustrate, it is difficult to be sure of the real extent of the problem as for obvious reasons abuse by staff is less likely to be reported. Abuse by fellow residents is fairly extensively documented (Ferrah et al., 2015; Lindbloom et al., 2007; McDonald et al., 2015; Payne & Fletcher, 2005). Many agencies which provide residential services in this field are likely to use internal safeguarding procedures to address these problems and may only be likely to involve police in more severe cases.

The foregoing is by no means an exhaustive summary of research on these issues, but there is a consensus across the findings of many reviews that there is an increased risk of victimization and other forms of maltreatment of people with disabilities of several kinds and of vulnerable older adults, as compared with the population in general. Note also that published reviews predominantly focus on incidents of a type that can be measured, such as recorded assault, but even with respect to those, available information may be unreliable and is probably an underestimate of actual incidents. As regards other forms of victimization, the scale of problems is extremely difficult to assess, and it seems likely that a large proportion of several forms of abuse and of vulnerability remains hidden or unknown. In a different domain, Manthorpe et al. (2017) reported a scoping review of the extent to which adults with needs for care and support were also at risk of involvement in gambling and susceptible to gambling-related harm, financial abuse or scams. Many other aspects of vulnerability and the need for protection, such as motives for abuse or neglect, are investigated in some of the studies included here but remain under-researched.

### *7.2.2 Formal Policies and Guidelines*

In recognition of the marked level of need in this area, some of it often unmet, both the national statutory agencies and the relevant professional bodies which have responsibilities within it have produced official policy or guidance statements concerning the protection of vulnerable people. Key landmarks in legislation and in policy have included the inception of the *No Secrets* framework (Department of Health, 2000) which established the Disclosure and Barring Service (DBS), the introduction of the Safeguarding Vulnerable Groups Act 2006 and the Care Act 2014. Brammer (2009) illustrates the formidable body of relevant legislation that was passed in the period 2000–2008. Thus, policy and practice have both evolved over time and have been subject to some change relatively recently.

Government policy and recommendations and guidelines for practice have been published by the Department of Health (2011), NHS England (2015), the Office of the Public Guardian (2015), and the Home Office (2014) which produced a report on its *Multi Agency Working and Information Sharing Project*. Amongst professional bodies, the British Medical Association (2011) produced a *Tool Kit* for general practitioners; and the National Police Improvement Agency (2012), coordinated by the Association of Chief Police Officers, issued *Guidance on Safeguarding and Investigating the Abuse of Vulnerable Adults*. The Association of Directors of Social Services (2005) developed a framework of national standards for safeguarding, and the Association of Directors of Adult Social Services London (2015) produced its own set of practice guidelines for Multi-Agency Safeguarding in London.

Two books by Mandelstam (2013, 2017) were useful background sources for this review. The first provides a detailed discussion of legal frameworks governing the safeguarding process with vulnerable adults. That volume however preceded some legislative changes including the Care Act 2014 which introduced a number of new provisions in the area of safeguarding. The second book takes the form of a dictionary explaining numerous terms employed in the field of adult care. According to this source (Mandelstam, 2017), the Care Act 2014 more often uses the terminology of *protecting people* rather than *safeguarding*. Local authorities are required to establish a Safeguarding Adults Board (SAB). Under certain circumstances the SAB can require other agencies or persons to provide information to it, and they must comply. The handling of any such information must also however accord with the provisions of the Data Protection Act 1998 and the European Convention on Human Rights. The SAB has both the duty and the power to convene a Safeguarding Adults Review, the objective of which is to learn lessons from any problem that has arisen in the process of safeguarding in individual cases. This may be done not only in cases of death where it is suspected that it may have resulted from abuse or neglect but also where an adult is still alive but there is suspected serious abuse or neglect or reasonable cause for concern regarding the possibility that one or other may be occurring.

A few of the journal articles that were found in this review focused on research ethics and knowledge transfer where this raised issues of safeguarding, for example, those by Bellman et al. (2010), Lyketsos et al. (2004) and Randall et al. (2015). While clearly important, this was regarded as a separate issue and was not addressed in the present review. The sources found were in any case formal statements of principles or procedures or analytic discussions rather than empirical studies.

## 7.3 Previous Reviews

No prior reviews of this exact field were found that had the same central aim as the present one. A few reviews were found of adjoining areas which have some bearing on the issues addressed here, for example, one by Baker et al. (2016) on interventions to prevent abuse in older adults was valuable (Table 7.1) but found only seven eligible studies: Its results were inconclusive and its relevance to safeguarding is unclear. No review was found that collated studies of evaluations of outcomes effectiveness or compared different forms of practice or changes within safeguarding practice. This is in marked contrast to the adjacent field of child protection which has been extensively researched and documented.

A very wide-ranging, integrative meta-review has been reported by Dickson et al. (2017, based on a fuller report by Sutcliffe et al., 2012). The objective of what these authors called a meta-review of systematic reviews was to identify gaps in research literature on the improvement of outcomes of social care. The authors found a total of 43 reviews pertaining to different aspects of this. The majority of the reviews that were discovered dealt with the impact of interventions on quality of life or on delaying or reducing the need for support; only one review focused on what the authors considered as safeguarding. Given its breadth of compass, the meta-review by Dickson et al. (2017) has been excluded from Table 7.1. Of the numerous sources they cite, only the single review which was thought to include material on safeguarding, by Lindbloom et al. (2007), has been included. However, although described in that way in Dickson et al.'s review, the focus of Lindbloom et al. was on factors linked to abuse in adult residential care. Hence their work is partly relevant to the aims of the present review.

## 7.4 Method

As in other chapters, the present one employs the methodology of a rapid evidence review, which applies some elements of the methods used in a systematic review but entails less elaborate or detailed and time-consuming procedures. The material to be covered in the review was restricted to published studies (peer-reviewed journal articles or government reports) and to documents available in English and was planned as far as possible to be relevant to policing. Six databases were searched to locate potentially relevant research literature: PsycINFO, Scopus, Web of Science, the Cochrane Database of Systematic Reviews, the website of the Campbell

**Table 7.1** Previous reviews of related areas: safeguarding vulnerable adults

| Review | Focus | No. of studies | Findings |
|---|---|---|---|
| Baker et al. (2016) | Prevention of abuse of older adults | 7 | Cochrane systematic review: searched 19 databases. Required 12-week follow-up for inclusion. All retained studies had control conditions and 5/7 used randomization, but most were assessed as having high risk of bias. Overall authors concluded that there is "inadequate trustworthy evidence" regarding the effects of interventions to reduce abuse |
| Hutchinson and Stenfert Kroese (2015) | Causes of abuse of adults in residential care settings | 15 | The located studies employed diverse methodologies (eight quantitative, six qualitative, one mixed-methods) and so were appraised using a "cross-paradigm" framework for quality review. Risk factors for abuse were placed in two categories: organizational or cultural and individual/interpersonal. The mix of study types and abuse types made clear patterns hard to detect, but some trends emerged with reference to staff features, client characteristics and aspects of practice with services. Overall, it was concluded that research in this area "remains in its infancy" |
| Lindbloom et al. (2007) | Mistreatment of older adults in nursing homes: A review of prevalence but also of factors associated with maltreatment | n/a | The review located a large number of studies (324) but does not explicitly state how many were retained for review purposes. Groups were classed by types of abuse, focusing on characteristics of abusers, problems at both institutional and individual levels and features of interventions that reduced abuse |
| Manthorpe and Lipman (2015) | Prevention of abuse through pre-employment checks | 11 | Collated articles from Anglophone or Northern European countries, to investigate the extent of use of police vetting prior to employment in care roles. Large differences were found between jurisdictions. No evidence was found showing whether checks made safeguarding more effective |
| Moore and Browne (2017) | Systematic review of research evidence on protecting older adults from elder abuse and neglect | 67 | Searched 7 databases and located studies of evidence-based practice (28), "best practices" (22) and emerging/promising innovations in practice (17). This identified five risk assessment instruments considered reliable and valid for use in elder abuse and neglect. Evidence was found on education for perpetrators and professionals. Results for the effects of multidisciplinary teams were mixed, but there was some tentative support for use of "forensic centres" and a "combined social work/lawyer" model. No findings were obtained directly relevant to safeguarding in a UK context |

(continued)

**Table 7.1** (continued)

| Review | Focus | No. of studies | Findings |
|---|---|---|---|
| Stevens (2015) | Contribution of leadership to safeguarding within healthcare organizations | 18 | Thematic review of qualitative studies that focused on the part played by leadership in the safeguarding process. Studies were critically appraised and generated five core themes: concepts of leadership; agency and organizational culture; governance and accountability structures; training, procedures and policy; and values and ethics. Proposed a framework for establishing an effective leadership strategy drawing on the discovered themes |
| Viljoen et al. (2017) | Disability sensitivity training for police officers | 3 | Systematic review of 13 databases, located 19 studies but only 3 met eligibility criteria specified through the PICO framework. Excluded studies of mental health, suicide and substance abuse problems. Quality appraisal showed retained studies met 53–73% of criteria. Training included exercises such as role-play of investigative interviews. "Studies consistently reported statistically significant improvements in participants' attitudinal scores following training and in comparison with the control groups" (p. 151) |
| Wallcraft (2012) | Involvement of service users in safeguarding | 72 | Drew articles for review from a database provided by the Social Care Institute for Excellence, supplemented by a small-scale telephone survey ($n$ = 13 participants). Sources highlighted tensions between involvement and genuine empowerment. Identifies some problems with service user involvement, factors which promote it and aspects of good practice within it. Makes a set of recommendations concerning service user involvement in community outreach |

Collaboration and the National Criminal Justice Reference Service (NCJRS, US Department of Justice). No time limits were set for the search period. Reference lists of the above review articles (Table 7.1) were inspected for further sources.

The search terms used were various combinations of the words *safeguard**, *vulnerable adult*, *polic** and *effect**. As pilot searches created an impression that the volume of relevant research literature was likely to be limited, a decision was made not to restrict the search too much by adding additional words such as evaluation, results or outcomes. While the number of records identified was larger than expected, only a small portion of them consisted of empirical research. One atypical outcome was that by far the majority of the documents located were based on work carried out in the UK. Comparatively few documents were located that were based on work carried out in other countries, possibly because the terminology used elsewhere differs in key ways from that used in the UK.

### *7.4.1 Inclusion and Exclusion Criteria*

To be retained for inclusion in the initial review, studies had to meet the following inclusion criteria. First, it was necessary for them to report research concerned with the protection or safeguarding of vulnerable adults, regardless of the factors that were considered to be associated with that vulnerability. They could comprise a study of factors that were thought to influence the effectiveness of safeguarding or evaluation of the effectiveness of different approaches to ensuring it. Alternatively, they could be studies of the perspectives of different professionals on factors or processes that influence the effectiveness of safeguarding policies or procedures.

For the initial searches, they could have been published at any point up to 30th of June 2017 (no start dates were set for searches). They had to be published in the English language, as facilities were not available for translation; and they had to be contained in a peer-reviewed publication such as a scientific journal or government report. Research degree dissertations or unpublished reports were excluded from consideration.

Conversely therefore, studies were excluded if they were concerned with child protection, if they were not available in English or if they consisted of conference presentations and dissertations or were published in a source without peer review. It is also important to note that the focus of the review was not on any approaches to reducing harm at an individual level (such as by education or counselling) but on effectiveness of multi-agency safeguarding.

Searches located an initial total of 614 records (PsycINFO 192, Scopus 77, Web of Science 37, NCJRS 102, Cochrane database 183, Campbell Library 0, found in reference lists 23). Figure 7.1 presents a diagrammatic summary of the numbers of records removed or retained at each stage. After removal of duplicates and screening of abstracts according to inclusion criteria, this was reduced to a set of 109 potentially relevant documents which were downloaded. Fuller screening of these

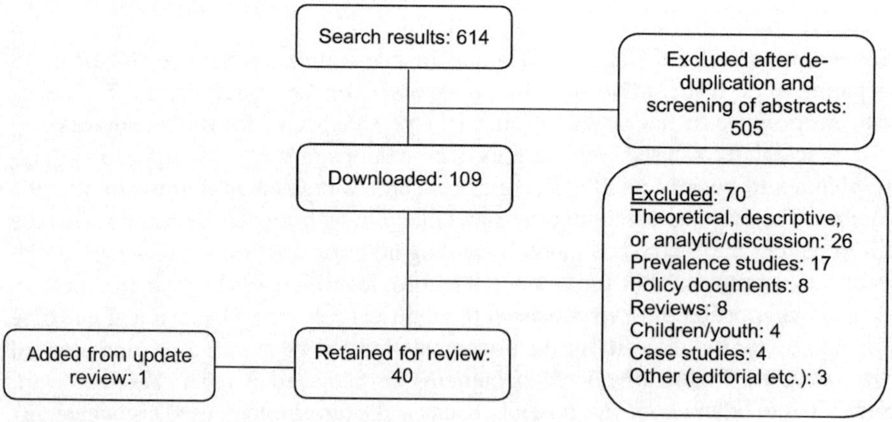


**Fig. 7.1** Flowchart of search and screening process: safeguarding vulnerable adults

reduced the number of reports to be retained for detailed review to a final set of 39, to which 1 was added from the updating review. A large proportion of the documents removed were overviews of policy issues, descriptions of interventions or discussions of or guidelines for practice, but not containing any empirical data. A small proportion were case studies, which can be very informative for some purposes, but unless they are based on single-case experimental designs, their findings are difficult to synthesize.

## 7.5 Findings

This section presents the findings from this review. The 40 reports that were retained covered a wide range of issues and employed a variety of research methods. Key areas of information from the research studies that were retained are summarized in Table 7.2.

The first point to note is that very few studies were found that used typical evaluation designs. For example, only one of the located studies compared the outcomes of an intervention after it had been introduced, with "business as usual" that preceded it (before-and-after studies). Only four compared the relative effectiveness of different procedures or approaches in adult protection. For practical and ethical reasons and given the complexity of this area, evaluations of those kinds may be very difficult to conduct, and the use of robust design features, such as random allocation, may not even be viable. Almost all studies focused instead on processes of decision-making, investigating the extent to which policies were put into practice or guidelines were observed or examining the relative influence of different factors on safeguarding. Researchers often employed qualitative methodology, but some studies involved surveys of service provision or analysis of case files.

The studies retained from the searches show a variety of patterns in terms of methodology, with respect to both design and data collection. One large group involves analysis of case files or of reports on serious case reviews. A second group consists of interviews or discussions (e.g. focus groups) with key personnel. Both of these types of study are predominantly qualitative and use some form of thematic analysis to elicit core themes related to safeguarding practice. A third group, mainly conducted in the USA, involved measurement of quantifiable outcomes and statistical analysis of results. Combining these different approaches, the following is an overview of the main findings to emerge.

First, there is a moderate amount of evidence on the effectiveness of some forms of multidisciplinary team working in the area of reducing abuse of older adults. Community-based multidisciplinary teams are widely employed and ubiquitously perceived as the preferred model of working in a number of areas. But as Rizzo et al. (2015, pp. 3–4) remark, although "…the rationale for advocating for this preferred model is strong, empirical evidence from research supporting a multidisciplinary model is weak". Research located here remedies this to some, albeit limited, extent.

**Table 7.2** Studies of aspects of adult safeguarding[a]

| Study | Methodology/data collection | Samples/data sources | Focus and findings |
|---|---|---|---|
| Alon and Berg-Warman (2014) | Prospective, before-and-after evaluation using questionnaires, interviews and observations | 558 older adults in 3 locations in Israel; 10 social workers; 9 other professionals including police | Evaluation of the Israeli multisystem model for prevention of elder abuse. Involved staff from several agencies. Psychological abuse was the most prevalent form. Social workers recorded types of intervention used. With legal interventions alone (court order or police referral), there was an 82% improvement rate; for support alone, 65%. Police raised priority of abuse complaints |
| Aylett (2016) | Thematic analysis of reports, qualitative analysis | 114 summaries of Serious Case Reviews (SCRs) from 2000 to 2012 | Extracted data from SCRs and tabulates types of vulnerability, perpetrators and location of abuse. Noted information missing and lack of consistency in reports and practice. Collates a core list of the seven recommendations most often made: staff training, policy review, facilitate information sharing, develop governance systems, holistic multi-agency assessment, dynamic risk assessment and management and engagement with a wide range of agencies |
| Braye et al. (2012) | Thematic analysis of 44 research studies + survey and analysis of documents | Reports on 13 CQC inspections; 203 SAB reports; feedback from 7 staff workshops | Study objective was to identify best practice in the governance of adult safeguarding, combining information from different sources. Proposed that there are five key features of SABs: (a) strategic goals, purpose and leadership; (b) structure and composition; (c) membership and network patterns, including inter-agency collaboration; (d) clear specification of seven board functions; and (e) accountability |

(continued)

**Table 7.2** (continued)

| Study | Methodology/data collection | Samples/data sources | Focus and findings |
|---|---|---|---|
| Brownell and Wolden (2003) | Cross-sectional, non-equivalent comparison study, testing hypotheses | 29 CVB cases<br>27 ES cases randomly selected from 700 | Compared two types of community services for reducing elder abuse: justice-based Crime Victims Board (CVB), and social work based Elder Services (ES). Overall, no significant differences in outcomes were found between the two services, with one exception: CVB resulted in more safety and successful resolutions of the situation for victims of financial abuse |
| Clawson (2016) | Exploratory national survey (16 questions)<br>+ 2 interviews | 58/127 SABs in England (46%); data collected in 2012–2013 | Application of safeguarding procedures to avoiding forced marriage amongst people with intellectual disabilities. Findings showed a "lack of engagement" with the issue: 71% of SABs define forced marriage as abuse, but only 33% included guidance on it in the area of ID; only 22% had data on the extent of any risk in their area, and only 14% could name a lead specialist with knowledge of the issues, though 58% said it was an area of concern. (Note that new statutory guidelines were issued in 2014) |
| Cooper et al. (2015) | Analysis of reports | Impact statements on work undertaken and changes made by 43 local authorities | Examination of effects of "Making Safeguarding Personal" policy and the reported impact of changes made in the years 2013–2014. The personalization approach entails moving emphasis from procedures to engagement. Adoption of this was reported as making safeguarding more effective, but this was not independently verified. Presents 16 key findings from impact statements, overall positive effects from using person-centred outcomes as a "cultural change", also found to be more helpful to partner agencies including police |

(continued)

**Table 7.2** (continued)

| Study | Methodology/data collection | Samples/data sources | Focus and findings |
|---|---|---|---|
| Cummins (2007) | Small-scale pilot study based on a series of semi-structured interviews | 10 custody officers from one police area | Examined the decision-making processes of custody officers assessing vulnerable adults manifesting mental health problems, following PACE 1984 guidelines. Findings suggested officers had only minimal training on mental health issues and this concerned them, leading them to rely on their own experience, and they felt frustrated when the police station had to be used as a place of safety due to lack of other resources or to cases being given low priority elsewhere |
| Cummins (2012) | Analysis of cases of arrested persons having a mental health assessment | 58 cases where a forensic physician was called to examine person in police custody in Lancashire | Analysed features of cases where following an arrest, custody sergeants requested a mental health assessment. This occurred in only 1.5% of cases in custody. Most of those assessed had no contact with community mental health services, and 16 (27%) were not registered with a GP. Although forensic physician assessment found no mental health problem in 21 of the cases, the study indicates ways in which such problems may be missed leaving individuals vulnerable. Recommended use of street triage |
| Ernst and Smith (2012) | Cross-sectional comparison, retrospective analysis of secondary data | 869 case files from 2 similar counties in Maryland | Compared two approaches in adult protection: a multidisciplinary team with nursing and social work or the latter acting alone. Measured case disposition, risk identification and reduction, recidivism and cost-effectiveness. Lone workers confirmed more types of abuse, but MDTs achieved greater risk reduction. There were no differences in recidivism rates. MDTs were less cost-effective |

(continued)

**Table 7.2** (continued)

| Study | Methodology/data collection | Samples/data sources | Focus and findings |
|---|---|---|---|
| Fanneran et al. (2013) | Survey questionnaire | 33 NHS mental health trusts (41% of 79 invited to take part) | National survey of adult safeguarding (NHS England and Wales). Found large variations in how the DoH "No Secrets" policy was implemented: 82% had a lead post, and 81% were linked to local multi-agency policies, but 48% did not have a safeguarding team, and patterns for monitoring staff were very variable. Replies identified many barriers to practice; there were "crucial discrepancies" in some organizational arrangements |
| Farquharson (2016) | Quantitative analysis of a sample of case referrals | Analysis of referrals from three local authorities to a rural police force over a 12-month period | Examined outcomes of referrals to police to increase understanding of barriers to prosecution of suspects. Of 858 referrals, a crime was established in only 108. Thus 87% of cases did not meet the threshold for prosecution. Numbers who were cautioned or prosecuted and found guilty were very low. The paper analyses and reports the reasons why referrals were not prosecuted |
| Fyson and Kitson (2012) | Completion of short pro formas, analysed both quantitatively and qualitatively | Information on 42 cases from 12 teams in 1 local authority | Factors influencing the course of adult safeguarding alerts; in 36% of cases, it was substantiated that alleged abuse had occurred, 43% were unsubstantiated, and the rest were not determined or ongoing. Identified some differences between groups; only one factor was close to significance: whether or not there was a safeguarding plan meeting. High value was placed on inter-professional collaboration. Police were involved in 19% of cases, though accounts of this were very variable |

(continued)

**Table 7.2** (continued)

| Study | Methodology/data collection | Samples/data sources | Focus and findings |
|---|---|---|---|
| Gassoumis et al. (2015) | Quasi-experimental comparison of treated cases with propensity score-matched sample | 472 victims of financial abuse: 235 EAFC cases<br>237 "usual care" cases,<br>Los Angeles | Evaluation of a multidisciplinary team, an EAFC in protecting older adults from financial abuse. Outcome variable was referral to the Public Guardian (PG) for "conservatorship". The EAFC made significantly more PG referrals, resulting in more being protected, but the latter difference was not significant. The strongest predictor of referral was suspected cognitive impairment |
| Gough (2016) | Analysis of electronic case records using a critical theory perspective | 109 recorded outcomes of safeguarding enquiries within 1 local authority | Evaluation of "Making Safeguarding Personal" (MSP) policy. Analysed recordings of enquiries to establish to what extent individuals' own wishes were reflected in the process. A key finding was that desired outcomes were not achieved in 74 of 109 cases (a 2:1 ratio). Results found the majority of outcomes were service- rather than client-centred |
| Heath and Phair (2009) | Qualitative, hermeneutic analysis of written statements, interviews and observations | 130 participants: nurses, care assistants, care residents, relatives, home managers and other staff | Examined the contribution of nursing staff and care assistants to outcomes of care for older adults, evaluated with reference to an outcomes framework containing five domains, which the authors proposed can improve safeguarding. The study illustrates how this can operate, but the process by which the data analysis supports the conclusions drawn is not however very clear |
| Horspool et al. (2016) | Small-scale cross-sectional, qualitative study using semi-structured topic guide + textual analysis | 14 staff: 9 police officers and 5 mental health practitioners in 2 UK locations | Investigated perceptions of street triage in a service jointly run by police and NHS. Found three emergent themes: key aspects of triage, perceived benefits and how it could be further developed. Triage was thought to facilitate better use of local services. It was concluded that the study provides additional evidence for positive perceptions of triage |

(continued)

**Table 7.2** (continued)

| Study | Methodology/data collection | Samples/data sources | Focus and findings |
|---|---|---|---|
| Hussein et al. (2007) | Large-scale telephone survey, data analysis logistic regression | Representative sample of 1000 people aged ≥16 | Surveyed public perceptions of maltreatment of older people. Analysed associations between respondent characteristics and opinions about elder mistreatment and neglect. Some links to demographic variables were found, but trends were difficult to interpret. There were 245 respondents who knew someone who had experienced mistreatment, and their views were analysed separately |
| Hussein et al. (2009) | Multi-method study with quantitative and qualitative components | Secondary analysis of 5294 referrals to POVA in 2004–2006 + detailed analysis of 298 cases | Analysis of staff referrals to the POVA list which contains names of care workers who have been dismissed for misconduct. Paper provides detailed analysis of demographic data of referrals, types of abuse allegedly committed, over-representation of males. Results show large differences in types of abuse committed in care home versus domiciliary settings. Some differences were significant, many others not and the overall implications of the results are unclear |
| Hussein et al. (2009/10) | Mixed-methods design: quantitative survey + focus groups and interviews | 144/172 (84%) of Councils with Social Services Responsibilities (local authorities) in England and Wales | Examination of patterns of multi-agency working in local authorities. Used pre-designed *Partnership Assessment Tool* for survey. One hundred twenty-three areas had Adult Protection Committees; police were members of 94%. Twenty different agencies contributed in various places. Strengths seen as shared expertise, more effective approach, sense of shared responsibility and strategic effectiveness. Barriers included: commitment difficulties, agency discrepancies in priorities, lack of clarity about roles, time/resource pressures, decision delays, uneven leadership |

(continued)

**Table 7.2** (continued)

| Study | Methodology/data collection | Samples/data sources | Focus and findings |
|---|---|---|---|
| Jessiman and Cameron (2017) | Perceptions of the roles of appropriate adults, studied in interviews and focus groups | 25 professionals interviewed + 2 two focus groups with 13 service users | Under the Police and Criminal Evidence Act (1984), it is a legal duty of police custody sergeants in England and Wales to ensure an appropriate adult (AA) is present when a vulnerable person is detained for questioning. The study investigated how AAs are perceived by professionals and service users. Researchers found some confusion over how the role is defined and what AAs are expected to do. While the professional respondents placed more emphasis on the processes involved, the service user groups regarded the skills of the AA in enabling them to communicate with police as the crucial consideration |
| Lawrence and Banerjee (2010) | In-depth interviews + qualitative analysis using grounded theory | 14 managers + 24 members of staff from 14 care homes in Croydon | Evaluation of a care home support team (CHST) set up in response to reports of abuse. The CHST ran a series of training interventions with care home staff at numerous sites. The study was designed to assess its perceived impact. Themes that emerged in analysis of outcomes included improved staff communication, staff development and confidence and improved quality of care. The major strength of the CHST was perceived as being its collaborative, non-judgemental approach |
| Manthorpe and Martineau (2010) | Qualitative study with face-to-face or telephone interviews | 4 chairpersons of SCRs 10 members of SABs | Focused on what can be learned from the reflections of those who have chaired or commissioned SCRs that could be used to improve safeguarding. Key themes emerged including specifying aims of reviews, role of independent chairs, value of current official guidance and of national collation of SCR recommendations. Also an emphasis on inter-agency communication in recognizing vulnerability |

(continued)

**Table 7.2** (continued)

| Study | Methodology/data collection | Samples/data sources | Focus and findings |
|---|---|---|---|
| Manthorpe and Martineau (2011) | Documentary analysis of sample of reports | 22 SCR reports (15 full, 7 summary)<br>13 involving fatalities | Analysis of reports of SCRs on a variety of cases using a set of 11 predetermined categories. Provides summaries of key features of cases. Lists issues identified in reports related to inter-agency communication, absence of a lead agency, need for training, definition of thresholds, adequacy of advocacy. Extracts a list of recommendations made in reports |
| Manthorpe and Martineau (2015) | Documentary analysis of sample of reports | 18 SCR reports where harmed person had ID + 3 SCRs where status is unclear | Analysis of reports of SCRs using a similar procedure to Manthorpe and Martineau (2011), but with additional qualitative analysis to identify themes. Key points in the latter were distortions of power and control in relationships and influences of long-term biographical knowledge of service users. Authors also raise issue of "interfaces with criminal justice systems" |
| Manthorpe and Samsi (2013) | Thematic "framework analysis" of telephone interviews | 15 Adult Safeguarding Coordinators, third interviews following earlier occasions by Manthorpe et al. (2013) | Explored personal budgets and financial abuse of vulnerable adults who have dementia, to assess any requirements for further safeguarding. Applied a specially devised coding framework. Use of budgets evoked anxiety in most interviewees given known high rate of financial abuse, and they saw a need for stronger protocols, but also considered direct payments could be empowering and giving people choices |

(continued)

**Table 7.2** (continued)

| Study | Methodology/data collection | Samples/data sources | Focus and findings |
|---|---|---|---|
| Manthorpe et al. (2013) | Thematic analysis of interviews (telephone or in-person) | ASCs:<br>15 in 2008<br>12 in 2010 | Interviews at two time points as part of a larger study to examine the impact of the MCA. Initially interviewees had favourable views of the MCA; at second interview concerns were expressed about how to assess the best interests of vulnerable adults, given the interface between safeguarding and "personalization". Effective working relationships with police were viewed as crucial in safeguarding investigations. ASCs hoped case law would develop to a stage where it could strengthen the safeguarding role. But the MCA was still seen positively |
| Medford et al. (2003) | Single-cohort correlational study including subgroup comparisons | 501 audio-recorded police interviews in London; 365 with adults | Evaluated the effectiveness of the *appropriate adult* (AA) safeguards, and also of legal representatives (LRs), during police interviews with vulnerable people. AAs were present in 212 (58%) of adult interviews. Details are provided on how AAs behaved during interviews. Presence of an AA was associated with increased likelihood of LRs being present, of their playing a more active part, and with less "interrogative pressure" in the interview |
| Navarro et al. (2013) | Quasi-experimental evaluation with logistic regression | 476 victims of financial abuse: 237 EAFC cases<br>239 "usual care" cases<br>Los Angeles | Earlier report on the same project described by Gassoumis et al. (2015) of an EAFC with different outcome variables and analysis. Referral of cases to the district attorney was best predicted by the case being seen by the EAFC and co-occurring physical abuse, while co-occurring self-neglect decreased the odds of referral. The same variables predicted whether charges were filed and whether or not there was a guilty plea or conviction for elder abuse |

(continued)

**Table 7.2** (continued)

| Study | Methodology/data collection | Samples/data sources | Focus and findings |
|---|---|---|---|
| Norrie et al. (2015) | Scale development, testing questions stage, interviews + focus group | 10 adults at risk<br>20 relatives<br>12 LA staff<br>10 agency staff | Feasibility study forming part of the development of an adult safeguarding outcome measure as no such instrument is available. Interviews were used to establish whether questions were appropriate and could be understood. The study led to some revisions in the scale questions and in the guidance that would be given to staff users |
| Olivier et al. (2016) | Exploratory qualitative study, thematic analysis of semi-structured interviews | 4 professionals involved in adult safeguarding | Police, trading standards and voluntary sector perspectives on safeguarding vulnerable adults from mass-market fraud. Main aim was to gain insight into the impact of fraud on older people. Themes identified included fraudster manipulation, scams appearing legitimate and personal motives for accessing money. Other data emerged on how individuals can remain susceptible to scams, due to loneliness/isolation and the "morphing" of scams over time |
| Oxburgh et al. (2016) | Single-cohort questionnaire and interview-based study, grounded theory analysis | 35 police officers from 6 forces | Focused on police officers' perceptions of offenders with mental disorders, on support provided for them and on their training. Qualitative analysis identified 9 conceptual categories and 21 sub-categories within the data. Developed an understanding of this in terms of a Police Experience Transitional Model, specifying factors that influence changes in officers' perceptions over time. Most (74.3%) officers had negative perceptions of suspects with mental disorders. Details are given of how this impacted the communication process within interviews and officers' strategies for gaining investigation relevant information |

(continued)

**Table 7.2** (continued)

| Study | Methodology/data collection | Samples/data sources | Focus and findings |
|---|---|---|---|
| Phair (2009) | Audit and content analysis within a specific "reflective framework" | 250 individual investigation assessments from 4 nursing homes + 2 care homes | Used analysis of case assessment documents as a basis for development of a risk assessment tool relating to neglect in residential units. File analysis was used to extract examples of neglectful practice which were then formatted according to a formula to devise an assessment protocol in the form of a *risk matrix*. The use of this is then illustrated with three case examples |
| Phair and Manthorpe (2012) | Thematic analysis of interviews and discussions, including use of a case vignette | Survey of 42 hospital staff<br>Interviews with 12 staff<br>Focus groups with 13 staff | Examined knowledge and experience of use of the MCA. The overall objective was to improve how the act is implemented. Only one respondent knew ill-treatment and wilful neglect are criminal offences. Themes emerged related to how the MCA could be more instilled into staff thinking; suggestions were also made concerning changes in NHS trust policies to take account of consent and capacity |

(continued)

**Table 7.2** (continued)

| Study | Methodology/data collection | Samples/data sources | Focus and findings |
|---|---|---|---|
| Rizzo et al. (2015) | Analysis and hypothesis testing with a cohort of case file data using logistic regression | Random sample of 250 closed case records from 3 sites in New York City | Evaluation of the Jewish Association Serving the Aging and Legal/Social Work Elder Abuse Prevention Program. Extracted data from case files using a pre-designed system and with reliability checks. The key outcome variable was mistreatment status at case closure. Analysis indicated that client retention in Jewish Association Serving the Aging and Legal/Social Work Elder Abuse Prevention Program was linked to better outcomes, i.e. lowered mistreatment status at case closure, as was higher treatment fidelity (intervention carried out as planned), and use of a multidisciplinary legal/social work team model. Some risk of selection bias could not be entirely eliminated from the analyses |
| Sengstock et al. (1991) | Cross-sectional comparison of four service delivery conditions | Levels of services provided to 136 abuse victims at 2 rural and 2 suburban sites, run by Illinois Department on Aging | Describes "model projects" for responding to allegations of elder abuse within 24 hours. Two were "law oriented" (mandatory reporting and legal intervention) and one an "advocacy model". There were 20 separate types of service that could be accessed. The highest level of services occurred in one of the law-oriented programmes. There were no between-site differences in levels of legal service provided. But unexpectedly, there was a higher level of other services at law-oriented than at advocacy sites |

(continued)

**Table 7.2** (continued)

| Study | Methodology/data collection | Samples/data sources | Focus and findings |
|---|---|---|---|
| Stevens and Cook (2015) | Thematic analysis of written assignments; development of quality checklist; audit of sample of assignments in next cohort | Student nurses: In cohort 1, randomly chosen 10% sample of work In cohort 2, randomly chosen 35% of work ($N = 59$) | Approached the question of how to identify safeguarding concerns by reviewing the reflective assignments of student nurses and locating learning points that could be addressed in their preregistration training. Assignments focused on a critical incident in safeguarding. Analysis of the first sample of assignments made it possible to produce a quality checklist that could then be used to appraise the second sample. This yielded results relating both to how much students had learned and where there were gaps in knowledge and understanding of safeguarding processes that needed to be addressed. On this basis recommendations were made concerning nurse training |
| Trainor (2015) | File search and quantitative analysis + semi-structured interviews | 50 service user file referrals + 6 Designated Officers (case coordinators) in Northern Ireland | Study objective was to review factors that influence decisions made in safeguarding investigations for adults. Developed a file tool to analyse information recorded on a series of cases. In addition, interviews were conducted with six professionals making safeguarding decisions. Factors thought to influence decisions included profession of Designated Officer; training; type of abuse; client group; frequency, seriousness and impact of abuse; process issues; and aspects of alleged perpetrator. Findings led to some redesign procedures within the host trust |

(continued)

**Table 7.2** (continued)

| Study | Methodology/data collection | Samples/data sources | Focus and findings |
|---|---|---|---|
| Twomey et al. (2010) | Descriptive and comparative study | Multidisciplinary teams working with older adults in California | Essentially a descriptive study which was on the borderline for inclusion. Examined similarities and differences of seven multidisciplinary teams to identify effective features of practice. Teams included medicine, psychology, law, adult protective services and police. Concluded that team working showed clear advantages in the process of safeguarding vulnerable adults |
| Wiglesworth et al. (2006) | Mixed quantitative (survey) and qualitative design (interviews) | Survey of 52 EAFC team members and external professionals on 114 cases; + interviews with an unstated number on specific cases | Evaluation of efficiency and effectiveness of collaboration at an EAFC. Examined perceptions of the EAFC's performance by analysing survey responses in terms of levels of agreement on whether cases were better dealt with than without the team. Results showed EAFC was considered to deal with cases in less time and was handled more effectively, but that the same conclusion would have been reached without the EAFC |
| Young et al. (2013) | Single-cohort screening and clinical interview study, quantitative analysis | 200 persons detained in police custody in London over a 12-week period | Investigated prevalence of three kinds of vulnerability amongst detained suspects, effects on police resources, effectiveness of assessments and use of appropriate adults. Prevalence rates were ID 6.7%, ADHD 23.5% and childhood CD 76.3%, all higher than general population. Previous CD or ADHD, current ADHD but not ID were associated with higher consumption of police time |

[a]The following abbreviations are employed in this table: *AA* appropriate adult, *ADHD* attention deficit hyperactivity disorder, *ASC* Adult Safeguarding Coordinator, *CD* conduct disorder, *CHST* care home support team, *CQC* Care Quality Commission, *DoH* Department of Health, *EAFC* Elder Abuse Forensic Center, *ID* intellectual disability, *LA* local authority, *LR* legal representative, *MSP* Making Safeguarding Personal, *MCA* Mental Capacity Act 2005, *MDT* multidisciplinary team, *PACE* Police and Criminal Evidence Act 1984, *POVA* Protection of Vulnerable Adults, *SAB* Safeguarding Adults Board, *SCR* Serious Case Review

Examples of this include the work of Elder Abuse Forensic Centers (EAFCs) in the USA (Gassoumis et al., 2015; Navarro et al., 2013; Wiglesworth et al., 2006). Similarly, the Jewish Association Serving the Aging and Legal/Social Work Elder Abuse Prevention Program service demonstrated good outcomes (Rizzo et al., 2015; for a fuller account of the functioning of this project, see Schecter & Dougherty, 2009); as did a service run along similar multisystem lines in Israel (Alon & Berg-Warman, 2014). In their comparison of multidisciplinary teams with lone workers, Ernst and Smith (2012) found the former produced better results in terms of reduction of risk of harm. Twomey et al. (2010) found that the ethos of team working was highly valued, in a study based on staff reports and perceptions rather than outcome data. All these studies were conducted in the USA and often used measurable outcomes taken from case records or other sources.

In contrast in England and Wales, most studies have taken a different form and have used qualitative methodology, more often relying on thematic analysis of reports or perceptions rather than on more robust or independently obtained measurements of change. Support was found for the value of a care home support team for staff working in residential nursing units (Lawrence & Banerjee, 2010).

The earliest study located in the review, by Sengstock et al. (1991), found slightly better results for services with a *law-oriented* rather than a *social work-oriented* programme. Brownell and Wolden (2003) also obtained results slightly favouring a legally oriented Crime Victims Board. Results tentatively paralleling this were obtained in some other studies, but these effects are not entirely clear-cut and could be attributed to a number of factors, making firm conclusions difficult to draw.

Analysis of various aspects of serious case reviews has succeeded in identifying some elements of safeguarding which could have been done better. This emerges amongst other studies in those by Manthorpe and Martineau (2010, 2011, 2015). On this basis these and other authors (e.g. Braye et al., 2012; Manthorpe & Martineau, 2011, p. 235) extract and offer sets of recommendations that could improve safeguarding practice. There is a consensus on the need for more standardization of practice and closer adherence to published guidelines. Given that the latter have often been based on scrutiny of system errors or failures (resulting in case reviews), that proposal appears to be soundly based. Teams and multi-agency collaboration are regarded as indispensable, and while that seems self-evident, other than in the studies cited earlier, as noted then it is difficult to demonstrate it clearly in outcome research. Hence the basis for promoting guidelines is more often to be found in examination of why in some cases events took an adverse course.

Another generally agreed conclusion from the file-based studies is that there is a marked disparity between standards and possibly also in resources in child and adult safeguarding. That also corresponds to and may partly explain the difference noted earlier in the amounts of research available on the two areas. In addition, there is preliminary evidence to support adoption of what has been called a more "personalized approach", an emphasis on client-centred rather than service-centred thinking, which also appears to improve the safeguarding process (Cooper et al., 2015; Gough, 2016). Doing this also helps to improve implementation of the Mental

Capacity Act 2005 (Manthorpe et al., 2013), amongst other ways in facilitating the vulnerable person's control of budgets (Manthorpe & Samsi, 2013).

While the number of findings on this aspect is very small, there is provisional support for the value of disability sensitivity training for police officers, incorporating focused role-play exercises (Viljoen et al., 2017). However, the outcomes measured were mainly of attitudinal change with no evaluation of skill acquisition or other attributes.

Much of the time, the results appear to suggest that things would have worked satisfactorily if existing guidelines and specified procedures had been followed or if components of services were in place as guidelines suggested. That applies, for example, where recommendations had not been implemented properly (Fanneran et al., 2013; Farquharson, 2016), where there is no safeguarding planning meeting (Fyson & Kitson, 2012), where the Mental Capacity Act 2005 is not understood or implemented (Phair & Manthorpe, 2012) or where an issue such as forced marriage of people with intellectual disabilities has received only marginal attention (Clawson, 2016). All of these disparities could of course be the result of difficult choices having been made to prioritize some areas of service over others.

In a separate strand of research, concerned with police assessments of vulnerable individuals following arrest, several studies point towards the need for more training in this area. This is identified in the study by Medford et al. (2003) on use of appropriate adults and in the work of Cummins (2007, 2012), of Young et al. (2013 see also Young et al., 2011) on identification of some long-term disorders and of Cummins and Edmondson (2016) and Horspool et al. (2016) on street triage. Some of these issues might be better grasped applying a model such as that of Oxburgh et al. (2016) concerning how police officers' perceptions evolve as experience accumulates. This work may also highlight the need for more extensive joint working between police and mental health professionals. More widely, that may be of direct relevance for the composition of community-based multi-agency safeguarding teams.

With regard to community safeguarding therefore, overall, it is difficult to avoid the broad conclusion that many services would probably perform better and many difficulties and possible crises could be averted if there were simply closer adherence to existing guidelines. But this is in a context of services under pressure of limited and in some cases diminishing resources.

Accompanying this perhaps somewhat bleak picture, there are some potentially promising developments from the use of other approaches that represent innovations in this field and so to date have been little used. They include a project to develop a standardized scale for assessing extent of vulnerability (Norrie et al., 2015; Phair, 2009). There are numerous suggestions about ways in which staff training requires improvement (see, e.g. Domac & Haider, 2013; Stevens & Cook, 2015). One aspect of this might focus on the question of how to influence the decisions made in safeguarding investigations (Trainor, 2015) and how staff could acquire the skills for doing so. In a separate strand of work, Tapper (2010) outlined the possibility that family group conferences, a model used in work with young offenders and other groups, could potentially be used in work on elder abuse. She described the pilot phase of a planned 3-year trial of this in Hampshire with good feedback. However, it is not clear whether this was successfully carried out as no other literature could be located on the project, and the recent systematic review by Moore and Browne (2017) reports no subsequent study linked to this work. There are also other plausible models not supported to date by outcome evidence. They include, for example, the community-based elder mistreatment response programme described by Burnes (2017). In many respects this reflects an operationalization of the list of good practice criteria proposed by Manthorpe and Martineau (2011).

### 7.5.1 Police in a Multi-agency System

With regard to what can be learned from this review concerning priorities for policing, clear conclusions are difficult to draw beyond the statutory responsibilities of responding to evidence of maltreatment, of abuse or neglect. But many safeguarding failures may never be made known to the police, and unless police services also had a role as overseers of the implementation of policy in other services, that may remain the position. In this connection however it may be that police could have a role in bringing agencies together, specifying team structures, establishing networks and monitoring their operation, leaning towards the more law-oriented position described in some of the research studies reviewed. Yet, police services too are under pressure in terms of existing commitments and resource limitations.

Possible directions in which the police could extend their work in this respect were outlined by Shearlock and Cambridge (2009) with reference to changing safeguarding practices in the English county of Somerset. This specifies possible roles for police in enabling staff of other agencies to develop their abilities in identifying when cases should be brought to police attention, in understanding decisions about whether prosecution is or is not in the public interest and in asking questions of involved parties and collecting information that can produce evidence that would sustain a prosecution where appropriate. Teams involved in Protection of Vulnerable Adults seek collaboration with police and rely on them in the process of securing justice when difficult issues arise (Giordano & Neville, 2015). Thus, police could have both a generic role as coordinators of multi-agency systems and a number of specific roles as providers of interview training or of advice and consultation to strengthen decision-making practice inside other agencies. There are unfortunately limits to what police can achieve in multi-agency systems that are already overburdened. A study in one area of Wales with a population of 350,000 found that police submitted almost 3500 notifications of need for safeguarding in a single year (Ford et al., 2020). While over half (57%) were referred for social services intervention, only a small proportion (8.7%) of the adults referred received any form of "direct action or input" (p. 100).

## 7.6 Discussion

The research identified in this scoping review addresses a number of important problems in relation to safeguarding, for example, on whether different authorities have in place the kinds of provision that are stipulated in national guidelines. However, in the absence of studies with different designs from the ones discovered here, it is difficult to draw clear or reliable conclusions regarding its effectiveness. Alongside this it is important to keep in mind that the statutory frameworks governing safeguarding and adjacent areas have developed over time and continue to be discussed and evaluated from a legal viewpoint (Brammer, 2009; Campbell, 2016; Keywood, 2017). While the present review did not have any immediate or concrete impact on practice or policy, its content and findings were shared with the regional multi-agency safeguarding hubs and appointed Safeguarding Boards in the commissioning police areas. Hence it was believed likely to have had some subtle influence on practitioners' knowledge and perspectives.

### *7.6.1 Strengths and Limitations of the Research*

The volume of research found relevant to this review question is slightly larger than was expected, but given its disparate nature, it is still unlikely to be enough to permit any clear conclusions to be drawn or recommendations to be made. As part of a project designed to identify features of best practice in adult safeguarding, Braye et al. (2012) carried out a literature review. Their conclusion was that "…the effectiveness of adult safeguarding governance arrangements has not been subject to prior formal evaluation and thus the literature provided little research-led evidence of good practice"; they found "…no evidence in the literature that particular forms of governance lead directly to improvements in safeguarding" (pp. 55, 68). More broadly Sutcliffe et al. (2012, p. 118) pointed to the "…severe lack of evidence on the efficacy of safeguarding interventions". In the 5 years since then, it does not appear that a great deal has changed with respect to the availability of evaluation research. Overall, therefore, in a sense all that has been possible here has been simply to map out in general terms the kinds of work reported in the area, although there have been some modest advances in a few segments of it.

While that may sound tentative or even pessimistic, the research that has been done has been anchored in close examination of practice arrangements, including detailed scrutiny of pitfalls and omissions, thereby highlighting the challenges of this work. The majority of the studies of this kind were carried out in agencies directly engaged in safeguarding and were predominantly based in England and Wales. A large proportion of the located studies appeared fairly recently: Of 39 studies, approaching three-quarters (72%) were published from 2010 onwards and 14 in the period 2014–2017 and so may be expected to reflect recent or current practice. Arguably therefore, while this research may fall short in terms of *internal validity* as defined in experimental evaluations, it may achieve greater *external validity* in being closely linked to everyday service settings.

Any review exercise in this field such as the present one is likely to be subject to several limitations. One is uncertainty over whether there are potentially eligible reports that could not be found and accessed. For example, there may be internal reports prepared by police research departments that are not available on external databases but which contain valuable information. That could apply also to unpublished conference contributions and degree dissertations and to studies not published in English. However, the likelihood of large tracts of research having been missed is lower than in some other areas, as the use of the term safeguarding and the law and practice associated with it are specific to the UK context.

Another limitation in this field is the diversity of work undertaken and the unevenness of research methods used. Experimental or quasi-experimental studies of the kinds undertaken in other areas were unlikely to have been conducted on an issue as complex as safeguarding. In addition, where the number of studies is not large and they are divided into sets by focus or method, the number in each resultant subgroup can be very small.

A weakness in how the present review was conducted is that there was no second rater or adjudicator of the studies in making inclusion/exclusion decisions or in deriving information from them. This is one of the ways of simplifying the review process and saving time, but it is an important deficit, and it would be preferable if a proportion of the work could be checked by a second reviewer.

There is also further work that could be done with some of the documents that were located. A number of case studies were found that have the potential to throw light on disruptions that occurred in individual case management, sometimes with the most serious consequences (Draper et al., 2009; Nash et al., 2010; Olubokun, 2008; Simcock & Manthorpe, 2014). But generalizing from these instances without a more methodical framework for doing so presents a number of interpretative challenges. Finally, many other proposals for service improvement have been made, for the most part plausible and potentially valuable. But it is unclear how many are followed up in practice, and little research is available to illuminate whether or not they add to service effectiveness. Examples include the work of Clawson and Kitson (2013), Collins (2010), Galpin and Hughes (2011), Hough (2012), Phair and Health (2009), Stevens (2013), and Williams (2000, 2011).

## 7.7 Conclusions

While a sizeable amount is known about the needs of adults identified as vulnerable and in need of multi-agency safeguarding, less is known about effective methods of achieving that end. Examining the findings of the present review, no studies were found that can provide a clear indication of the most effective way to carry out safeguarding of vulnerable adults. No evaluative studies were found showing outcomes of procedures or comparing different approaches with one another. In any case the room for manoeuvre within the existing statutory framework, developed in response to serious problems that have arisen, is fairly limited. Simultaneously, current guidance provides a clear and workable framework that should help agencies make appropriate decisions; though some surveys suggest, it is not uniformly implemented. The research that was located yields provisional evidence that there are features of good practice that do appear to be associated with satisfactory levels of effective service.

On the basis of this, it is difficult to make any firm, specific and unambiguous recommendations, but the following are offered as tentative suggestions as to courses of action worthy of consideration. First, it is vital to ensure that local provision complies with requirements and standards specified in official (state-wide or national) statutory documents. There may be a role for policing the system, which may sound rather daunting from some perspectives, especially as there are inspectorial procedures already in existence, but there may be scope and possibly a need for some form of monitoring role. Second, alternatively or in addition, police services could have an influence in fostering the emergence of a law or justice-oriented model of inter-agency working, given some evidence supporting this as a method of working, which would also entail closer affiliation with police. Third, within police services themselves, it is preferable that there are designated roles for liaison and coordination with multiple agencies in the area of adult safeguarding, with a named senior officer and good lines of communication to agency partners. Fourth, it is advisable for police to communicate with other agencies in the local area and offer provision related to a range of difficulties they face when cases arise that could potentially be referred to the police. This may involve seminars on how decisions are made to proceed with investigation or prosecution or training in interviewing or in gathering evidence. Fifth and finally, it is recommended that police develop a decision-making flowchart or algorithm for use in this context, potentially applying the model suggested for GPs by Gibson et al. (2016). Clearly where emergencies arise, the police response would be as for other situations, but it is likely that a majority of issues that arise in this area both require and also allow for more reflective consideration. Disseminating something similar to partner agencies could lead to improved efficiency in identifying instances where fuller consultation is needed.

Adopting any of the above would understandably place additional demands on police time and resources. However, implementation of them could potentially lead to savings in other respects. To enable senior staff to make decisions in regard to this, a study could be undertaken to compare relative benefits and costs of a more proactive and preventative as opposed to what might be characterized as a solely responsive approach.

In collaboration with other agencies and, if possible, in conjunction with academic researchers, it may be possible to develop and to test a scale for assessment of vulnerability or at-risk status for adults in the key spheres that have been discussed at various points in this review.

When this review was first being researched, the Metropolitan Police and other forces were reportedly facing difficult choices in relation to how best to allocate resources (Rawlinson, 2017). The position is unlikely to have improved significantly since then. One implication may be a need to concentrate on the more vulnerable members of the community, and given evidence reviewed here that this group is at greater risk of becoming victims of crime, an increased proportion of face-to-face visits to them could be a valuable strategy in strengthening the effectiveness of safeguarding.

Overall, the above suggestions could be seen as forming part of an approach based on activating "the principles of community policing to develop a scientific and systematic approach to effective community engagement" (Paterson & Best, 2015, p. 156).

## References

Alon, S., & Berg-Warman, A. (2014). Treatment and prevention of elder abuse and neglect: Where knowledge and practice meet – A model for intervention to prevent and treat elder abuse in Israel. *Journal of Elder Abuse & Neglect, 26*, 150–171.

Aylett, J. (2016). Universal learning: Findings from an analysis of serious case review executive summaries. *Journal of Adult Protection, 18*, 28–39.

Association of Directors of Social Services. (2005). *'Safeguarding Adults': A National Framework of Standards for good practice and outcomes in adult protection work*. Association of Directors of Social Services.

Association of Directors of Adult Social Services London. (2015). *London multi-agency adult safeguarding policy and procedures*. ADASS.

Baker, P. R. A., Francis, D. P., Hairi, N. N., Othman, S., & Choo, W. Y. (2016). Interventions for preventing abuse in the elderly. *Cochrane Database of Systematic Reviews*, (8), CD010321.

Beadle-Brown, J., Mansell, J., Cambridge, P., Milne, A., & Whelton, B. (2010). Adult protection of people with intellectual disabilities: Incidence, nature and responses. *Journal of Applied Research in Intellectual Disabilities, 23*, 573–584.

Bellman, L., Webster, J., & Jeanes, A. (2010). Knowledge transfer and the integration of research, policy and practice for patient benefit. *Journal of Research in Nursing, 16*, 254–270.

Biggs, S., Manthorpe, J., Tonker, A., Doyle, M., & Erens, B. (2009). Mistreatment of older people in the United Kingdom: Findings from the First National Prevalence Study. *Journal of Elder Abuse & Neglect, 21*, 1–14. https://doi.org/10.1080/08946560802571870

Boland, B., Burnage, J., & Chowhan, H. (2013). Safeguarding adults at risk of harm. *British Medical Journal, 346*, f2716. https://doi.org/10.1136/bmj.f2716

Brammer, A. (2009). Legal developments since *No Secrets*. *Journal of Adult Protection, 11*, 43–53.

Braye, S., Orr, D., & Preston-Shoot, M. (2012). The governance of adult safeguarding: Findings from research. *Journal of Adult Protection, 14*, 55–72.

British Medical Association. (2011). *Safeguarding vulnerable adults – A tool kit for general practitioners*. British Medical Association.

Brownell, P., & Wolden, A. (2003). Elder abuse intervention strategies. *Journal of Gerontological Social Work, 40*, 83–100.

Burnes, D. (2017). Community elder mistreatment intervention with capable older adults: Toward a conceptual practice model. *The Gerontologist, 57*, 409–416.

Campbell, M. (2016). Adult protection in Scotland in 1857 and in 2015: What have we learned? *Journal of Adult Protection, 18*, 96–108.

Clawson, R. (2016). Safeguarding people with learning disabilities from forced marriage: The role of Safeguarding Adult Boards. *Journal of Adult Protection, 18*, 277–287.

Clawson, R., & Kitson, D. (2013). Significant Incident Learning Process (SILP) – The experience of facilitating and evaluating the process in adult safeguarding. *Journal of Adult Protection, 15*, 237–245.

Collins, M. (2010). Thresholds in adult protection. *Journal of Adult Protection, 12*, 4–12.

Cooper, C., Selwood, A., & Livingston, G. (2008). The prevalence of elder abuse and neglect: A systematic review. *Age and Ageing, 37*, 151–160.

Cooper, A., Lawson, J., Lewis, S., & Williams, C. (2015). Making safeguarding personal: Learning and messages from the 2013/14 programme. *Journal of Adult Protection, 17*, 153–165.

Cummins, I. (2007). Boats against the current: Vulnerable adults in police custody. *Journal of Adult Protection, 9*, 15–24.

Cummins, I. (2012). Mental health and custody: A follow on study. *Journal of Adult Protection, 14*, 73–81.

Cummins, I., & Edmondson, D. (2016). Policing and street triage. *Journal of Adult Protection, 18*, 40–52.

De Donder, L., Luoma, M.-L., Penhale, B., Lang, G., Santos, A. J., Tamutiene, I., Koivusilta, M., Schopf, A., Alves, J. F., Reingarde, J., Pertttu, S., Savola, T., & Verté, D. (2011). European map of prevalence rates of elder abuse and its impact for future research. *European Journal of Ageing, 8*, 129–143.

Department of Health. (2000). *No secrets: The development of multi-agency responses to the abuse of vulnerable adults*. The Stationary Office.

Department of Health. (2011). *Statement of government policy on adult safeguarding*. https://www.gov.uk/government/uploads/system/uploads/attachment_data/file/215591/dh_126770.pdf

Dickson, K., Sutcliffe, K., Rees, R., & Thomas, J. (2017). Gaps in the evidence on improving social care outcomes: Findings from a meta-review of systematic reviews. *Health and Social Care in the Community, 25*(4), 1287–1303.

Domac, S., & Haider, S. (2013). Interagency safeguarding adults training for protection and prevention. *Journal of Interprofessional Care, 27*, 520–522.

Draper, T., Roots, S., & Carter, H. (2009). Safeguarding adults: Perspectives from primary care trusts in Kent and Medway. *Journal of Adult Protection, 11*, 6–11.

Ernst, J. S., & Smith, C. A. (2012). Assessment in adult protective services: Do multidisciplinary teams make a difference? *Journal of Gerontological Social Work, 55*, 21–38.

Fanneran, T. B., Kingston, P., & Bradley, E. (2013). A national survey of adult safeguarding in NHS mental health services in England and Wales. *Journal of Mental Health, 22*, 402–411.

Farquharson, J. A. (2016). Referrals to the police of vulnerable adult abuse. *Journal of Adult Protection, 18*, 119–127.

Ferrah, N., Murphy, B. J., Ibrahim, J. E., Bugela, L. C., Winbolt, M., LoGiudice, D., Flicker, L., & Ranson, D. L. (2015). Resident-to-resident physical aggression leading to injury in nursing homes: A systematic review. *Age and Ageing, 44*, 356–364.

Fisher, M. H., Baird, J. V., Currey, A. D., & Hodapp, R. M. (2016). Victimisation and social vulnerability of adults with intellectual disability: A review of research extending beyond Wilson and Brewer. *Australian Psychologist, 51*, 114–127.

Ford, K., Newbury, A., Meredith, Z., Evans, J., Hughes, K., Roderick, J., Davies, A. R., & Bellis, M. A. (2020). Understanding the outcome of police safeguarding notifications to social services in South Wales. *The Police Journal: Theory, Practice and Principles, 93*(2), 87–108.

Fyson, R., & Kitson, D. (2012). Outcomes following adult safeguarding alerts: A critical analysis of key factors. *Journal of Adult Protection, 14*, 93–103.

Galpin, D., & Hughes, D. (2011). A joined up approach to safeguarding and personalisation: A framework for practice in multi-agency decision-making. *Journal of Adult Protection, 13*, 150–159.

Gassoumis, Z. D., Navarro, A. E., & Wilber, K. H. (2015). Protecting victims of elder financial exploitation: The role of an Elder Abuse Forensic Center in referring victims for conservatorship. *Aging & Mental Health, 19*, 790–798.

Gibson, J., Nicol, B., Ronayne, E., & Grant, M. (2016). Safeguarding adults in primary care: Making a safeguarding adults referral. *British Journal of General Practice*, e454–e456. https://doi.org/10.3399/bjgp16X685525

Giordano, A., & Neville, A. (2015). Collaborating across health and social care: Joint funding an adult protection coordinator post in Caerphilly, UK. *Journal of Adult Protection, 17*, 139–147.

Gough, M. (2016). An evaluation of adult safeguarding outcomes' focused recording in the context of making safeguarding personal. *Journal of Adult Protection, 18*, 240–248.

Heath, H., & Phair, L. (2009). Shifting the focus: Outcomes of care for older people. *International Journal of Older People Nursing, 4*, 142–153.

Home Office. (2014). *Multi agency working and information sharing project: Final report*. Home Office.

Horner-Johnson, W., & Drum, C. E. (2006). Prevalence of maltreatment of people with intellectual disabilities: A review of recently published research. *Mental Retardation and Developmental Disabilities Research Reviews, 12*, 57–69.

Horspool, K., Drabble, S. J., & O'Cathain, A. (2016). Implementing street triage: A qualitative study of collaboration between police and mental health services. *BMC Psychiatry, 16*, 313. https://doi.org/10.1186/s13888-016-1026z

Hough, R. E. (2012). Adult protection and 'intimate citizenship' for people with learning difficulties: Empowering and protecting in light of the no secrets review. *Disability & Society, 27*, 131–144.

Hughes, K., Bellis, M. A., Jones, L., Wood, S., Bates, G., Eckley, L., McCoy, E., Mikton, C., Shakespeare, T., & Officer, A. (2012). Prevalence and risk of violence against adults with disabilities: A systematic review and meta-analysis of observational studies. *Lancet*. https://doi.org/10.1016/S0140-6736(11)61851-5

Hussein, S., Manthorpe, J., & Penhale, B. (2007). Public perceptions of the neglect and mistreatment of older people: Findings of a United Kingdom survey. *Ageing & Society, 27*, 919–940.

Hussein, S., Manthorpe, J., Reid, D., Penhale, B., Perkins, N., & Pinkney, L. (2009/10). Working together in adult safeguarding: Findings from a survey of local authorities in England and Wales. *Research, Policy and Planning, 27*(3), 163–176.

Hussein, S., Stevens, M., Manthorpe, J., Rapaport, J., Martineau, S., & Harris, J. (2009). Banned from working in social care: A secondary analysis of staff characteristics and reasons for their referrals to the POVA list in England and Wales. *Health and Social Care in the Community, 17*(5), 423–433.

Hutchinson, A., & Stenfert Kroese, B. (2015). A review of literature exploring the possible causes of abuse and neglect in adult residential care. *Journal of Adult Protection, 17*, 216–233.

Jessiman, T., & Cameron, A. (2017). The role of the appropriate adult in supporting vulnerable adults in custody: Comparing the perspectives of service users and service providers. *British Journal of Learning Disabilities, 45*, 246–252.

Keywood, K. (2017). The vulnerable adult experiment: Situating vulnerability in adult safeguarding law and policy. *International Journal of Law and Psychiatry*. https://doi.org/10.1016/j.ijlp.2017.05.011

Latalova, K., Mamaradova, D., & Prasko, J. (2014). Violent victimisation of adult patients with severe mental illness: A systematic review. *Neuropsychiatric Disease and Treatment, 10*, 1925–1939.

Lawrence, V., & Banerjee, S. (2010). Improving care in care homes: A qualitative evaluation of the Croydon care home support team. *Ageing & Mental Health, 14*, 416–424.

Lindbloom, E. J., Brandt, J., Hough, L. D., & Meadows, S. E. (2007). Elder mistreatment in the nursing home: A systematic review. *Journal of the American Medical Directors Association, 8*, 610–616.

Lyketsos, C. G., & and the Medical and Scientific Advisory Board of the Greater Maryland Chapter of the Alzheimer's Association. (2004). Research consent for cognitively impaired adults: Recommendations for Institutional Review Boards and Investigators. *Alzheimer Disease and Associated Disorders, 18*, 171–175.

Mandelstam, M. (2013). *Safeguarding adults and the law* (2nd ed.). Jessica Kingsley Publishers.

Mandelstam, M. (2017). *Care Act 2014: An A-Z of law and practice*. Jessica Kingsley Publishers.

Manthorpe, J., & Lipman, V. (2015). Preventing abuse through pre-employment checks: An international review. *Journal of Adult Protection, 17*, 341–350.

Manthorpe, J., & Martineau, S. (2010). 'In our experience': Chairing and commissioning serious case reviews in adult safeguarding in England. *Journal of Social Work, 12*, 84–99.

Manthorpe, J., & Martineau, S. (2011). Serious case reviews in adult safeguarding in England: An analysis of a sample of reports. *British Journal of Social Work, 41*, 224–241.

Manthorpe, J., & Martineau, S. (2015). What can and cannot be learned from serious case reviews of the care and treatment of adults with learning disabilities in England? Messages for social workers. *British Journal of Social Work, 45*, 331–348.

Manthorpe, J., & Samsi, K. (2013). 'Inherently risky?': Personal budgets for people with dementia and the risks of financial abuse: Findings from an interview-based study with Adult Safeguarding Coordinators. *British Journal of Social Work, 43*, 889–9031.

Manthorpe, J., Samsi, K., & Rapaport, J. (2013). "Capacity is key": Investigating new legal provisions in England and Wales for adult safeguarding. *Journal of Elder Abuse & Neglect, 25*, 355–373.

Manthorpe, J., Bramley, S., & Norrie, C. (2017). Gambling and adult safeguarding: Connections and evidence. *Journal of Adult Protection, 19*(6), 333–344.

McDonald, L., Sheppard, C., Hitzig, S. L., Spalter, T., Mathur, A., & Mukhi, J. S. (2015). Resident-to-resident abuse: A scoping review. *Canadian Journal on Aging, 34*, 215–236.

Medford, S., Gudjonsson, G. H., & Pearse, J. (2003). The efficacy of the appropriate adult safeguard during police interviewing. *Legal and Criminological Psychology, 8*, 253–266.

Meijward, S. C., Kikkert, M., de Mooij, L. D., Lommerse, N. M., Peen, J., Schoevers, R. A., Van, R., de Wildt, W., Bockting, C. L. H., & Dekker, J. J. M. (2015). Risk of criminal victimisation in outpatients with common mental health disorders. *PLoS One, 10*(7), e0128508. https://doi.org/10.1371/journal.pone.0128508

Moore, C., & Browne, C. (2017). Emerging innovations, best practices, and evidence-based practices in elder abuse and neglect: A review of recent developments in the field. *Journal of Family Violence, 32*, 383–397.

Nash, C., Shipwright, D., & Smeaton, M. (2010). The triggers protocol. *Journal of Adult Protection, 12*, 19–27.

National Policing Improvement Agency. (2012). *Guidance on safeguarding and investigating the abuse of vulnerable adults*. National Policing Improvement Agency and Association of Chief Police Officers.

Navarro, A. E., Gassoumis, Z. D., & Wilberm, K. H. (2013). Holding abusers accountable: An Elder Abuse Forensic Center increases criminal prosecution of financial exploitation. *The Gerontologist, 53*, 303–312.

NHS England. (2015). *Safeguarding vulnerable people in the NHS – Accountability and assurance framework*. NHS England.

Norrie, C., Cartwright, C., Rayat, P., Grey, M., & Manthorpe, J. (2015). Developing an adult safeguarding outcome measure in England. *Journal of Adult Protection, 17*, 275–286.

Office of the Public Guardian. (2015). *Safeguarding policy*. Office of the Public Guardian.

Olivier, S., Burls, T., Fenge, L.-A., & Brown, K. (2016). Safeguarding adults and mass marketing fraud – Perspectives from the police, trading standards and the voluntary sector. *Journal of Social Welfare and Family Law, 38*, 140–151.

Olubokun, J. (2008). The vulnerable adult in police custody: Lessons from the case of *R* v *Paul James Aspinall. Medicine, Science and the Law, 48*, 199–202.

Oxburgh, L., Gabbert, F., Milne, R., & Cherryman, J. (2016). Police officers' perceptions and experiences with mentally disordered suspects. *International Journal of Law and Psychiatry, 49*, 138–146.

Paterson, C., & Best, D. (2015). Policing vulnerability through building community connections. *Policing, 10*(2), 150–157.

Payne, B. K., & Fletcher, L. B. (2005). Elder abuse in nursing homes: Prevention and resolution strategies and barriers. *Journal of Criminal Justice, 33*, 119–125.

Phair, L. (2009). The development of the West Sussex institutional care neglect risk assessment tool: A reflective analysis using Mezirow's transformative learning framework. *International Journal of Older People Nursing, 4*, 132–141.

Phair, L., & Health, H. (2009). Neglect of older people in formal care settings part one: New perspectives on definition and the nursing contribution to multi-agency safeguarding work. *Journal of Adult Protection, 12*, 5–13.

Phair, L., & Manthorpe, J. (2012). The use of the Mental Capacity Act among hospital patients: Findings from a case study of one Acute Hospital Trust in England. *Journal of Adult Protection, 14*, 259–270.

Randall, D., Childers-Buschle, K., Anderson, A., & Taylor, J. (2015). An analysis of child protection 'standard operating procedures for research' in higher education institutions in the United Kingdom. *BMC Medical Ethics, 16*, 66. https://doi.org/10.1186/s12910-015-0058-0

Rawlinson, K. (2017). Met police cuts will mean fewer face-to-face visits, says senior officer. *The Guardian*, 25th August. https://www.theguardian.com/uk-news/2017/aug/25/police-budget-cuts-to-reduce-face-to-face-visits

Rizzo, V. M., Burnes, D., & Chalfy, A. (2015). A systematic evaluation of a multidisciplinary social work–lawyer elder mistreatment intervention model. *Journal of Elder Abuse & Neglect, 27*, 1–18. https://doi.org/10.1080/08946566.2013.792104

Schecter, M., & Dougherty, D. (2009). Combating elder abuse through a lawyer/social worker collaborative team approach: JASA legal/social work elder abuse prevention program (LEAP). *Care Management Journals, 10*, 71–76.

Sengstock, M. C., Hwalek, M., & Stahl, C. (1991). Developing new models of service delivery to aged abuse victims: Does it matter? *Clinical Sociology Review, 9*, 142–161.

Shearlock, L., & Cambridge, P. (2009). Working effectively with the police in safeguarding vulnerable adults: Sharing experience from Somerset. *Journal of Adult Protection, 11*, 6–19.

Simcock, P., & Manthorpe, J. (2014). Deafblind and neglected or deafblindness neglected? Revisiting the case of Beverley Lewis. *British Journal of Social Work, 44*, 2325–2341.

Stevens, E. (2013). Safeguarding vulnerable adults: Exploring the challenges to best practice across multi-agency settings. *Journal of Adult Protection, 15*, 85–95.

Stevens, E. L. (2015). How does leadership contribute to safeguarding vulnerable adults within healthcare organisations? A review of the literature. *Journal of Adult Protection, 17*, 258–272.

Stevens, E. L., & Cook, K. (2015). Safeguarding vulnerable adults: Learning from the reflective assignments of pre-registration students in the adult field of nursing practice. *Journal of Adult Protection, 172*, 31–40.

Sutcliffe, K., Rees, R., Dickson, K., Hargreaves, K., Schucan-Bird, K., Kwan, I., Kavanagh, J., Woodman, J., Gibson, K., & Thomas, J. (2012). *The adult social care outcomes framework: A systematic review of systematic reviews to support its use and development*. EPPI-Centre, Social Science Research Unit, Institute of Education, University of London.

Tapper, L. (2010). Using family group conferences in safeguarding adults. *Journal of Adult Protection, 12*, 27–31.

Trainor, P. (2015). A review of factors which potentially influence decisions in adult safeguarding investigations. *Journal of Adult Protection, 17*, 51–61.

Trevillion, K., Oram, S., Feder, G., & Howard, L. M. (2012). Experiences of domestic violence and mental disorders: A systematic review and meta-analysis. *PLoS One, 7*(12), e51740. https://doi.org/10.1371/journal.pone.0051740

Twomey, M. S., Jackson, G., Marino, T., Melchior, L. A., Randolph, J. F., Retselli-Deits, T., & Wysong, J. (2010). The success and challenges of seven multidisciplinary teams. *Journal of Elder Abuse & Neglect, 22*, 291–205.

Viljoen, A., Bornman, J., Wiles, L., & Tonsing, K. M. (2017). Police officer disability sensitivity training: A systematic review. *The Police Journal: Theory, Practice and Principles, 90*(2), 143–159.

Wallcraft, J. (2012). Involvement of service users in adult safeguarding. *Journal of Adult Protection, 14*, 142–150.

Wiglesworth, A., Mosqueda, L., Burnight, K., Younglove, T., & Jeske, D. (2006). Findings from an elder abuse forensic center. *The Gerontologist, 46*, 277–283.

Williams, J. (2000). The inappropriate adult. *Journal of Social Welfare and Family Law, 22*, 43–57.

Williams, S. (2011). Safeguarding adults at risk in the community through inter-agency working. *Journal of Adult Protection, 13*, 100–113.

World Health Organisation (WHO). (2015). *WHO global disability action plan 2014–2021: Better health for all people with disability*. WHO. http://apps.who.int/iris/bitstream/10665/199544/1/9789241509619_eng.pdf?ua=1

Yon, Y., Mikton, C. R., Gassoumis, Z. D., & Wilber, K. H. (2017). Elder abuse prevalence in community settings: A systematic review and meta-analysis. *Lancet Global Health, 5*, e147–e156.

Young, S., Goodwin, E. J., Sedgwick, O., & Gudjonsson, G. H. (2013). The effectiveness of police custody assessments in identifying suspects with intellectual disabilities and attention deficit hyperactivity disorder. *BMC Medicine, 11*, 248. https://doi.org/10.1186/1741-7015-11-248

# Chapter 8
# People with Mental Health Problems: A Systematic Review of Policing Interventions

## 8.1 Overall Aims

There are three commonly used MH interventions associated with policing: liaison and diversion (L&D), street triage (ST) and having specialist MH staff embedded in police command and control rooms (CCRs). In addition, the Memphis model of Crisis Intervention Teams (CITs), already used in the USA, is now attracting wider interest, including in the UK. Investment in these interventions is growing, so it is important to have systematic evidence of their effectiveness. The overall aim of the original review (Kane et al., 2017) which has been updated for this chapter is to provide police, health providers and commissioners and policymakers with a rigorous and systematic digest of the available evidence to help shape service design, investment and decision-making.

Search keywords were collected through canvassing expert opinion and a review of key documents. This was operationalized using a Population/Participant, Intervention/Indicator, Comparator/Control, Outcome(s) (PICO) search framework. The content of this framework is outlined in Table 8.1.

## 8.2 Background, Scene Setting: Key Issues, Major Developments and Landmark Studies

Individuals experiencing mental health problems often fare poorly in the justice system (Pettitt et al., 2013). First contact is not uncommonly with the police, and some studies have found that criminalization may result if this policing role is not performed appropriately (Lamb & Weinberger, 2002). Indeed, for offences of equal severity, studies have found that a person with mental illness can be twice as likely to be arrested (Charette et al., 2014). Other studies however have found suspects



J. McGuire et al., *Evidence-Based Policing and Community Crime Prevention*, Advances in Preventing and Treating Violence and Aggression,
https://doi.org/10.1007/978-3-030-76363-3_8

**Table 8.1** A summary of the PICO strategy used to search the literature on the police and people with mental health problems

| | |
|---|---|
| Population/ participants | People with mental health problems, symptoms or diagnoses coming into contact with the police (target population)<br>Police officers and practitioners from other agencies who deal with the target population whether in person or by telephone, partner agencies: the range of mental health practitioners and agencies providing any relevant generic or specialist service |
| Intervention/ indicator | Basing mental health practitioners in contact and control rooms, police stations or custody suites or embedding them with other police teams to ensure appropriate treatment and/or referral, including assessments; partnerships for diverting people with mental health problems away from any criminal justice setting at any stage of the process when appropriate, to ensure relevant treatment; and any similar approaches with similar aims |
| Comparison groups or controls | Any comparison group not receiving the intervention, or only receiving it after a delay, providing for comparison, pre-/post-type comparisons |
| Outcome(s) | Outcomes were treated as primary – those likely to be directly affected by the intervention – or secondary, those on which the interventions may have an effect, but which may also be affected by other factors. Primary included improved assessment, referral and treatment (quality and timeliness) of mentally ill people, reduced demand on police forces and officer time, improved mental health outcomes and service engagement and reduced use of mental health-specific police detention powers. Secondary included increased demand on community mental health services and reductions in reoffending or arrest |

with mental disorders to be significantly less likely to be arrested compared to those without, after controlling for other factors known to affect officer decision-making in statistical models (e.g. Engel et al., 2000; Novak & Engel, 2005).

Police officers themselves are often troubled by encounters with people with mental illnesses – for example, they take much more time than other calls for service, typically involve repeat contacts with the same individuals mostly in response to minor or "nuisance" offences and occasionally involve volatile situations, risking the safety of all involved (Reuland et al., 2012). Police are not formally trained to recognize, assess and treat mental illness; the knowledge and skills they have are mostly acquired through on-the-job experience (Green, 1997) or limited awareness training. Furthermore, they may depend on the availability of community MH resources for successful outcomes.

Such calls for service may also require the use of police powers under Section 136 (s136) of the Mental Health Act 1983; this section gives the police the power to remove a person from a public place, when they appear to be suffering from a mental disorder, to a place of safety. The person needs to be deemed by the police to be in immediate need of care and control as their behaviour is of concern. It is important to point out that a person is not under arrest when the decision is made to remove the person to a place of safety. The police power is to facilitate assessment of their health and well-being as well as the safety of other people around them. For many people with MH issues, these encounters are influenced by having previously had a negative experience with the police or fear of being blamed or not believed because they have MH problems. Individuals may also fear being sectioned under the Mental Health Act (Pettitt et al., 2013). Taken together, these studies highlight the inherent difficulties faced by both police officers and individuals experiencing MH problems when they encounter each other in stressful situations and emphasize the importance of appropriate and evidence-based support from mental health professionals being available to support the police in this work.

Our aim was to conduct a systematic literature review to answer questions about the effectiveness of currently available police-mental health service interventions for responding to people with mental disorder and suspected offending or public safety problems. First, it is necessary to define the interventions. As above there are four groups of internationally commonly used interventions: L&D, street triage with mental health specialists, embedded mental health specialists in police control rooms (CCRs) and CITs. Mental health courts are excluded from this review as they involve a limited role for the police.

L&D services have the aim of diverting individuals with vulnerabilities, including mental health problems, at their earliest possible contact with the justice system. They may also support the individual while she/he remains in the criminal justice system if the index offence or risk means they cannot be diverted immediately. Such services have existed in various locations and forms for over 30 years in England and Wales. In April 2014, the National Health Service in England introduced a standard model of operation, which will be available in all police custody suites and courts by 2021. This provides for a core team, which is almost always entirely staffed by psychiatric nurses, and an extended team with staff from various agencies that play key roles in diversion, including housing and welfare specialists (Kane et al., 2017).

Street triage is a joint mental health service and policing approach to crisis care. Based on locally agreed protocols, the aim is to support access to appropriate crisis care and to provide more timely access to other health, social care and third sector services (Reveruzzi & Pilling, 2016).

CCRs have become one of the primary referral agencies for psychiatric assistance in the community (Pogrebin, 1986). The CCR is a main open access point for the public. Mental health specialists are embedded in some CCR teams, advising call handlers and dealing with individual callers (Kane et al., 2017).

CITs require police officer training and changes in police procedures as well as collaboration with mental health providers. This model was initially developed in 1988 in Memphis, Tennessee, after a police officer fatally shot a man with a history of mental illness and substance abuse and is designed to increase the safety of encounters with the police (Dupont & Cochran, 2000). In the basic model, police call centre dispatchers are trained to identify calls that may relate to a mental state issue and assign them to CIT-trained officers; these have access to a designated psychiatric emergency drop-off site that operates a no refusal policy. Over the years since the model was first developed, it has been further shaped to adapt to the demands of different areas during implementation.

## 8.3 Specific Objectives of Review

The specific objective of the review was to conduct a systematic literature review to address questions about the effectiveness of police-mental health service models aimed at responding to people with mental disorder and suspected offending or public safety problems.

## 8.4 Method

Our literature search was conducted in June 2019 (updating a previous search conducted in 2016, see Kane et al., 2017) and covered 29 databases and sources. We used the following inclusion criteria. To be retained, a study had to relate to an intervention for those with a MH problem; it should have an objective outcome measure(s) regarding offending or MH; it must involve participants aged over 18. The design was required to be experimental or quasi-experimental and to include an intervention and comparison group(s) or a pre/post comparison. Members of the comparison group should have been individually matched to intervention participants, or baseline comparability was demonstrated, or allocation of participants was random. We excluded PhD theses and articles written in non-English languages, on time and resource grounds. Papers published before 1980 were excluded either because the interventions did not exist (CIT, ST and CCR embedded staff) or had no broadly standardized model (L&D) before that date.

The elements of the PICO framework (see Table 8.1) were broken into search terms to conduct the review. In order to avoid publication bias and selective reporting, we included grey literature and unpublished reports. We contacted authors for more information where necessary. Studies of varying quality were retained in the review and differentiated in the discussion.

Due to the limited and varied nature of the research evidence in this field, it was not appropriate to produce a GRADE table of findings to identify relevant results, nor was it possible to pool data from included studies or conduct a meta-analysis. We conducted a narrative synthesis of included studies. Relevant studies were assessed for risk of bias using the Cochrane tools for RCT and non-RCT designs, RoB 2.0 and ROBINS-I, respectively (http://www.riskofbias.info/).

The search results generated were saved in EndNote X7. The results of this search were sent to the two lead researchers for independent screening and reviewing, with discussions on any disagreements and recourse to a third party.

## 8.5 Results

Thirty-one studies were selected for inclusion in this review; 11 concerned L&D (8 using a control group design, 3 a pre/post design), 7 related to street triage (4 using a control group design and 3 a pre/post comparison), and 11 considered CIT interventions (2 using a pre/post design, 1 being a meta-analysis and the rest using a control group). In addition, two studies, by the same team, compared approaches to mentally ill people by the police (both of which used a control group design). Tables 8.2 and 8.3 summarize the overall results and then present findings for each model in turn. None of these studies specifically considers embedding mental health practitioners in police CCRs; however, some of the street triage and CIT studies contain elements of this model.

### *8.5.1 Liaison and Diversion*

A number of these studies show a positive impact of liaison and diversion on various criminogenic outcomes, including a decrease in arrests (Bonkiewicz et al., 2014; Council of State Governments Justice Center, 2007; Rivas-Vazquez et al., 2009; Steadman & Naples, 2005) and days spent in jail or prison (Case et al., 2009; Council of State Governments Justice Center, 2007) as well as contact with appropriate services (Broner et al., 2004; Steadman & Naples, 2005). Two of the studies evaluate the L&D service in Cornwall, England (Earl et al., 2015, 2017), and report positive effects on both primary health outcomes, such as identification of illness (Earl et al., 2015), and on police contact and offending, following contact with the service. These studies found that post-contact individuals were significantly less

**Table 8.2** Resources searched and results: people with mental health problems

| Resource | Search interface | # of hits |
|---|---|---|
| Campbell Library | – | 86 |
| Cochrane Library (including CDSR, CENTRAL, HTA, NHS EED) | – | 80 |
| EMBASE [excluding MEDLINE journals] | Ovid SP | 148 |
| MEDLINE | Ovid SP | 995 |
| National Police Library Catalogue | – | 1073 |
| ProQuest databases | ProQuest | 427 |
| PsycINFO | Ovid SP | 864 |
| PubMed [excluding MEDLINE] | – | 28 |
| Scopus | – | 398 |
| Web of Science databases | – | 309 |
| *Integration of results* | | |
| Subtotal | 4408 | |
| Duplicates | 1173 | |
| *Total (for screening)* | *3235* | |

**Table 8.3** Outcome of screening of results: people with mental health problems

| | |
|---|---|
| Total, from Table 8.2 | 3235 |
| Excluded on title/abstract | 3176 |
| Excluded based on full text review | 23 |
| Included in review | 31[a] |

[a]In addition, eight systematic reviews of the subject area were returned in the search and reviewed. Any relevant studies they returned included in this review are noted in the total above

likely to be in subsequent contact with criminal justice agencies in any capacity (whether a suspect, victim or witness) and a highly significant reduction in the number of proven offences (Earl et al., 2017).

However, the benefits of L&D were not consistent across all studies. Kane et al. (2018) reported that compared to offenders not referred to L&D, those who had been referred spent significantly longer in custody, this being due, possibly, to delays in L&D staff assessing offenders. Furthermore, Shafer et al. (2004) reported no significant differences between those study participants diverted and not regarding further offending or mental health with both groups generally showing an improvement on these measures over time (see also Scott et al., 2016). This points to the limitations of what is a brief intervention which relies on individuals following up with the services recommended. Indeed, Earl et al. (2017) reported that the significant reduction in proven offences observed following a referral to the L&D services occurred whether or not the individual was offered any action or onward referral which the authors suggest indicates that this reduction is a result of other processes rather than by meeting previously unmet mental health need.

### 8.5.2 Street Triage

Overall, these studies show that street triage teams provide a quicker and more appropriate response to incidents (Kisely et al., 2010; Scott, 2000; The Allen Consulting Group, 2012), for example, reducing presentations at hospital emergency departments with people instead routed directly to inpatient units (McKenna et al., 2015). There is also evidence that street triage can improve outcomes, such as reducing the use of formal detention (Dyer et al., 2015) and arrest (McKenna et al., 2015) or increasing use of health-based places of safety (Reveruzzi & Pilling, 2016) and reducing contact time with treatment services (Kisely et al., 2010; McKenna et al., 2015).

### 8.5.3 *Crisis Intervention Teams*

The findings of these studies suggest that CIT-certified officers differed regarding primary outcomes from those officers not trained. For example, they directed a greater proportion of persons with mental illness to MH services than their non-CIT-certified peers (Broner et al., 2004; Compton et al., 2014a; Teller et al., 2006; Watson et al., 2010, 2011), and encounters were less likely to end in arrest (Compton et al., 2014a). However, this is influenced by the nature of the incident, its severity and whether those involved were considered to be suffering mental ill health alone or to also be affected by drugs or alcohol and the local services available. In addition, these officers demonstrated different approaches towards individuals encountered with mental illness (Bahora et al., 2008; Compton et al., 2011a, b, 2014b; Morabito et al., 2012). For example, Compton et al. (2014b) found that CIT-trained officers scored more highly on attitudinal surveys on empathy and lower on fear and anger. These have been found most likely to be an existing difference, influencing their decision to take up such training (Davidson, 2016; Taheri, 2016). There is some suggestion in these studies that the effect of CIT training is persistent, with trained officers showing differences in self-efficacy, de-escalation skills and referral decisions pertaining to psychosis, key skills for such officers, persisting for a median of 22 months post training (Compton et al., 2014b). Furthermore, there was evidence of a diffusion of benefit from CIT- to non-CIT-trained officers regarding knowledge of mental health and approaches to such incidents (Herrington & Pope, 2014).

### 8.5.4 *Comparison of Approaches*

Steadman et al. (1999, 2000) compared three different approaches to police involvement with persons with MH problems: (1) involving civilian police employees with additional training to assist police officers in mental health emergencies and difficult-to-resolve calls in Birmingham, Alabama; (2) a CIT-style intervention in Memphis, Tennessee; and (3) a Mobile Crisis Unit staffed by social workers or registered nurses who respond to calls in the community and local jails without in-house support in Knoxville, Tennessee. At each site, a sample of around 100 cases was examined in which a specialized response occurred using the 3 approaches outlined above and compared to 100 police dispatch calls where the police responded as usual to a situation that may have involved a mentally ill person. The variations in these three programmes were found to reflect differences in the structure, approach and resources of each programme, suggesting that while such approaches can be effective, not all are equally effective. They found statistically significant differences across the three sites examined in the proportion of mental disturbance calls eliciting a specialized response (Birmingham 28%, Knoxville 40%, Memphis 95%). The dispositions of cases handled by the specialized response personnel were found to be related to the programme type. All three programmes had relatively low rates of arrest for these types of calls (average 7%). Two key factors of success were identified: first, the existence of a psychiatric triage or drop-off centre where police can transport individuals in crisis (reiterated in Steadman et al., 2001) and, second, community partnerships, ensuring that the police response formed part of a wider response involving relevant agencies.

## 8.6 Discussion

Overall, the studies included showed a positive impact of the various interventions for those with mental illness or in a MH crisis where police are involved. The reported effects were not consistent, but the presence or contact availability of MH professionals appears beneficial to both officers and suspects. This is variously reported as decreasing arrests, reducing jail time, providing a route into mental health treatment services and the identification of other unmet needs. While this gives cause for a level of optimism, more and wider-ranging research is needed to justify the continued level of investment in individual interventions. The studies reviewed offer some positive evidence for the interventions. However, the research base remains underdeveloped needing more large-scale, well-designed trials. Only two studies looked at the differences between approaches, and neither is conclusive. This should give some pause for thought to policymakers, service commissioners, police and providers. The profile of public investment in these interventions has tended to be compartmentalized, and that in turn has led to limitations in access to services based not on evidence but on local preferences or targeted national funding programmes.

The twin policy objectives of each of the interventions included in this review are to reduce reoffending and improve MH outcomes. It is not clear from the studies included the extent to which these headline objectives are being achieved. In addition, there is limited evidence on the cost-effectiveness of these interventions; generally diversion interventions result in lower criminal justice costs and greater health-funded intervention costs. This makes sense at one level as costs are being allocated more appropriately between public bodies. However, it also introduces financial disincentives particularly for service providers such as the police and health and social care agencies to act in concert if it damages their budget bottom lines. A comprehensive economic evaluation that includes a rigorous examination of not only direct financial costs and shifts but also the societal economic costs and benefits of investment in these services and how they are currently deployed is urgently needed.

While still under-researched, the intervention that stands out is CIT. This is to some extent a function of being more systematically evaluated over time. However, key to its reported effectiveness is that it offers an integrated service combining initial call and response triage with specialist-trained officer and MH professional interventions. This integrated provision and training approach contrasts with the current profile of investment in England and Wales, for example, where non-evidence-based decisions are made to select one individual intervention option over another. In addition, if more than one intervention is available in a locality, they are rarely designed into an integrated model of service. Perhaps the biggest gap that this review points to, beyond that of systematic integration, is the training of police officers and especially joint training of police and MH professionals to deliver an integrated service. Ongoing training is also a key; there is a measurable decay in the reported self-efficacy of officers and perceptions of verbal de-escalation, suggesting that training can have a short period of effectiveness if not refreshed. The specific experiential training, core to CIT, is not generally and systematically available because of competing policing and healthcare demands on human and financial resources. Individuals with mental health problems, whether diagnosed or not, fitting the *Diagnostic and Statistical Manual of Mental Disorders* or International Classification of Diseases classification or at a sub-clinical level, continue to fare poorly in the justice system.

## 8.7 Implications for Practice

Police officers and staff often manage the critical gateway that determines whether an individual experiencing MH problems enters the justice system or not. While courts and prisons offer later opportunities for diversion, this initial interaction can be the most critical and merits a well-designed, integrated and funded service. While there remains much work to be done in all aspects of evaluating these intervention models, it is clear that the cycle of arrest, charge, conviction, prison, release and re-arrest is unlikely to be the most beneficial model from an economic, ethical or service effectiveness perspective. The position that there is no time for training needs to be challenged robustly; there is ample evidence from across the public and private sectors that not training in key areas carries costs that exceed, by a significant margin, the investment in delivering high-quality training. Over time, commentators in academe, policy and practice have identified the need for service integration, adequate training and coordinated and evidence-based investment in diversionary services. It is important that those experiencing MH problems and who are involved in the justice system have a rational system in place to ensure they are treated fairly and reasonably. The services at the police and MH interface should not be hostage to budget disagreements especially between public bodies whose funding largely derives from the same sources. Services should not be shaped by local adherence to rival and non-integrated service models. The evidence in this review, while based on limited research, prompts at least material to stimulate fresh thinking and debate and move towards a more integrated service and a better trained workforce.

Concerning the use of these findings in the police areas that commissioned the review, there were indicators of impact in several areas: Mental health training was improved with lived experience trainers becoming involved. Street triage was funded in one county, mental health incidents involving the police were subject to joint police and National Health Service audit weekly, and this continued at the time of writing. The review influenced the redesigning of the partnership between the two police areas, the Health Service Trusts in their respective areas and the then Police and Crime Commissioners.

## 8.8 Implications for Policy

The Memphis model of CIT is the intervention with most robust evidence underpinning it but is not widely used outside the USA. In England and Wales, although not operating with any design fidelity to the Memphis CIT model, there is some local integration of approaches that are elsewhere delivered as discrete interventions. The next generation of services should take note of the current research and seek to capitalize on what works and further build the evidence to refine and develop integrated interventions. It is recommended that new services start from the position of the individual experiencing mental health problems and involved in the justice system, rather than the structural limits of organizations or funding structures currently in place.

## 8.9 Future Developments/Prospects

L&D services are due to be available across the whole of England in 2020/2021 which will offer at least one element of what should be an integrated service available to all who are in contact with the justice system either when arrested or at court hearings when they are experiencing MH issues. However, these are not the majority of individuals that the police officers and staff report encountering on a day-to-day basis and which police often report feeling overwhelmed by. Whether the police are the right agency to fill what appear to be substantial gaps in service is doubtful, but there is no doubt that many officers feel the need to do so. This is probably the result of a number of converging issues such as a genuine shortfall in NHS and social care investment, reduction in police officer numbers, lack of effective training for police officers and a lack of experience in dealing with what can often be difficult and regular encounters with the same distressed individuals. The introduction of Crisis Cafes[1] and similar community-based models of diversion and support appear to be an answer to some of these service shortfall issues, but they are not yet a fully tested model of intervention and support. Triage services, which in some form or another are present in virtually every police force, are under review. There have been questions raised around their effectiveness, and following a report from Her Majesty's Inspectorate of Constabulary, Fire and Rescue Services (HMICFRS,

[1] https://www.england.nhs.uk/2020/03/mental-health-crisis-services-rolled-out-across-england/

2018), all forces have been asked to carry out an evaluation of their triage services. Some forces have already begun to disinvest in these services and others are planning to do. MH and other health professionals being based in control rooms, while heavily invested in, in some areas, they are not yet present in the majority of forces. The overall picture remains one of poorly coordinated services with police feeling overwhelmed by demand and individuals experiencing MH problems and distress still faring poorly in the justice system.

## References

Bahora, M., Hanafi, S., Chie, V. H., & Compton, M. T. (2008). Preliminary evidence of effects of crisis intervention team training on self-efficacy and social distance. *Administration and Policy in Mental Health and Mental Health Services Research, 35*(3), 159–167. https://doi.org/10.1007/s10488-007-0153-8

Bonkiewicz, L., Green, A. M., Moyer, K., & Wright, J. (2014). Left alone when the cops go home: Evaluating a post-mental health crisis assistance program. *Policing: An International Journal of Police Strategies & Management, 37*(4), 762–778. https://doi.org/10.1108/PIJPSM-04-2014-0035

Broner, N., Lattimore, P. K., Cowell, A. J., & Schlenger, W. E. (2004). Effects of diversion on adults with co-occurring mental illness and substance use: Outcomes from a National Multi-Site Study. *Behavioral Sciences & the Law, 22*(4), 519–541. https://doi.org/10.1002/bsl.605

Case, B., Steadman, H. J., Dupuis, S. A., & Morris, L. S. (2009). Who succeeds in jail diversion programs for persons with mental illness? A multi-site study. *Behavioral Sciences & the Law, 27*(5), 661–674. https://doi.org/10.1002/bsl.883

Charette, Y., Crocker, A. G., & Billette, I. (2014). Police encounters involving citizens with mental illness: Use of resources and outcomes. *Psychiatric Services, 65*(4), 511–516. https://doi.org/10.1176/appi.ps.201300053

Compton, M. T., Demir Neubert, B. N., Broussard, B., McGriff, J. A., Morgan, R., & Oliva, J. R. (2011a). Use of force preferences and perceived effectiveness of actions among crisis intervention team (CIT) police officers and non-CIT officers in an escalating psychiatric crisis involving a subject with schizophrenia. *Schizophrenia Bulletin, 37*(4), 737–745. https://doi.org/10.1093/schbul/sbp146

Compton, M. T., Broussard, B., Munetz, M., Oliva, J. R., & Watson, A. C. (2011b). *The Crisis Intervention Team (CIT) Model of collaboration between law enforcement and mental health*. Nova Science Publishers, Inc..

Compton, M. T., Bakeman, R., Broussard, B., Hankerson-Dyson, D., Husbands, L., Krishan, S., Stewart-Hutto, T., D'Orio, B. M., Oliva, J. R., Thompson, N. J., & Watson, A. C. (2014a). The police-based crisis intervention team (CIT) model: I. Effects on officers' knowledge, attitudes, and skills. *Psychiatric Services, 65*(4), 517–522.

Compton, M. T., Bakeman, R., Broussard, B., Hankerson-Dyson, D., Husbands, L., Krishan, S., Stewart-Hutto, T., D'Orio, B. M., Oliva, J. R., Thompson, N. J., & Watson, A. C. (2014b). The police-based crisis intervention team (CIT) model: II. Effects on level of force and resolution, referral, and arrest. *Psychiatric Services, 65*(4), 523–529.

Council of State Governments Justice Center. (2007). *Increasing collaboration between corrections and mental health organizations: Orange county case study*. Council of State Governments Justice Center.

Davidson, M. L. (2016). A criminal justice system–wide response to mental illness: Evaluating the effectiveness of the memphis crisis intervention team training curriculum among law enforcement and correctional officers. *Criminal Justice Policy Review, 27*(1), 46–75. https://doi.org/10.1177/0887403414554997

Dupont, R., & Cochran, S. (2000). Police response to mental health emergencies – Barriers to change. *The Journal of the American Academy of Psychiatry and the Law, 28*(3), 338–344.

Dyer, W., Steer, M., & Biddle, P. (2015). Mental health street triage. *Policing, 9*(4), 377–387. https://doi.org/10.1093/police/pav018

Earl, F., Cocksedge, K., Rheeder, B., Morgan, J., & Palmer, J. (2015). Neighbourhood outreach: A novel approach to liaison and diversion. *The Journal of Forensic Psychiatry & Psychology, 26*(5), 573–585. https://doi.org/10.1080/14789949.2015.1045428

Earl, F., Cocksedge, K., Morgan, J., & Bolt, M. (2017). Evaluating liaison and diversion schemes: An analysis of health, criminal and economic data. *Journal of Forensic Psychiatry & Psychology, 28*(4), 562–580. https://doi.org/10.1080/14789949.2017.1308539

Engel, R. S., Sobol, J. J., & Worden, R. E. (2000). Further exploration of the demeanor hypothesis: The interaction effects of suspects' characteristics and demeanor on police behavior. *Justice Quarterly, 17*(2), 235–258. https://doi.org/10.1080/07418820000096311

Green, T. M. (1997). Police as frontline mental health workers: The decision to arrest or refer to mental health agencies. *International Journal of Law and Psychiatry, 20*(469–486), 1997.

Her Majesty's Inspectorate of Constabulary and Fire & Rescue Services. (2018). *Policing and mental health: Picking up the pieces*. HMICFRS.

Herrington, V., & Pope, R. (2014). The impact of police training in mental health: An example from Australia. *Policing and Society: An International Journal of Research and Policy, 24*(5), 501–522. https://doi.org/10.1080/10439463.2013.784287

Kane, E., Evans, E., & Shokraneh, F. (2017). Effectiveness of current policing-related mental health interventions in England and Wales and Crisis Intervention Teams as a future potential model: A systematic review. *Systematic Reviews, 6*(85). https://doi.org/10.1186/s13643-017-0478-7

Kane, E., Evans, E., Mitsch, J., Jilani, T., Quinlan, P., Cattell, J., & Khalifa, N. (2018). Police interactions and interventions with suspects flagged as experiencing mental health problems. *Criminal Behaviour and Mental Health, 28*, 424–432. https://doi.org/10.1002/cbm.2078

Kisely, S., Campbell, L. A., Peddle, S., Hare, S., Pyche, M., Spicer, D., & Moore, B. (2010). A controlled before-and-after evaluation of a mobile crisis partnership between mental health and police services in Nova Scotia. *The Canadian Journal of Psychiatry, 55*(10), 662–668. https://doi.org/10.1177/070674371005501005

Lamb, R. L., & Weinberger, L. E. (2002). The police and mental health. *Psychiatric Services, 53*(10), 1266–1271. https://doi.org/10.1176/appi.ps.53.10.1266

McKenna, B., Furness, T., Brown, S., Tacey, M., Hiam, A., & Wise, M. (2015). Police and clinician diversion of people in mental health crisis from the Emergency Department: A trend analysis and cross comparison study. *BMC Emergency Medicine, 15*, 14. https://doi.org/10.1186/s12873-015-0040-7

Morabito, M. S., Kerr, A. N., Watson, A., Draine, J., Ottati, V., & Angell, B. (2012). Crisis intervention teams and people with mental illness: Exploring the factors that influence the use of force. *Crime & Delinquency, 58*(1), 57–77. https://doi.org/10.1177/0011128710372456

Novak, K. J., & Engel, R. S. (2005). Disentangling the influence of suspects' demeanor and mental disorder on arrest. *Policing: An International Journal of Police Strategies & Management, 28*(3), 493–512. https://doi.org/10.1108/13639510510614573

Pettitt, B., Greenhead, S., Khalifeh, H., Drennan, V., Hart, T., Hogg, J., Borschmann, R., Mamo, E., & Moran, P. (2013). *At risk, yet dismissed: The criminal victimisation of people with mental health problems*. Victim Support, Mind.

Pogrebin, M. R. (1986). Police responses for mental health assistance. *Psychiatric Quarterly, 58*(1), 66–73.

Reuland, M., Schwarzfeld, M., & Draper, L. (2012). *Law enforcement responses to people with mental illnesses: A guide to research-informed policy and practice*. Council of State Governments Justice Center.

Reveruzzi, B., & Pilling, S. (2016). *Street triage: Report on the evaluation of nine pilot schemes in England*. University College London.

Rivas-Vazquez, R. A., Sarria, M., Rey, G., Rivas-Vazquez, A. A., Rodriguez, J., & Jardon, M. E. (2009). Jailing is failing people with mental illness. *Psychiatric Services, 60*(6), 766–771. https://doi.org/10.1176/ps.2009.60.6.723

Scott, R. L. (2000). Evaluation of a mobile crisis program: Effectiveness, efficiency, and consumer satisfaction. *Psychiatric Services, 51*(9), 1153–1156. https://doi.org/10.1176/appi.ps.51.9.1153

Scott, D., McGilloway, S., & Donnelly, M. (2016). A prospective comparative evaluation of a Criminal Justice Liaison and Diversion Service in Belfast. *Journal of Forensic Psychiatry and Psychology, 27*(2), 198–214. https://doi.org/10.1080/14789949.2015.1102313

Shafer, M. S., Arthur, B., & Franczak, M. J. (2004). An analysis of post-booking jail diversion programming for persons with co-occurring disorders. *Behavioral Sciences & the Law, 22*, 771–785. https://doi.org/10.1002/bsl.603

Steadman, H., & Naples, M. (2005). Assessing the effectiveness of jail diversion programs for persons with serious mental illness and co-occurring substance use disorders. *Behavioral Sciences and the Law, 23*(2), 163–170. https://doi.org/10.1002/bsl.640

Steadman, H. J., Morrissey, J. P., Deane, M. W., & Borum, R. (1999). *Police response to emotionally disturbed persons: Analyzing new models of police interactions with the mental health system*. National Institute of Justice.

Steadman, H. J., Deane, M. W., Borum, R., & Morrissey, J. P. (2000). Comparing outcomes of major models of police responses to mental health emergencies. *Psychiatric Services, 51*(5), 645–649. https://doi.org/10.1176/appi.ps.51.5.645

Steadman, H., Stainbrook, K., Griffin, P., Draine, J., Dupont, R., & Horey, C. (2001). The need for a specialised crisis response location for effective police-based diversion programs. *Psychiatric Services, 52*(2), 219–222. https://doi.org/10.1176/appi.ps.52.2.219

Taheri, S. A. (2016). Do crisis intervention teams reduce arrests and improve officer safety? A systematic review and meta-analysis. *Criminal Justice Policy Review, 27*(1), 76–96. https://doi.org/10.1177/0887403414556289

Teller, J. L. S., Munetz, M. R., Gil, K. M., & Ritter, C. (2006). Crisis intervention team training for police officers responding to mental disturbance calls. *Psychiatric Services, 57*(2), 232–237. https://doi.org/10.1176/appi.ps.57.2.232

The Allen Consulting Group. (2012). *Police, ambulance and clinical early response (PACER) evaluation, final report to Department of Health, Victoria*. The Allen Consulting Group.

Watson, A. C., Ottati, V. C., Morabito, M., Draine, J., Kerr, A. N., & Angell, B. (2010). Outcomes of police contacts with persons with mental illness: The impact of CIT. *Administration and Policy in Mental Health and Mental Health Services Research, 37*(4), 302–317. https://doi.org/10.1007/s10488-009-0236-9

Watson, A. C., Ottati, V. C., Draine, J., & Morabito, M. (2011). CIT in context: The impact of mental health resource availability and district saturation on call dispositions. *International Journal of Law and Psychiatry, 34*(4), 287–294. https://doi.org/10.1016/j.ijlp.2011.07.008

# Chapter 9
# Victim and Witness Retraction and Disengagement: A Systematic Review of Contributing Factors

## 9.1 Questions and Objectives

The core questions of concern in this area centre first on trying to establish which factors influence victims and witnesses during investigation or prosecution of criminal cases that result in them retracting evidence or withdrawing from the process and, second, testing whether there are any approaches to this problem that can effectively reduce it. Hence, the overall objective of this work was to conduct an evidence review with the principal purpose of summarizing what is known about the factors that contribute to *attrition*, in which during the process of investigating a case or preparing it for prosecution, victims or witnesses retract their evidence or withdraw entirely from proceedings. Two supplementary objectives were to take account of the views of different professionals on why retraction occurs and to explore whether any effective remedies have been found for this problem. A third related objective was to identify appropriate steps that could be taken by police, which could be tested on an experimental basis and their effectiveness evaluated. Any such experimental testing would need to be done in a way that did not interrupt the regular flow of criminal justice processing. It was expected that most research on these questions would involve analysis of criminological data or case material or be based on interviews with victims or witnesses.

From the outset it was considered that the review would focus on serious crimes of violence or sexual assault committed against adult victims. However, a small number of studies covered a wider age range and included victims under 16. Coverage of issues of disclosure and/or recantation in cases of child sexual abuse per se would have entailed a larger-scale review, as there is a considerable volume of literature on that topic. Moreover, it is interwoven with other complex questions concerning the nature of children's evidence and their testimony which would have entailed a significantly more extensive review.



J. McGuire et al., *Evidence-Based Policing and Community Crime Prevention*, Advances in Preventing and Treating Violence and Aggression,
https://doi.org/10.1007/978-3-030-76363-3_9

**Table 9.1** PICO framework: victim and witness retraction and disengagement

| | |
|---|---|
| Population/ participants | Persons engaged in police investigations or legal proceedings, who have been either (alleged) victims of crime or witnesses to it<br>Potentially all crime types but with specific reference to violence, sexual violence, partner violence<br>Partner agencies: Crown Prosecution Service, probation, social services, children's services, young offender teams, solicitors, Law Society<br>Police officers involved in investigation and in compiling witness statements and other evidence<br>Other known parameters influencing retraction, e.g. organized crime, gang involvement, criminal histories/individual notoriety<br>Persons with known histories of victim/witness intimidation |
| Intervention/ indicator | Any known intervention or procedure that will reduce the extent of retraction of evidence and of witness statements or disengagement from investigations or legal proceedings<br>Extent of provision of victim support or witness protection<br>Forms of communication between police and victims/witnesses<br>Modes of conducting police interviews or other elements of investigation<br>Extent of media exposure |
| Comparison/ control | Baseline information on levels of retraction or disengagement in relation to (a) different attributes of victims/witnesses (demographic or other variables), (b) types and seriousness of crime, (c) aspects of police investigating team (size, composition, resources)<br>Comparisons between different forces nationally or different jurisdictions internationally |
| Outcome(s) | Comparisons between outcomes of different procedures or mechanisms<br>Rates of successfully completed cases and of cases halted or suspended as a result of retraction/disengagement<br>Reduced duration of time to case clearance<br>Savings of police time<br>Alterations in rates over time or in cross-sectional comparisons |

Prior to commencing the review, the initial phase of the work was planned using the PICO framework. This assists in generating a set of terms or combinations of them that can be used to search electronic databases of research literature and other sources of information. The framework that was devised for the present review is shown in Table 9.1. The items in Table 9.1 were supplemented through consultation with police, and a set of terms devised which were used to search a number of databases and websites as detailed below.

## 9.2 Background

It is well established that many more crimes are committed than are reported to the police. In criminology the difference between the two has traditionally been called the *dark figure* of crime. In England and Wales, the figure can be defined as the difference between the numbers of crimes recorded by the police and the number that are estimated to have been committed on the basis of surveys of victims or of the general public. For example, in the 12 months to the end of June 2020, the Crime Survey for England and Wales estimated that there was a total of 11.5 million crime incidents. The number recorded by the police by contrast was 5.8 million. The gap between the two figures is markedly lower now than in some earlier years, but still quite substantial (Office for National Statistics, 2020).

However, even after offences are reported to the police, many other decisions take place in a lengthy sequence of events which can be spread over an extended period. This means that the anticipated end-point of the process, where defendants appear in court, is not guaranteed to happen. Whether an offence is reported, under which category it is recorded and whether a suspected offender is apprehended, charged and prosecuted are all complex decisions. Given those complexities, the reversals that can occur – such as retraction of evidence – are not well understood. There are many factors thought to influence them, and the rationale underpinning this review is to ask what if anything can be learned from research studies in this area.

Data on sexual offences in England and Wales illustrate patterns of attrition in a striking way. Table 9.2 shows figures for the flow of sexual offences through the criminal justice system averaged across a 3-year period (Ministry of Justice, Home Office, & Office for National Statistics, 2013). A later report examining reasons for the last stage of attrition found that victim retraction, victim non-attendance in court or evidence of the victim not supporting the prosecution prevented 16% of "rape-flagged" cases and 13% of other sexual offence cases from proceeding any further through the criminal justice process (Office for National Statistics, 2018).

Clearly, very large numbers of crimes are not reported to the police, and by far the largest portion of attrition takes place at that stage. Studies show that rates of initial reporting of domestic abuse/intimate partner violence (DA/IPV) to police are also very low (e.g. Glass et al., 2010). But even after complaints and initial allegations are made, there are further progressive drops in the numbers of offences that eventually result in court appearances and – where the evidence confirms it – findings of guilt. For rape, the next largest drop occurs during the police investigation (Feist et al., 2007; Kelly et al., 2005; Munro & Kelly, 2009). We should keep in mind that this happens too with other types of offences including so-called volume crimes, such as house burglary and thefts from and of motor vehicles (Burrows et al., 2005). There is a major difference of course in that for those offences, the main reason for attrition is that there is usually no identified suspect.

**Table 9.2** Flow of sexual offences through the criminal justice system

| | Estimated number of victims | Police-recorded crimes | Detections | Court proceedings (persons) | Convictions (persons) |
|---|---|---|---|---|---|
| Sexual offences | 430,000–517,000 | 54,310 | 16,450 | 9950 | 5620 |
| Rape | 60,000–95,000 | 15,670 | 3850 | 2910 | 1070 |

Lea et al. (2003), p. 583) defined *attrition* as "...the process whereby cases drop out of the CJS [Criminal Justice System] at one of a number of potential points of exit". This then is the reverse of *participation*, continuing involvement in or cooperation with the legal process. There can be many reasons for the attrition that occurs during each phase of that process. The present review is concerned only with what we can learn about the proportion of it that appears to be due to retraction, disengagement or withdrawal on the part of victims and witnesses.

It is of course a core part of the responsibilities of police and prosecutors to decide whether cases proceed beyond each decision point. There have been many studies on the factors that influence those decisions. The present review is concerned only with that portion of attrition that is a result of decisions made by victims and witnesses themselves or with circumstances or events that appear to precipitate their withdrawal. However, there are also cases in which it is not possible to be sure who initiated a withdrawal decision. It may sometimes be a product of exchanges between victims or witnesses and justice system personnel. It can then be difficult to apportion the extent to which disengagement is a result of decisions made by different stakeholders in the process.

### *9.2.1 Attrition Early in the Justice Process*

Kelly et al. (2005) analysed the UK crime statistics for rape reporting and attrition. There was a clear trend over the preceding 20-year period whereby the rate of reporting had substantially increased, and the number of prosecutions had gone up slightly, but the number of convictions remained static. This produced what they called a steadily widening justice gap between reporting rates and conviction rates (see also Temkin & Krahé, 2008, who examine this more closely in the judicial context, but also on wider public attitudes). The largest loss of cases was at the early stage of the process, with between one-half and two-thirds of cases dropping out before referral to prosecutors which was also found by Hohl and Stanko (2015).

Kelly et al. (2005) attributed this to two principal causes, police designation of complaints as false allegations and withdrawals by victims/complainants. Regarding the first of these, there are studies of the variables that influence charging decisions in cases of alleged sexual assault. These are influenced by the victim-perpetrator relationship (i.e. whether partner, acquaintance or stranger) and in some circumstances by reports of the victim's character (Spohn & Holleran, 2001). In a survey of police officers and prosecutors carried out in Sweden, Ask (2010) noted that the former will see some cases that are retracted and as a result do not go to court. Prosecutors therefore see fewer of them and thereby may be more inclined to accept the ones they see as valid. This study found that police officers often had greater doubts about the veracity of victim complaints, but as there was no analysis of the possible relationship between this and case retraction, this study was not included for full analysis.

Comparisons with some other countries have suggested that attrition is a problem in many places but that rates are higher in England and Wales than in most other jurisdictions with comparable features such as Denmark (Hansen et al., 2015), New South Wales (Fitzgerald, 2006) and Alaska (Snodgrass, 2006). Aspects of this position with regard to rape and in seeking to understand what causes attrition have been critically analysed by authors from the different perspectives of law (Koss, 2006), criminology (Spohn et al., 2014), psychology (Brown, 2011; Jordan, 2011) and policing (Maddox et al., 2011). With reference to policing in London, a major report by Angiolini (2015) sought to identify the mechanisms that produced attrition in rape cases at each stage of the investigative process.

The figures shown earlier notwithstanding, according to the Crown Prosecution Service (2013), conviction rates for rape rose by a modest 5.5 percentage points over the 6 years between 2007–2008 and 2012–2013. For domestic violence there was a more impressive increase of 14 percentage points over an 8-year period, between 2005–2006 and 2012–2013. These figures refer of course to the final stage of the system, when cases come to court.

### 9.2.2 Factors Influencing Victims

Guidance on the prosecution of domestic violence cases issued by the Crown Prosecution Service (2014) lists a number of possible reasons for retractions and withdrawals. This is presumably based on the reported experiences of prosecutors but no specific source is cited for the information. Reasons given include pressure from the defendant, a wish to be reconciled, that the relationship had ended, fear for the safety or possible removal of children, fear of the impact of family break-up on children, loss of income if the defendant is imprisoned, feelings of responsibility, embarrassment and self-blame, fear of not being believed or that the complainant will end up isolated and vulnerable or when the victim is involved in prostitution and does not expect her story to be taken seriously. Many of these issues have been examined in the research studies reviewed here, and each has been found to be operating in some cases. Other reasons the CPS document suggests, such as fear of immigration status becoming known, fear of being "outed" in a same-sex relationship or cultural barriers to complaining of partner abuse, while likely to be valid, have not been investigated in the studies reviewed here.

Researchers have examined other factors in specific studies. At an early stage, victims must make statements to the police, and there is evidence that this is particularly challenging for some. For example, in a study of women with intellectual disabilities in New South Wales, Keilty and Connelly (2001) described a number of difficulties that arose when reporting and describing what happened in a sexual assault. Having made a complaint to police, it is by no means uncommon for female victims of domestic violence to be harassed and victimized again in other ways once police attention reduces (Meyer, 2014). There is evidence that victims and suspects who partially or entirely retract their evidence statements are seen by prosecutors and juries as inconsistent and therefore unreliable (Malloy & Lamb, 2010). In an analysis of 50 cases of domestic abuse recorded by the Thames Valley Police, Barrow-Grint (2016) found that the largest single proportion of withdrawals occurred during the first 5 days after the incident that led to initially contacting the police. Based on a study of victim's statements of their reasons for withdrawal, Barrow-Grint proposed a *temporal sequence model* of the process in which individuals perceived their position at each point as a means of managing the entire situation of experiencing abuse.

Some studies in this area touch upon the possible relationship between a victim's experience of police interviewing and her or his subsequent willingness to continue participating in the legal process (e.g. Holmberg, 2004). However, in the present review, no study was found in which this relationship was directly analysed. Other research has focused on the responses of victims of domestic abuse to their predicament and examined their coping styles. We might expect that those exercising what are assessed as more *problem-focused* coping styles, which entail seeking help, staying away from the abusive partner and pursuing retraining or protection orders, would also be more likely to pursue other legal processes including following through to prosecution. However, this was not studied directly, and how problem-solving is applied in practice may depend on what the individual defines as the problem or objective; for example, a victim may want the partner to be warned or restrained but not prosecuted. In a study by Sabina and Tindale (2008), only 40% of the participants regarded as active problem-solvers sought help from the police. Other studies have reported lower rates than this (e.g. 14% in a study in Nicaragua by Ellsberg et al., 2001).

As already noted, the process that leads from an alleged criminal act involving a victim to an eventual appearance by a defendant in court involves a series of decisions, each with its own kind of complexity. Victim or witness withdrawal is only one factor in the chain of events. There are several unanticipated complexities within this. We might expect that women who were more afraid of their abuser and who considered abuse more likely to recur would be more likely to contact the police. However, a study by Apsler et al. (2003) runs counter that expectation. These authors did not however study retraction or withdrawal as such, focusing more on initial police contacts. There is evidence that some women describe themselves as stupid for remaining in abusive relationships. This emerged, for example, in a qualitative study conducted in Sweden (Enander, 2010). Unfortunately, this study did not report data on whether the women's views of themselves and their circumstances played a part in decisions as to whether to proceed in or withdraw from criminal justice processes.

While the focus here is on disengagement from legal processing of cases in the course of criminal investigations or on the way to court, looking more widely victims of partner violence also sometimes disconnect themselves from other legal frameworks such as protection orders (Mele et al., 2011; Roberts et al., 2008). This has been found to be associated with the age and employment status of victims, but also with reasons they gave such as perceptions that the perpetrator had changed or was undergoing counselling. Similarly, a proportion of women who sought an emergency restraining order against a violent partner (usually imposed for a period of 1 year) did not complete the process, in some cases because of attachment to the partner, but in others because of threats to their children's safety (Zoellner et al., 2000). As neither of these studies dealt directly with the process of following through to prosecution, they were excluded from the present review.

In a still broader context, that of justice policy and practice, there is also a recurrent dispute running through this area, and research reflects that context. This is in relation to whether or not the courts or state should pursue policies of prosecuting IPV cases regardless of victims' wishes (Hoyle, 1998). On the one hand, such a policy could be seen as offering victims greater protection (Lewis, 2004). From another perspective, it can be viewed as paternalistic, and the decision should remain in the complainant's hands. Furthermore, as most spousal assaults are by male upon female partners and with increasing severity that ratio expands markedly, it is argued that this discussion also raises fundamental issues of gender and power. What is more empowering for the (by no means exclusively, but predominantly female) victims of IPV? That question and others remain unanswered and research in the field often takes different directions as a result.

Attrition is a ubiquitous problem across many public services, even where people are seeking help and presumably motivated to attend appointments. It can also be a major obstacle in background research on the issues that services are intended to address intimate partner violence (Dutton et al., 2003, p.3). Studies have also shown that there are often high levels of dropout in research on therapy for post-traumatic stress disorder, which many victims of serious crimes experience (Matthieu & Ivanoff, 2006).

## 9.3 Method

To recapitulate, the objectives of this rapid evidence review were as follows:

1. To locate research on what is known about the factors that contribute to attrition, loss of victim or witness evidence due to retraction, disengagement or withdrawal during the course of police investigations and legal proceedings.
2. To include direct studies of victims and witnesses themselves and of the views of different professionals on the factors associated with attrition.
3. To explore whether any effective remedies have been found for this problem.
4. To identify potential methods for police-based research, which could be piloted on an experimental basis to address this problem.

### 9.3.1 Search Strategy

In carrying this work forward, care had to be taken to ensure the focus remained on the selected search terms as used in the present context. A difficulty in reviewing this area is that many of the words listed earlier in Table 9.1 have multiple meanings in criminal justice and in psychological research. For example, the word *withdrawal* sometimes occurs in victim studies in relation to emotional reactions following the traumatic experience of the crime itself, associated with depression (e.g. Relyea & Ullman, 2015). Most of the words used here have several different meanings even within research on issues related to crime and justice. Another example is *moral disengagement*, a concept that has generated extensive research on the factors that influence criminal offending itself (Bandura, 1999). There are also studies of "engaged versus disengaged coping" (Taft et al., 2007a, b). A disengaged coping style is associated with passivity, avoidance, self-criticism or the use of denial, wishful thinking, or escapist strategies, sometimes accompanied by substance misuse (Calvette et al., 2007; Iverson et al., 2013; Scarpa & Haden, 2006). All of these researchers have studied this form of coping amongst crime victims, an area reviewed by Waldrop and Resick (2004). Disengagement has also been used to refer to a phase of recovery from the experience of being in an abusive relationship. Landenburger (1989) formulated a model of entrapment in such situations, from which some women find it impossible to escape. Thus, there are several separate but partially overlapping terms as follows:

1. *Victim participation*: this refers to the victim's ongoing involvement in the criminal justice progress from initial complaint to providing evidence in court.
2. *Attrition*: generally defined as the proportion of total cases lost during the legal process, for all reasons combined, and the amount of it that occurs at each stage.
3. *Retraction*: where a victim or witness alters or withdraws a statement or part of a statement made to police that would be used in prosecution, to an extent whereby it no longer constitutes evidence sufficient to sustain the initial accusation.
4. *Disengagement* and *withdrawal* in which the victim or witness ceases to cooperate with police or prosecution and refuses to proceed further or contact is lost. This is usually contrasted with *engagement coping* which refers to proactive steps to manage stressful events or consequences employing strategies such as problem-solving, cognitive restructuring, emotional expression and seeking social support (Tobin et al., 1989).
5. *Recantation*: used in one sense, this means the same as retraction. However, in some studies it is used to refer to situations in which victims redefine an event in such a way that their evidence no longer implicates the accused. This term appears more commonly in the investigation of allegations of child sexual abuse.

Traditionally, police and court officials have often viewed victim withdrawal as a kind of failure as opposed to their own decisions to discontinue a case which would be based on its limited likelihood of successful prosecution, for example, because of having insufficient evidence. However, there is also a concept of *supportive retraction* in which a victim, supported by an advocate, decides to retract for constructive reasons (Robinson, 2006).

A preliminary search of PsycINFO on 21st of July 2016 using a combination of the terms *victim* and *disengagement* located 93 items. More thorough searches were then designed and conducted using a more elaborate procedure and set of terms. Initial searches covered the period from first of January 2000 up to September 2016. The following databases and websites were electronically searched for that period: PsycINFO, Scopus, Web of Science, Ministry of Justice, Interpol, Europol, the National Criminal Justice Reference Service (NCJRS) and the Netherlands Institute for the Study of Crime and Law Enforcement (NISCALE). The update searches employed only the PsycINFO, NCJRS, Scopus and Web of Science and websites for the period up to November 2020. From an initial set of 33 records downloaded, there were no further reviews, but 7 additional studies were located.

### 9.3.2 Inclusion and Exclusion Criteria

To be retained for inclusion in the review, studies had to meet the following criteria. They had to be published (1) between January 2000 and November 2020, (2) in the English language (facilities were not available for translation) and (3) in a peer-reviewed publication such as a scientific journal or government report. Research degree dissertations or unpublished reports were excluded. They also had (4) to consist of a study of patterns, correlates or causes of victim or witness disengagement from an investigation or prosecution, or withdrawal of evidence, or (5) to be a study of the perspectives of different professionals on factors or processes involved in disengagement and withdrawal.

A few studies that were located dealt with the problem of victim or witness intimidation. These were excluded from the review as this was considered a separate problem. Intimidation or other forms of perverting the course of justice constitute offences in themselves, and where it is established that they are occurring, police can take direct action against them by arresting those responsible or by protecting victims and witnesses. In many cases, however, it cannot be clarified whether an individual's reluctance to proceed is caused by this or other factors. The latter cases were the focus of the review. Intimidation raises a number of other issues in which it was beyond the scope of the present review to address.

Decisions as to whether to include or exclude studies were difficult in some cases. The following are some examples to clarify the application of the selection criteria. Some very large-scale projects that evaluated provision of services to victims were excluded, as they did not report on the effects of those services on participation in or disengagement from the legal process (e.g. Fugate et al., 2006). A difficult decision arose in relation to possibly the largest study found that was potentially relevant to this area, that of Belknap et al. (2000). However, despite extensive data collection, the study contained no detailed analysis that allowed any detailed conclusions to be drawn about factors which influence victims' disengagement. Similarly, studies that evaluated the effect of an intervention on rates of prosecution for partner abuse, but which did not analyse levels of participation or disengagement as part of that, were also excluded (e.g. Salazar et al., 2007).

There were other difficult inclusion/exclusion decisions. One arose in relation to a study by Spohn et al. (2014). This was concerned with recantation of allegations of sexual assault, where analysis of the case material indicated that the offence was unlikely to have occurred, and cases were "unfounded", that is, considered probably to be false reports, by the investigating police (Los Angeles Police Department). This was a marginal decision, as in a small proportion of cases (12.3%), there were indications that the offence had genuinely occurred. Nevertheless, as the study was primarily focused on decisions to "unfound" and threw little light on the process of recantation in cases that should have been prosecuted, it was decided to exclude the study. A study by Bailey (2010) appeared directly relevant as it analysed the failure of efforts by Northamptonshire Police to reduce their rate of attrition in domestic violence cases, but the analysis of the material was based in a Foucauldian framework that does not entail methodical presentation of data collection or analysis.

Several other studies which at first seemed relevant to the review were excluded as on closer inspection they were focused on decisions made by the criminal justice gatekeepers – police and prosecutors – and often on the reasons why they rejected cases from further processing (e.g. Beichner & Spohn, 2005). These decisions were often based on information about victims but sometimes on perceived victim characteristics, including, for example, judgements of their credibility or "blame and believability" (Holleran et al., 2010) or alternatively about the perceived "blameworthiness" of suspects (O'Neal & Spohn, 2016). Thus, they were not about victims' own decisions to decline to cooperate and were therefore excluded. On the other hand, a Canadian study of prosecutors' decisions showed that they were influenced by a victim's cooperation with the authorities (Dawson & Dinovitzer, 2001). That was however influenced by whether victims had met with staff of the Victim/Witness Assistance Program; cases were more likely to proceed if they had. If a victim has not done this, does that mean she has disengaged? In these circumstances it is not clear whether the disengagement decision is the victim's or the prosecutor's. Another even more marginal case was a study by Hirschel and Hutchison (2003) which involved direct interviews with victims. This focused on their decision to call police and what they wanted to achieve by doing so. This too did not address the issue of retraction or disengagement beyond that point. Both of these studies were therefore excluded. A study by Hall (2007) which examined the effects of social measures taken in trials, which were designed to facilitate evidence-giving by vulnerable and intimidated witnesses, appeared to focus on the possibility that such measures led to a risk that such witnesses might withdraw from cases. However, the study presented no data with a direct bearing on this. The net effect of these decisions resulted in a pattern of study inclusion or exclusion as shown in the flowchart in Fig. 9.1.

Searches produced a total of 4416 results which after removing duplicates meant a total of 3241 unique documents was located via databases. These were placed in

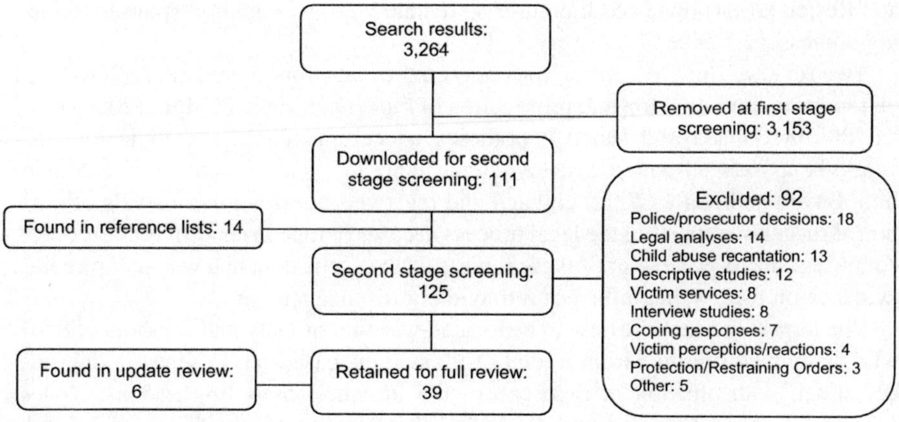


**Fig. 9.1** Flowchart of search results: victim and witness retraction and disengagement

an *Endnote* file. Website searches produced a further 25 documents, 2 of which were also in the *Endnote* file. Thus, there was a total of 3264 documents available for first-stage screening. The screening process resulted in removal of 3153 documents, many for the range of reasons listed earlier deriving from the multiple meanings of some key terms. This produced a set of 111 documents that were downloaded for more detailed, second-stage screening, to which were added a further 14 documents obtained from reference lists. In second-stage screening of the resultant 125 reports, 92 documents were excluded for the reasons listed in Fig. 9.1. After updating, the final tally was a set of 39 documents retained for full review.

## 9.4 Previous Reviews

As far as could be ascertained from the literature searches, so far in this field, there has been no published review of studies on victim retraction and disengagement with the same objectives as the present one. It is a standard practice in journal articles and research reports to carry out a brief review of previous relevant work, to provide a rationale for the study being reported. But no article or other document was found that explicitly set out to conduct and report an evidence review of this area as its main objective.

A large review of the research literature on non-reporting of sexual assault by Lievore (2003) although wide-ranging discusses withdrawal only briefly and contains very little information on factors that may influence it. A report and set of recommendations by Dedel (2006), part of an important series of publications on problem-oriented policing, contains a brief overview of the factors thought to influence witness intimidation. However, this did not employ any formal review procedures and cites only a few relevant studies and does so only very briefly. Waldrop and Resick (2004) reviewed literature on female victims' coping responses following domestic violence.

Two reviews were located on the patterning of attrition in general, both focused on reporting, investigation and prosecution of rape. Du Mont and Myhr (2000) studied this in Canada and tested hypotheses concerning client-related factors that would be associated with a case being less likely to result in a charge or a conviction. Lovett and Kelly (2009) collated and reviewed information on levels of attrition at successive stages of the legal process in cases of rape in ten different European countries. However, neither of these reports analyses the data in a way that provides evidence on factors that influence retraction or disengagement.

The largest literature review to be located was that of Daly and Bouhours (2010) who assembled findings from a total of 90 studies, based on 75 separate datasets, concerned with attrition in rape cases in 5 jurisdictions – England and Wales, Scotland, Canada, the USA and Australia. The majority of studies covered a wide age range, and only 17% were focused solely on adults, with 54% containing mixed-age samples. Studies were divided into two periods (1970–1989 and 1990–2005) to test whether patterns had changed over time. Their analyses confirmed that amongst the five jurisdictions, England and Wales showed the highest degree of attrition over time. They also reported some detailed analysis of the factors influencing attrition at the investigation stage, from the perspective of factors affecting police decisions, but there are no data on victim retraction or withdrawal.

These reviews are clearly relevant to the present one but only moderately so as they do not include any detailed analysis of the likely reasons for disengagement, and they did not examine it with reference to the perspectives or motives of victims and witnesses. Thus, despite the very thorough and extensive analysis reported by Daly and Bouhours (2010), in a sense it remains on the surface of the issues of concern here and leaves the causes of disengagement unexplained.

## 9.5 Results

The studies located in the review have been arranged into four sections with information from the included studies presented in a series of four tables.

### *9.5.1 Analyses of Case File Information and/or Interviews*

The first group focused on analysis of patterns of victim disengagement or on studies of interviews with victims and consisted of 31 studies. They came from 8 different countries – the USA (14), the UK (10), Denmark (2), and Canada, Israel, Nicaragua, Singapore and Spain (1 each). The located studies fell into two groups. Amongst them 19 were concerned with victims of domestic abuse/partner violence. Information from them is presented in Table 9.3. Twelve studies focused on victims

**Table 9.3** Information from included studies: disengagement in domestic abuse/partner violence cases

| Author(s), (date), country | Design and methodology | Samples/data sources | Focus and findings |
|---|---|---|---|
| Boivin and Leclerc (2016) Canada | Statistical analysis of a cohort of police case reports and inter-group comparisons | From 967 DV incidents reported to police in a city in Quebec, classified 815 into 4 groups, reduced to 665 with full data available | The study objective was to investigate whether there was an interdependent relationship between the decision to call the police and willingness to press charges against the assailant, expressed to police at the time of the incident. It was thought that different motives influenced these two actions but that they are related. The study cohort was divided into four groups each with a different profile: (a) victim reported incident and wanted to press charges (390), (b) victim reported incident but did not want to press charges (196), (c) third party reported incident and victim wanted to press charges (64), and (d) third party reported incident and victim did not want to press charges (165). No single variable significantly differentiated all four groups. The variables associated with sustained willingness to press charges were incident reported within 24 hours, previous incidents of DV, victim determined to denounce abuser and the presence of children. Group (4) appeared to present "situational couple violence" that was accepted as ordinary by both parties, and both were more likely to be intoxicated. The most common reason for calling police was to stop the incident, but victims who called police themselves were nearly 5 times more likely to want to press charges. The study does not however contain any data on victims' reasons for their decisions |
| Bonomi et al. (2011) USA | Qualitative analysis of telephone conversations | 25 heterosexual couples; men in a detention facility, women in community (all victims recanted evidence) | Analysed phone calls between couples during the pre-prosecution phase. Callers were informed that calls were recorded and researchers obtained the institution's permission to analyse them. Talking time ranged from 30 to 192 minutes. Analysed features of the calls in terms of interpersonal processes and how couples constructed decisions to recant evidence. Used the qualitative analysis method of *constructivist grounded theory*. Devised a five-stage conceptual model of the process by which women arrived at a point where they withdrew their evidence. Dominant patterns that emerged were the perpetrator's appeals to the victim's sympathy for his plight, progressive minimization of the abusive events and redefining the "abuse narrative", activating fears of life apart and reinvigorating images of the couple's life together, development of a picture of the couple against others and culminating in a stance in which they blamed the state for their problems. The overall process was classed as "witness tampering" at work in relation to IPV |

(continued)

**Table 9.3** (continued)

| Author(s), (date), country | Design and methodology | Samples/data sources | Focus and findings |
|---|---|---|---|
| Cala et al. (2016) Spain | Single-cohort survey analysed using logistic regression | Data from 345 women who had instigated legal proceedings for IPV in Andalusia | Of 806 women who agreed to participate, only 2% withdrew, but others' cases were still in progress. Women were accessing a range of IPV victim services. Extensive data were collected using a questionnaire jointly developed by legal professionals, police and women citizens. This covered sociodemographic, psychosocial, emotional and motivational variables: The last category inquired about reasons for pressing charges. Comparisons were made between 214 (62%) of the sample who continued cases and 131 (38%) who disengaged (dropped charges). The groups differed on educational level, amount of psychological support, support from relatives/friends, contact with the aggressor, thoughts of returning to him, fear of danger to self and children, fear of aggressor going to prison and guilt. Motives also differed (in declining order of effect size): Give him a scare, get protection, stop the abuse, separation and incarceration. In regression analysis, lack of psychological support, contact with the aggressor, fear of abandonment and guilt were the strongest predictors |
| Camacho and Alarid (2008) USA | Statistical analysis of case file information | 384 case files of victims of IPV (334 female, 50 male) given advice by a court advocate | The study objective was to examine the impact of shelter court advocates on the progress of IPV victims through the legal system and their attendance at court dispositions. The cases examined were classed as misdemeanours (less serious level than felonies). One dependent variable in analyses was the level of participation at the concluding stage of the legal process (case outcomes of guilt and sentence were also studied). Cooperation was significantly predicted by having made a victim impact statement at the initial interview with the advocate and by having victim services provided, i.e. contacts made with sources of help such as victim education, information on shelters, counselling, legal assistance, protection, etc. however, notification or reminder letters sent to victims were negatively associated with participation |

(continued)

**Table 9.3** (continued)

| Author(s), (date), country | Design and methodology | Samples/data sources | Focus and findings |
|---|---|---|---|
| Davis et al. (2008) USA | Cross-sectional comparison of two districts of New York City with different DV prosecution policies | 211 DV cases in Brooklyn<br>272 DV cases in the Bronx | Although part of the same unified court system, district attorneys in Brooklyn and Bronx applied different practices in DV cases. In the former most cases are "filed" for charging and prosecution, while in the latter cases are not filed where the victim does not want to proceed. In the Bronx, an assessment is made to ascertain whether the victim is being coerced to drop the case. In Brooklyn, victims were not offered the opportunity to drop the case. An initial part of the study compared declined with prosecuted cases. In the main study, files and outcomes were compared, and a small proportion of victims was interviewed. No difference was found between districts in rates of re-arrest of DV defendants at 9 months after the initial arrest. There were slightly more complaints of inappropriate treatment amongst Bronx than Brooklyn interviewees and some dissatisfaction over lack of arrests. The findings of the study are difficult to interpret as few differences emerged from the two sets of case file data and possibly too much reliance is placed on interviews with only a small proportion of the respective samples. Legal staff in Brooklyn spent a far larger amount of time than those in Bronx processing cases. "The study did not produce a definitive picture of which prosecution policy is superior… however, victims expressed a preference for being relieved of the responsibility of prosecuting …based on an objective assessment of the potential benefits and costs of doing so" (p.658) |

(continued)

**Table 9.3** (continued)

| Author(s), (date), country | Design and methodology | Samples/data sources | Focus and findings |
|---|---|---|---|
| Fleury-Steiner et al. (2006) USA | Statistical analysis of interview data from a study cohort | 178 female victims of IPV from 3 sites, interviewed on 3 occasions | The study formed part of a larger longitudinal project on battered women's safety. Participants were interviewed shortly after closure of legal cases and 6 and 12 months later (times 1, 2 and 3). The main outcome of interest was women's expressed willingness to use the CJS again in the event of further violence and which factors influenced this. Background, offence-related and other kinds of data were collected, plus information on experience of the legal system, recent case disposition and whether it was what they had wanted to happen. Women were asked how likely they were to call the police again and to want court action taken. Answers remained highly consistent across times 1, 2 and 3. Most women (70%) had been victims of a severe assault. Four models were tested using hierarchical regression analysis, with more variables controlled at each stage. Women who were living with the assailant at the time of the index offence and who said the assailant contributed the household showed lower intent to reuse the CJS. Women who were employed and who thought the community was more supportive of them had stronger intent. Women who were assaulted again before the first case was resolved had lower intent. Initial intent to have cases proceed against abusers was associated with future intent to do so if needs be. If women had wanted charges to be dropped and they were, they intended to sue the system again (i.e. if court actions were consistent with their wishes). Finally, with other variables controlled, women's experiences with the CJS had a significant impact on their willingness to reuse it. If she herself had called the police; if she had been given information by the responding police; and if she described her treatment by police, prosecutors and victim advocates in positive terms, she was more likely to use the CJS again. She was less likely to do so if she had been pressured towards prosecution and if she had several times gone to court to find proceedings were cancelled |

(continued)

**Table 9.3** (continued)

| Author(s), (date), country | Design and methodology | Samples/data sources | Focus and findings |
|---|---|---|---|
| Ganapathy (2006) Singapore | Qualitative in-depth interview study and observation of police-victim encounters | 26 female victims of IPV recruited via 1 police division | IPV victims were interviewed in police stations, social work units or family service centres. All three agencies worked in a coordinated way on IPV. Only 6 of the victims had reported IPV to the police; in other cases, the incident had been reported by someone else. The police official policy was to pursue charges after they were filed regardless of whether victims withdrew or requested dropping the case. Officers then had to negotiate entry to the household. In some instances, they classed incidents as "no offence disclosed" or "police assistance required" but did not record an offence unless there was "grievous hurt". All but two of the interviewed victims did not want their husbands arrested; some had obtained protection orders but did not want their abusers prosecuted (it was "the last thing on their minds"); some respondents said they would simply like their husbands removed for a while. But they did not want to embark on a lengthy legal process. They considered that the costs of prosecution outweighed its benefits and feared they could end up isolated. They also feared the "disgrace" of police involvement |
| Hare (2006) USA | Mixed-methods study based on both quantitative and qualitative analyses | 94 battered women, cases randomly selected from prosecution files in Indiana | The study focused on different reasons why women may favour or oppose prosecution of men who have assaulted them in close relationships. Interviews were retrospective, conducted approximately 2 years after case closure. Comparisons of demographic and offence-related data were made between those who had (70.2%) and had not want prosecution. Background and demographic factors were mostly non-significant. Variables which emerged significantly linked to favouring prosecution were being aged <30, having previously had a protective order against the abuser, being emotionally attached to property that was damaged and being in a dating rather than marital relationship. Although over 70% of women in both subgroups were injured, this was not associated with seeking prosecution. Qualitative analysis yielded 26 separate reasons for decisions. Ones given by those opposing prosecution included offence being minor (38%), prosecution was going too far; being committed to the defendant (23%); wanting help rather than punishment (11%); and wanting to be left alone (11%). Only a small number feared retaliation. Those favouring prosecution gave as reasons seeking retribution (40%), to deter the abuser (29%) and wanting the defendant locked up (incapacitated, 21%) |

(continued)

**Table 9.3** (continued)

| Author(s), (date), country | Design and methodology | Samples/data sources | Focus and findings |
|---|---|---|---|
| Hare (2010) USA | Mixed-methods study based on both quantitative and qualitative analyses | 94 female IPV victims, cases randomly selected from prosecution files in Indiana | The study is linked to that by Hare (2006). The focus here is on what factors influence victims to favour or oppose going for a trial of their case. 37.2% of participants wanted a trial, with most preferring other legal steps. Being less likely to support a trial was associated with being still married to the defendant, being younger, having substantial injuries and higher medical costs; having found the crime-scene police helpful; having had a history of victimization (as level of this rose, so did support for a trial); having previously obtained a protection order; being afraid of the defendant; and having negative interactions with the defendant during the legal process. Only some of these variables emerged as significant in multivariate as opposed to bivariate analysis. Those opposed to trial gave a total of 71 reasons; the most frequent one was that the incident was not serious enough to warrant it. Others included not wanting to experience the strain, concerns over mental health, fear of retaliation of things went that far, financial and emotional dependence on defendants, concerns over children and family support. Those in favour of a trial cited the need for retribution as a principal reason, wanting a public acknowledgement of the crime, and some sought rehabilitation of the offender, while others sought incapacitation. The findings were used to test the validity of two different models of victims' reactions to the legal process |
| Hester (2005) UK | Multi-methods study: Statistical analysis of police files; qualitative analysis of interviews; observations of cases in court | 291 DV incident arrest reports by Northumbria Police. Interviews with 26 police officers and civilian staff and with 74 DV victims. Observations of 25 court cases. Interviews with staff of 30 other agencies | Initial data showed that of 869 DV incidents in a 3-month period, 222 resulted in arrest (26%) and 31 led to convictions (14% of arrests, 4% of incidents), mostly resulting in fines. There was extensive support for victims, and many police officers were frustrated by their unwillingness to provide statements. Cases were often managed via a *public order* approach: Some arrests were for breach of the peace, though this varied across three command areas. There was a high proportion of repeat offenders amongst the incidents (70%). Prosecutors usually discontinued cases when statements were retracted, or when a couple were back together, where cases were seen as unreliable. However, there was also often a lack of other evidence such as photographs which other sources indicated as increasing the likelihood of conviction. Victims described their main needs as being for violence to stop and for steps to be taken to ensure it did not continue. It appeared as if they used the CJS up to a point where those goals seemed likely to be achieved. They were satisfied when police arrived quickly and brought situations under control. Those seeking longer-term protection were less satisfied and were dismayed by plea bargaining and other elements of the legal process. However, women with children were less likely to give statements, whereas contact with children was "exploited" by defence solicitors in obtaining more lenient sentences |

(continued)

**Table 9.3** (continued)

| Author(s), (date), country | Design and methodology | Samples/data sources | Focus and findings |
|---|---|---|---|
| Hoyle and Sanders (2000) UK | Qualitative, in-depth interview-based study | 53 female victims of IPV; cases reported to the Thames Valley Police | The research is framed in the context of changing legal policies in England and Wales and also draws on a larger study reported in an earlier book by the first author (Hoyle, 1998). It also evaluates different models of police response to IPV ("victim choice", "pro-arrest" and "victim empowerment" positions). Most women (31) wanted abusers to be arrested, whereas 22 did not. However, most of the former did not want the abuser to be prosecuted. Thirty wanted the man "removed from the scene" in order to obtain some respite from aggression and wanted the justice system to "teach him a lesson", but did not appear to want the process to go much farther. A smaller number (7) wanted the police just to calm the situation. Only a minority of those wanting arrest also wanted retribution. Others saw police as a way to get the man help and to protect their children. Most police attending incidents saw them as criminal matters and asked most women to make a statement. The main reasons given by women for not seeking prosecution were that the arrest itself was effective so no further action was necessary and that the costs of going further outweighed the benefits. Some saw arrest as a kind of "summary justice". But the main reason for refusing to provide a statement was fear of retaliation and also that the CJS could not solve the problem |
| Kingsnorth and Macintosh (2004) USA | Statistical analysis of case file information | 5272 cases of DV processed through the district attorney's office in Sacramento over an 18-month period | The main objective of the study was to investigate which factors influenced victim support for prosecution, by analysing victim behaviour at earlier stages of the legal process and attitudes to calling for assistance and towards arrest. Numerous variables were analysed as potential predictors including the alleged offender's history, actions in the incident, victim's pattern of contacts, victim characteristics and the victim-offender relationship. Overall, 74.8% of victims wanted arrest to be made but only 28.6% wanted prosecution. Logistic regression showed a number of factors were predictors at each stage of the process. There were some differences between ethnic groups. Cohabitation reduced support for arrest and prosecution; having children increased the likelihood of prosecution; a more severe assault increased support for arrest and prosecution. Occurrence of prior incidents increased support for arrest. Supports for both arrest and prosecution were lower if the victim had been using substances at the time of the incident. When more services were provided to the victim in the early stages, there was more support for prosecution later. When a case was filed as more serious, odds of supporting prosecution went down significantly |

(continued)

**Table 9.3** (continued)

| Author(s), (date), country | Design and methodology | Samples/data sources | Focus and findings |
|---|---|---|---|
| Robinson and Chandek (2000) USA | Statistical analysis of a large sample of police records | Data on 471 DV complaints from a total of 1313 made to a Midwestern Police Department in a 5-month period. The department operated Domestic Abuse Response Teams (DART) | Analysed the relationships between data from three sources: Case summaries prepared by officers visiting DV incidents, police records of the history of the victim and case details and characteristics of responding officer and detectives assigned to each case. The dependent variable was victim participation in the criminal justice process. Independent (predictor) variables were arranged in three categories: Characteristics of disputants, of police and of situations. Seventy-five percent of victims chose not to pursue cases. Victims were less likely to participate when the suspect was black and when the assigned detective was female. They were more likely to participate when a weapon was used, when they had already experienced DV or had existing proceedings against the suspect, when an arrest was made at the scene and when children were present at the incident. Only the last variable was significant in multivariate analysis |
| Robinson and Cook (2006) UK | Mixed-methods study with analysis of quantitative data and informant interviews | 216 DV cases from 5 sites (4 England, 1 Wales) with Specialist Domestic Violence Courts | The objective was to examine the relative roles of features of victims (nature of relationship, abuse history, children present, vulnerability), offences (injury, alcohol use, etc.) and case processing (admission of guilt, witness available, medical statement, etc.), and also case file information, on decisions to retract. Exactly 50% of cases were retracted. Reasons given for retraction included couple reconciled, wanting rehabilitation, concern for children, incident seen as "one-off", self-blame, wanting to move on, stress/fear and others. In bivariate analyses, victims were significantly less likely to retract if the offender was an ex-partner/ spouse, if there was an initial plea of guilty and if other witness statements were available. They were more likely to retract if there had been previous DV, they had been injured and the offender had been drinking at the time. In addition, in multivariate analysis, victims were less likely to retract if they had made a victim personal statement and if the case had been sent for pre-trial review. The highest rates of *increase* in retraction were linked with victim injury (+186%), previous DV (+149%) and offender drinking before incident (+98%). The highest rates of *decrease* in retraction were for assault by ex-partner (−77%), initial guilty plea (−67%), having a victim personal statement (−54%), other witness statement (−50%) and case sent for pre-trial review (−47%) |

(continued)

**Table 9.3** (continued)

| Author(s), (date), country | Design and methodology | Samples/data sources | Focus and findings |
|---|---|---|---|
| Shoham (2000) Israel | Single-cohort questionnaire study | 90 women who had complained of IPV at 5 police stations in Central Israel | Analysed the experiences of women victims in encounters with police and their perceptions of the process of investigation. Used a questionnaire including rating scales and open-ended questions. Earlier research by the author suggested some officers believed women had an ulterior motive for making complaints and that some were incited to do so by lawyers or social workers. In this study half of the respondents thought the police officer sided with their abusive husbands, and only 37% believed the officer understood their situation. A majority of women who withdrew complaints thought that police officers did not take the complaint seriously, a significantly higher proportion than those who did not withdraw. Police were perceived as "professional and business-like but not as understanding" (p. 253) |
| Sleath and Smith (2017) UK | Mixed methods: Cross-sectional analysis of case reports with qualitative study of accounts of retraction | 524 case reports of police-recorded IPV analysed statistically Statements or accounts of retraction analysed qualitatively | Collected data from police reports on a set of victim, perpetrator and offence characteristics with the aim of testing hypotheses about their relationship to the likelihood of retraction and disengagement. Overall, 113 cases (21.6%) were formally retracted and 140 cases (26.7%) disengaged (defined as uncontactable on several occasions). The factors having the strongest association with outcomes were, for retraction, higher level of community deprivation and higher scores on *Domestic Abuse, Stalking, and Harassment and Honour Based Violence* risk assessments (Richards, 2009) and, for disengagement, absence of use of alcohol or drugs, involvement of children and lower *Domestic Abuse, Stalking, and Harassment and Honour Based Violence* risk assessments. Several reasons emerged for withdrawal but could not distinguish between retraction and disengagement. They included reconciliation, victim pregnancy, victim loved perpetrator, couple working on issues and wishing to avoid distress to children. A list of reasons and their frequencies is given in the journal paper |

(continued)

**Table 9.3** (continued)

| Author(s), (date), country | Design and methodology | Samples/data sources | Focus and findings |
|---|---|---|---|
| Smith (2000) USA | Single-cohort questionnaire survey | 241 women victims of domestic violence living in shelters for battered women in 8 states | The objective of the study was to survey the views of female IPV victims on their use of the legal system, different resources (e.g. contacting police, seeking restraining order) and interventions including mandatory arrest and prosecution laws. Data were also collected on their personal histories of abusive relationships. A small proportion of abusers (5%) were female. Most participants supported mandatory arrest, "no drop" and compulsory medical examination policies. However sizeable minorities did not, and slightly larger proportions were unsure, e.g. while 56.7% thought "no drop" policies were beneficial, 19.3% did not, 16% were unsure and 8% had no opinion. Also, while 56% said that policy would make them more likely to report future violence, 14.5% said they would be less likely to do so, 14.5% said it would make no difference, and 14.9% were not sure. As women victims do not wholly endorse mandatory prosecution (the no drop policies), the findings may be part of the explanation why a proportion of victims disengages from legal processes, as they anticipate the likelihood of negative effects. The author suggests mandatory laws may have "the unintended consequence of deterring victims from initiating legal or medical interventions" (p. 1398) |
| Vásquez et al. (2018) Nicaragua | Comparison between women who retracted a complaint of IPV and those who did not | 136 female victims of IPV in the city of León; all from a poor neighbourhood and with family incomes of less than US $100 per week | Access to interviewees was via the commissariat for women of the Nicaraguan National Police and women's support networks. Most women had begun living with their attackers from an early age and had been with them for an average of 9.16 years. Data were collected by structured interview. Only 6.6% of the group had taken their complaint to its conclusions. Five variables were found to significantly differentiate those who retracted from those who did not. The latter had slightly lower family income and higher (daily) abuse frequency and were less likely to prefer to stay with the perpetrator and children despite everything else, less likely to believe that men must take responsibility for family expenses and more likely to agree with the view that women have a role of educating and improving men |

(continued)

**Table 9.3** (continued)

| Author(s), (date), country | Design and methodology | Samples/data sources | Focus and findings |
|---|---|---|---|
| Weisz (2002) USA | Statistical analysis of telephone survey data | 207 African American women victims of domestic violence in Detroit | An initial part of the study involved random selection of 1057 police incident reports and development of an interview schedule. 65.2% of the study sample said it was a good idea to press charges against abusers. Some variables were not related to views for or against prosecution. They include the victim's age, income level, employment, education or marital status; number of times her abuser had been arrested for DV in the past 6 months; duration of relationship with the abuser; and other factors. Women were more likely to oppose prosecution if it had not been initiated or if they had been pressured to either pursue or drop charges. They were more likely to support it if they were separated from the partner, if the partner had used alcohol or drugs during an assault in the past 6 months and if they had left home or called police more often in the past 6 months. In open-ended questions, the reasons most commonly given for supporting prosecution were that the behaviour was unacceptable and, for opposing prosecution, that the incident was not regarded as sufficiently serious, that it was the first time something like it had happened or that the abuser was no longer thought to be dangerous. There are several other detailed findings contained in the report |

of rape, attempted rape or other serious sexual assaults. Information extracted from them is contained in Table 9.4.

### 9.5.2 *Perceptions of Professionals*

A second category involved studies of the accounts given by professionals of what they considered to be the barriers in the criminal justice system that led to victim or witness disengagement. This was a much smaller group containing only two studies and information from them is shown in Table 9.5. One of these studies came from the USA, and the other from Canada.

### 9.5.3 *Interventions to Reduce Retraction/Disengagement*

It had been hoped that the review would include studies of steps taken to reduce the extent of the problems of retraction and disengagement, ideally with well-conducted outcome evaluations. However, no studies were found that had been specifically or

**Table 9.4** Information from included studies: disengagement in serious sexual offence cases

| Author(s), (date), country | Design and methodology | Samples/data sources | Focus and findings |
|---|---|---|---|
| Feist et al. (2007) UK | Statistical analysis of case file information | Information on 676 cases of rape of a female recorded in 1 April 2003 to 31 March 2004 Data obtained from 8 police forces | An intensive analysis of all stages of the process of investigating and prosecuting rape of a female (of any age). Of the cases examined, 15% were "no crime". Of the remainder, victims withdrew support in 39% of cases, mainly at the police investigation stage, and 58% of withdrawals took place before the suspect was arrested. Reasons for victim withdrawal, in 142 cases where they were stated, were not wanting to go through with the court process (20%), wanting to "move on" (20%), impact on Well-being of self or others (12%), concern over impact of proceedings on suspect (10%), pressure from others to withdraw (10%), refusal to cooperate (6%), concerns over reprisal (5%), doubt over success of court outcome (4%), victim stopped believing crime took place (3%), victim just wanted to talk to suspect (2%) and others (9%). Withdrawal was 70% more likely if the offence was reported to police on the same day as it had occurred. It was 90% less likely if the investigation was linked to that of another sexual offence, 80% less likely if the offender was a parent or other relative or acquaintance and 50% less likely if the victim was injured. Withdrawal was less likely if a specially trained officer was involved in the case (though this was not entered in the regression analysis due to the number of missing cases). There were also significant differences between police areas |
| Hansen et al. (2015) Denmark | Analysis of case file information | 282 cases of rape or attempted rape reported to 1 police department; in 138 cases victims were seen in a regional Center for Rape Victims | Data suggest that the rate of reporting of rape as a proportion of the estimated total number of rapes is far higher in Denmark than in England and Wales. This study focused on reasons for attrition following reports to the police. Note that though the average victim age was 23, the study included victims as young as 12. Of the total cases, 174 cases were closed by police and 59 by prosecutors. Reasons for the former were insufficient evidence (37.4%), lack of a suspect (33.3%), victim unwillingness (26.4%) and smaller proportions for legal reasons. Reasons for the latter were insufficient evidence (76.3%), other legal reasons (18.6%) and victim unwillingness (5.1%). There were no differences between those in contact with the Center for Rape Victims and those not with respect to reasons for case closure. No more detail is given on why victims wanted charges dropped |

(continued)

**Table 9.4** (continued)

| Author(s), (date), country | Design and methodology | Samples/data sources | Focus and findings |
|---|---|---|---|
| Hansen et al. (2018) Denmark | Analysis of case file information + interview and psychological assessment of participants using clinical scales | 64 victims of rape or attempted rape, comparing cases where prosecution was recommended with those not and those willing or not willing to participate | All but one of the victims was female, and all suspected perpetrators were male. Assessments were undertaken of levels of psychological distress, including depression, anxiety, sleep disturbance and other variables including acute stress disorder as defined in DSM-IV. Authors tested the hypothesis that decisions to prosecute and willingness to proceed would be associated with presence of acute stress disorder and levels of social support. Higher levels of acute stress disorder and other distress, and lower levels of social support, were more likely amongst cases where prosecution was not recommended (Cohen's *d* effect sizes 0.39 and − 0.25); higher levels of depression and anxiety, and lower levels of social support, were found in cases closed because of unwillingness to proceed (respective Cohen's *d* 0.86, 0.91 and − 0.47) |
| Hohl and Stanko (2015) UK | Statistical analysis of case file information | 587 case file reports of rape allegations in a 2-month period in 2012 in London | Analysis of reports of attrition in cases of rape. All victims were female but 33% were aged under 16. Using a series of regression analyses, the study compares the effects of different factors on three types of attrition: Victim withdrawal, police "no crime" decisions and police "no further action" decisions. The first accounted for 48% of the attrition in the sample and was highest during the police investigation phase (67% of it occurring then). Variables significantly associated with a greater likelihood of victim withdrawal were cooperation or communication problems, a history of consensual sex with the accused and an intimate relationship with the accused. Victim variables significantly associated with a greater likelihood of continuing with the case were making a video-recorded statement, involvement of the child protection unit investigating the case, victim being aged under 13, suspect having a police record, victim had attended a haven[a] and when the suspect was identified. Victims classified as vulnerable through mental health problems or learning difficulties were no more likely to withdraw than others but were more likely to have cases withdrawn by police or prosecutors |

(continued)

**Table 9.4** (continued)

| Author(s), (date), country | Design and methodology | Samples/data sources | Focus and findings |
|---|---|---|---|
| Kelley and Campbell (2013) USA | Cross-sectional content analysis of a set of police reports | 266 police reports of sexual assault cases from 3 midwestern police departments | The objective was to identify whether different factors influenced three outcomes of police reports on sexual assault cases: Police referral for prosecution, police decision not to proceed and victim withdrawal from the case. Data extracted from police reports included demographic information on victims and alleged offenders, assault descriptions and details of evidence collected on the incidents. Some factors showed differences in "paired contrasts", notably the size of the police departments (smaller department made more prosecution decisions). But in the full multinomial regression analysis, the factors that emerged were victims being unconscious at the time of the assault due to alcohol/drug use and "detective effort" (meaning the number of suspects interviewed, range of evidence gathered and the time and resources invested in the case). It was not possible to say whether victim withdrawal was wholly voluntary or based on police advice |
| Kelly et al. (2005) UK | Cross-sectional and longitudinal design, case file analysis | Rape victims: 480 completed questionnaires at 3 time points; +80 interviewed | As part of a larger study using multiple methods of data collection at multiple sites, analysed the levels of attrition at six stages of the investigative and legal process and, where known, the reasons for its occurrence. They present some data on 40 cases who did not report rapes to the police (but sought help at a sexual assault referral Centre). Attrition point 4 was "early withdrawal" and accounted for 34% of cases (633 individuals). Approximately half of these (315) declined to complete the initial process of making statements or being examined; some withheld information, refusing to name a known attacker. The remainder (318) completed that process but withdrew shortly afterwards. They were more likely to be aged 16–35, currently in a relationship, and there were both drugs and alcohol involved. Others expressed fear of the court process; some expressed uncertainty over whether they had been raped. Several other reasons were given for withdrawal but in 21% of cases, there was no reason recorded |

(continued)

**Table 9.4** (continued)

| Author(s), (date), country | Design and methodology | Samples/data sources | Focus and findings |
|---|---|---|---|
| Lea et al. (2003) UK | Descriptive analysis of questionnaires on case file reports | 379 cases of rape or attempted rape of an adult reported in 1 police area over a 5-year period | Case files were not accessed directly but via a questionnaire sent to senior investigating officers. The article provides detailed information on the pattern of offences in the police area involved. Most of the offences (66%) were reported within 24 hours. Examining current status of cases at the time of writing, 61% were subject to "no further action" (NFA) by police or CPS; 11% were "no crime"; 10% were pending; and in 7% victims refused to assist or retracted. Eleven percent resulted in a conviction and 5% resulted in a conviction of rape. Reasons for discontinuation were available for 191 cases. While the largest proportion were due to lack of evidence, 38% were due to retraction or refusal to assist. Police recorded that victims were too afraid to proceed, had reunited with the accused, "wanted to spare him the ordeal of court" or were under pressure from their families to give up. In 3% of cases, victims were thought unreliable as they had been inconsistent. Officers thought just below 10% of cases were false allegations. Statistical analysis indicated that the only variable significantly associated with current case status was the victim's prior relationship with the accused: If they had a sexual relationship, retraction was more likely. The only variables significantly associated with reasons for current status were the place of initial contact and location of the offence |
| Lea et al. (2016) UK | Matched-pairs group comparison design | Of 1146 rapes in a city over a 21-year period, analysed 67 where victims were sex workers | As part of a larger project, researchers analysed reported rapes or attempted rapes of 67 sex workers (SWs) and compared 62 of that group with a matched sample of 62 non-sex workers (non-SWs) drawn from the rest of the study population. (Part of the article reports a profile of the 21-year study population.) Most SW rapes (66%) were by strangers, the remainder by a partner or ex-partner. Twenty-five percent of cases were discontinued by the CPS and 26% by police; 19% of cases went to trial; 16% resulted in a conviction for rape as opposed to 2% of non-SW cases. Complaints were withdrawn by 6% of SWs and 11% of non-SWs. SWs reportedly experience higher levels of violence in rape and sexual assaults, and the two samples were matched for violence levels: But overall attrition was lower in the SW group. This was thought to be because of the close link between rape and IPV in non-SW cases |

(continued)

**Table 9.4** (continued)

| Author(s), (date), country | Design and methodology | Samples/data sources | Focus and findings |
|---|---|---|---|
| Maddox et al. (2011) UK | Single-cohort correlational study | 22 victims of rape (21 women, 1 man) recruited online or from a Sexual Assault Referral Centre | Investigated psychological factors thought likely to influence willingness of rape victims to take their cases to court. Participants completed a series of self-report scales designed to assess severity of trauma, experiences of shame and self-blame, perceptions of police interviewers' levels of empathy and reported likelihood of proceeding with or retracting from the case. All participants reported elevated levels of post-traumatic stress disorder, shame and self-blame, which were negatively correlated with perceptions of police interviewer empathy. Intention to go to court was positively associated with perceived police empathy. It is not suggested that there is a causal connection between variables as the direction of any influence could be either way. There was no direct association between experiencing the consequences of rape and likelihood of going to court. The authors suggested however that "…the police interview may provide a key pathway to reducing attrition in rape cases" (p. 116) |
| Murphy et al. (2014) USA | Content analysis of a sample of police reports of sexual assaults | 125 incidents of sexual assaults on female victims | Previous data suggested that after reporting sexual assaults, 25% to 36% of victims chose to drop cases. This study examined the possible effect of police decision-making at an early stage on the rate of attrition in reports of sexual assault. There was a 97.5% level of agreement between those who coded the interviews. The dependent variables were the frequency with which police recorded that victims chose to drop cases and what reasons were given for doing so. Of 125 cases, police reported that 41 victims chose not to pursue cases. In 30.2% of those cases, an explicit reason was given: Including stress/distress, pregnancy, hospitalization, fear of the suspect, desire for the police to warn or monitor the suspect and self-blame. In 36.6% of cases, no explicit reason for dropping charges was given, but in $\frac{2}{3}$ of those cases, the victim failed to attend an appointment or did not answer phone calls and was uncooperative, or their credibility was doubted. In the remaining 31.7% of cases, no reason was given for dropping charges. The authors concluded that reasons were often not sufficiently clear and it was difficult to say whether the victim or the reporting officer had led the withdrawal decision |

(continued)

**Table 9.4** (continued)

| Author(s), (date), country | Design and methodology | Samples/data sources | Focus and findings |
|---|---|---|---|
| Patterson and Campbell (2010) USA | Qualitative, interview-based study using grounded theory | 20 female survivors of rape, mean age 28 | Examined reasons given by rape victims for participating in the criminal justice system. Almost half of the respondents said they wanted the offender stopped from harming other women or themselves; roughly a quarter were encouraged by others to report the rape; and in the remaining cases, someone else contacted police without their permission. Thus, over half were hesitant to call police because they were unsure that they would be believed and were also unsure if they could claim to be raped because they had offered only verbal rather than physical resistance. The study results include accounts of the circumstances in which women made decisions to contact police. Women who reported rape were not primarily interested in offenders being charged; rather they wanted physical and sexual violence to stop and/or relationships to end. Willingness to continue the legal process was influenced by multiple factors, but mainly by a wish to prevent the perpetrator from raping again, and most became more confident in pursuing the case following interactions with a nurse examiner, a victim advocate or the police; almost a quarter said they were influenced by being treated respectfully by system personnel. But some others were upset by the way they were treated |

(continued)

**Table 9.4** (continued)

| Author(s), (date), country | Design and methodology | Samples/data sources | Focus and findings |
|---|---|---|---|
| Tellis and Spohn (2008) USA | Statistical analysis of a database of sexual crimes | 1452 cases of rape of a female aged 14 or older or related offences reported to the Sex Crimes Unit of San Diego Police from 1991 to 2002 | The study was designed to test the hypothesis that what has been called "real rape" is treated differently by the justice system compared to far more numerous "simple rape". The former is the concept of rape as an attack by a stranger, using a weapon, where the victim resists and is injured. In legal terms it would usually be called aggravated rape. It has been argued that the authorities have difficulty accepting that rape has occurred when it does not fit this pattern. The *sexual stratification hypothesis* states that rapes of White women by Black or Hispanic mean will be more likely to result in prosecution than in other victim-offender combinations. The study tested a number of specific hypotheses derived from these two concepts. The dependent variable of most relevance to this review was whether victims declined prosecution – Which would signal the end of the case as there was no mandatory prosecution policy. Other dependent variables analysed were whether the case was "unfounded" (closed) by police and whether the district attorney filed charges. Police unfounded 11% of cases; victims declined 36% of those remaining; the DA filed charges in 48% of the remainder. Victims' declining prosecution significantly increased if the accused was an acquaintance or dating partner. The authors viewed this as partly supporting the aggravated rape hypothesis. But the presence of a weapon and sustaining injury were non-significant. Victims were more likely to decline prosecution if they were under the influence of alcohol or drugs, but more likely to proceed with it if the suspect was under such influence. Victims aged under 16 were less likely to refuse to cooperate than those ≥16. No demographic variables emerged as significant |

[a]Formally called Sexual Assault Referral Centres (SARCs), a series of projects set up jointly by the Metropolitan Police and King's College Hospital, initially at three sites in London, now also available in other locations

**Table 9.5** Information from included studies: perceptions of professionals

| Author(s), (date), country | Design and methodology | Samples/data sources | Focus and findings |
|---|---|---|---|
| Gauthier (2010) Canada | Qualitative, interview-based study | 22 officials from two Montreal courts:<br>6 judges<br>7 prosecutors<br>4 defence attorneys 5 victim advocates | In-depth interviews focused on the consequences for different parties involved of decisions to drop domestic violence cases from further action. Earlier research showed that 52.8% of cases in Montreal were withdrawn, for a range of reasons (victim requested it, refused to testify, failed to appear in court, recanted statement). On the basis of earlier studies, factors influencing this were thought to include fear of spousal retaliation, having forgiven the spouse, reconciled with the spouse or being dependent on him. Interviews explored in depth the consequences of those decisions for victims themselves and for others involved. Victims often believed the court system trivialized IPV, and, when they withdrew, they believed it destroyed their credibility in future. Dropping cases was also thought to have a demotivating effect on police officers and on prosecutors. To reduce these effects, participants suggested prosecutors should meet victims, to explain why they had agreed to drop proceedings, and that judges should communicate that they would still take future cases seriously and that advocates should try to slow down decisions when complainants appeared about to withdraw. Only 3/22 respondents saw dropped cases as a failure |
| Patterson and Tringali (2015) USA | Qualitative, interview-based study using grounded theory | 13 victim advocates<br>10 forensic nurses based in a sexual assault nurse examiners programme | Studied the views of victim advocates and of forensic nurses on barriers experienced by female IPV victims in the criminal justice system (CJS). None of the participants saw it as their role to persuade women to pursue cases, but rather to support the decisions women made. Many of the points that emerged in interviews underlined the daunting challenges women victims said they faced in pursuing prosecution against an abusive partner and suggested there was insufficient awareness of this throughout the CJS. For example, women did not expect to be believed, and so often withheld offence details, and often blamed themselves. It was stated that when they had an impression of being believed, they were more likely to remain in the CJS process |

*CJS* criminal justice system

primarily designed to test and evaluate interventions with this explicitly stated as a sole or major objective. The only relevant findings came from a small number of studies that had broader aims of developing ways to improve victim welfare through increasing their take-up of services. A number of studies incorporated feedback on how services were perceived. However only two studies involved well-designed interventions and evaluations. Information about them is presented in Table 9.6. Both are from the USA. Three other studies which mentioned these kinds of outcomes but in a more fleeting or incidental way will be briefly described but not set out in tabular form as they contained only minimal relevant information.

The two studies by Campbell and her colleagues described in Table 9.6 were part of a larger ongoing project with different facets. Implementing changes such as the ones tested in that work would be an elaborate process as it would entail either the introduction of a new group of personnel in the investigatory process or the provision of additional training to existing staff. As the studies by Campbell et al. deal with sexual assault, thought would need to be given as to how it might be possible to address parallel kinds of problems in other areas such as domestic violence. However as found in some of the studies listed in Tables 9.3 and 9.4, eliciting victim statements, taking photographs, doing medical tests or gathering forensic evidence at the scene of offences would increase the probability of ongoing victim participation and possible eventual convictions. Two other studies described in Table 9.6 were controlled experimental tests of the possible effect of mobile telephone text reminders or prompts on the rate of attendance at court hearings by defendants, victims and witnesses. Both of these interventions are viewed as part of what is known as *nudge strategy*, in which attempts are made to influence behaviour through unobtrusive means (Halpern, 2015). In these studies, however, the intervention did not prove to be effective.

Possibly the most encouraging results come from the research of Vallely et al. (2005), in which the impact of particular compositions of staff and practices was piloted at two sites in the UK – Caerphilly in Wales and Croydon, part of the London conurbation. As shown in Table 9.6, the outcomes at both sites were very favourable, with lowered rates of retraction and withdrawal and increased rates of progression to court, and of findings of guilt, conjoined with improved perceptions of the quality of service provided to IPV victims. The central process that appeared to lead to these benefits was the integrated and well-coordinated approach offered from the earliest stage of case appraisal in which police officers had either a focused and dedicated role or were provided with specialist training for participation in a domestic violence court.

Three other studies provided tentative indicators of possible methods of increasing participation, that is, of reducing retraction and withdrawal. Best et al. (2006) examined the impact of a multimedia programme including a 12-minute DVD for use with crime victims with serious injuries, with the objective of helping them to "understand and navigate" the criminal justice system. This was not formally evaluated, but preliminary feedback from victims indicated that it had held their attention, imparted useful information and did not increase their anxiety, and these and

**Table 9.6** Information from included studies: studies of interventions to reduce retraction or disengagement

| Author(s), (date), country | Design and methodology | Samples/data sources | Focus and findings |
|---|---|---|---|
| Campbell, Bybee, et al. (2012) USA | Content analysis of case reports | 343 reports of sexual assault cases from 3 police departments | This is an indirect evaluation of the effects of using SANE, specially trained forensic nurses, to work with victims. It examines the relationship between different police actions and the eventual effect on victims. File reports on case examinations were analysed under ten separate headings to investigate the relationship between different features of each case. The dependent variable was whether police referred the case to prosecutors. Mediational analysis (using multi-level logistic regression) showed that with involvement of a SANE specialist, additional evidence was collected, victims were 40% less likely to disengage, and cases were 5 times more likely to be forwarded to prosecutors. Police were also more likely to collect other kinds of information to support the case, also leading to greater likelihood of prosecution and higher rates of conviction in other research |
| Campbell, Patterson, and Bybee (2012) USA | Quasi-experimental, non-equivalent but longitudinal design | 146 victims participating in the SANE programme in the years 1999–2005. 171 adult sexual assault victims from the years 1994–1999 (comparison group). Checks were carried out on equivalence of cases | Focusing on sexual assaults, the dependent variable was whether or not cases were referred for prosecution of perpetrators, whether prosecution took place and whether there was a finding of guilt. The study covered 5 years before and 7 years after the introduction of the SANE model (see previous entry). Case progression was divided into four phases: Whether police referred to prosecutor, whether prosecutor warranted for prosecution, whether case was dropped/acquitted or proceeded and whether there was a plea of guilt or conviction at trial. Statistical analysis found that there was a significant increase in case progression following the introduction of SANE. Multivariate regression showed that cases processed after then had on average a 70% higher likelihood of proceeding to the next phase. This was moderated by differences between the five police departments involved in the study, with one showing a lower rate of onward referral than the four others; it too however showed an increase |
| Chivers and Barnes (2018) UK | Randomized controlled trial: Random assignment to one of two conditions, using intention-to-treat analysis | 946 defendants in court cases over a 6-month period in 1 English county | Tested whether being sent a reminder text message 1 day before a magistrates' court hearing would result in a higher rate of attendance, and a lower rate of fail-to-appear warrants, than the standard procedure of being sent a postal notification 14–28 days in advance. No statistically significant difference was found between groups on either outcome variable. No moderating influence was observed for any other variables (e.g. distance to travel to court or history of prior failure to appear). However, a large proportion of mobile phone numbers (62%) were found to be invalid. Limiting analysis to only telephone numbers checked as valid showed a trend towards higher attendance, but the difference was statistically non-significant |

(continued)

**Table 9.6** (continued)

| Author(s), (date), country | Design and methodology | Samples/data sources | Focus and findings |
|---|---|---|---|
| Cumberbatch and Barnes (2018) UK | Randomized controlled trial: Random assignment to one of two conditions, using intention-to-treat analysis | 811 crime victims or witnesses in court cases over a 6-month period in 1 English county | Tested whether being sent a reminder text message 2–3 days before a magistrates' court hearing would result in a higher rate of attendance than the standard procedure of being sent a postal notification. However, the non-attendance rate amongst the treatment group was slightly higher than amongst the controls, though the difference was not statistically significant. There was a slightly higher proportion of victims than witnesses in the treatment as compared to the control group. Moderator analysis according to rated crime severity was also non-significant. There was a marginally significantly higher rate of findings of guilt amongst treatment (text reminder) than amongst control (postal letter) group members (58% vs. 51%). This was difficult to explain, but it was speculated that it may have been connected to a relationship between information technology and the manner in which individuals testified in court |
| Monnington-Taylor et al. (2019) UK | Randomized controlled trial | 36 witness care officers (WCOs), 1507 victims and 1009 witnesses assigned to treatment and control conditions | An intervention was designed with three components: (1) a new conversation guide for WCOs to use when discussing court attendance with victims or witnesses, (2) a redesigned warning letter prior to the court hearing and (3) a reminder call and SMS 1 week before the trial. This was compared with business-as-usual procedures. There were small increases in court attendance for both victims and witnesses, and a slightly larger increase (3.2%) for a subgroup involved in domestic violence cases, in the treatment groups as compared to the controls, but none of the differences was statistically significant |
| Vallely et al. (2005) | Process and outcome evaluation with staff interviews and analysis of case results, using both qualitative and quantitative data | Study conducted at two sites with differing models. Analysis of case progression: Site 1: 127 cases Site 2: 164 cases Interviews with key stakeholder staff and with 22 IPV victims | Project undertaken by the crown prosecution service (England and Wales) to test a pilot project for increasing rates of progression to court hearings. This involved a specialist domestic violence coordinator based in a police station, advocate and dedicated police officer (site 1) or specially trained police officers working in a specialist domestic violence court (site 2). Training was found to lead to improved evidence collection. At both sites, over 12 months of data collection, there were increases in rates of guilty pleas and in eventual findings of guilt There were large reductions in the rate of retraction (from 53% to 27%) and of withdrawals (from 32% to 25% and from 36% to 20%). There were also improved perceptions of the quality of service to victims and reductions in numbers of adverse outcomes |

Abbreviations used in the tables correspond to the terms used in the original studies. Thus *CJS* criminal justice system, *DV* domestic violence, *IPV* intimate partner violence, *SANE* Sexual Assault Nurse Examiner.

other indicators suggested it may be one part of a package that could increase individuals' rate of participation in the legal process.

Glass et al. (2010) developed a computerized "safety decision aid" for use with women victims of IPV, the majority of whom reported high levels of current danger in their relationships. They experienced decisional conflict over whether to stay or leave and other issues. This guided women through an on-screen self-assessment of risk of their current circumstances. Doing so enabled them to gain greater clarity about the decisions they were trying to make. A pilot study with 90 English- and Spanish-speaking women found that they experienced reduced conflict at the end of the session. Used in conjunction with access to advocacy services, this could assist victims in making decision that would increase their likelihood of participating in legal cases where that would be the best course of action for their own safety.

Finally, Reid-Howie Associates (2002) prepared a review for the Scottish Executive Central Research Unit, concerned with identifying best practices for enhancing the participation of vulnerable victims in the justice system. This included consideration of a range of possible provisions, including changing court requirements that would enable more witnesses to testify; widening the framework of acceptable evidence; increasing flexibility in how evidence could be presented in court; witness preparation measures; additional steps to preserve anonymity; and restricting the kinds of questions that could be asked of vulnerable witnesses. The key aspect of this for present purposes is the possibility that, if any such steps were taken, victims could be made aware of them and potentially feel less apprehension about the prospect of testifying. However, this review was prepared some time ago, and no other studies have been found of follow-up actions taken in response to it. The review does not include any outcome data on any of the proposals made.

These findings appear broadly encouraging, although as they stand, they might seem only tangentially relevant to the problem of trying to reduce victim and witness withdrawal from the CJS. In addition, it is difficult to be confident about whether the approaches that have been studied work consistently or would be applicable in other circumstances. None of the latter three reports achieves the status of a formal evaluation with a type of research design that would permit the drawing of firm conclusions about the effectiveness of the methods involved for the purposes of interest here.

### 9.5.4 Summary of Results

Overall, the studies retained in the review present a complex picture. They show that a large number of factors, or several different kinds, can have an effect on the various forms of victim or witness attrition, disengagement and withdrawal. They include features of both victims and offenders, the nature of their relationship, the offence incident(s), the initial police response, subsequent encounters between police and the victim, police decision-making processes and decision-making by prosecutors or other legal professionals. In some cases, there is an interaction between these factors. For example, even victims who want to proceed to court may decide to withdraw from the process based on their perception that police or prosecutors think that there is insufficient evidence to secure a conviction, before that decision has been made by CJS personnel.

Distilling patterns from the wide range of findings located, the following conclusions are offered concerning the factors that contribute, respectively, to either increase the likelihood of retraction, disengagement and withdrawal or to reduce them. First, there are no firm or clear-cut relationships between demographic or other background factors and rates of withdrawal. Some studies found that younger adult victims of partner violence or of sexual violence were more likely to remain involved with cases, but others found older ones did. In the few studies that involved victims younger than 16, there was a trend for their cases to be more likely to be sustained. There is some evidence that being in employment, and with more years of education, makes withdrawal less likely, but those results are not uniform. Some North American studies found Black suspects more likely to be convicted and for rape cases less likely to be pursued where there were female detectives. Second, the factors that most frequently appear to be associated with retraction and withdrawal in cases of domestic abuse include where a couple are living together, where despite conflicts they have apparently reconciled, where the victim wants the partner to be rehabilitated rather than punished, where the abuser agrees to have counselling or other help and where the victim engages in self-blame or feels ashamed. Third, some victims want, and some are determined, to ensure that their abuser or attacker is prosecuted and if possible is found guilty and seek retribution and deterrence. In those instances, they want to be separated from abusing partners or to be protected from ex-partners. In these cases, risks of retraction or withdrawal are likely to be low. Fourth, many victims do not wish to pursue prosecution, and a large number seek other objectives likely to include for the abuse to stop; to be protected from assault; for children to be protected; and, if possible, for the abuser to be given a scare of future more serious consequences. But they are less likely to wish for the abuser to be convicted, partly because of shame and embarrassment and partly because of the possible separation from family or loss of resources. In those cases, victims often consider that the costs of pursuing investigation and prosecution outweigh the benefits and mainly may just want to move past the incident. On the basis that arrival of the police brings incidents under control, they may hope that police involvement will in itself be enough to stop them recurring and not want any further action taken. They may not want an abuser arrested; or, they may want an arrest but no further action. These variables are in turn associated with the nature of the pre-existing relationship. Many women victims describe offences as minor and it is not worth taking further action. Fifth, many female victims of rape and sexual assault fear that they will not be believed and fear going to court and having to give evidence and be cross-examined, especially if that can be done by the defendant. Retraction is more likely and prosecution less likely when there has been a prior relationship and previous consensual sex. Sixth, women are more likely to disengage from rape cases if they are more highly distressed, engage in self-blame, have become pregnant or have been hospitalized. Finally, seventh, prosecutions are more likely to happen if suspects have previous histories of having committed domestic abuse or sexual offences; if there has been a previous restriction or protection order; if attacks included damage to property which victims regarded as personal or precious; if children were directly involved or witnessed incidents; and if sexual assaults were by strangers or ex-partners, rather than by dating partners or acquaintances.

Several other findings from this area of research are also worth keeping in mind though they are not always in line with what we might expect. For example, evidence on the severity of injury was mixed, with some studies finding more serious injury was associated with retraction, rather than the reverse.

There is clearer evidence that crime investigations that include taking photographs, gathering forensic evidence, making a video-recorded statement, making a victim impact statement, where more possible suspect people are interviewed and where victims are speedily put in contact with support services are more likely to be followed through to prosecution. Clearly if there is supporting witness evidence, a prosecution is more likely to take place and to be successful, but that does not guarantee it will not be withdrawn if the victim feels pressured by others to continue, especially where others had called the police.

There is also evidence that participation is sustained where victims found the initial police contact more helpful, if information was given and contacts made with support agencies. The likelihood of this appeared to be maximized when there were dedicated or specially trained police officers working alongside prosecuting staff, as shown in the research by Vallely et al. (2005), which reported the strongest results amongst the intervention studies located here. Other studies found that police contacts were less likely to lead to ongoing participation if there were communication problems between police and victim, if the police did not appear empathic, if victims believed that their complaints had not been taken seriously and if they gained a sense that police were on the side of the aggressor. There is evidence that police may misinterpret some evidence such as victims making inconsistent statements as being indicators of false allegations.

The findings on the possible roles of alcohol and drugs are mixed. But there are trends in which, if victims or both victim and offender were intoxicated, retraction is more likely. If abusive partners are intoxicated, there too retraction may be more likely, but there are also findings counter to this. Evidence on the use of weapons, like that on extent of injury, is also somewhat mixed.

Vulnerable victims, such as people with intellectual disabilities, are no more likely to withdraw cases than others, but are more likely to have cases withdrawn by the CPS.

The review has not specifically focused on the problems of victim or witness intimidation, or the problem of false allegations, which would require separate evidence reviews. Some evidence emerged concerning those issues but is not available in a sufficiently large quantity to permit any clear conclusions to be drawn.

## 9.6 Discussion

### 9.6.1 *Strengths and Limitations*

This area of research literature has a number of strengths. One is the variety of methods used. There is a healthy mixture of both quantitative and qualitative research and several mixed-methods studies. Some studies have reported complex analysis of large datasets using multivariate statistics. Others have made use of in-depth interviews and have applied various forms of content analysis, thematic analysis or grounded theory. Case files have directly reflected the work of police, victim advocates and prosecutors. So, the research could be claimed to reflect the real workings of the justice system. Questionnaire or telephone surveys and interview-based studies have sought the views and responses of victims themselves. Many different aspects of the process have been investigated, from initial decisions to call police, through the interview process, to deliberations over arrest, charge, prosecution, trial and even what to do if the scenario is repeated. There are some very innovative and revealing studies, such as the analysis of telephone conversations by Bonomi et al. (2011) or Hester's (2005) observational work in courtrooms. Also, a fairly large proportion of the located studies were carried out in England and Wales.

A difficulty in all such research, in common with many other areas of crime, policing and justice, is the lack of trust that often exists between those who come into contact with the CJS either as victims or offenders and those who hold official status as workers within that system. Some of the research reviewed here has addressed that issue directly. But it is difficult to be sure how far the gaps that remain are bridged by the answers victims give to the questions put to them.

The findings of this review had an impact on the work of serious sex offending teams within both of the police forces who commissioned the study. The review report became part of the stimulus for another commissioned piece of empirical research examining why victims disengaged from police investigations and also from the Sexual Assault Resource Centre (SARC). This in turn led to several changes in the way the respective teams worked, which was given more impetus by later unrelated work concerned with Crown Prosecution Service lawyers being embedded in the Rape and Serious Sexual Offences specialist teams.

### 9.6.2 *Quality Appraisal*

Given the diversity of research methods used in the studies reviewed and the sometimes marked differences between them, it was not possible to identify any single standard approach to quality appraisal that could be applied to make comparisons between them. It would be preferable if there could be a further phase of work to identify a number of quality appraisal procedures that could be applied as appropriate to different segments of the studies located. Doing so could allow a further section to be incorporated in reviews, such as that reported in this chapter, comparing the relative strengths of different study designs, methods of data collection or types of analysis conducted.

### 9.6.3 Future Prospects: Research and Practice Possibilities

It is difficult to discuss how to address the issues raised in this review without making reference to the legal framework within which they arise. With reference to DA/IPV, the current legal framework is outlined by Starmer (2011), but practices in relation to both this and to the investigation and prosecution of rape have been subject to regular review, as having procedures employed by police in responding to these kinds of offences and to the needs of victims.

Many different types of solutions have been forwarded in response to the above problems, often in the context of more far-reaching policy changes designed to address the under-reporting of family violence and of rape, alongside arguments that the justice system does not adequately provide for the needs of female victims of male aggression. Initiatives to solve the problems of disengagement and withdrawal, and to influence the levels of participation of crime victims in the justice process, have resulted in a number of changes in legal practice and policy.

Setting this in a wider context, many legal discussions have taken place about the value of coerced prosecution, what in the USA have been called "no drop" or "hard drop" policies (Kuennen, 2007). But many lawyers and others see this as problematic in other ways. Smith (2000) examined why advocates of better services for women are not sure about taking this direction because of the potential unintended consequences. Explanations include the idea that it induces *learned helplessness*, in which individuals feel they have no power over events that affect them. Mandatory arrest and prosecution may not be congruent with victims' goals. They may want medical treatment for injuries but nothing more, i.e. for there to be no legal repercussions from having called the police to calm a situation down. There is a widespread view that "…victims' perceptions and responses to the laws are necessary to develop laws that improve the criminal justice responses to victims' needs" (Smith, 2000, p. 1399). Koss (2006) cites evidence that rape survivor/victims whose cases were prosecuted experience more trauma than those whose cases were not, that the justice system leads to re-traumatization of victims. Koss argued therefore for a range of civil alternatives.

Another proposal is a resort to what is called victimless prosecution (Ellison, 2003) as has been practised in some American states. This entails coercing participation by applying "no drop" policies in which victims are not allowed to drop charges once made (Ford, 2003). These policies have been controversial in that, given a range of unintended consequences, their net effect may be a disservice to victims (Hoyle & Sanders, 2000).

Another more radical strategy that has been used by some criminal justice agencies in the USA is that of *exceptional clearance*. This occurs with the agreement of prosecution agencies at early stages of the legal process. Pattavina et al. (2016) describe what this involves. At an early stage, a decision is made regarding a case as to whether it will be cleared by *arre*st or by *exceptional means*. The latter can occur if four criteria are met: (1) the police know the identity of the offender; (2) there is enough information to support an arrest, charge and referral for prosecution; (3) the location of the offender is known and he/she could be taken into custody; however, (4) there is some reason outside law enforcement control that precludes arresting, charging and prosecuting the offender. A common reason that meets criterion (4) is that the victim has declined to cooperate. The police then "clear" the case but may set in motion other actions that can address the problems arising in it. This does not reduce disengagement; rather we might say it bypasses or neutralizes it. It does not solve the problems relating to individual cases, which would require referral to other agencies.

Attempts to increase participation that entail changes in the law itself are outside the scope of this review. An issue worth considering however is the extent to which the legal context may allow scope for some discretion in the kinds of decisions police services can make, and some suggestions concerning this are offered below.

There are many questions remaining unanswered in this area, and it would be possible to design research projects to answer some of them. Taylor and Gassner (2010), respectively, an academic and a police officer, have emphasized the need for collaborative research combining theoretical, methodological and operational perspectives. Applying that standpoint the following suggestions can be made. One type of project that could be conducted would be an in-house analysis of data already collected, using information recorded on serious cases over a specified period (e.g. 1 year or longer if resources permitted). Compare those where there was a form of disengagement or discontinuation with those that carried through to completion. This replicates some of the kinds of work reviewed here, but it is nevertheless important to check whether similar patterns as found elsewhere emerge at local level. The published studies illustrate the range of variables that would be worth measuring, but others could be added covering areas that have been missed.

A second possibility is to conduct an exploratory, open-ended interview study of those who withdraw. This may be a highly sensitive undertaking and some would probably decline to participate, but others might agree if approached by victim advocates or support services. Something could however be learned from those who do agree, and if compared with non-participants, it would be possible to test their representativeness.

Further training could benefit police officers interviewing victims who claim they have been raped or who are victims of DA/IPV. There is evidence that the behavioural signs of trauma or verbalizations of shame shown by such victims can be misinterpreted as indicators of unreliability or dishonesty (Maddox et al., 2012). Some authors have specifically recommended that more training should be developed and delivered for this kind of work (Westera et al., 2016).

In the concept of victim-centred justice and as found in many of the studies discussed in this chapter, especially in relation to DA/IPV, there is an emphasis on discovering what victims want to happen or want not to happen. It might be feasible to incorporate those views into initial decisions taken when attending incidents, repeated on subsequent occasions, and factor them into the broader legal decision process. That would entail judgements as to whether victims were being intimidated or coerced. But it could be done alongside a process, discussed in a previous review on DA/IPV, of carrying out on-site risk assessments of perpetrators. Case review could combine the two sets of judgements to arrive at a more realistic decision as to how best to proceed in the case. Given certain parameters (e.g. seriousness of offence), gatekeeper decisions to proceed with charge and prosecution could still prevail, but some discretion could be applied that was based on evidence concerning how to achieve the most suitable outcomes. If such a departure was made, it would be important to monitor its progress using several kinds of data.

More generally, if any of these changes were introduced and additional training were to be developed and delivered, it would be essential to carry out appropriately designed evaluation of its reception and its effects. That could be based first on the levels of skill acquisition by trainee participants and second on an experimental trial to evaluate changes in victim response at different stages of investigations and in later phases of the legal decision process.

Another option already available could be extended, involving the increased use of various civil orders as an alternative to justice or penal-based processes. Some experts have proposed making available a menu of options both within and also outside the penal system (Daly & Bouhours, 2010, p. 625). Many of those involved in current debates in this area argue for different strategies of penal reform, and some moves in that direction have taken place. Discussion of those questions in any detail requires legal expertise however and is outside the scope of this review.

For offences of rape, a larger-scale departure could be undertaken with the introduction of an equivalent to the Sexual Assault Nurse Examiners employed by some agencies in the USA or by other specially trained personnel focused on specific issues that arise in sexual assaults and partner violence. This would entail significant investment of resources but might offset other costs of policing or of other components of the justice process.

There have been ongoing debates about the principles in legal and moral terms, and the advantages and disadvantages in practical terms, of pursuing policies that might conflict with each other. For example, "bringing offenders to justice" versus "victim-centred justice" can have diametrically opposed results (Robinson & Cook, 2006). These issues are outside the scope of this review, but there might be value in setting up a series of seminars in which the implications of such diverse policies were discussed. Some of the outcomes of that could have an impact on decisions about what kinds of action to take concerning victim retraction and withdrawal.

## References

Angiolini, E. (2015). *Report of the independent review into the investigation and prosecution of rape in London*. Crown Prosecution Service. https://www.cps.gov.uk/Publications/equality/vaw/dame_elish_angiolini_rape_review_2015.pdf

Apsler, R., Cummins, M. R., & Carl, S. (2003). Fear and expectations: Differences among female victims of domestic violence who come to the attention of the police. *Violence and Victims, 17*, 445–453.

Ask, K. (2010). A survey of police officers' and prosecutors' beliefs about crime victim behaviors. *Journal of Interpersonal Violence, 25*, 1132–1149.

Bailey, M. (2010). Understanding attrition in domestic violence cases. *International Journal of Interdisciplinary Social Sciences, 5*, 377–387.

Bandura, A. (1999). Moral disengagement in the perpetration of inhumanities. *Personality and Social Psychology Review, 3*, 193–209.

Barrow-Grint, K. (2016). Attrition rates in domestic abuse: Time for a change? An application of temporal sequencing theory. *Policing, 10*(3), 250–263.

Beichner, D., & Spohn, C. (2005). Prosecutorial charging decisions in sexual assault cases: Examining the impact of a Specialized Prosecution Unit. *Criminal Justice Policy Review, 16*, 461–498.

Belknap, J., Graham, D. L. R., Hartman, J., Lippen, V., Allen, G., & Sutherland, J. (2000). *Factors related to domestic court dispositions in a large urban area: The role of victim/witness reluctance and other variables, executive summary*. US Department of Justice.

Best, C. L., Acierno, R. E., & Resnick, H. S. (2006). *A multimedia program to improve criminal justice system participation and reduce distress among physical injured crime victims*. Office of Justice Programs, US Department of Justice.

Boivin, R., & Leclerc, C. (2016). Domestic violence reported to the police: Correlates of victims' reporting behaviour and support to legal proceedings. *Violence and Victims, 31*, 402–414.

Bonomi, A. E., Gangamma, R., Locke, C. R., Katafiasz, H., & Martin, D. (2011). "Meet me at the hill where we used to park": Interpersonal processes associated with victim recantation. *Social Science & Medicine, 73*, 1054–1061.

Brown, J. (2011). We mind and we care but have things changed? Assessment of progress in the reporting, investigating and prosecution of allegations of rape. *Journal of Sexual Aggression, 17*, 263–272.

Burrows, J., Hopkins, M., Hubbard, R., Robinson, A., Speed, M., & Tilley, N. (2005). *Understanding the attrition process in volume crime investigations*. Home Office Research, Development and Statistics Directorate.

Cala, M. J., Trigo, M. E., & Saavedra, F. J. (2016). Women's disengagement from legal proceedings for intimate partner violence: Sociodemographic and psychological variables. *European Journal of Psychology Applied to Legal Context, 8*, 35–42.

Calvette, E., Corral, S., & Estévez, A. (2007). Cognitive and coping mechanisms in the interplay between intimate partner violence and depression. *Anxiety, Stress, & Coping, 20*, 369–382.

Camacho, C. M., & Alarid, L. F. (2008). The significance of the victim advocate for domestic violence victims in municipal court. *Violence and Victims, 23*, 288–300.

Campbell, R., Bybee, D., Kelley, K. D., Dworkin, E. R., & Patterson, D. (2012). The impact of sexual assault nurse examiner (SANE) program services on law enforcement investigational practices: A mediational analysis. *Criminal Justice and Behavior, 39*, 169–184.

Campbell, R., Patterson, D., & Bybee, D. (2012). Sexual assault cases: A longitudinal analysis of the impact of a sexual assault nurse examiner program. *Violence Against Women, 18*, 223–244.

Chivers, B., & Barnes, G. (2018). Sorry, wrong number: Tracking court attendance targeting through testing a "nudge" text. *Cambridge Journal of Evidence Based Policing, 2*, 4–34.

Crown Prosecution Service. (2013). *Violence against women and girls*. Public Accountability and Inclusion Directorate.

Crown Prosecution Service (2014). *The Prosecution of Domestic Violence Cases*. London: Crown Prosecution Service. DVConsultation2014@cps.gsi.gov.uk

Cumberbatch, J. R., & Barnes, G. C. (2018). This nudge was not enough: A randomised trial of text message reminders of court dates to victims and witnesses. *Cambridge Journal of Evidence Based Policing, 2*, 35–51.

Daly, K., & Bouhours, B. (2010). Rape and attrition in the legal process: A comparative analysis of five countries. *Crime and Justice, 39*, 565–650.

Davis, R. C., O'Sullivan, C. S., Farole, D. J., & Rempel, M. (2008). A comparison of two prosecution policies in cases of intimate partner violence: Mandatory case filing versus following the victim's lead. *Criminology and Public Policy, 7*, 633–662.

Dawson, M., & Dinovitzer, R. (2001). Victim cooperation and the prosecution of domestic violence in a specialized court. *Justice Quarterly, 18*, 593–622.

Dedel, K. (2006). *Witness Intimidation*. Problem-Oriented Guides for Police, Problem-Specific Guides Series No. 42. Washington, DC: Office of Community Oriented Policing Services, US Department of Justice.

Du Mont, J., & Myhr, T. L. (2000). So few convictions: The role of client-related characteristics in the legal processing of sexual assaults. *Violence Against Women, 6*, 1109–1136.

Dutton, M. A., Holtzworth-Munroe, A., Jouriles, E., McDonald, R., Krishnan, S., McFarlane, J., & Sullivan, C. (2003). *Recruitment and retention in intimate partner violence research*. National Institute of Justice, US Department of Justice.

Ellison, L. (2003). Responding to victim withdrawal in domestic violence prosecutions. *Criminal Law Review, 760*.

Ellsberg, M., Winkvist, A., Peña, R., & Stenlund, H. (2001). Women's strategic responses to violence in Nicaragua. *Journal of Epidemiology and Community Health, 55*, 547–555.

Enander, V. (2010). "A fool to keep staying": Battered women labelling themselves stupid as an expression of gendered shame. *Violence Against Women, 16*, 5–31.

Feist, A., Ashe, J., Lawrence, J., McPhee, D., & Wilson, R. (2007). *Investigating and detecting recorded offences of rape*. Home Office online report 18/07. London: Home Office Research Development and Statistics Directorate.

Fitzgerald, J. (2006). The attrition of sexual offences from the New South Wales criminal justice system. *Contemporary Issues in Crime and Justice*, Number 92. Sydney: NSW Bureau of Crime Statistics and Research.

Fleury-Steiner, R. E., Bybee, D., Sullivan, C. M., Belknap, J., & Melton, H. C. (2006). Contextual factors impacting battered women's intentions to reuse the criminal legal system. *Journal of Community Psychology, 34*, 327–342.

Ford, D. A. (2003). Coercing victim participation in domestic violence prosecutions. *Journal of Interpersonal Violence, 18*, 669–684.

Fugate, M., George, C., Haber, N., & Stawiski, S. (2006). *Providing a system of single point access to domestic violence information, resources and referrals to a diverse population: An evaluation of the City of Chicago Domestic Violence Help Line*. National Institute of Justice, US Department of Justice.

Ganapathy, N. (2006). Between the devil and the deep-blue sea: Conceptualising victims' experiences of policing in domestic violence in the Singaporean context. *Australian and New Zealand Journal of Criminology, 39*, 90–108.

Gauthier, S. (2010). The perceptions of judicial and psychosocial interveners of the consequences of dropped charges in domestic violence cases. *Violence Against Women, 16*, 1375–1395.

Glass, N., Eden, K. B., Bloom, T., & Perrin, N. (2010). Computerized aid improves safety decision process for survivors of intimate partner violence. *Journal of Interpersonal Violence, 25*, 1947–1964.

Hall, M. (2007). The use and abuse of special measures: Giving victims the choice? *Journal of Scandinavian Studies in Criminology and Crime Prevention, 8*, 33–53.

Halpern, D. (2015). *Inside the nudge unit: How small changes can make a big difference*. W. H. Allen.

Hansen, N. B., Hansen, M., Nielsen, L. H., Bramsen, R. H., Elklit, A., & Campbell, R. (2018). Rape crimes: Are victims' acute psychological distress and perceived social support associated with police case decision and victim willingness to participate in the investigation? *Violence Against Women, 24*(6), 684–696.

Hansen, N. B., Nielsen, L. H., Bramsen, R. H., Ingemann-Hansen, O., & Elklit, A. (2015). Attrition in Danish rape reported crimes. *Journal of Police and Criminal Psychology, 30*, 221–228.

Hare, S. C. (2006). What do battered women want? Victims' opinions on prosecution. *Violence and Victims, 21*, 611–628.

Hare, S. C. (2010). Intimate partner violence: Victims' opinions about going to trial. *Journal of Family Violence, 25*, 765–776.

Hester, M. (2005). Making it through the criminal justice system: Attrition and domestic violence. *Social Policy and Society, 5*, 79–90.

Hirschel, D., & Hutchison, I. W. (2003). The voices of domestic violence victims: Predictors of victim preference for arrest and the relationship between preference for arrest and revictimization. *Crime & Delinquency, 49*, 313–336.

Hohl, K., & Stanko, E. A. (2015). Complaints of rape and the criminal justice system: Fresh evidence on the attrition problem in England and Wales. *European Journal of Criminology, 12*, 324–341.

Holleran, D., Beichner, D., & Spohn, C. (2010). Examining charging agreement between police and prosecutors in rape cases. *Crime & Delinquency, 56*, 385–413.

Holmberg, U. (2004). Crime victims' experiences of police interviews and their inclination to provide or omit information. *International Journal of Police Science and Management, 6*, 155–170.

Hoyle, C. (1998). *Negotiating domestic violence: Police, criminal justice and victims*. Oxford University Press.

Hoyle, C., & Sanders, A. (2000). Police response to domestic violence: From victim choice to victim empowerment? *British Journal of Criminology, 40*, 14–36.

Iverson, K. M., Litwack, S. D., Pineles, S. L., Suvak, M. K., Vaughn, R. A., & Resick, P. A. (2013). Predictors of intimate partner violence revictimization: The relative impact of distinct PTSD symptoms, dissociation, and coping strategies. *Journal of Traumatic Stress, 26*, 102–110.

Jordan, J. (2011). Here we go round the review-go-round: Rape investigation and prosecution – Are things getting worse not better? *Journal of Sexual Aggression, 17*, 234–249.

Keilty, J., & Connelly, G. (2001). Making a statement: An exploratory study of barriers facing women with an intellectual disability when making a statement about sexual assault to police. *Disability and Society, 16*, 273–291.

Kelley, K. D., & Campbell, R. (2013). Moving on or dropping out: Police processing of adult sexual assault cases. *Women & Criminal Justice, 23*, 1–18.

Kelly, L., Lovett, J., & Regan, L. (2005). A gap or a chasm? Attrition in reported rape cases. In *Home Office research study 293*. Home Office Research, Development and Statistics Directorate.

Kingsnorth, R. F., & Macintosh, R. C. (2004). Domestic violence: Predictors of victim support for official action. *Justice Quarterly, 21*, 301–328.

Koss, M. P. (2006). Restoring rape survivors: Justice, advocacy, and a call to action. *Annals of the New York Academy of Sciences, 1087*, 206–234.

Kuennen, T. L. (2007). Analyzing the impact of coercion on domestic violence victims: How much is too much? *Berkeley Journal of Gender, Law & Justice, 22*, 2–30.

Landenburger, K. (1989). A process of entrapment in and recovery from an abusive relationship. *Issues in Mental Health Nursing, 10*, 209–227.

Lea, S. J., Callaghan, L., Grafton, I., Falcone, M. A., & Shaw, S. (2016). Attrition and rape case characteristics: A profile and comparison of female sex workers and non-sex workers. *Journal of Interpersonal Violence, 31*, 2175–2195.

Lea, S. J., Lanvers, U., & Shaw, S. (2003). Attrition in rape cases: Developing a profile and identifying relevant factors. *British Journal of Criminology, 43*, 583–599.

Lewis, R. (2004). Making justice work: Effective legal interventions for domestic violence. *British Journal of Criminology, 44*, 204–224.

Lievore, D. (2003). *Non-reporting and hidden recording of sexual assault: An international literature review*. Commonwealth of Australia.

Lovett, J., & Kelly, L. (2009). *Different systems, similar outcomes? Tracking attrition in reported rape cases across Europe*. Child & Woman Abuse Studies Unit, London Metropolitan University.

Maddox, L., Lee, D., & Barker, C. (2011). Police empathy and victim PTSD as potential factors in rape case attrition. *Journal of Police and Criminal Psychology, 26*, 112–117.

Maddox, L., Lee, D., & Barker, C. (2012). The impact of psychological consequences of rape on rape case attrition: The police perspective. *Journal of Police and Criminal Psychology, 27*, 33–44.

Malloy, L. C., & Lamb, M. E. (2010). Biases in judging victims and suspects whose statements are inconsistent. *Law and Human Behavior, 34*, 46–48.

Matthieu, M., & Ivanoff, A. (2006). Treatment of human-caused trauma: Attrition in the adult outcomes research. *Journal of Interpersonal Violence, 21*, 1654–1664.

Mele, M., Roberts, C. J., & Wolfer, L. &. (2011). Characteristics of women who withdraw from the protection order process and their decisions for withdrawal. *Journal of Current Issues in Crime, Law and Law Enforcement, 3*, 1–11.

Meyer, S. (2014). Victims' experiences of short- and long-term safety and wellbeing: Findings from an examination of an integrated response to domestic violence. *Trends & Issues*, No. 478. Canberra: Australian Institute of Criminology.

Ministry of Justice, Home Office & Office for National Statistics. (2013). An overview of sexual offending in England and Wales. In *Statistical Bulletin*. Office for National Statistics.

Monnington-Taylor, E., Bowers, K., Hurle, P. S., Ward, L., Ruda, S., Sweeney, M., Murray, A., & Whitehouse, J. (2019). Testimony at court: A randomised controlled trial investigating the art and science of persuading witnesses and victims to attend trial. *Crime Science, 8*, 10. https://doi.org/10.1186/s40163-019-0104-1

Munro, V. E., & Kelly, L. (2009). A vicious cycle? Attrition and conviction patterns in contemporary rape cases in England and Wales. In M. Horvath & J. Brown (Eds.), *Rape: Challenging contemporary thinking* (pp. 281–300). Willan Publishing.

Murphy, S. B., Edwards, K. M., Bennett, S., Bibeau, S. J., & Sichelsteil, J. (2014). Police reporting practices for sexual assault cases in which "the victim does not which to pursue charges". *Journal of Interpersonal Violence, 29*, 144–156.

O'Neal, E. N., & Spohn, C. (2016). When the perpetrator is a partner: Arrest and charging decisions in intimate partner sexual assault cases – A focal concerns analysis. *Violence Against Women*. https://doi.org/10.1177/1077801216650289

Office for National Statistics. (2018). *Sexual offending: Victimization and the path through the criminal justice system*. Office for National Statistics.

Office for National Statistics. (2020). *Crime in England and Wales: Year ending June 2020*. Office for National Statistics.

Pattavina, A., Morabito, M., & Williams, L. M. (2016). Examining connections between the police and prosecution in sexual assault case processing: Does the use of exceptional clearance facilitate a downstream orientation? *Victims & Offenders, 11*, 315–334.

Patterson, D., & Campbell, R. (2010). Why rape survivors participate in the criminal justice system. *Journal of Community Psychology, 38*, 191–205.

Patterson, D., & Tringali, B. (2015). Understanding how advocates can affect sexual assault victim engagement in the criminal justice process. *Journal of Interpersonal Violence, 30*, 1987–1997.

Reid-Howie Associates. (2002). *Vulnerable and Intimidated Witnesses: Review of provisions in other jurisdictions*. Crime and Criminal Justice Research Findings No. 60. Edinburgh: Scottish Executive Central Research Unit.

Relyea, M., & Ullman, S. E. (2015). Unsupported or turned against: Understanding how two types of negative social reactions to sexual assault relate to postassault outcomes. *Psychology of Women Quarterly, 39*, 37–52.

Richards, L. (2009). *Domestic Abuse, Stalking, and Harassment and Honour Based Violence (DASH, 2009) risk identification and assessment and management model.* http://www.dashrisk-checklist.co.uk/wp-content/uploads/2016/09/DASH-2009.pdf

Roberts, J. C., Wolfer, L., & Mele, M. (2008). Why victims of intimate partner violence withdraw protection orders. *Journal of Family Violence, 23*, 369–375.

Robinson, A. L. (2006). Reducing repeat victimization among high-risk victims of domestic violence: The benefits of a coordinated community response in Cardiff, Wales. *Violence Against Women, 12*, 761–788.

Robinson, A. L., & Chandek, M. S. (2000). Philosophy into practice? Community policing units and domestic violence victim participation. *Policing: An International Journal of Police Strategies and Management, 23*, 280–302.

Robinson, A. L., & Cook, D. (2006). Understanding victim retraction in cases of domestic violence: Specialist courts, government policy, and victim-centred justice. *Contemporary Justice Review, 9*, 189–213.

Sabina, C., & Tindale, R. S. (2008). Abuse characteristics and coping resources as predictors of problem-focused coping strategies among battered women. *Violence Against Women, 14*, 437–456.

Salazar, L. F., Emshoff, J. G., Baker, C. K., & Crowley, T. (2007). Examining the behaviour of a system: An outcome evaluation of a coordinated community response to domestic violence. *Journal of Family Violence, 22*, 631–641.

Scarpa, A., & Haden, S. C. (2006). Community violence victimization and aggressive behavior: The moderating effects of coping and social support. *Aggressive Behavior, 32*, 502–515.

Shoham, E. (2000). The battered wife's perception of the characteristics of her encounter with the police. *International Journal of Offender Therapy and Comparative Criminology, 44*, 242–257.

Sleath, E. & Smith, L. L. (2017). Understanding the factors that predict victim retraction in police reported allegations of intimate partner violence. *Psychology of Violence, 7*(1), 140–149.

Smith, A. (2000). It's my decision, isn't it? A research note on battered women's perceptions of mandatory intervention laws. *Violence Against Women, 6*, 1384–1402.

Snodgrass, G. M. (2006). Sexual assault case processing: A descriptive model of attrition and decision making. *Alaska Justice Forum, 23*, 1 & 4–8.

Spohn, C., & Holleran, D. (2001). Prosecuting sexual assault: A comparison of charging decisions in sexual assault cases involving strangers, acquaintances and intimate partners. *Justice Quarterly, 18*, 651–688.

Spohn, C., White, C., & Tellis, K. (2014). Unfounding sexual assault: Examining the decision to unfound and identifying false reports. *Law & Society Review, 48*, 161–192.

Starmer, K. (2011). Domestic violence: The facts, the issues, the future. *International Review of Law, Computers & Technology, 25*, 9–15.

Taft, C. T., Resick, P. E., Panuzio, J., Vogt, D. S., & Mechanic, M. B. (2007a). Examining the correlates of engagement and disengagement coping among help-seeking battered women. *Violence and Victims, 22*(1), 3–17.

Taft, C. T., Resick, P. E., Panuzio, J., Vogt, D. S., & Mechanic, M. B. (2007b). Coping among victims of relationship abuse: a longitudinal study. *Violence and Victims, 22*(4), 408–418.

Taylor, S. C., & Gassner, L. (2010). Stemming the flow: Challenges for policing adult sexual assault with regard to attrition rates and under-reporting of sexual offences. *Police Practice and Research, 11*, 240–255.

Tellis, K. M., & Spohn, C. C. (2008). The sexual stratification hypothesis revisited: Testing assumptions about simple versus aggravated rape. *Journal of Criminal Justice, 36*, 252–261.

Temkin, J., & Krahé, B. (2008). *Sexual assault and the justice gap: A question of attitude*. Hart Publishing.

Tobin, D. L., Holroyd, K. A., Reynolds, R. V., & Wigal, J. K. (1989). The hierarchical factor structure of the coping strategies inventory. *Cognitive Therapy and Research, 13*, 343–361.

Vallely, C., Robinson, A., Burton, M., & Tredidga, J. (2005). *Evaluation of domestic violence pilot sites at Caerphilly (Gwent) and Croydon 2004/05: Final report*. Crown Prosecution Service.

Vásquez, J. J., Rivas, E., Suarez, A. C., & Panadero, S. (2018). Retraction of complaints among female victims of intimate partner violence living in poverty in Nicaragua. *International Journal of Offender Therapy and Comparative Criminology, 62*(10), 3151–3167.

Waldrop, A. E., & Resick, P. A. (2004). Coping among adult female victims of domestic violence. *Journal of Family Violence, 19*, 291–302.

Weisz, A. (2002). Prosecution of batterers: Views of African American battered women. *Violence and Victims, 17*, 19–34.

Westera, N. J., Kebbell, M. R., & Milne, B. (2016). Want a better criminal justice response to rape? Improve police interviews with complainants and suspects. *Violence Against Women, 22*, 1748–1769.

Zoellner, L. A., Feeny, N. C., Alvarez, J., Watlington, C., O'Neill, M. L., Zager, R., & Foa, E. B. (2000). Factors associated with completion of the restraining order process in female victims of partner violence. *Journal of Interpersonal Violence, 15*, 1081–1099.

# Chapter 10
# Victim Counselling and Support: A Review of Police, Community and Therapeutic Interventions

## 10.1 Questions and Overall Aim

This is concerned with the question of which methods or approaches, if any, have been found to be effective in providing counselling or other forms of support to victims of crime, with particular reference to serious offences including domestic abuse, rape and other sexual assault? The overall aim of the review described was therefore to collate evidence pertaining to that question, to provide a summary of what is known about the effectiveness of victim counselling and support.

It was our initial hope that it would be feasible to compare different approaches to this and to draw conclusions about their relative effectiveness. On that basis it was also hoped it would be possible to offer recommendations or guidelines that can enable police departments to commission support services. At present, the state of knowledge does not appear to be sufficient to provide grounds for arriving at any firm conclusions or clear recommendations. It was therefore thought that a review of evidence would locate research that could better inform this kind of work and the decisions to be made concerning it.

Preliminary searches of this area suggested that the volume of information directly relevant to its aims was likely to be limited. It was thought that a probable reason for this is that the majority of victim counselling is fairly brief, often consisting of a single meeting, or of a very small number of sessions, and that the work done is well contained, with an attempt to keep formal demands to a minimum and making no attempt at evaluation. Elaborate and costly research is unlikely to be directed towards evaluation of fairly short-term procedures such as this, but even small-scale evaluation did not seem to have been done very often. There may be unpublished reports of work done in local centres, but they are unlikely to be found in electronic searches or through other methods used in research reviews.



J. McGuire et al., *Evidence-Based Policing and Community Crime Prevention*, Advances in Preventing and Treating Violence and Aggression,
https://doi.org/10.1007/978-3-030-76363-3_10

## 10.2 Specific Objectives of the Review

The following more specific objectives were set for the present evidence review: (1) to carry out a literature search using selected terms to locate studies focused on evaluating interventions designed to provide effective support to victims of crime; (2) to summarize the findings from the located studies, with a view to identifying possible options for action that could be taken by police services; and (3) to locate any research study or resource that could be employed as a guideline or framework for commissioning victim support services.

## 10.3 Background

Being a victim of any crime is an unpleasant experience. In the case of minor offences, that feeling may wear off in a short while. But as the seriousness of crimes escalates and the amount of harm is increased, the effects can be profound and enduring. If individuals already felt vulnerable beforehand for some other reason, the impact of victimization may be substantially greater, for example, for people with disabilities (Bellis et al., 2012) or those experiencing mental illness (de Mooij et al., 2015; Khalifeh et al., 2015). Both of these groups have a higher risk of victimization than the general population average.

The annual reports of the Crime Survey for England and Wales (CSEW) provide a wide range of statistics on volumes of crimes of different types and in some years provide additional details on crime effects. For example, data for the year ending March 2015 indicated that, in addition to physical injuries sustained, most respondents (81%) were emotionally affected by violent incidents.

The CSEW for 2011/2012 gave some details on the nature of those effects. This kind of information is not routinely contained in annual CSEW reports. In descending order of frequency, they included anger, annoyance, shock, fear and loss of confidence, crying, difficulty sleeping, depression and anxiety or panic attacks. Nearly a quarter (24%) of reported violent incidents were repeat victimizations (Office for National Statistics, 2013, 2016). It has long been recognized that crime has multiple effects on victims (Maguire, 1980, 1991). Its impact is not confined to being a victim of violent crime, but the effects are most marked following serious crimes such as rape or robbery. Increasingly throughout the 1970s and 1980s, there was growing awareness of the needs of crime victims and development of services to address them (e.g. Ben-Zvi & Horsfall, 1985; Burgess & Holmstrom, 1974; Goodwin & Holmes, 1987). This arose especially in relation to the problems faced by victims of rape and other sexual assault and of domestic violence. More recently Miller (2008) has summarized research showing the impact of violent assault on victims and the extent to which it produces not only acute short-term distress but can also have longer-lasting effects, some of which are sufficiently severe as to be classified as mental disorders.

The recognition that victims of crime require help in addition to the efforts of police in investigating the crime and arresting offenders led to the establishment of Victim Support, a voluntary organization, in Bristol in 1964. Since then, its work has expanded to cover locations throughout the UK. According to the agency's Annual Report for 2018-19, during the preceding year information and specialist support was offered to 849,236 victims of crime (among them 297,304 victims of violence), of whom 86% felt better informed about the support available to them and 76% felt safer following the provision of support. The USA has a network of State Victim Service Academies which provide training for designated roles such as that of Victim Services Practitioner (Doerner & Lab, 2015).

Probably the most extensively developed network of support services has been created in response to violence against female partners in close relationships (domestic or intimate partner violence). The Vienna-based organization WAVE (Women Against Violence Europe), housed by the Austrian Women's Shelter Network, has produced a series of reports on aspects of the provision of support services in 46 countries. Stelmaszek and Fisher (2012; see also Logar et al., 2016) provided a Europe-wide, country-by-country summary of what services are available. Across the 46 European countries surveyed, with a combined population of 831 million people, there are 2937 women's centres. The majority (92%) of these centres are in the 28 European Union member countries.

However, there are many other types of service in operation. In England and Wales, the police provide victims with information on how to access a variety of services, and that can include a range of specialist help (Ministry of Justice, 2014). The revised and updated *Code of Practice for Victims of Crime* (Ministry of Justice, 2020) sets out a series of 12 victims' rights and explains the types of services to which individuals have access and what they can expect from each stage of the processing of their case through the criminal justice system. It identifies a series of entitlements, how they can be accessed, and the duties of service providers.

Linked to this, many victims are also directly referred to Victim Support in local areas. Services may range from short-term counselling and support comprising just a few contacts to onward referral to mental health services and extending to management of high-risk situations by providing protection or enabling victims to move to refuges. Alongside this, efforts are made to secure victim and witness statements and other evidence that will increase the likelihood of successful prosecution of the perpetrator. Victims can also be supported in making victim personal statements that may be used in court following a finding of guilt.

The relationship between crime seriousness and the magnitude of effects on victims is complex. But the impact on individuals of crime victimization can be extensive and pervasive and can entail mental health problems such as debilitating anxiety, depression, anger, irritability, severe reactions including post-traumatic stress disorder (PTSD) and a range of other psychological outcomes (Miller, 2008). Victims may also have been physically injured or may have incurred financial loss of money or property, with repercussions across other areas of their lives (Doerner & Lab, 2015). In a recent survey in Sheffield, 86% of those who reported having been victims of crime described experiencing at least one form of psychological or behavioural change, and effects were more marked for those who had been victims of violence (Tan & Haining, 2016).

For the most serious personal crimes, the impact on victims and witnesses can be overwhelming. It is well known that individuals can experience severe emotional reactions as a result of any event perceived as life-threatening, such as involvement in road traffic accidents (Mayou et al., 2000), losing a loved one through homicide (Connolly & Gordon, 2014; Rynearson, 2012), from being victims of torture (McColl et al., 2010) or being victims of or witnesses to terrorism incidents or other forms of mass violence (Miller, 2002). The last necessitates both an individual-level and a system-wide response, as occurred following the 2001 terrorist attacks on New York (Donahue et al., 2006) and following the 2011 massacre committed by Anders Breivik in Norway (Kärki, 2015). Police services are amongst the first responders to all such incidents, and alongside responsibilities for control of the situation and for law enforcement, they also coordinate the work of other agencies. Finally, there are instances in which police officers themselves are witnesses to or victims of serious crimes and may require assistance and support to manage the impact of such experiences. Clearly, a review of evidence pertaining to all of these areas could be a potentially large-scale undertaking. The present chapter is therefore confined to examining studies of support for victims of offences within the range of severity that most frequently leads to provision of counselling or other forms of personal or mental health services.

The most widely delivered services for victims of crime involve a process of listening and relatively informal one-to-one counselling. There are reasonable grounds for claiming that short-term counselling (comprising up to a maximum of 12 sessions) can be shown to be effective for a range of problems, as attested by several reviews of its use in general practice (primary medical care) settings. Bower et al. (2003, 2011; Rowland et al., 2001) and Brettle et al. (2008; Hill et al., 2008) have each reviewed this area, including a number of randomized controlled trials, which show modest but statistically significant gains in relation to symptom reduction and other types of benefit. That applies also to other brief therapies employed in primary care settings (Cape et al., 2010). It should be noted that the follow-up period in most of the studies included in these reviews was comparatively short (usually a maximum of 4 months). The key question of interest here, therefore, is whether such interventions also produce evidence of effectiveness in work with victims of crime.

## 10.4 Method

At the outset of this review, it was considered that the search terms could be relatively simple in construction, as there was a clear and fairly well-specified focus of the area to be reviewed. It was also thought that there might be many unpublished reports on this area that would be unlikely to be of high quality, making it difficult to draw any clear conclusions. Search strategies were therefore devised to locate only published research consisting of evaluations of victim counselling or other forms of support provided either directly by police or by adjunct agencies to whom police would refer crime victims or other community agencies that provided services to victims on a self-referred basis (e.g. healthcare, social services or voluntary organizations). A key step within this was to locate previous reviews of the topic and of adjoining areas, to discover what has been learned to date and whether a general picture had emerged of the outcomes of victim counselling.

### 10.4.1 Search Strategy

Tracking down research relevant to the objectives of the present review was done in a series of steps. First, a pilot, exploratory search of the PsycINFO database was carried out in 2016 using the simple terms *victim support* and *polic**. This yielded a total of only 38 items but was useful in developing a clearer perspective on how to search this field and in giving a preliminary indication of the range and types of study that might be discovered in a fuller review.

A search of the Cochrane Database of Systematic Reviews and the Campbell Systematic Reviews library using the terms *crime victim/victim of crime* or *victimization* yielded only a few items. Similarly, the research section of the Victims Support website was searched, and although it listed 17 reports, none was focused on evaluation of services. A major volume on the methods used in counselling crime victims, while covering many aspects of this – including discussion of clinical interventions for severe trauma reactions – contained no information on evaluation of victim services (Miller, 2008). Subsequently the following five other databases were searched employing a more detailed search strategy: PsycINFO, EBSCOhost, Scopus, National Criminal Justice Reference Service (NCJRS), and Web of Science.

Electronic searches of these databases were carried out in mid-2016. To maximize the likelihood of capturing potentially relevant material, the timeframe was left open, that is, no start date was set for any searches. Several of the library resources listed above are large-scale electronic literature databases that incorporate many other more specialized databases across the fields of medicine and healthcare and the social, physical and biological sciences. The NCJRS is maintained by the US Department of Justice and collates research work carried on both by government departments and academic institutions around the world. Searches were updated in November 2020 using Scopus, PsycINFO and NCJRS.

### 10.4.2 Inclusion and Exclusion Criteria

The detailed list of search terms used for the review is shown in Table 10.1. Given the objectives of this review, studies were retained if they met the following inclusion criteria: (1) The study was published in a peer-reviewed journal or as a

**Table 10.1** Search summary on victim counselling and support

| Databases or websites | Search term(s) | Number of items located | Number retained after screening |
|---|---|---|---|
| PsycINFO | *victim support evaluation*<br>*victim counsel* AND evaluat* AND polic**<br>*victim counsel* AND effectiveness or efficacy AND review* | 468<br>55<br>95 | 23 |
| EBSCOhost | *crime victim AND support services AND evaluation or review* | 482 | 5 |
| NCJRS | *"victims of crime" AND support AND evaluation* | 450 | 22 |
| Scopus | *victim counsel* AND evaluat* AND review*<br>*crime victim* AND police AND counsel**<br>*victim support AND effectiveness AND evaluation* | 226<br>66<br>88 | 19 |
| Web of Science | *crime victim OR victim of crime AND counsel* AND evaluat** | 38 | 5 |
| Total | | 1968 | 74 |

government report. (2) The study described a process or outcome evaluation of counselling, therapy, crisis intervention or other form of support or service provided to victims of crime. (3) Data were collected on variable(s) that reflected impact on victims' well-being, sense of safety and willingness to report further crimes or to provide evidence to the police. (4) An evaluation had to report either quantitative or qualitative data (or both), informing some aspect of the effectiveness of the intervention or how it was perceived.

Studies also had to be published in English, as timescales and resources did not permit the possibility of translation. Dissertations were excluded, partly as they were unpublished and, although examined, had not been peer-reviewed and partly because their larger format required more time in reading and data extraction. Studies were also excluded from the final analysis if they addressed issues which, although closely related with the study of victims and services provided to them, were not focused on evaluation of those services as such, even if they took place in the context of counselling (e.g. King & Woollett, 1997). For example, many studies were found of risk factors for becoming a victim of crime; of victim-offender interaction processes; of victims of school bullying; of the long-term effects and treatment of childhood sexual abuse or other kinds of child maltreatment; of the effects of victim personal impact statements in court; and of the use of restorative justice, mediation or reconciliation procedures. All of these were excluded from further consideration.

What effects might be expected or hoped for in providing services to crime victims? At a general level, crime victims might view such services as an expression of the community's concern for their welfare. Victim groups have often drawn attention to the considerable resources deployed towards working with offenders as compared with the sums available for victim support. We might therefore evaluate victims' overall reported satisfaction with types and levels of support being seen as appropriate to individual experiences of victimization. More specific objectives of such support services could include one or more of the following: improvement in victim well-being, reduction in feelings of fear or vulnerability and, conversely, enhanced feelings of personal safety; restoring the confidence to resume normal life activities; lowering the risk of victims developing more serious or long-term mental health problems such as PTSD; greater willingness to report further offences in future; more willingness to cooperate with police in giving evidence statements and testifying in court; and more globally improved perceptions of the police. The results of the searches that were undertaken are also shown in Table 10.1.

Some initial searches in the Scopus databases using very broad terms (*victim counsel* AND evaluat** and *crime victim* AND police*), respectively, produced 1722 and 1686 items, but many of these were not directly relevant; therefore the searches were narrowed to the sets of terms shown in Table 10.1. More focused searches still located many hundreds of research articles and other documents at this stage, resulting in a total of 1968 hits which were screened online. Those eligible for full review were then identified through a two-stage selection process. In Stage 1, titles and where necessary abstracts were read for relevance to the review objectives, resulting in a narrowing down to 97 items. For example, studies that were found of the effects of school bullying were removed, as this is generally managed by schools themselves, and even when police become involved, victim support is likely to be provided internally. In Stage 2, abstracts and in some cases electronic documents were read in more detail, to identify research that entailed evaluation of a service for victims as defined for the review, yielding 74 items. Two review articles found in reference lists were added to this total ($N = 76$). Numerous research studies were found on factors influencing well-being in victims, but only those entailing an intervention that had been methodically evaluated were retained for full review, resulting in a final set of 37 studies. To these a further 18 items were added, mainly found in reference lists of other sources, making a final total of 55 items for full review, to which 3 were added after updating to 2020. The process of selection with numbers of items discarded and retained at each phase is presented in Fig. 10.1.

At Stage 2, a few studies were excluded that focused on victimization amongst known offenders who had themselves also been victimized (Golder et al., 2015; Taylor, 2015), as they did not contain any account of service provision focused on those specific needs. However, they did indicate the role of prior victimization and of family support as factors influencing subsequent criminal recidivism.

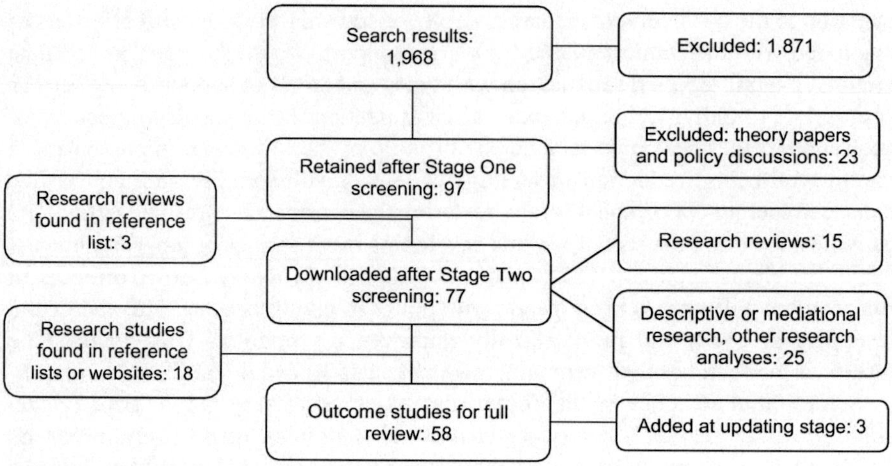


**Fig. 10.1** Flowchart of search results: victim counselling and support

## 10.5 Previous Reviews

No review was found which covered exactly the area focused on here. An early attempt to draw conclusions about the effectiveness of victim services found that evaluations "...were still in their infancy" (Maguire, 1991, p.410). At that stage there was little evidence to review, and what was available was methodologically rather weak. Research suggested that victims regarded the emotional impact as the worst aspect of their plight. Most victim support, which consisted of relatively brief visits by volunteers lasting on average only half an hour, appeared to be highly appreciated. But as some victims also became more anxious through discussing their experiences, overall findings were regarded as inconclusive. There was a wide range of approaches to helping victims of rape, but insufficient evidence to decide whether any specific approach produced better effects than others.

One more recent document that was located appeared to have objectives very similar to, and to cover almost the same ground as, the present review (Marandos & Perry, 2009). However, when retrieved it was found to be a protocol only, i.e. an outline of a review that was planned, giving details of the work to be done, but there was no information on whether it had been completed. Fortunately, it proved possible to contact the second author, who explained that the review planned for the Campbell Collaboration had been withdrawn but that there was a literature review included in the first author's PhD dissertation (Marandos, 2005).[1] Although unpublished dissertations were not to be included, because of the close relevance of this work and because it had initially been identified as a Campbell Collaboration protocol, it was decided to include it amongst the list of previous relevant reviews. Sixteen

[1] The authors thank Dr Amanda Perry, University of York, for making this thesis available.

references not found elsewhere were located via this review. However, three of them could not be accessed as two proved to be unobtainable and one was published in French. All but one were published prior to 2000, as contrasted with those found in database searches of which 32/37 were published after 2000. Five additional studies were obtained via a website dedicated to *cognitive processing therapy for post-traumatic stress disorder* (http://cptforptsd.com/).

Alongside this, there have been other reviews of closely adjacent areas or of related aspects of the general issue of counselling, therapy or other support following distressing events, including being a victim of crime. Table 10.2 provides basic information from a total of 15 relevant reviews of research on interventions designed to provide support or treatment of reactions to crime victimization. As we might expect, most focus on the impact of serious crimes, entailing some kind of personal violence, including physical assault, intimate partner violence, other forms of domestic abuse, rape or other sexual assault.

There is also a separate review examining the status of a theoretical model of reactions following victimization (Van Reemst et al., 2016). This tests the validity and explanatory power of the *social information processing* model. The authors found 64 studies, but this is primarily of academic interest and is not included in Table 10.2 as it is not an outcome review, i.e. it is not examining the effectiveness of interventions. Another review not included in Table 10.2, by Finkelhor et al. (2001), was concerned with factors that influence the under-reporting of offences against children. While this has relevance when considering potential interventions for child victims, again it does not contain information on outcomes or evaluations and therefore was also excluded. A third review, by Petrak (1996), was excluded as its account of research was too brief and now surpassed by more recent review work.

It was noted earlier that there is evidence for the effectiveness of counselling in general practice but that research in that area does not separately identify those who are seeking help after having been victims of crime. The literature reviews listed in Table 10.2 show that numerous approaches have been tried and tested in seeking to address the specific problem of providing support to that group. Interventions covered in these reviews show remarkable variety, and it is difficult in a limited space to do justice to the ground covered in them. Some of the above reviews address closely related topics, and there are overlaps in the studies retained, but also some differences. Several of the same studies appear in more than one review, but others do not as the specific aims differ slightly between the reviews. Outcome variables amongst the studies included in these reviews also showed considerable variety.

The following are some of the key findings and trends that emerged from these 14 reviews. This attempts to take account of the consistency with which findings were obtained, alongside the strength of the research designs that were employed. First, there is moderate to strong support for the use of psychological therapy for victims of rape, sexual assault and domestic abuse (Hackett et al., 2016; Regehr et al., 2013; Taylor & Harvey, 2009; Vickerman & Margolin, 2009). Second, the review of methods of reducing negative effects of victimization by Marandos (2005) indicated a clear difference between the effectiveness of more intensive interventions and that of brief, short-term interventions, which yielded little evidence of

**Table 10.2** Previous reviews of related areas: victim counselling and support

| Review | Focus | No. of studies | Findings |
|---|---|---|---|
| Arroyo et al. (2017) | Systematic review and meta-analysis of short-term interventions for survivors of intimate partner violence | 21 | Searched 12 databases with terms designed to locate brief, short-term or time-limited forms of psychological therapy. Reports a narrative review (summary of each located study) and a meta-analysis. Analysed nine categories of outcome variable. The mean effect size was in the range considered large (Hedges' $g$ statistic = 1.02), representing a "34% advantage". There were large positive effects for PTSD, self-esteem, depression, general distress and life functioning and moderate positive effects for substance misuse, emotional well-being, feelings of safety and recurrence of violence |
| Campbell et al. (2005) | SANEs | 10 | Specially trained forensic nurses provide 24-hour support, including medical, psychological, legal and other services to victims of sexual assault. Narrative review of ten studies conducted at various sites in the USA and Canada. All found evidence of positive benefits but most reported on only a single type of impact of SANEs. Few studies had robust designs, and most were small-sample case studies or before-and-after designs |
| Forneris et al. (2013) | Effectiveness of methods for prevention of PTSD | 19 | Systematic review of RCTs but 12/19 did not use blinded conditions. Several methods produced positive results, but overall pattern was regarded as insufficient to demonstrate any single treatment as best practice. Included two studies of pharmacological interventions. Meta-analysis of one subset of studies showed brief CBT more effective than supportive counselling in reducing PTSD symptoms |
| Hackett et al. (2016) | Efficacy of interventions for victims of domestic violence | 17 | Meta-analysis comparing several interventions including advocacy, empowerment, parent-child work, play therapy and CBT. Examined effects on both women and children. Found a large mean effect size (0.812) from uncontrolled studies and a moderate effect size (0.518) from seven RCT designs. Results were positive across a range of outcome variables (psychological adjustment, behaviour problems, alcohol use, family relations, maltreatment events, etc.) |

(continued)

**Table 10.2** (continued)

| Review | Focus | No. of studies | Findings |
|---|---|---|---|
| Jonker et al. (2014) | Efficacy of interventions during and after shelter residence | 10 | Meta-analysis of the effectiveness of residence in women's shelters following domestic abuse. Included eight RCTs and two uncontrolled trials. Periods spent in shelters improved mental health (reduced depression), decreased abuse and improved social outcomes (levels of support, access to resources). All mean effect sizes were also statistically significant |
| Marandos (2005) | Systematic review of the effectiveness of methods for reducing negative psychological effects of victimization | 20 | The objectives and methodology of this review were the closest found to those of the present evidence review. Its focus was on "what works" in reducing negative psychological correlates of having been a crime victim. All but one of the located studies were published before 2000. They were subject to quality appraisal and divided into two groups:<br>10 of "intensive" interventions (entailing ≥2 sessions in a structured format) (8 RCTs)<br>10 of "short-term" interventions (an average of 1 unstructured session) (4 RCTs)<br>The former had higher design quality, and 7/10 yielded evidence of improvement in intervention groups as compared to controls. The latter produced very little evidence of effectiveness. This group included five studies of police-based programmes, but none was found to have positive effects |
| Martin et al. (2007) | Healthcare interventions for victims of sexual assault | 30 | The majority of studies reviewed consisted of analyses or surveys of the perceived training needs of staff involved in working with victims, or detailed descriptions of modes of service delivery. Only nine studies involved some attempt at evaluation, but most reported data at post-intervention only, with only two reporting any follow-up on a subset of participants. No clear conclusions could be drawn about the effects of services for victims |
| O'Reilly et al. (2010) | Systematic review of screening and interventions with pregnant women victims of domestic violence | 9 | Of the nine studies included, five were studies of screening to identify occurrence of domestic violence, and only four were concerned with evaluation of interventions. The latter mainly compared counselling with other interventions (e.g. mentoring) or with no treatment. Results were mixed with no intervention proving superior to standard care in terms of preventing further violence |

(continued)

**Table 10.2** (continued)

| Review | Focus | No. of studies | Findings |
|---|---|---|---|
| Price et al. (2001) | Psychotherapy for adult survivors of childhood sexual abuse | 8 | Located studies of experiential therapy (4), cognitive-behavioural therapy (2), psycho-dynamic therapy (1) and psycho-education (1). Most reported pre-post changes, and only one involved a comparison with a no-treatment control group. Outcome variables were self-reports on psychometric scales. All studies found improvements on most variables assessed, some with up to 9-month follow-up. However, the weak designs alongside limited descriptions of samples and procedures made drawing of clear conclusions difficult |
| Regehr et al. (2013) | Meta-analysis of interventions to reduce distress in victims of rape and sexual violence | 6 | Restricted to RCTs (4) and quasi-experiments (2) only. Dependent variables were PTSD, anxiety and depression. All six studies found improvements in PTSD and depression and three in anxiety, with changes also in guilt and dissociation. Largest effects were obtained for cognitive processing and prolonged exposure therapies and EMDR |
| Rivas et al. (2015) | Advocacy interventions to reduce violence against women victims of partner abuse | 13 | Cochrane systematic review of RCTs and quasi-experimental designs, but studies were very varied in other features. Analysed evidence on a range of variables (levels of physical, sexual or emotional abuse; quality of life; and depression). Found few indications that advocacy produced significant benefits. Minimal gains were found in some studies, but none in most, and little evidence of gains being maintained at follow-up |
| Shorey et al. (2014) | CCR for victims of IPV | 13 | Narrative review of studies of the effectiveness of multi-agency integrated responses to IPV with an emphasis on results for victims. The article places more emphasis on the components of CCR than on its outcomes but does report some results for advocacy, criminal justice, counselling and healthcare services. There were positive results on emotional state, self-esteem, coping, social support and other factors for advocacy and counselling. However, there were also some results showing no between-group differences and a lack of clarity on which CCR components generated changes. Findings for criminal justice and healthcare-led services were more equivocal |

(continued)

**Table 10.2** (continued)

| Review | Focus | No. of studies | Findings |
|---|---|---|---|
| Taylor and Harvey (2009) | Meta-analysis of therapy effects for victims of sexual assault showing symptoms of rape trauma or PTSD | 15 | Reported two meta-analyses, one of eight studies using independent sample (group comparison, mostly RCT) designs and one of seven pre-post studies (repeated measures). Most studies evaluated behavioural or cognitive-behavioural therapies. Mean effect sizes for both sets of studies were large (0.91 and 0.90, respectively) with effects maintained at 12-month follow-up (based on ten studies). Better effects were found with 10–16 than with <10 sessions |
| Vickerman and Margolin (2009) | Review of effectiveness of treatments for post-traumatic stress (PTSD) in victims of rape | 20 | Located 32 articles based on 20 research samples; 11 studies used random allocation. Describes a range of therapeutic approaches employed in treatment of serious trauma reactions to rape. They include stress inoculation training, prolonged exposure therapy, cognitive processing, EMDR, supportive counselling and CBT. Strongest support was found for cognitive processing and prolonged exposure with stress inoculation training also producing positive outcomes. In the only direct comparisons between active treatments CBT was found superior to supportive counselling. On average, one-third of treated participants still had severe symptoms following treatment |
| Wathen and MacMillan (2003) | Review of interventions for violence against women and prevention of abuse | 22 | This review includes a mixture of studies focused on work with victims and/or perpetrators of IPV. Of the 22 studies retained, only 5 were focused on services for women victims, and the remainder dealt with interventions for perpetrators or couples. Services included advocacy, shelter residence, personal and vocational counselling and prenatal counselling. The principal focus was on prevention of further abuse, but only one study found evidence of reduced physical abuse but not of other forms of abuse. There was some evidence that interventions enabled victims to make better use of services, but no evidence of changes in depression or other health outcomes |

*CBT* cognitive-behavioural therapy, *CCR* coordinated community response, *IPR* intimate partner violence, *RCT* randomized controlled trial, *SANEs* Effectiveness of Sexual Assault Nurse Examiners, *PTSD* post-traumatic stress disorder

positive outcomes. Third, there was moderately good evidence for the effectiveness of domestic violence shelters in improving mental health, decreasing abuse and enabling women victims to access other services (Jonker et al., 2014). By contrast there was only minimal evidence for the effectiveness of advocacy for victims of domestic abuse/intimate partner violence (Rivas et al., 2015; Wathen & MacMillan, 2003). Fourth, while there are some demonstrable positive effects for coordinated community response approaches, other results are ambivalent (Shorey et al., 2014). Fifth, there is positive evidence concerning the value of Sexual Assault Nurse Examiners with victims (Campbell et al., 2005), though this comes from relatively weak studies. Sixth, where side-by-side comparisons were possible, CBT secured better outcomes than supportive counselling in preventing symptoms of post-traumatic stress (Forneris et al., 2013; Vickerman & Margolin, 2009). CBT and interpersonal therapy proved particularly helpful for victims of partner violence when they were "IPV-tailored" (Arroyo et al., 2017, p.167). Seventh, interventions to address the long-term effects of child sexual abuse produced equivocal results (Price et al., 2001) though this review may now require updating as other research may have accumulated since its publication. Eighth and finally, very little research was found evaluating specific actions taken by police services in addressing victims' problems, and the few studies that were found did not produce positive results (Marandos, 2005). Findings in several other areas were unclear and difficult to interpret, partly because of inconsistencies amongst study outcomes and partly because of weaknesses in the types of research that had been conducted.

Within this mixed picture, some results were particularly striking. Hackett et al. (2016) calculated a *failsafe number* of 4478 for their review. That is the estimated number of unpublished studies with zero effects that would be needed to undermine the positive effect size they obtained. It is extremely unlikely that such a large number of studies have been carried out but then not published. This increases confidence that the reported findings are meaningful and reliable. Evaluations of the impact of shelter residence were also impressive: although mean effect sizes were smaller, they were all statistically significant. Taylor and Harvey (2009) found large average effect sizes for the studies included in their meta-analyses, focused on therapeutic interventions for traumatized sexual assault victims. For example, in the studies that involved comparisons between treatment and control groups, the success rate in terms of symptom reduction for the former was 70.8%, while for the latter it was 29.2%. The failsafe number of studies needed to reduce the observed effect sizes to 0.20 were 50 and 38 for the independent-sample and repeated-measures studies, respectively.

It is important to recognize however that studies carried out in healthcare settings, challenging though they may be, often lend themselves to the use of more tightly controlled research designs than it is possible to implement in community settings where different kinds of services are being compared and where there is often a very high rate of attrition (dropout). The proportion of well-designed trials tends to be higher in clinical settings; therefore the results of studies in that area can often be easier to interpret. An issue for the present evidence review was to establish whether the same trends emerge in the research studies located here as can be seen in pre-existing reviews.

## 10.6 Research Designs and Quality Appraisal

It has to be kept in mind that the quality of the research found in these reviews is very variable. There are regular criticisms made by reviewers, both here and in related areas, to the effect that many research projects have methodological shortcomings, which can render it difficult to draw clear conclusions from them. Part of this derives from the challenges of conducting well-controlled research when trying to address human problems within agencies and organizations that exist mainly to provide services. The complexity of the systems within which the work is done makes the design of sound evaluations difficult. This issue rose in importance when considering the individual studies retained for full review.

For quality appraisal of the majority of the studies retained in the present review, each was allocated a score on the Maryland Scale Scientific Methods Score according to the research design employed, as outlined in Chap. 6. Those scores are included in the summary results of each study which are reported in Tables 10.3, 10.4 and 10.5 further. However, some studies could not be allotted scores, as their methodology did not belong in any of the categories defined by the Maryland Scale Scientific Methods Score. That was the case for a small number of qualitative studies, for several studies that employed survey methodology to obtain user feedback or to review service case files and for the single study that was found evaluating cost-effectiveness (Table 10.6). In those cases, the Maryland Scale Scientific Methods Score was recorded as not applicable (n/a).

## 10.7 Results

Regarding the locations of the 58 studies by country, more than two-thirds of them (40 studies, 68%) were carried out in the USA. Others originated from the UK (11 studies), Canada (3 studies), the Netherlands (3 studies) and Spain (1 study). As found in the research reviews listed earlier, there was a wide variety of services, procedures and interventions examined within them. In some respects, this is an impressive array of projects and shows the breadth of thought that has been applied to addressing the immense problems that can be produced by crime victimization. In a few cases, the located studies were separate outputs from the same long-term project (notably the studies by Campbell and by Resick), but in each case it was clear that they reported independent datasets. In one set of two studies (Zweig et al., 2002, 2003), the extent of possible overlap between the sources of material that was presented in each report was not made clear, but they appeared to focus on distinct aspects of the data collected.

The 58 studies included in this review were divided into 3 categories. Since some studies have multiple aims and sometimes examine more than one type of service, these groups were loosely defined, with permeable and by no means watertight divisions between them. They were police and criminal justice, access to community resources and therapeutic interventions. There were 19 studies on police and criminal justice including initiatives or actions instigated by police services themselves, but also including their patterns of response to victims, and the potential influence on victims of decisions taken at crime scenes, or evidence about whether or not aspects of contact with victims during initial investigation help victims at that time or subsequently. Information extracted from these studies is presented in Table 10.3. There were 17 studies on access to community resources. This included research evidence about a variety of approaches in which different forms of community resources are harnessed to provide a range of support and services to victims, with varying levels of strategic coordination. It includes studies of the value of advocacy, support groups and helplines, either separately in themselves or reached through service brokerage in which victims are linked up to various kinds of support through a coordinated system. Information extracted from these studies is presented in Table 10.4. Finally, there were 21 studies of therapeutic Interventions. This included on different kinds of more formalized help provided to individuals (or sometimes small groups), usually to those who are experiencing more marked emotional needs or mental health problems as a result of violent or sexual assaults. It includes counselling, debriefing, psycho-education and psychological therapy. Information extracted from these studies is presented in Table 10.5.

Note once again that there were some studies in each of the categories that included similar elements such as counselling, which was often provided as a component in other types of services, sometimes evaluated separately and sometimes not. One report could not be placed under any of the above headings as it was a study in health economics, estimating the cost-effectiveness of training for general practitioners to improve their skills in identifying victims of domestic violence. Enabling GPs to do this could potentially result in costs savings in other areas of healthcare and adjoining agencies. This was the only study of its type found in the searches. Information taken from it is shown in Table 10.6.

### *10.7.1 Police and Criminal Justice (19 studies)*

Table 10.3 shows studies placed under this heading, which included a variety of approaches. Studies show the importance of the first and immediate police contact on some of the patterns that happen afterwards and their effects on victims (e.g. Rosenbaum, 1987). Other studies (not reviewed here as they contained no formal evaluative component) showed that police patterns of questioning have a significant impact on victims' perceptions of them (e.g. Apsler et al., 2003). The studies included in Table 10.3 can be divided into a number of subgroups. They include research on police-based crisis teams which undertook speedy intervention with victims of domestic abuse, including counselling arranged directly through police services (Young et al., 2008) or referring them to a Victim Support Team.

Another procedure that was examined was police *re-contact* or *callback* after a crime event, usually taking place 2 weeks after the incident as a form of follow-up.

**Table 10.3** Information from included studies: police and criminal justice

| Study: author(s), (date), country | Design and SMS | Samples/data sources | Interventions and outcomes |
|---|---|---|---|
| Bryce et al. (2016) UK | Qualitative study SMS = n/a | Semi-structured interviews with 17 victims of violent crime | Study designed to obtain deeper insight into victim experiences and access to support services. Contacts were made through a police area and Victim Support agency. Interview responses subjected to thematic analysis. Though given contact information, levels of engagement with support services were fairly low. Several felt able to cope without help. Others felt overwhelmed by too many offers of support and suggested leaving a gap before contact was furthered, as their initial reactions meant they could not benefit from help. The small proportion who did accept further service contact described "extremely positive experiences" of it (p.249) |
| Campbell et al. (2008) USA | Post-intervention feedback survey SMS = n/a | 52 sexual assault victims referred to SANE services | The paper provides details of the stages of the process of evaluating the development and delivery of Sexual Assault Nurse Examiner (SANE) services. In this part of the study, feedback was collected from participants in SANE to judge whether the "empowering care" model (seen as central to the service) was being successfully implemented. This involved provision of healthcare, support and access to resources. Almost all feedback ratings were very high |

(continued)

**Table 10.3** (continued)

| Study: author(s), (date), country | Design and SMS | Samples/data sources | Interventions and outcomes |
|---|---|---|---|
| Campbell et al. (2012a) USA | Content analysis of case reports SMS = 1 | 343 reports of sexual assault cases from 3 police departments | This is an indirect evaluation of the effects of using SANE to work with victims. Examines the relationship between different police actions and the eventual effect on victims. File reports on case examinations were analysed under ten separate headings to investigate the relationship between different features of each case. The dependent variable was whether police referred the case to prosecutors. Mediational analysis (using multi-level logistic regression) showed that with involvement of a SANE specialist, additional evidence was collected, victims were 40% less likely to disengage and cases were 5 times more likely to be forwarded to prosecutors. Police were also more likely to collect other kinds of information to support the case, also leading to greater likelihood of prosecution and higher rates of conviction (in other research) |
| Campbell et al. (2012b) USA | Quasi-experimental, non-equivalent, longitudinal SMS = 4 | 146 victims helped by the SANE programme in the years 1999–2005. 171 adult sexual assault victims from the years 1994–1999 (comparison) | Dependent variable was whether or not cases were referred for prosecution of perpetrators, whether prosecution took place and whether there was a finding of guilt. Statistical analysis (using multi-level regression) found that there was a significant increase in case progression following the introduction of SANE. This was moderated by differences between the five police departments involved in the study. Cases processed in the month of December were less likely to be progressed |

(continued)

**Table 10.3** (continued)

| Study: author(s), (date), country | Design and SMS | Samples/data sources | Interventions and outcomes |
|---|---|---|---|
| Corcoran and Allen (2005) USA | Group comparison SMS = 3 | Cases of family violence involving both female and male victims and abusers: 96 referred to crisis team; 80 randomly drawn from non-referred cases | Six-month evaluation of a victim crisis intervention service focusing on its impact on police-related outcomes. Numbers of arrests were higher in the crisis team referrals than non-referrals (82% versus 49%). In many other respects, the groups were similar, though a slightly higher proportion of the crisis referrals went to shelters (7% versus 1%). Non-cooperation with the police was higher amongst the crisis referrals (15% versus 4%) |
| Irazola et al. (2015) USA | Survey SMS = n/a | Crime victims: 723 Service providers: 1246 | Evaluated the use of automated notification systems, in which victims are provided with information about court events and status changes as the person who offended against them moves through the criminal justice system. Notification was by phone, post, e-mail or text. Large majorities of both service providers and victims reported benefits of the system including increased sense of safety, feeling empowered and feeling more involved in the legal case; it was also perceived as beneficial to the justice system. However, there were large numbers of non-responders and it is not clear how representative the sample is |

(continued)

**Table 10.3** (continued)

| Study: author(s), (date), country | Design and SMS | Samples/data sources | Interventions and outcomes |
|---|---|---|---|
| Kernic and Bonomi (2007) USA | Got SMS = n/a | 2092 female victims of male IPV referred to Seattle Police Department in years 2000–2002<br>415 referred on to a specialized support team<br>1677 not referred | Examined which factors increased the likelihood of police referral to Victim Support Team (VST, crisis intervention services). This is not an outcome evaluation but was retained as it included information on how decisions were made by police services. Compared those referred or not referred to the VST. Data analysed using multiple regression showed that referral was more likely if women were married, pregnant, Latina, Asian and with severe injury or minor visible injury and if the abuser was arrested. These differences emerged in four of five precincts but in the fifth no differences emerged |
| Kerr et al. (2003) UK | Case file review SMS = n/a | Records of 676 cases of women victims referred to The Haven, London, in the period May 2000 to May 2001 | The Haven was a project set up jointly by King's College Hospital and the Metropolitan Police to meet the needs of women who had been sexually assaulted. The study does not report a formal evaluation but provides data on the take-up of different aspects of the service by referred women. Most (79%) were referred by the police. Of the total referrals, 12% declined further appointments and 33% did not attend appointments offered |

(continued)

**Table 10.3** (continued)

| Study: author(s), (date), country | Design and SMS | Samples/data sources | Interventions and outcomes |
|---|---|---|---|
| Madoc-Jones et al. (2015) UK | Qualitative study SMS = n/a | 33 members of staff in agencies working with victims of crime in 1 police area | Study funded by the Office of Police and Crime Commissioner (OPCC) to improve understanding of victims' needs. Interviews were conducted with police services, victim support probation trust, Crown Prosecution Service, advocacy services and staff of a range of other provider agencies. Analysis of interviews highlighted a number of issues arising in the process of service delivery, from referral and assessment processes to the need for more thorough integration and clarification regarding oversight |
| McKee et al. (2020) UK | RCT SMS = 5 | Uniformed officers: 50 urban, 50 rural Rape detectives: 40 Student officers: 53 | Given evidence that rape victims may not be regarded by some police officers as credible, the study evaluated whether a 4-hour in-service training programme provided to four groups of police (student officers, uniformed officers in urban vs. rural areas and specialist rape investigators) could influence attitudes concerning this. Participants were randomly allocated to the training programme or a no-training control condition. The main outcome variable was degree of rape myth acceptance (RMA), measured at baseline (pre-training), immediately after training and 6 weeks later. Analysis showed the training programme had a positive effect in reducing levels of RMA amongst all groups of qualified officers but not amongst police students |

(continued)

**Table 10.3** (continued)

| Study: author(s), (date), country | Design and SMS | Samples/data sources | Interventions and outcomes |
|---|---|---|---|
| Resnick et al. (1999) USA | Group comparison SMS = 4 | 80 adult female victims of rape; pseudo-random assignment:<br>13 in experimental group<br>33 in standard condition | Evaluated the effect of a 17-minute video presented immediately before forensic examination of rape victims on their levels of distress and the relationship to later risk of PTSD. The video gave information about the examination and showed individuals coping successfully and calmly with the procedures. Used structured scales to assess distress, anxiety and PTSD. Level of distress prior to the examination was strongly correlated with subsequent PTSD. At post-test there were significantly lower scores on distress and anxiety for those shown the video than for those in the standard condition |
| Rosenbaum (1987) USA | Group comparison SMS = 3 | 122 police recruits:<br>Experimental group<br>Control group<br>105 at follow-up (86%)<br>Subgroup numbers not given; victim numbers not given | Detroit Victims Experiment. Tested hypotheses that police-victim interactions in the period after victimization mediate the psychological impact of having been a victim and that training can be trained to improve how police act in that situation. New police recruits were given special training prior to interviewing victims of aggravated assault, robbery or residential burglary. Their attitudes were assessed and they rated the importance of different aspects of the crime scene. Victims took part in a 30-minute telephone survey. There was evidence the training influenced the amount of information officers recorded about victims. However, there was no evidence the training had any effect on victims' psychological and behavioural reactions, on their fear of crime or on their attitudes to police or the courts |

(continued)

**Table 10.3** (continued)

| Study: author(s), (date), country | Design and SMS | Samples/data sources | Interventions and outcomes |
|---|---|---|---|
| Skogan and Wycoff (1987) USA | RCT SMS = 5 | Crime victims aged 13 or over; excluded rape and relatives of homicides<br>235 treatment group<br>250 controls | Programme designed by Houston police to address the needs of crime victims, by re-contacting them 1–4 weeks after the crime (*callback*). They checked for any further incidents, offered crime prevention advice and made referrals to other agencies for support. Seventy-four percent of the treatment group and 70% of control cases were interviewed at end. Only one between-group difference was found post-intervention, and it was counter to expectations: the treatment group perceived property crime as a larger problem in their locality than did the controls. Multiple regression analysis controlling for features of crimes and other variables enhanced this unanticipated effect. A second analysis showed these effects were particularly strong amongst Hispanic and Asian participants. The main unanticipated effect was difficult to explain but may be due to the gap between crime and contact |

(continued)

**Table 10.3** (continued)

| Study: author(s), (date), country | Design and SMS | Samples/data sources | Interventions and outcomes |
|---|---|---|---|
| Srinivas and DePrince (2015) USA | Correlational + regression design SMS = 4 | 265 female victims of IPV:<br>135 experimental<br>130 control<br>236 at 2-year follow-up | Examined the relationship between police response and extent of PTSD symptoms, taking account of background variables and examining several aspects of participants' reactions. Unmet expectations of police (arresting/not arresting offender against victim's wishes, not providing desired services) were associated with higher PTSD symptom severity with a trend towards greater anger. Other factors, e.g. social support, moderated outcomes. At post-test between-group differences were significant, favouring the advocacy programme, except for psychological abuse. At follow-up, fewer differences were significant but trends still favoured the advocacy group |
| Stafford (2018) UK | Providing information to crime victims via call handlers SMS = n/a | 12 non-emergency call handlers from 1 police area in England<br>Analysis of 55 calls from crime victims | Contents of exchanges between crime victims and call handlers were studied using thematic analysis. Records were also kept of call handlers' post-call activity related to the information given in the call. Data were examined in the context of the *National Call handling Standards* (2005, updated 2016) and the *Code of Practice for Victims of Crime* (2020). These specify the steps that should be taken, but the study found that call handlers rarely followed the prescribed format completely. Some steps were missed, or information given was vague. Accurate information was provided in only 15/55 calls yet still often had some missing elements. The author regarded the study as preliminary and stated that more research is required |

(continued)

**Table 10.3** (continued)

| Study: author(s), (date), country | Design and SMS | Samples/data sources | Interventions and outcomes |
|---|---|---|---|
| Winkel (1989) Netherlands | RCT SMS = 3 | 115 victims of burglary: 58 experimental group 57 control group (randomly assigned) | Presents and seeks to test a *re-contact* model of responses to crime victimization. Devised a 3-day training programme for police, enabling them to provide sessions of emotional, informational and practical support to victims. This took place sometime after the burglary ("victim re-contact"). Its impact was tested with an experimental group; the control group did not take part. This re-contact was perceived as very useful in almost all cases, but its impact varied according to victim characteristics, such as level of stress in the preceding year and severity of reaction to the burglary. For some participants, the police visits had a negative effect |
| Winkel (1991) Netherlands | RCT SMS = 5 | 250 victims of burglary over an 18-month period from 3 municipalities 92 experimental group 158 control group (randomly assigned) | Burglary victims in the experimental group were visited on a series of occasions by two uniformed police officers who provided extensive information on burglary, crime prevention and increased safety. The control group received no visits. The first group were more satisfied with police action, saw police more positively and were more willing to take preventive action to reduce burglary recurring. However, the groups did not differ on fear of crime. Women and victims with an external risk orientation became more fearful, while men and victims with internal risk orientation became less fearful. However there was no evidence of "generalization", meaning that the effect of police communication would be to induce people to take extreme measures to protect themselves and their property |

(continued)

**Table 10.3** (continued)

| Study: author(s), (date), country | Design and SMS | Samples/data sources | Interventions and outcomes |
|---|---|---|---|
| Winkel and Vrij (1993) Netherlands | Case-control comparison of police areas SMS = 3 | 53 police officers Burglary victims: 64 in experimental area 101 in control area | Tested a specially designed intervention to help victims cope with burglary, improve perceptions of police and support crime prevention. Two police forces served as experimental and control areas, respectively. In the former, two officers visited a victim's home within half an hour of a call to police; one focused on evidence gathering, while the other focused on the victim. Training was provided for these roles. Measured police- and victim-related variables, for the latter including capacities for emotion-focused and problem-solving coping. Victims in the experimental area had more favourable attitudes to police, felt more protected against burglary and showed a stronger belief in being able to take preventive measures (problem-solving) |
| Young et al. (2008) USA | Survey of victims' responses SMS = n/a | Survey participants were 91 police officers of whom 73 had called the Crisis Team in the period 2000–2007, from 285 potential 25 victims from 190 who were contacted | Evaluation of a police-based Crisis Team which involved on-scene counselling by volunteer mental health professionals who travelled in police cars on Friday and Saturday nights (7:00 pm to 2:00 am). Calls were made for a wide range of usually serious crimes, and over the study period, the range of crimes gradually extended. A total of 768 Crisis Team calls made during the study period was analysed. Ninety-four percent of responding officers wanted the department to retain the Crisis Team; victims also regarded it as very helpful. Descriptions of the service were predominantly positive but there were also some critical comments. However, the overall low rate of response makes it difficult to draw conclusions about its value |

This appears to produce mixed results as some victims feel reassured, but others worry that such visits signify that the police have become concerned that crime is rising in their area. Some studies focused on notification arrangements – procedures by which police keep victims updated concerning the progress of cases through the courts (Irazola et al., 2015); outcome evaluation however shows no clear effects of these arrangements. Finally, there was evidence for the effectiveness of the Sexual Assault Nurse Examiners (SANE) programme, which was developed by the nursing profession in the USA in the 1970s and subsequently spread to many locations in the 1990s (Campbell et al., 2012b). Nursing staff were given additional training to work with victims of rape, provide emotional support, make contact with other services and collect evidence that may be useful in prosecution. Several positive effects have been found as a result of the involvement of these professionals in examining victims after sexual assaults.

### *10.7.2 Access to Community Resources (17 Studies)*

Table 10.4 shows studies placed under this heading which included the following approaches: advocacy, helplines, support services and other efforts to link crime victims to a range of community resources through brokerage of services. Some studies compared the effectiveness of these kinds of provision with or without a coordinated strategy for linking them together. Advocacy was defined by Bell and Goodman (2001) as having four components: (a) assistance in personal safety planning, (b) provision of emotional support, (c) provision of information about access to community resources and (d) providing information about and accompanying an individual through the legal process.

There is evidence that advocacy, hotline and other community services can be both highly valued by victims and may have measurable effects. However, a key study in this area (Bennett et al., 2004) had a relatively weak methodology, and a later study obtained more varied outcomes (Bennett & O'Brien, 2007).

Structured, multi-agency, community interventions (e.g. ECARE, for victimized older adults) or coordinated community responses combining police, legal, health and social care components, usually have a lead agency which acts as a gatekeeper or plays a pivotal brokerage role in making contact with other services. Individual counselling provided by independent victim support agencies often formed part of these networks of services: it was usually relatively brief (one to two sessions) but sometimes entailed a longer series of contacts.

**Table 10.4** Information from included studies: accessing community resources

| Study: author(s), (date), country | Design and SMS | Samples/data sources | Interventions and outcomes |
|---|---|---|---|
| Bell and Goodman (2001) USA | Pre-post single-cohort design SMS = 2 | 81 women victims of IPV: 22 in advocacy group 59 in comparison group 70.4% attended follow-up at 6 weeks | Evaluation of a victim advocacy service provided through two law schools. Used structured measures of depression, perceived emotional support and levels of physical and psychological abuse and re-abuse (including revised Conflict Tactics Scales). Members of both groups showed improvement on most measures, with some evidence of differential effects favouring the advocacy condition: there were significantly lower rates of psychological and physical re-abuse amongst women in the advocacy condition. But there was significantly higher attrition in the comparison group than in the advocacy group |
| Bennett et al. (2004) USA | Survey and pre-post designs SMS = 2 | 5260 women victims of domestic violence across 54 programmes in Illinois; 638 women in pre-post counselling study | Evaluation containing two components: (a) a survey of service users' responses regarding five areas of service: hotline, brief advocacy, extended advocacy, shelter and counselling. Self-ratings of service effects across a series of specially constructed scales were uniformly positive and very high (close to maximum on almost all scales). (b) Computed a composite Counselling Outcomes Index for responses to counselling sessions and found a highly significant pre-post difference, modest effect size of 0.25 |
| Bennett and O'Brien (2007) | Pre-to-post, repeated measures SMS = 2 | Women victims of IPV attending 4 agencies: 255 at programme entry 128 at 4–6 months later | Described as a demonstration project evaluating "integrated service models" or coordinated multi-agency arrangements for women with multiple problems: as victims of IPV who also had had previous treatment for substance/alcohol abuse problems. Collected self-report data on victim experience, ability to manage IPV and substance use. On average women received 22.2 counselling sessions within helping agencies. From baseline to follow-up, there were a small but significant reduction in abuse, increase in reported self-efficacy and large reduction in substance use. There were however some differences between those who did and those who did not complete follow-up |

(continued)

**Table 10.4** (continued)

| Study: author(s), (date), country | Design and SMS | Samples/data sources | Interventions and outcomes |
|---|---|---|---|
| Campbell et al. (2001) USA | Community sample survey SMS = n/a | 102 female victims of rape recruited via a community survey | Retrospective open community survey of victims of rape asking them to describe their experiences of services since the crime incident, which had occurred on average 8.25 years earlier. Data were collected regarding five possible sources of help: legal, medical, mental health, rape crisis centres and religious communities. Participants were interviewed for an average of 2.27 hours. They rated how different agencies helped them and completed an adapted health inventory. Few variables were shown to differentiate those who sought help from different sources. Those raped by strangers were more likely to report the offence to the police. The study reports comparisons between reports of how helpful different agencies were considered to be. Analysis showed that those whose cases were not prosecuted reported higher rates of physical and psychological distress |
| Campbell et al. (2004) USA | Survey of evaluation processes SMS = n/a | 20 victim services and rape prevention programmes in Michigan | Describes the Sexual Assault and Rape Prevention (SARP) project and the "empowerment evaluation" model and presents some data from the latter. Sets out the phases of the evaluation model and the eight components of a structured interview for collecting data from stakeholders (= programme staff). Used a multi-method approach to data collection including staff ratings of training they had received in evaluation from the SARP team. Presents data on the extent to which projects were in the process of being evaluated by applying the model. Follow-up interviews after 1 year found that 90% of victim services programmes were evaluating their work, though only three were combined process and outcome evaluations |

(continued)

**Table 10.4** (continued)

| Study: author(s), (date), country | Design and SMS | Samples/data sources | Interventions and outcomes |
|---|---|---|---|
| DePrince et al. (2012) USA | Longitudinal RCT with intent-to-treat analysis SMS = 5 | 236 women abused by partners (reported to police) in 2 groups at 0, 6 and 12 months: Outreach condition: 79 → 70 → 66 Referral condition: 50 → 40 → 39 | Evaluative comparison of two programmes with the same goal but different components: (a) a confidential outreach service incorporating community-coordinated victim advocacy services and (b) referral via non-confidential system-based criminal justice advocates to community agencies. Several psychometric assessments were administered to participants at three time points. Results showed outreach led to reductions in depression, fear and PTSD symptoms that remained at follow-up. Referral led to larger short-term gains but then reversal to intermediate levels of problems. The two conditions led to similar results in ethnic minority women but divergent results for white women: Outreach showed better trends for both. There were no group differences in reports of subsequent safety (violent events) |
| Dillenburger et al. (2008) UK | Time-series study of single cohort SMS = 2 | 75 (29 men, 46 women) victims of traumatic events linked to community violence in Northern Ireland | Administered several structured questionnaires and one specially designed for the context of the NI troubles. These were administered on four occasions each 3–4 months apart. Comparisons were made between users of different mental health, alternative therapy or other community services, though the majority did not access any. The numbers declined sharply at successive measurement points (75 → 25 → 20 → 13). The high attrition makes it difficult to draw any firm conclusions |
| Gibbs et al. (2015) USA | Survey of needs and usage SMS = n/a | 201 young people (age < 18) victims of sexual trafficking seen across 3 agencies | Evaluated the uptake and use of three services for victims of sexual trafficking. Intake assessments showed high levels of needs across a wide range of problem areas. Results reported consist only of levels of service received according to ten main areas of need, including support or crisis intervention, food or clothing, safety planning, mental healthcare, sexual healthcare, education, family reunification, assistance with benefits, employment/ vocational assistance and housing. It was noted that the highest rates of service utilization occurred where the appropriate help was provided on-site (where young people were located) |

(continued)

**Table 10.4** (continued)

| Study: author(s), (date), country | Design and SMS | Samples/data sources | Interventions and outcomes |
|---|---|---|---|
| Madoc-Jones and Roscoe (2010) UK | Qualitative study SMS = n/a | Face-to-face or telephone interviews with 13 women victims of domestic abuse | A qualitative study of women victims whose abusing partners were attending a probation-run programme for domestic abuse perpetrators (the Integrated Domestic Abuse Programme (IDAP))[a]. In conjunction with this, women were offered services concerned with personal safety, and the objective of the research was to explore their perceptions of them. Using a grounded theory approach, this generated key themes from the interview material. Women evaluated services offered to them very positively, having at first felt abandoned by the criminal justice system. Key issues they identified included need for support, victim-focused contact, empathy, negative experiences of criminal justice and specific challenges that arose for women living in rural communities |
| Part (2006) UK | Survey of participant feedback SMS = n/a | Families experiencing DA in Tayside, Scotland: 37 respondents to a survey questionnaire and some were also interviewed | Describes and evaluates a DA support project developed by police and Barnardo's. Rejected use of term "victim". 259 women, 13 men and 446 children were seen in the project but evaluation was based on smaller numbers. DA had occurred over extended periods. Results showed a wide range of help was received (information and support of several kinds) and participant ratings and comments suggested high levels of satisfaction. Services were made available over lengthy periods: exact time is not clear but one respondent mentions 15 months |

(continued)

**Table 10.4** (continued)

| Study: author(s), (date), country | Design and SMS | Samples/data sources | Interventions and outcomes |
|---|---|---|---|
| Smith et al. (1985), Cook et al. (1986) USA | Quasi-experimental SMS = 4 | 323 victims of a variety of crimes including assault, sexual assault, domestic assault, robbery or burglary:<br>109: crisis intervention<br>114: delayed intervention<br>100: no services<br>258 followed up 4–6 months later | A large-scale study with two components, an evaluation of victim services and an investigation of the social-psychological effects of victimization. For the former, three groups were compared: those who received crisis intervention, those who received delayed services and others who received no formal services. Interviews were also conducted with police officers and prosecutors (attorneys). Victim interviews covered several areas concerning their reactions and included use of psychometric assessments and perceptions of police and other services. Participants regarded the victim services in very positive terms and described them as very helpful and praised the police. All groups showed reduced anxiety and stress at follow-up, and there were no differences between them in measured anxiety or stress levels. Levels of fear of crime did not reduce in any group. It was considered that the level of trauma following a crime was largely influenced by its severity and the groups were not matched with reference to this: crisis intervention was most often requested for the most traumatized group. Severity of reaction was also correlated with stress levels in the year preceding victimization. Police and attorney views also expressed positive views of the services, but the services nevertheless remained very under-utilized |
| Sullivan and Bybee (1999) USA | RCT SMS = 5 | 278 women victims of domestic abuse | Evaluation of the effectiveness of a 10-week community-based advocacy programme provided to women following shelter residence. Trained advocates provided individual session to women, enabling them to access community resources. Women were interviewed at 6 time points over the 2-year project period, with a very low rate of attrition (5%). Rates of physical violence, psychological abuse and depression all decreased significantly, and quality of life and social support ratings all improved significantly |

(continued)

**Table 10.4** (continued)

| Study: author(s), (date), country | Design and SMS | Samples/data sources | Interventions and outcomes |
|---|---|---|---|
| Sullivan et al. (2002) USA | Longitudinal experimental SMS = 5 | 80 female victims of domestic abuse 80 children | Long-term evaluation of an advocacy intervention and its effectiveness for battered women and for their children (age range 7–11). The intervention involved a mean of 8.95 hours of advocacy per week over 16 weeks for mothers and a support and education group for children. Project had high retention rates. Effects on mothers' well-being over time were significant for depression and self-esteem and marginally significant for quality of life. Some variables for children showed significant change, while others did not |
| Tutty (1996) Canada | Exploratory research with some pre-post data SMS = 2 | 60 women who left abusive partners and were followed up after shelter residence Interviews with 31 women Pre- and post-test measures with 28 women | Evaluation of two post-shelter follow-up programmes, one in a small town and one in a large city. Women completed measures of social support, stress/coping and self-esteem on entry and after 3 months. There were significant changes on scales for appraisal support (availability of someone to talk to) and self-esteem (completed by 12 women only) but none on other scales. Workers rated participants as having changed far more. Analysis of interviews showed areas of main concern to the women and their description of the support they had received. The amount of contact time with staff is not reported |
| Wasco et al. (2004) USA | Survey of service users + pre-post analysis SMS = n/a | A total of 771 adult women provided with services following sexual assault at 1 of 33 programmes in Illinois | Evaluated three kinds of services, a crisis hotline (259 users), advocacy (281 users) and counselling (231 users), using self-report survey methods. A majority of participants (50.9% to 79.4%) responded that they had gained a lot of information, support and help in making decisions via hotline and advocacy services. Also, a pre-to-post study of 76 counselling clients (usually involving >10 sessions) showed significant gains on all self-report scales and on reduced symptoms of PTSD. However, only a proportion of the prospective participants responded to the survey |

(continued)

**Table 10.4** (continued)

| Study: author(s), (date), country | Design and SMS | Samples/data sources | Interventions and outcomes |
|---|---|---|---|
| Zweig et al. (2002) USA | Telephone interview survey SMS = n/a | 20 agencies from a larger number participating in a national evaluation study | Focused on a small proportion of 4433 programmes across the USA that provide services to women victims facing multiple barriers (e.g. substance abuse, mental illness, learning disability, prostitution) in addition to having been victims of violent/sexual assault. The study reports different ways in which those barriers were addressed in the responding agencies, which included advocacy, substance abuse/mental health treatment, problem-specific support, outreach services, staff training and inter-agency collaboration (30% with law enforcement). However, only 55% reported that collaborations were successful, and most reported the weakest link was criminal justice. The paper documents perceived reasons for this |
| Zweig et al. (2003) USA | Community survey SMS = n/a | 1509 women using victim services following sexual or domestic violence in 26 communities across 8 states: 890 victim service users 619 randomly selected community sample | Large-scale study collecting data from multiple sites. It is not clear how this study relates to the work described in Zweig et al. (2002). But this report refers to 1936 projects focused on victim services, run by nonprofit agencies. There were two phases to the project: a survey of representatives from victim programmes and an evaluative study with victims themselves, addressing the additional question of whether community coordination enhances service effects. Female victims were recruited from two groups, "help seekers" (users of victim services) and a wider community sample. Several kinds of information were collected through a lengthy survey instrument. The report gives detail analysis of women's knowledge of services and how they find out about them and what factors affect their use of them. A model was developed of how to predict service outcomes. Data are reported on the perceived helpfulness of different services, based on rating scales used in telephone interviews. Analysis demonstrated that women benefitted from the services and the benefit increased when the provider agencies worked together and in conjunction with the legal system. Such coordination also increased the likelihood of perpetrators being arrested and convicted |

[a]The IDAP programme has demonstrated effectiveness in reducing recidivism of domestic violence perpetrators (Bloomfield & Dixon, 2015)

### 10.7.3 Therapeutic Interventions (21 Studies)

Table 10.5 shows studies placed under this heading which included a variety of approaches. This includes studies of counselling, debriefing, psycho-education and psychological therapies mainly employing cognitive-behavioural approaches and methods.

*Counselling* is conceptualized here as a process of helping troubled individuals by developing a trusting relationship with them and enabling them to harness their own personal resources to address and, if possible, overcome their difficulties. *Debriefing*, in contrast, is an intervention provided soon after a traumatic event in which the victim or witness is asked to recall and describe the event in some detail. Somewhat different again, *psycho-education* is an intervention with a partly educational and partly therapeutic focus, to enable people in distress or with significant challenges in their lives to acquire information or skills to enable them to solve their problems.

*Cognitive-behavioural therapies* or variants of them are usually provided for individuals with higher levels of distress and in some cases with diagnostic features of post-traumatic stress disorder (PTSD). These approaches ranged from more behaviourist, learning-based interventions such as prolonged exposure to others that focused more on patterns of thinking, such as self-instructional training, cognitive processing therapy or Eye Movement Desensitization and Reprocessing (EMDR), designed to alleviate depression, anxiety and symptoms of traumatic stress.

Studies that were located of counselling and therapy with crime victims can be divided into two broad groups. One is based on evaluations of brief or short-term services offered to victims, usually of less serious crimes and entailing supportive counselling or a similar approach, provided by voluntary or other community-based organizations. The other includes interventions that are more often provided for victims of serious sexual or other violent crimes, who are more severely affected, and which involved some form of structured psychological therapy. These involve a larger number of sessions and are provided by healthcare agencies. Evaluation of the latter is usually of a more a formalized nature, involving stronger designs and larger samples.

Apart from the types of studies included here, there are also evaluation studies of longer-term treatment provided for children who have been sexually abused, but those children are not usually seen by victim services, and services for them are not contracted by Police and Crime Commissioners but provided by mental healthcare professionals usually working in the NHS (or their equivalents in other countries). As noted earlier, while one review of this field was included in the set of previous reviews (Price et al., 2001), individual studies in this area were not retained in the present review.

**Table 10.5** Information from included studies: therapeutic interventions for victims of crime

| Study: author(s), (date), country | Design and SMS | Samples/data sources | Interventions and outcomes |
|---|---|---|---|
| Brownell and Heiser (2006) Canada | Pilot RCT SMS = 5 | 15 female older adult victims of family mistreatment: 9 intervention group 6 control group | Evaluated a psycho-educational support group for older adult victims provided in a shelter programme in Manitoba. The group comprised eight 2-hour weekly sessions. Employed structured assessments of depression, locus of control, self-esteem, social support, anxiety and guilt. Participants had similar characteristics at the outset but there were no differences obtained at post-test. Authors questioned the effectiveness of the psycho-educational approach with this group but also considered other factors |
| Davis (1987) USA | RCT SMS = 5 | Victims referred by police in 8 New York precincts 249 pre-test, 181 post-test Victims of burglary (39%), robbery (34%), assault (24%) and rape (2%) | Evaluation of three kinds of treatment: crisis intervention with brief counselling, or with cognitive restructuring; material assistance; plus a "no services" condition. Counselling consisted of one session only. Used structured assessments (Symptom Check-List-90, Affect Balance Scale, the Impact of Events Scale) and ratings of numbers of problems. Victims improved across all four conditions (with or without treatment), and there were no pre-post between-group differences on any of the scores |
| Echeburúa et al. (1997) Spain | Group comparison design SMS = 3 | 20 female victims of sexual assault | Comparison of two types of therapy for PTSD for victims of sexual aggression: exposure with cognitive restructuring and relaxation training. Follow-up at 1, 3, 6 and 12 months. No untreated control. There was a significantly greater change amongst those in the exposure/restructuring condition; all became symptom-free at follow-up ("disappearance of PTSD"). This was found across all measures at all stages of the study |

(continued)

**Table 10.5** (continued)

| Study: author(s), (date), country | Design and SMS | Samples/data sources | Interventions and outcomes |
|---|---|---|---|
| Foa et al. (1991) USA | RCT SMS = 5 | 45 female victims of rape or attempted rape suffering from PTSD | Clinical experiment with four conditions: stress inoculation training, PE, supportive counselling and waiting-list control group. All data collection was blind. Groups were followed up for 3.5 months. There were positive changes (reductions in PTSD) over time across all groups, strongest for stress inoculation training in the short term but for PE in the longer term. Both were more effective than supportive counselling |
| Foa et al. (1995) USA | Group quasi-experimental comparison SMS = 4 | 20 female assault victims: 10 brief prevention programme and 10 assessment controls. Tested at pre-, post- and 5-month points | Designed and evaluated a brief prevention programme to arrest the development of PTSD. Tested with matched group allotted to an assessment-only condition, using structured measures and self-report ratings of distress and symptom severity. Both groups improved, but there were larger changes in the brief prevention programme than the assessment controls condition, but they were non-significant given low sample size |
| Foa et al. (1999) USA | RCT SMS = 5 | 96 female assault victims meeting PTSD criteria assigned to 4 conditions: given pre- and post-test, 3-, 6 + 12-month follow-up | Experimental comparison of four conditions: PE, self-instructional training, combined treatment and waiting-list control. Evaluated using structured psychometric and self-report data. All treatments reduced PTSD symptom severity but no change observed in control group. Measured gains were maintained at follow-up for three treatment groups. Largest effect sizes were for PE on all measures |

(continued)

**Table 10.5** (continued)

| Study: author(s), (date), country | Design and SMS | Samples/data sources | Interventions and outcomes |
|---|---|---|---|
| Foa et al. (2006) USA | RCT<br>SMS = 5 | 90 female victims of assault (57 sexual, 33 non-sexual); all met criteria for PTSD<br>Pre-test, post-test, 3- and 9.5-month follow-up | Experimental evaluation of brief CBT, an assessment-only condition and structured counselling (each four sessions). Assessment and evaluation (blind) used established clinician-administered interviews and validated self-report measures. Trends varied slightly over time but at final follow-up there were no significant differences between the groups. Some participants were also diagnosed with antisocial personality disorder, but this bore no relation to outcomes |
| Howard et al. (2003) USA | Group comparison<br>SMS = 3 | 500 female victims:<br>(a) 357 victims of battery<br>(b) 143 victims of rape and battery | Compared the effects of counselling on two groups of women victims seen across 54 domestic violence agencies. Measures were self-report ratings of self-blame, self-efficacy, control and social support. Group (b) had lower scores at both pre- and post-test. Both groups showed significant improvement through counselling, group (b) showing the largest change. Group (b) however had significantly more sessions of counselling than (a) |
| Ironson et al. (2002) USA | RCT<br>SMS = 5 | 22 patients (17 women, 5 men) in a specialized trauma clinic; 19 direct victims of sexual or violent assault, 3 indirect. Randomly allocated to therapy groups | Comparison between EMDR and PE as treatments for PTSD. Treatment consisted of six sessions. Follow-up was 3 months later. There was higher dropout in PE. Members of both groups showed significant improvement at both post-test and 3 months, but symptom reduction happened faster with EMDR. However, data collection was not blind; the PE group had higher clinical scores at pre-test; there was no untreated control group |

(continued)

**Table 10.5** (continued)

| Study: author(s), (date), country | Design and SMS | Samples/data sources | Interventions and outcomes |
|---|---|---|---|
| Johnson et al. (2011) USA | Pilot RCT (developmental trial) SMS = 5 | Women with IPV-related PTSD residing in battered women's shelters: 35 experimental 35 standard control | Tested the feasibility and efficacy of an intervention, Helping to Overcome PTSD through Empowerment, a series of up to 12 biweekly CBT-based sessions provided in a shelter. Follow-up at 1 week and 3 and 6 months. Used Conflict Tactics Scales and measures of PTSD symptoms, depression, empowerment, support and other variables. Attrition was very low. Both groups showed reduction in PTSD; the Helping to Overcome PTSD through Empowerment group reported significantly less abuse at follow-up and also lower depression and higher empowerment. Results were better for those who attended at least five sessions of the Helping to Overcome PTSD through Empowerment programme |
| Maguire and Corbett (1987) UK | Group comparison SMS = 3 | Compared 26 victims who were visited by staff of VSS with 26 who were not. Groups matched on key variables but no statistical controls | Brief counselling visits by Victim Support Services staff. At 3–6 weeks after the offence, there were small but consistent group differences noted on self-reported change in how much the offence still affected them, in feeling frightened or at a low point, in scores on the General Health Questionnaire and on expression of punitive attitudes towards offenders and willingness to take part in mediation. No statistical tests reported |
| Mariam et al. (2015) USA | Pre-to-post intervention comparison SMS = 2 | 175 adult victims of elder abuse (all age > 55, mean age 79), amongst which: 26 given brief intervention 47 given full intervention | Evaluation of the Eliciting Change in At-Risk Elders programme designed to reduce risk of elder abuse for vulnerable older adults. Results are only reported pre-post for what was defined as the "full intervention" group. There were a significant improvement in working alliance, significant reduction in overall risk factors and progression in stages of change. However, data were based on assessments of outreach workers |

(continued)

**Table 10.5** (continued)

| Study: author(s), (date), country | Design and SMS | Samples/data sources | Interventions and outcomes |
|---|---|---|---|
| McNamara et al. (2008) | Pre-to-post intervention design<br>SMS = 2 | 121 women in a domestic violence shelter (41 who completed all measures) | Evaluation of short-term counselling. Hypothesized that women who received at least three sessions would benefit. Evaluated using measures of distress, relationships, Life Coping Inventory given at the time of four counselling sessions and participant feedback afterwards. There were significant changes across four time points, and 68% of women achieved clinically meaningful change scores; there was also a high degree of satisfaction with services. However only 41 women completed all assessments |
| Resick et al. (1988)<br>USA | Group comparison<br>SMS = 3 | 45 victims of rape divided into 4 groups:<br>12 stress inoculation<br>13 assertion training<br>7 supportive therapy<br>13 waiting-list control<br>37 completed treatment | A small-scale pilot experimental trial with non-equivalent groups. Each intervention involved six 2-hour sessions, with follow-up at 3 and 6 months. Evaluated using self-report psychometric scales. However, no differences were found between the effects of the three treatment conditions, and it is not stated whether any difference was observed between them and the waiting-list control condition at post-test or at either of the follow-up points |
| Resick and Schnicke (1992)<br>USA | Quasi-experimental design<br>SMS = 4 | Victims of rape:<br>19 therapeutic CPT<br>20 waiting-list control<br>3- and 6-month follow-up | First of a series of publications testing CPT, developed by the authors for the treatment of PTSD in victims of rape, delivered in group format using a specially prepared written manual. Evaluated by comparison with untreated comparison group, using self-report psychometric scales. The CPT groups showed substantial and significant reductions in PTSD symptoms and other distress measures, maintained at 6 months. Almost all women met criteria for PTSD pre-treatment, but at post-treatment none did. It is stated that there was no similar improvement in the control group, but data on this are only presented for one measure, the Symptom Check-List-90 (SCL-90) |

(continued)

**Table 10.5** (continued)

| Study: author(s), (date), country | Design and SMS | Samples/data sources | Interventions and outcomes |
|---|---|---|---|
| Resick et al. (2002) USA | RCT with intent-to-treat analysis SMS = 5 | 171 female rape victims 121 completers: 41 CPT 40 PE 40 attention control | An experimental trial of CPT compared to another therapy, PE and a minimal attention condition as a control group. Assessed using structured interviews with inter-rater reliability, plus structured psychometric inventories: 3- and 9-month follow-up. Waiting-list group were phoned every 2 weeks. Both treatment groups showed similar significant change at post-treatment, maintained to follow-up, with moderate to large effect sizes compared to the minimal attention condition. No such change was observed in the minimal attention condition |
| Resick et al. (2008) USA | RCT with intent-to-treat analysis SMS = 5 | Community sample of women sexually or physically assaulted, meeting criteria for PTSD: 53 CPT 47 CPT-cognitive only 50 "written accounts" | A type of research called a *dismantling* study, to examine which components of a therapy were the most prominent or active in bringing about change. Compared CPT with two variants of it, one focusing only on written accounts of traumatic events and the other excluding such accounts and containing cognitive therapy methods alone. All therapies consisted of 12 sessions (2 per week for 6 weeks). Used structured interviews and psychometric assessments for assessment and evaluation. All forms of the intervention were equally successful in reducing PTSD symptoms and other symptoms of distress at post-test and 6-month follow-up. However, the speed of change during therapy was faster than for written accounts |
| Resick et al. (2012) USA | RCT with intent-to-treat analysis SMS = 5 | Follow-up of participants in the Resick et al. (2002) study (see above): 63 CPT (46 completers) 63 PE (44 completers) | Long-term follow-up evaluation of individuals who had received CPT, 5–10 years (mean = 6) after the original study. Because follow-up time varied across individuals, it was factored in as a variable in the analyses. Twelve percent of the groups had some other treatment for trauma in the intervening period. There was a slight advantage for PE over CPT at follow-up (17.5% versus 22.2% still suffering from PTSD). Other results were more mixed |

(continued)

**Table 10.5** (continued)

| Study: author(s), (date), country | Design and SMS | Samples/data sources | Interventions and outcomes |
|---|---|---|---|
| Rose et al. (1999) UK | RCT SMS = 5 | 157 victims, mainly (94%) of physical assault: Education: 52 Education + debriefing: 54 Assessment only: 51 (control group) 138 at 6-month follow-up 92 at 11-month follow-up | Tested the effectiveness of debriefing on the experience of trauma amongst victims of crime. One group was assessed only and acted as controls; a second group had a 30-minute educational session; a third had education plus a 1-hour psychological debriefing session. The latter entailed asking for a narrative account of reactions to the crime and to express the feelings experienced. Equal proportions were lost to follow-up across groups. Used structured psychometric assessments of depression and post-traumatic stress. There was no evidence of any significant impact of debriefing on any of the outcome measures |
| Rothbaum (1997) USA | RCT SMS = 5 | 21 adult female victims of rape: 10 treatment (EMDR) 11 waiting-list control 3-month follow-up Control group given EMDR in second phase | EMDR was compared with waiting-list control group. EMDR involved assessment plus three weekly sessions of 90 minutes. Several structured psychometrics were used to monitor progress and outcomes, with "blind" administration. EMDR participants improved more from pre- to post-test on PTSD and depression scores, but differences on general anxiety were non-significant. However, at post-test only one EMDR participant met criteria for PTSD, while 88% of the control group did so. Gains were maintained at follow-up. Waiting-list controls then received EMDR and were followed for 3 months showing improvement. However, only four of the group were available at follow-up |

(continued)

**Table 10.5** (continued)

| Study: author(s), (date), country | Design and SMS | Samples/data sources | Interventions and outcomes |
|---|---|---|---|
| Tutty et al. (1993) Canada | Pre-post group evaluation SMS = 2 | 76 women IPV victims seen before and after 12 support groups and at 6-month follow-up | Evaluation of the Family Violence Coordinated Treatment Program in Waterloo, Ontario. Support groups entailed 10–12 sessions of 2–3 hours each. Psycho-educational model with future planning. Employed a series of psychometric and self-rating scales on 11 variables. Positive pre-to-post change was found on locus of control, self-esteem, "belonging support", lower stress, less stereotyped role beliefs, perceptions of marital relations, less controlling behaviour, reductions in reported physical abuse and verbal and physical abuse components of the Conflict Tactics Scale. A small number of dependent variables showed no change. Thirty-two women who attended follow-up showed maintenance of gains, but they had shown better outcomes at post-test, and the remainder did not attend |

*CPT* cognitive processing therapy, *EMDR* Eye Movement Desensitization and Reprocessing, *IPV* intimate partner violence, *SMS* Maryland Scientific Methods Scores

## 10.7.4 Economic Evaluation: Cost-Effectiveness

Only one study was found that reported an economic analysis of the provision of services to crime victims, but this was based in a healthcare setting and employed models used in the econometric evaluation of the relationship between health benefits and the investments needed to obtain them. This involves applying formulae used in other areas of health service planning. Details of the study by Norman et al. (2010) are shown in Table 10.6. The large study by Smith et al. (1985; Cook et al., 1986; see Table 10.4) also reported unit costs for service provision, but the data cannot be interpreted as some users of the same services were not crime victims as the agencies also provided family and neighbourhood dispute resolution services, and the other information needed for conducting a cost-effectiveness study is not reported.

**Table 10.6** Cost-effectiveness study

| Study: author(s), (date), country | Design and SMS | Samples/data sources | Interventions and outcomes |
|---|---|---|---|
| Norman et al. (2010) UK | Cost-effectiveness study SMS = n/a | Four general practice sites in London (one control, three experimental), testing a GP-based intervention Prevention of Domestic Violence | Evaluation of cost-effectiveness using a complex mathematical model (Markov model). Calculated the costs of a GP referring a female patient thought to be experiencing IPV for appropriate help and the costs of providing that help, as compared to not doing so, based on assumptions about the rates of undiscovered IPV. Tested in three GP clinics, estimated that the incremental cost-effectiveness ratio for making such assessments and referrals per quality-adjusted life year was £2450, considerably below what is regarded as a standard threshold of £30,000 per annum |

## 10.8 Discussion

The largest single group of studies that were retained for full review were of the effects on victims of serious physical or sexual assaults, including rape, and domestic/intimate partner violence. There were three studies of burglary, all from the Netherlands (Winkel, 1989, 1991; Winkel & Vrij, 1993), but all done over 20 years ago. A few studies included victims of other crimes such as robbery (Davis, 1987; Rosenbaum, 1987; Smith et al., 1985), but as can be seen, that research too was done some time ago. Only one study was found of services for victims of stalking, but was in German and had to be excluded, though an English abstract indicated some positive effects (Gallas et al., 2009).

Overall, on the basis of the evidence collected here, several conclusions can be offered, but they can only partially answer the questions that were set for the review. The studies reported a wide range of outcomes, and the general trend of this research supports the expectation that it is possible to provide a number of kinds of effective assistance and support to victims of crime. However, there were some marked contrasts and variations in the findings obtained. Some approaches were found to be only minimally helpful and a few may even be counterproductive, and if we contemplate the full scope of the types of work located in this review, a vivid picture appears of the efforts that have been made to address the problems faced by crime victims. On the other hand, if we apply strict criteria and focus on only those research studies that reported well-designed trials of interventions to evaluate their effectiveness, the remaining batch of studies becomes fairly sparse.

### 10.8.1 Strengths and Limitations

The present review like any work of its kind has some limitations.

#### 10.8.1.1 Literature Search

An unusually large number of studies were located in an unpublished review (Marandos, 2005), reference to which was first discovered via a review protocol for a planned study that was not then completed. At a later stage, some studies were located on a website concerned with cognitive processing therapy, a type of therapy devised for the treatment of PTSD by Dr Patricia Resick, a well-established researcher in that field. That a sizeable proportion of the located studies were not found through direct searches raises the possibility that other relevant studies may exist that have not been located and suggests there may have been inadequacies in the search strategy, and as a result the review may be incomplete. However, given the relatively dispersed nature of the located studies, it seems unlikely that there would be a large number of missing studies. There are few examples of rolling research programmes. The only ones that emerged were the work of Dr Patricia Resick and her group on cognitive processing therapy, that of Dr Rebecca Campbell and her group on Sexual Assault Nurse Examiners (SANE) and, some years earlier, that of Dr Edna Foa and her colleagues on therapies for trauma symptoms following rape. In addition, it is possible that the inclusion criteria were too wide, in that some studies were retained that consisted mainly of victim or practitioner feedback on perceptions of a service, using surveys or qualitative methodology, rather than more formal evaluations employing rigorous research designs.

#### 10.8.1.2 Inclusion/Exclusion Decisions

Some decisions as to inclusion or exclusion were straightforward and easy to make. Studies of victims attending for counselling sessions that produced only descriptive data were excluded as they contained no evaluative information (e.g. King & Woollett, 1997), whereas studies that contained outcome data analysis were definitively included (e.g. Davis, 1987). Other cases however were more marginal. Where studies contained information on the delivery of services, they were retained, even if they did not report outcomes, as they were considered to be useful as process evaluations (e.g. Campbell et al., 2008). Considerable thought had to be given when deciding to include some studies that were eventually retained (Campbell et al., 2004, 2012a; Madoc-Jones et al., 2015; Rosenbaum, 1987). The single study that provided cost-effectiveness estimates was also retained (Norman et al., 2010). On the other hand, where studies reported perceptions of police or court processes (e.g. a study by Laxminarayan et al. (2012) which compared such procedures in the Netherlands and Australia), they were discounted. Similarly studies which reported analysis of police decision-making as to whether victims should receive specific forms of assistance, *prior to* any such services being received, were also excluded (e.g. Apsler et al., 2003).

#### 10.8.1.3 Methodological Quality

A third limitation arose from the weakness of primary research studies themselves. There is considerable heterogeneity amongst the located studies in terms of the issues they addressed, and the methodology they adopted, which was often relatively weak. This results in two related difficulties, one of attempting to draw conclusions from evaluations of limited quality and another of there being few examples of consolidated work, i.e. where there are several interconnected projects allowing accumulation of findings. These two difficulties limit the confidence with which conclusions can be drawn. In addition, some studies, even when randomized trials, had very small sample sizes and comparatively short follow-up periods (often only 3 months). Thus, even with satisfactory designs, studies sometimes offered limited scope for drawing more generalizable conclusions.

Almost all of the better-designed evaluations that were found dealt with the more serious problems of trauma and focus on psychological interventions delivered in mental health services. Inspection of the Maryland Scientific Methods Scores (SMS) showed a far higher proportion within this category obtaining a score of 5. By contrast, the studies which focused on more immediate responses to crime scenes, whether they were centred on victim requests for assistance or on innovative projects designed by police forces, had very varied methods of evaluation that were low in internal validity. That is, they were open to a risk of bias calling into question the status of reported results.

#### 10.8.1.4 Assessment and Evaluation

Another important aspect of the work included here is the basis on which researchers draw conclusions about the effectiveness of services they evaluate. In Tables 10.3, 10.4, and 10.5, there is frequent reference to assessments employed with participants in this field of research. They are of three main kinds. In some studies, researchers devised their own quite elaborate data collection methods, often extensive semi-structured interview schedules, covering many areas of people's lives, which required training for their administration (sometimes done face-to-face, but in other studies by telephone). Some authors attached them as appendices to project reports, but they are often unique to specific study contexts and not really transportable for use elsewhere. In a second group, less formal self-report rating scales were used, covering a variety of subjective states including levels of distress, perceptions of help that was offered or attitudes to police or other agencies. However, it is often very difficult to be sure what can be concluded on the basis of these kinds of information. A third group consisted of standardized and what are regarded as well-established psychometric assessments, usually drawn from other areas of psychological or psychiatric research. Generally, these were used for the purpose of assessing symptoms before and after therapy. They included measures of anxiety, depression, substance use, coping skills, symptoms of PTSD and many other clinical variables. There are studies that include two or all three of these methods. A small number of studies used minimally structured, qualitative interviews, but these are typically employed in more exploratory or process research rather than for evaluating outcomes. But studies that employ methods in the third category are capable of generating more reliable and usable results than those in the two preceding categories.

## 10.9 Conclusions and Implications

Bearing in mind the above limitations, examination of the studies reviewed here does reveal some broad trends and patterns. Several key conclusions can be offered on the basis of the evidence that was located. First, debriefing for crime victims has been found to be ineffective and even potentially counterproductive and for some time has not been considered advisable for victims of any traumatic event. The only study that was located of its use with victims of crime did not yield positive results.

There is also some evidence that visits by the police to victims within a few weeks of a crime event can increase fear of crime, since although some people may be reassured, others appear to worry that the police have become concerned about crime in their area. Those studies were however done some years ago. There is a separate research literature on factors that influence fear of crime that it has not been possible to include in this review.

Counselling and several forms of individual and community support have been shown to produce benefits with a range of problems including crime victimization. Generally, victims are highly appreciative of the contacts that are made with them and are grateful that someone has made time available to listen to them. However, there is very little sound evidence that a single session or a small number of sessions provided to crime victims make a significant difference to their well-being or to their fear of crime.

The studies collected here do not provide sufficient information to inform commissioning decisions, without data on relative costs and benefits of different policy options. Only one study was found that reported an economic analysis, though in the area of general practice. It indicated, however, that earlier identification of victims of partner violence would likely be cost-effective. In that context, given the tentative nature of some of the findings obtained here, the present review formed part of the stimulus for a further review that was carried out for the regional Office of Police and Crime Commissioners on approaches to redesign their victim services and to modify the types of information collected and analysed in annual wider victim surveys.

If, however, individuals have been victims of serious crimes, they are likely to need more extensive support. For those with greater need, such as victims of domestic violence, rape or other serious physical or sexual assault, understandably they are likely to be seriously traumatized and may be likely to require professional therapeutic help. Extensive evidence illustrates this, and there is good evidence that provision of this kind is also helpful and results in meaningful change. However, research also suggests that a proportion, perhaps as many as a third of those treated, will continue to have severe problems. They are likely to need extended levels of service to be able to recover. Providing assurance that those services address victims' needs in an effective way depends not only on their being provided by appropriately trained and accredited professionals but also on the use of well-validated assessments and measurements of outcome and the production of evidence as to the effectiveness of the services provided.

### 10.9.1 Status of Victim Services

Some years ago, Devilly (2002) raised several crucial questions about the status of different approaches to helping crime victims and arrived at approximately similar conclusions to the above. Devilly argued that there was no evidence that supportive counselling or active listening undertaken by quasi-professionals had been shown to be effective. Where crime victims require meaningful help, which those subjected to violent or sexual assault are likely to do, such help should be provided by fully trained professional clinicians. That conclusion appears to emerge again from the evidence assembled in this chapter.

Subsequently Sullivan (2011) has questioned the value of domestic violence support programmes being delivered without proper evaluation, arguing that notwithstanding the challenges of embarking on this, there were no insurmountable reasons why it could not be done more often. She distinguished between satisfaction surveys (user feedback) and outcome surveys that can provide better tests as to whether an intervention is having worthwhile effects and advocated for more extensive use of the latter, offering guidelines for doing so.

Some recommendations for commissioning processes might draw on these proposals. The strongest evidence to emerge from this review concerned the provision of psychologically based therapies to the most seriously damaged victims of crime, usually of violent or sexual assaults. Ensuring work of that kind is appropriately delivered will depend on the setting of criteria for training of staff, assessment of individuals, evaluation of services and adoption of other procedures for quality assurance. Those suggestions accord with ones that have been made by other researchers who have proposed guidelines for the Ministry of Justice, concerning how victims' services might be designed (Callanan et al., 2012) and outlining a set of resources for putting this into effect (Callanan et al., undated). There is arguably a firm convergence of findings from these different directions of research.

## References


Apsler, R., Cummins, M. R., & Carl, S. (2003). Perceptions of the police by female victims of domestic partner violence. *Violence Against Women, 9*, 1318–1335.

Arroyo, K., Lundahl, B., Butters, R., Vanderloo, M., & Wood, D. S. (2017). Short-term interventions for survivors of intimate partner violence: A systematic review and meta-analysis. *Trauma, Violence, & Abuse, 18*(2), 155–171.

Bell, M. E., & Goodman, L. A. (2001). Supporting battered women involved with the court system: An evaluation of a law school-based advocacy intervention. *Violence Against Women, 7*, 1377–1404.

Bellis, M. A., Jones, L., Wood, S., Bates, G., Eckley, L., McCoy, E., Mikton, C., Shakespeare, T., & Officer, A. (2012). Prevalence and risk of violence against adults with disabilities: A systematic review and meta-analysis of observational studies. *The Lancet*. https://doi.org/10.1016/S0140-6736(11)81851-5

Bennett, L., & O'Brien, P. (2007). Effects of coordinated services for drug-abusing women who are victims of intimate partner violence. *Violence Against Women, 13*, 395–411.

Bennett, L., Riger, S., Schewe, P., Howard, A., & Wasco, S. (2004). Effectiveness of hotline, advocacy, counseling, and shelter services for victims of domestic violence: A statewide evaluation. *Journal of Interpersonal Violence, 19*, 815–829.

Ben-Zvi, R., & Horsfall, E. (1985). Adolescent rape: The role of rape crisis counselling. *International Journal of Adolescent Medicine and Health, 1*, 343–356.

Bloomfield, S., & Dixon, L. (2015). *An outcome evaluation of the Integrated Domestic Abuse Programme (IDAP) and Community Domestic Violence Programme (CDVP)*. Analytic Summary. London: National Offender Management Service.

Bower, P., Rowland, N., & Hardy, R. (2003). The clinical effectiveness of counselling in primary care. *Psychological Medicine, 33*, 203–215.

Bower, P., Knowles, S., Coventry, P. A., & Rowland, N. (2011). Counselling for mental health and psychosocial problems in primary care (review). *Cochrane Database of Systematic Reviews*, (9), Art. No.: CD001025. https://doi.org/10.1002/14651858.CD001025.pub3

Brettle, A., Hill, A., & Jenkins, P. (2008). Counselling in primary care; a systematic review of the evidence. *Counselling and Psychotherapy Research, 8*, 207–214.

Brownell, P., & Heiser, D. (2006). Psycho-educational support groups for older women victims of family mistreatment: A pilot study. In M. J. Mellor & P. Brownell (Eds.), *Elder abuse and mistreatment: Policy, practice and research* (pp. 145–160). The Haworth Press.

Bryce, J., Brooks, M., Robinson, P., Stokes, R., Irving, M., Graham-Kevan, N., Willan, V. J., Khan, R., & Karwacka, M. (2016). A qualitative examination of engagement with support services by victims of violent crime. *International Review of Victimology, 22*(3), 239–255.

Burgess, A. W., & Holmstrom, L. L. (1974). Crisis and counselling requests of rape victims. *Nursing Research, 23*, 196–202.

Callanan, M., Brown, A., Turley, C., Kenny, T., & Roberts, J. (2012). *Evidence and practice review of support for victims and outcome measurement*. Ministry of Justice Research Series 19/12.

Callanan, M., Turley, C., Brown, A., & Kenny, T. (undated). *Measuring outcomes for victims of crime: A resource*. Available on the Ministry of Justice website at: http://www.justice.gov.uk/publications/research-and-analysis

Campbell, R., Wasco, S. M., Ahrens, C. E., Sefl, T., & Barnes, H. E. (2001). Preventing the "second rape": Rape survivors' experiences with community service providers. *Journal of Interpersonal Violence, 16*, 1239–1259.

Campbell, R., Dorey, H., Naegeli, M., Grubstein, L. K., Bennett, K. K., Bonter, F., Smith, P. K., Grzywacz, J., Baker, P. K., & Davidson, W. S., II. (2004). An empowerment evaluation model for sexual assault programs: Empirical evidence of effectiveness. *American Journal of Community Psychology, 34*, 251–262.

Campbell, R., Patterson, D., & Lichty, L. F. (2005). The effectiveness of sexual assault nurse examiner (SANE) programs: A review of psychological, medical, legal, and community outcomes. *Trauma, Violence, & Abuse, 6*, 313–329.

Campbell, R., Patterson, D., Adams, A. E., Diegel, E., & Coats, S. (2008). A participatory evaluation project to measure SANE nursing practice and adult sexual assault patients' psychological well-being. *Journal of Forensic Nursing, 4*, 19–28.

Campbell, R., Bybee, D., Kelley, K. D., Dworkin, E. R., & Patterson, D. (2012a). The impact of sexual assault nurse examiner (SANE) program services on law enforcement investigational practices: A mediational analysis. *Criminal Justice and Behavior, 39*, 169–184.

Campbell, R., Patterson, D., & Bybee, D. (2012b). Sexual assault cases: A longitudinal analysis of the impact of a Sexual Assault Nurse Examiner program. *Violence Against Women, 18*, 223–244.

Cape, J., Whittington, C., Buszewicz, M., Wallace, P., & Underwood, L. (2010). Brief psychological therapies for anxiety and depression in primary care: Meta-analysis and meta-regression. *BMC Medicine, 8*, 38. https://doi.org/10.1186/1741-7015-8-38

Connolly, J., & Gordon, R. (2014). Co-victims of homicide: A systematic review of the literature. *Trauma, Violence, & Abuse, 16*, 494–505.

Cook, R. F., Smith, B. E., & Harrell, A. V. (1986). *Helping crime victims: Levels of trauma and effectiveness of services: Executive summary*. National Institute of Justice.

Corcoran, J., & Allen, S. (2005). The effects of a police/victim assistance crisis team approach to domestic violence. *Journal of Family Violence, 20*, 39–45.

Davis, R. C. (1987). Studying the effects of services for victims in crisis. *Crime & Delinquency, 33*, 520–531.

de Mooij, L., Kikkert, M., Lommerse, N. M., Peen, J., Meijward, S. C., Theunissen, J., Duurkoop, P. W. R. A., Goudrian, A. E., Van, H. L., Beekman, A. T. F., & Dekker, J. J. M. (2015). Victimisation in adults with severe mental illness: Prevalence and risk factors. *British Journal of Psychiatry, 207*, 515–522.

DePrince, A. P., Labus, J., Belknap, J., Buckingham, S., & Gover, A. (2012). The impact of community-based outreach on psychological distress and victim safety in women exposed to intimate partner abuse. *Journal of Consulting and Clinical Psychology, 80*, 211–221.

Devilly, G. J. (2002). Clinical intervention, supportive counselling, and therapeutic methods: A clarification and direction for restorative treatment. *International Review of Victimology, 9*, 1–14.

Dillenburger, K., Fargas, M., & Akhonzada, R. (2008). Evidence-based practice: An exploration of the effectiveness of voluntary services for victims of community violence. *British Journal of Social Work, 38*, 1630–1647.

Doerner, W. G., & Lab, S. P. (2015). *Victimology* (7th ed.). Routledge.

Donahue, S. A., Lanzara, C. B., Felton, C. J., Essock, S. M., & Carpinello, S. (2006). Project Liberty: New York's crisis counselling program created in the aftermath of September 11, 2001. *Psychiatric Services, 57*, 1253–1258.

Echeburúa, E., de Corral, P., Zubizarreta, I., & Sarasua, B. (1997). Psychological treatment of chronic posttraumatic stress disorder in victims of sexual aggression. *Behavior Modification, 21*, 433–456.

Finkelhor, D., Wolak, J., & Berliner, L. (2001). Police reporting and professional help seeking for child crime victims: A review. *Child Maltreatment, 6*, 17–30.

Foa, E. B., Rothbaum, B. O., Riggs, D. S., & Murdock, T. B. (1991). Treatment of posttraumatic stress disorder in rape victims: A comparison between cognitive-behavioral procedures and counselling. *Journal of Consulting and Clinical Psychology, 59*, 715–723.

Foa, E. B., Hearst-Ikeda, D., & Perry, K. J. (1995). Evaluation of a brief cognitive-behavioral programme for the prevention of chronic PTSD in recent assault victims. *Journal of Consulting and Clinical Psychology, 63*, 948–955.

Foa, E. B., Dancu, C. V., Hembree, E. A., Jaycox, L. H., Meadows, E. A., & Street, G. P. (1999). A comparison of exposure therapy, stress inoculation training, and their combination for reducing posttraumatic stress disorder in female assault victims. *Journal of Consulting and Clinical Psychology, 67*, 194–200.

Foa, E. B., Zoellner, L. A., & Feeny, N. C. (2006). An evaluation of three brief programs for facilitating recovery after assault. *Journal of Traumatic Stress, 19*, 29–43.

Forneris, C. A., Gartlehner, G., Brownley, K. A., Gaynes, B. N., Sonis, J., Coker-Schwimmer, E., Jonas, D. E., Greenblatt, A., Wilkins, T. M., Woodell, C. L., & Lohr, K. N. (2013). Intervention to prevent post-traumatic stress disorder: A systematic review. *American Journal of Preventive Medicine, 44*, 635–650.

Gallas, C., Bindeballe, N., Gass, P., & Dressing, H. (2009). Therapeutisches gruppenprogramm fur stalking-opfer: Pilotprojekt zur implementierung eines strukturierten therapeutischen gruppenprogramms. *Psychotherapeut, 54*, 199–2004.

Gibbs, D. A., Walters, J. L. H., Lutnick, A., Miller, S., & Kluckman, M. (2015). Services to domestic minor victims of sex trafficking: Opportunities for engagement and support. *Children and Youth Services Review, 54*, 1–7. https://doi.org/10.1016/j.childyouth.2015.04.003

Golder, S., Engstrom, M., Hall, M. T., Higgins, G. E., & Logan, T. K. (2015). Psychological distress among victimized women on probation and parole: A latent class analysis. *American Journal of Orthopsychiatry, 85*, 382–391.

Goodwin, L. R., & Holmes, G. E. (1987). Counseling the crime victim: A guide for rehabilitation counsellors. *Journal of Applied Rehabilitation Counseling, 19*, 42–47.

Hackett, S., McWhirter, P. T., & Lesher, S. (2016). The therapeutic efficacy of domestic violence victim interventions. *Trauma, Violence & Abuse, 17*, 123–132.

Hill, A., Brettle, A., Jenkins, P., & Hulme, C. (2008). *Counselling in primary care: A systematic review of the evidence*. British Association for Counselling and Psychotherapy.

Howard, A., Riger, S., Campbell, R., & Wasco, S. (2003). Counseling services for battered women: A comparison of outcomes for physical and sexual assault survivors. *Journal of Interpersonal Violence, 18*, 717–734.

Irazola, S. P., Williamson, E. J., Niedzwiecki, E., Debus-Sherill, S., & Sun, J. (2015). Keeping victims informed: Service providers' and victims' experiences using automated notification systems. *Violence and Victims, 30*, 533–544.

Ironson, G., Freund, B., Strauss, J., & Williams, J. (2002). Comparison of two treatments for traumatic stress: A community-based study of EMDR and prolonged exposure. *Journal of Clinical Psychology, 58*, 113–128.

Johnson, D. M., Zlotnick, C., & Perez, S. (2011). Cognitive behavioural treatment of PTSD in residents of battered women's shelters: Results of a randomized clinical trial. *Journal of Consulting and Clinical Psychology, 79*, 542–551.

Jonker, I. E., Sijbrandij, M., van Luijtelaar, M. J. A., Cuijpers, P., & Wolf, J. R. L. M. (2014). The effectiveness of interventions during and after residence in women's shelters: A meta-analysis. *European Journal of Public Health, 25*, 15–19.

Kärki, F. U. (2015). Norway's 2011 terror attack: Alleviating national trauma with a large-scale proactive intervention model. *Psychiatric Services, 66*, 910–912.

Kernic, M. A., & Bonomi, A. E. (2007). Female victims of domestic violence: Which victims do police refer to crisis intervention? *Violence and Victims, 22*, 463–473.

Kerr, E., Cottee, C., Chowdhury, R., Jawad, R., & Welch, J. (2003). The Haven: A pilot referral centre in London for cases of serious sexual assault. *British Journal of Obstetrics and Gynaecology, 110*, 267–271.

Khalifeh, H., Johnson, S., Howard, L. M., Borschmann, R., Osborn, D., Dean, K., Hart, C., Hogg, J., & Moran, P. (2015). Violent and non-violent crime against adults with severe mental illness. *British Journal of Psychiatry, 207*, 275–282.

King, M. E., & Woollett, E. (1997). Sexually assaulted males: 115 men consulting a counselling service. *Archives of Sexual Behavior, 26*, 579–588.

Laxminarayan, M., Henrichs, J., & Pemberton, A. (2012). Procedural and interactional justice: A comparative study of victims in the Netherlands and New South Wales. *European Journal of Criminology, 9*, 260–275.

Logar, R., & the WAVE Team. (2016). *WAVE report 2015: On the role of Specialist Women's Support Services in Europe*. WAVE.

Madoc-Jones, I., & Roscoe, K. (2010). Women's safety service within the Integrated Domestic Abuse Programme: Perceptions of service users. *Child & Family Social Work, 15*, 155–164.

Madoc-Jones, I., Hughes, C., & Humphries, K. (2015). Where next for victim services in England and Wales? *Journal of Adult Protection, 17*, 246–257.

Maguire, M. (1980). The impact of burglary upon victims. *British Journal of Criminology, 20*, 261–275.

Maguire, M. (1991). The needs and rights of victims of crime. *Crime and Justice: An Annual Review of Research, 14*, 363–433.

Maguire, M., & Corbett, C. (1987). *The effects of crime and the work of victims support schemes*. Gower.

Marandos, O. (2005). *The development of a psychometric scale for the assessment of emotional vulnerability in victims of crime*. Unpublished PhD dissertation, University of York.

Marandos, R., & Perry, A. (2009). *Assessing the effectiveness of interventions designed to support victims of crime: A systematic review of psychological outcomes*. [Protocol]. Campbell Collaboration. https://www.campbellcollaboration.org/library/assessing-the-effectiveness-of-interventions-designed-to-support-victims-of-crime-a-systematic-review-of-psychological-outcomes.html

Mariam, L. M., McClure, R., Robinson, J. B., & Yang, J. A. (2015). Eliciting change in at-risk elders (ECARE): Evaluation of an elder abuse intervention program. *Journal of Elder Abuse and Neglect, 27*, 19–33.

Martin, S. L., Young, S. K., Billings, D. L., & Bross, C. C. (2007). Health care-based interventions for women who have experienced sexual violence: A review of the literature. *Trauma, Violence & Abuse, 8*, 3–18.

Mayou, R. A., Ehlers, A., & Hobbs, M. (2000). Psychological debriefing for road traffic accident victims. *British Journal of Psychiatry, 176*, 589–593.

McColl, H., Higson-Smith, C., Gjerding, S., Omar, M. H., Rahman, B. A., Hamed, M., El Dawla, A. S., Fredricks, M., Paulsen, N., Shabalala, G., Low-Shang, C., Perez, F. V., Colin, L. S., Hernandez, A. D., Lavaire, E., Zuniga, A. P., Calidonio, L., Martinez, C. L., Jamei, Y. A., & Awad, Z. (2010). Rehabilitation of torture survivors in five countries: Common themes and challenges. *International Journal of Mental Health Systems, 4*, 1–10. http://www.ijmhs.com/4/1/16

McKee, Z., Mueller-Johnson, K., & Strang, H. (2020). Impact of a training programme on police attitudes towards victims of rape: A randomised controlled trial. *Cambridge Journal of Evidence Based Policing, 4*, 39–55.

McNamara, J. R., Tamanini, K., & Pelletier-Walker, S. (2008). The impact of short-term counselling at a domestic violence shelter. *Research on Social Work Practice, 18*, 132–136.

Miller, L. (2002). Psychological interventions for terroristic trauma: Symptoms, syndrome, and treatment strategies. *Psychotherapy: Theory, Research, Practice, Training, 39*, 283–296.

Miller, L. (2008). *Counseling crime victims: Practical strategies for mental health professionals*. Springer Publishing Company.

Ministry of Justice. (2014). *Victims of crime: Understanding the support you can expect*. Ministry of Justice.

Ministry of Justice. (2020). *Code of practice for victims of crime in England and Wales*. Ministry of Justice.

Norman, R., Spencer, A., Eldridge, S., & Feder, G. (2010). Cost-effectiveness of a programme to detect and provide better care of female victims of intimate partner violence. *Journal of Health Services Research and Policy, 15*, 143–149.

O'Reilly, R., Beale, B., & Gillies, D. (2010). Screening and intervention for domestic violence during pregnancy care: A systematic review. *Trauma, Violence, & Abuse, 11*, 190–201.

Office for National Statistics. (2013). *Focus on: Violent crime and sexual offences, 2011/12*. ONS Statistical Bulletin.

Office for National Statistics. (2016). *Chapter 1 – Overview of violent crime and sexual offences*. ONS Statistical Bulletin.

Part, D. (2006). A flexible response to domestic abuse: Findings from an evaluation. *Practice, 18*, 47–58.

Petrak, J. (1996). Current trends in the psychological assessment and treatment of victims of sexual violence. *Sexual and Marital Therapy, 11*, 37–45.

Price, J. L., Hilsenroth, M. J., Petretic-Jackson, P. A., & Bonge, D. (2001). A review of individual psychotherapy outcomes for adult survivors of childhood sexual abuse. *Clinical Psychology Review, 21*, 1095–1121.

Regehr, C., Alaggia, R., Dennis, J., Pitts, A., & Saini, M. (2013). Interventions to reduce distress in adult victims of rape and sexual violence: A systematic review. *Research on Social Work Practice, 23*, 257–265.

Resick, P. A., & Schnicke, M. K. (1992). Cognitive processing therapy for sexual assault victims. *Journal of Consulting and Clinical Psychology, 60*, 748–756.

Resick, P. A., Jordan, C. G., Girelli, S. A., Hutter, C. K., & Marhoefer-Dvorak, S. (1988). A comparative outcome study of behavioural group therapy for sexual assault victims. *Behavior Therapy, 19*, 385–401.

Resick, P. A., Nishith, P., Weaver, T. L., Astin, M. C., & Feuer, C. A. (2002). A comparison of cognitive-processing therapy with prolonged exposure and a waiting condition for the treatment of chronic posttraumatic stress disorder in female rape victims. *Journal of Consulting and Clinical Psychology, 70*, 867–879.

Resick, P. A., Galovski, T. E., Uhlmansiek, M. O., Scher, C. D., Clum, G. A., & Young-Xu, Y. (2008). A randomized clinical trial to dismantle components of cognitive processing therapy for posttraumatic stress disorder in female victims of interpersonal violence. *Journal of Consulting and Clinical Psychology, 76*, 243–258.

Resick, P. A., Williams, L. F., Suvak, M. K., Monson, C. M., & Gradus, J. L. (2012). Long-term outcomes of cognitive-behavioral treatments for posttraumatic stress disorder among female rape survivors. *Journal of Consulting and Clinical Psychology, 80*, 201–210.

Resnick, H., Acierno, R., Holmes, M., Kilpatrick, D. G., & Jager, N. (1999). Prevention of post-rape psychopathology: Preliminary findings of a controlled acute rape treatment study. *Journal of Anxiety Disorders, 13*, 359–370.

Rivas, C., Ramsay, J., Sadowski, L., Davidson, L. L., Dunne, D., Eldridge, S., Hegarty, K., Taft, A., & Feder, G. (2015). Advocacy interventions to reduce or eliminate violence and promote the physical and psychosocial well-being of women who experience intimate partner abuse. *Cochrane Database of Systematic Reviews*, (2), No: CD005043. https://doi.org/10.1002/14651858.CD005043.pub3

Rose, S., Brewin, C. R., Andrews, B., & Kirk, M. (1999). A randomized controlled trial of individual psychological debriefing for victims of violent crime. *Psychological Medicine, 29*, 793–799.

Rosenbaum, D. P. (1987). Coping with victimization: The effects of police intervention on victims' psychological readjustment. *Crime & Delinquency, 33*, 502–519.

Rothbaum, B. O. (1997). A controlled study of eye movement desensitization and reprocessing in the treatment of posttraumatic stress disordered sexual assault victims. *Bulletin of the Menninger Clinic, 61*, 317–334.
Rowland, N., Bower, P., et al. (2001). Effectiveness and cost effectiveness of counselling in primary care. *Cochrane Database of Systematic Reviews*, (3), CD001025.
Rynearson, E. K. (2012). The narrative dynamics of grief after homicide. *Omega, 65*, 239–249.
Shorey, R. C., Tirone, V., & Stuart, G. L. (2014). Coordinated community response components for victims of intimate partner violence: A review of the literature. *Aggression and Violent Behavior, 19*, 363–371.
Skogan, W. G., & Wycoff, M. A. (1987). Some unexpected effects of a police service for victims. *Crime & Delinquency, 33*, 490–501.
Smith, B. E., Cook, R. F., & Harrell, A. V. (1985). *Evaluation of victim services: Final report*. National Institute of Justice.
Srinivas, T., & DePrince, A. P. (2015). Links between the police response and Women's psychological outcomes following intimate partner violence. *Violence and Victims, 30*, 32–48.
Stafford, A. B. (2018). Providing victims of crime with information on police response activity: The challenges faced by the police non-emergency call-handler. *The Police Journal: Theory, Practice and Principles, 91*(4), 297–315.
Stelmaszek, B., & Fisher, H. (2012). *Country report 2012. Reality check on data collection and European Services for Woman and Children Survivors of Violence: A right for protection and support?* WAVE-office. Austrian Women's Shelter Network.
Sullivan, C. M. (2011). Evaluating domestic violence support service programs: Waste of time, necessary evil, or opportunity for growth? *Aggression and Violent Behavior, 16*, 354–360.
Sullivan, C. M., & Bybee, D. I. (1999). Reducing violence using community-based advocacy for women with abusive partners. *Journal of Consulting and Clinical Psychology, 67*, 43–53.
Sullivan, C. M., Bybee, D. I., & Allen, N. E. (2002). Findings from a community-based program for battered women and their children. *Journal of Interpersonal Violence, 17*, 915–936.
Tan, S.-Y., & Haining, R. (2016). Crime victimization and the implications for individual health and wellbeing: A Sheffield case study. *Social Science & Medicine, 167*, 128–139.
Taylor, C. J. (2015). Recent victimization and recidivism: The potential moderating effects of family support. *Violence and Victims, 30*, 342–360.
Taylor, J. E., & Harvey, S. T. (2009). Effects of psychotherapy with people who have been sexually assaulted: A meta-analysis. *Aggression and Violent Behavior, 14*, 273–285.
Tutty, L. M. (1996). Post-shelter services: The efficacy of follow-up programs for abused women. *Research on Social Work Practice, 6*, 425–441.
Tutty, L. M., Bidgood, B. A., & Rothery, M. A. (1993). Support groups for battered women: Research on their efficacy. *Journal of Family Violence, 8*, 325–343.
Van Reemst, L., Fischer, T. F. C., & Zwira, B. W. C. (2016). Social information processing mechanisms and violent victimization: A literature review. *Trauma, Violence & Abuse, 17*, 3–25.
Vickerman, K. A., & Margolin, G. (2009). Rape treatment outcome research: Empirical findings and state of the literature. *Clinical Psychology Review, 29*, 431–448.
Victim Support. (2018-2019). *Annual Report & Accounts. Derby*; Victim Support.
Wasco, S. M., Campbell, R., Howard, A., Mason, G. E., Staggs, S. L., Schewe, P. A., & Riger, S. (2004). A statewide evaluation of services provided to rape survivors. *Journal of Interpersonal Violence, 19*, 252–263.
Wathen, C. N., & MacMillan, H. I. (2003). Interventions for violence against women: Scientific review. *Journal of the American Medical Association, 289*, 589–600.
Winkel, F. W. (1989). Responses to criminal victimization: Evaluating the impact of a Police Assistance Program and some social psychological characteristics. *Police Studies, 12*, 59–72.
Winkel, F. W. (1991). Police communication programmes aimed at burglary victims: A review of studies and an experimental evaluation. *Journal of Community & Applied Social Psychology, 1*, 275–289.

Winkel, F. W., & Vrij, A. (1993). Facilitating problem- and emotion-focused coping in victims of burglary: Evaluating a police crisis intervention program. *Journal of Community Psychology, 21*, 97–112.
Young, A. T., Fuller, J., & Riley, B. (2008). On-scene mental health counseling provided through police departments. *Journal of Mental Health Counseling, 30*, 345–361.
Zweig, J. M., Schlichter, K. A., & Burt, M. R. (2002). Assisting women victims of violence who experience multiple barriers to services. *Violence Against Women, 8*, 162–180.
Zweig, J. M., Burt, M. R., & Van Ness, A. (2003). *The effect on victims of Victim Services Programs funded by the STOP Formula Grants Program*. National Institute of Justice.

# Chapter 11
# What Works in Public Awareness Campaigns? A Scoping Review

## 11.1 Overall Objective

The objective of the evidence review reported in this chapter is to provide an overall descriptive summary of the available research on the effectiveness of public awareness campaigns in the fields of policing and criminal justice. The review focuses specifically on published studies concerning campaigns that have been carried out by police departments, although such initiatives have often been taken on a multi-agency basis with the police as one of the partners. This is not a full systematic review but a *scoping review*, which is speedier and less rigorous as it is designed to provide a wide-ranging account of the work that has been done in an area rather than to establish what are the most effective interventions or to compare them with one another. The decision to adopt this approach was taken partly due to limitations of time and partly based on an expectation that the published research in the area was likely to be limited and also to be diverse with respect to both its focus and its methodology. In retrospect, both of those expectations transpired to be correct.

## 11.2 Background

Across the entire field of public policy, it is considered essential that efforts should be made to inform the public of matters of importance to them. In relation to numerous issues in criminal justice however, the public often appears to be misinformed. For example, a Home Office study found that many people believed crime was rising when it was actually falling, and their beliefs were linked to the type of newspaper they read (Lovbakke, 2007). Threat perceptions – individuals' subjective judgements of the likelihood of being a victim of crime – are often sharply at odds with more methodically derived risk estimates.



J. McGuire et al., *Evidence-Based Policing and Community Crime Prevention*, Advances in Preventing and Treating Violence and Aggression,
https://doi.org/10.1007/978-3-030-76363-3_11

Public awareness campaigns in policing and criminal justice are usually launched with the aim of achieving specific objectives, usually associated with crime reduction and neighbourhood safety. They can involve a wide variety of activities, from providing and distributing information leaflets, press releases, community meetings, school visits, poster displays, day events, radio or television broadcasts, liaison with licensed premises or other types of venue, setting up websites or helplines and other resources. They may be carried out by police in conjunction with a range of other agencies from the public, private and third (voluntary) sectors and often involve local media outlets. To attract attention and ensure maximum publicity, they may be endorsed by well-known figures or use other means of getting messages across.

As a result of the variety of methods that are used in such projects, however, their effects are difficult to evaluate, and efforts to do so present a "number of unique interpretive problems" (Sacco & Silverman, 1982, p. 264). One challenge within this is the selection and recording of outcomes that are the designated targets of a campaign: Many of what evaluators call *dependent variables* are very difficult to measure. Another challenge arises from the complexity of campaigns – to increase chances of success, several methods are usually involved, with the consequence that if a change is observed, it cannot usually be said with any certainty which element of a campaign or which combination of elements contributed to the outcome. That leaves questions unanswered about the best use of resources and regarding how to proceed in subsequent campaigns, especially when their objectives or the context in which they are run may be different.

## 11.3 Method

This report follows the methodology of a scoping review, which is a more limited form of research review process than a systematic review, designed primarily to obtain a broad picture of the kinds of research carried out on a given question (Arksey & O'Malley, 2005; Peters et al., 2015; Pham et al., 2014). The material to be covered in the review was restricted to published studies (peer-reviewed journal articles or government reports) and to documents available in English. Seven databases were searched to locate potentially relevant research literature: the National Criminal Justice Reference Service; the former Home Office Research, Development and Statistics Directorate; PsycINFO; Scopus; Web of Science; the Cochrane Database of Systematic Reviews and the website of the Campbell Collaboration. No time limits were set for the search. The search terms used were various combinations of the words *public awareness, campaign, police* and *criminal justice*. As it was anticipated that there was unlikely to be a large volume of research on this area and pilot searches confirmed that impression, a decision was made not to restrict the search any further by adding additional words such as evaluation, results, effect(s) or outcome.

In addition to electronic searches, a separate hand search was conducted. That is, the tables of contents were inspected of the following four leading journals in the field of police research: *Police Practice and Research: An International Journal*; *Policing: A Journal of Policy and Practice*; *Policing: An International Journal of Police Strategies and Management*; and *Policing and Society: An International Journal of Research and Policy*. Searches covered the period from 1st of January 2000 up to the present; that is, for the purpose of updating the original report and preparing this chapter, the journals were searched to November 2020.

There were many studies of different aspects of the relationship between the police and the public. They included studies of community policing and police-community relationships in different places, on public perceptions of the police, on fear of crime and on the nature of police-citizen encounters. The study of these however examined different questions from the evaluation of public awareness campaigns; therefore studies in these areas were excluded from consideration. Initial searches located a total of 551 records (Web of Science 260, National Criminal Justice Reference Service 241, Scopus 35, PsycINFO 7, Home Office RDS 3, Cochrane database 1, hand searches 4). After removal of duplicates, screening and updating, this resulted in a set of 56 relevant reports.

## 11.4 Previous Reviews

No prior reviews covering this exact field were found, although reviews were obtained of evaluation research on public awareness campaigns in the adjoining field of public health. There has been some discussion of the relation between the two fields to which we will return later in the chapter. However, two relevant reviews were found that bridged the gap between a health-related and a criminal justice mass media campaign. Elder et al. (2004) reported a systematic review of such campaigns concerned with reduction of drink-driving. They located and analysed eight studies of the effectiveness of such campaigns. On average they produced a reduction of 13% in alcohol-related collisions. Their findings show mass media campaigns can be effective in this area if they are well planned and delivered and also coordinated with other changes including law enforcement. Effective campaigns also had a positive return in terms of benefit-cost ratios. Thus, there are encouraging results relating to this specific problem, but whether that applies similarly to other areas requires more research.

More recently Anderson et al. (2009) reported an integrative summary of systematic reviews and meta-analyses across the entire field of attempts to reduce levels of alcohol consumption. This noted that several policies, practices and treatments in the field of alcohol have been found to be effective. However, by comparison there was little scientific research concerning the effectiveness of public information campaigns or on media-based advocacy. Nevertheless, they noted that the latter can lead to more attention being focused on alcohol-related policies. One policy proposal they forwarded was that educational programmes should not be used in isolation, but in combination with other initiatives that highlight the problems created by alcohol. They also recommend that alcohol advertising be banned.

In a quite different domain, Kemshall and Moulden (2017) undertook a wide-ranging narrative survey of efforts that have been made to raise public awareness of child sexual abuse, which have been become more prominent since the 1990s. Initiatives of this kind were launched in many countries, sometimes including telephone helplines which were rapidly inundated with calls. Thus, wider discussion appeared to increase awareness, but it was some time before any methodical attempts were made at evaluating whether this had any impact on the occurrence of abuse. This may have been partly due to the absence of any clear model of how to measure this and also to the remaining cultural barriers against discussion of this topic. Although awareness campaigns became progressively more complex and multi-layered, Kemshall and Moulden (2017, p. 133) concluded that "despite decades of public awareness campaigns there is surprisingly limited empirical evidence to conclude what works or what does not".

## 11.5 Results of the Present Review

This section presents the findings from this scoping review. The 52 reports that were considered relevant covered a wide range of areas and employed a considerable variety of research methods. The level of research activity in many fields fluctuates over time, and the patterning of it in this area has been fairly uneven. Both the quantity and the nature of research on this topic have changed markedly over recent decades. The research studies that were retained have been divided into three groups: those describing general public awareness campaigns, those dealing more specifically with public responses to particular methods of crime prevention and those focused more narrowly on specific types of offence.

### *11.5.1 General Public Awareness Initiatives*

Some research has addressed the broad question of how to raise public awareness of risks to property or personal safety or of the work of the police in general terms. Several issues have been considered within this. A sizeable amount of work on the usefulness of public awareness and mass media campaigns was conducted in the late 1970s and early 1980s. At that time there was a *National Citizens' Crime Prevention Campaign* in the USA. A series of reports prepared by the University of Denver Centre for Mass Communications Research and Policy evaluated its implementation and effects (Mendelsohn & Wilson, 1978; Mendelsohn et al., 1981; Mendelsohn et al., 1982; O'Keefe et al., 1985). This was characterized in terms of a metaphor of "taking a bite out of crime" and was designed to improve citizens' general understanding of the process of crime prevention. It was judged as having had marked and consistent effects and as having succeeded in that aim (O'Keefe et al., 1985).

Kuttschreuter and Wiegman (1998) described a multimedia campaign in the Netherlands designed to influence perceptions of both residential burglary and street-based violence. Methods of dissemination included articles in both local and national newspapers, items on radio and police "crime prevention vans" on tour in the community. This generated more positive views of the criminal justice system, but there was little evidence of other effects.

A more focused kind of campaign was conducted in Ventura County, California, directed towards a designated audience, senior citizens who were thought potentially at risk of frauds and scams (Velasco, 2000), and was associated with an increase in referrals for prosecution through the district attorney's office. Warning campaigns of this kind have become widespread since that time, linked to the now almost ubiquitous use of online banking and other financial management and the rapid accelerating growth in cybercrime.

Some of the documents located in the literature search consist of sets of advice or descriptions of resources that can be utilized in developing public awareness or in programmes to strengthen crime prevention. Barthe (2006) describes different types of publicity campaigns – victim- and offender-oriented – the elements to be considered when planning a campaign, the stakeholders to involve and differing formats for publicizing the campaign's message. Methods of deploying media and community awareness strategies for addressing social problems including crime and truancy from school are summarized in information sheets prepared by the Development Services Group (2009, Development Services Group, 2010). Cordner (2010) has written a manual on aspects of the phenomenon of fear of crime and lists tools and techniques that police can use to target and reduce it, seeking to identify best practices for this purpose.

The role of awareness campaigns in influencing public perceptions of the police needs to be set alongside other factors that may be more pivotal. They include individuals' experiences of direct contact with the police. On the basis of two surveys conducted by Myhill and Bradford (2012), there is evidence that such contacts may be more important than criminal justice outcomes in maintaining confidence in the police.

In general terms however, the proposal that the police could benefit from improved communication with the public is questioned in a study reported by Choi et al. (2020), within the US Korean community. This suggested that citizens' confidence in the police is not influenced in a direct or simple manner by their levels of crime-related media consumption. Choi et al. examined the latter, alongside mediating variables of *fear of crime* and *perceived incivility* of police behaviour in participants' local neighbourhoods. Thus, "those who were more afraid of crime and who perceived more incivilities in their neighborhood were more likely to have fewer positive perceptions of the police compared with their counterparts" (2020). The latter variable accounted for much more of the variance than the former. Higher consumption of crime-related media was associated with greater fear of crime, which in turn was associated with lower confidence in the police.

## *11.5.2 Public Awareness Linked to Forms of Crime Prevention*

A second, smaller group of studies described approaches to crime or selected aspects of crime which were not offence-specific but were centred on a particular crime prevention method or an initiative designed to influence a particular category of crime opportunities.

### 11.5.2.1 Neighbourhood Policing

Bullock and Sindall (2014) reported on the extent of public participation in locally based crime prevention measures based on a community policing model, i.e. collaboration between police and members of the public. Obviously for this to work, the public need to be made aware of the operation of it. The study was based on analysis of data from two waves of the annual Crime Survey for England and Wales with a total of over 90,000 participants. The focus was on whether the public were aware of community policing and had some knowledge of it and whether or not they proactively made contact with local police. The proportions answering "yes" to these questions were respectively 42%, 32% and 7%. The study reports analysis of the factors associated with these three outcome variables.

### 11.5.2.2 Rail Network Safety

Power et al. (2016) described the role of the British Transport Police in alleviating fear of crime on the UK rail network, with particular reference to risk of terrorism incidents. This involved interviews with members of the public and of the BTP, asking them to compare different initiatives taken by the BTP, including police presence, visibility of armed officers, police dogs, stop and search and awareness campaigns. The presence of armed police emerged as providing the greatest sense of safety while awareness campaigns were the least effective. However, appearance of armed police without steps making the public aware of the reasons gave rise to alarm rather than providing reassurance.

### 11.5.2.3 Gun Markets

Ridgeway et al. (2011) reported an experiment in which they sent a letter, signed by prominent law enforcement officials, to those who purchased guns on odd-numbered but not even-numbered days, making them aware of the formal rules of gun ownership (e.g. to notify changes of address and of ownership). The letter had no effect on later rates of gun purchases, but it led to a significantly higher rate of reporting thefts of guns. This is potentially valuable as a large proportion of crimes are committed using stolen guns.

## 11.5.3 *Offence-Specific Awareness Campaigns*

Other public awareness initiatives have involved focusing on particular types of offence, in which case the methods used can be tailored in a more precise way to the context in which offences are likely to be committed.

### 11.5.3.1 Wearing Bicycle Helmets

As wearing helmets greatly reduces the risk of head injury following bicycle accidents, Huybers et al. (2017) evaluated the effects of a change in the law in Canada regulating helmet use. The legal change was accompanied by an educational and awareness campaign. Follow-up at 9, 11 and 14 years afterwards showed a significantly increased rate of helmet use (75–94%), sustained throughout the study period.

### 11.5.3.2 Shoplifting

McNees et al. (1976) compared the relative effects of two types of in-store messages about shoplifting: signs that warned of the penalties and identifiers that were attached to known frequently stolen items drawing attention to them and so increasing probability of detection. While both reduced the shop theft rate, the latter proved more effective. This supports findings elsewhere that likelihood of arrest is a stronger deterrent than severity of penalty.

### 11.5.3.3 Property Crime

Regarding property crime as a general category, Weatherburn and Grabosky (1999) expressed criticism of an approach to prevention that relies too heavily on more severe penalties and additional policing. They proposed a more strategic approach involving analysis of crime patterns and development of strategic public-private partnerships that would connect different government departments with each other. While they do not specifically refer to awareness campaigns, their approach would evidently require extensive communication of objectives and activities to the public if it was to be effective.

### 11.5.3.4 Burglary

In England and Wales, first in the 1980s and later under the Crime Reduction Programme from 1998 onwards, a number of large-scale crime prevention projects were undertaken which included some form of public awareness aspect (Hamilton-Smith, 2004). Examples from the earlier phase include the Kirkholt Burglary

Prevention Project (Rochdale: Forrester et al., 1988; Forrester et al., 1990) and from the Crime Reduction Programme the Hartlepool Strategic Development Project (Sturgeon-Adams et al., 2005). These were successful in reducing burglary rates, in reducing costs, and feedback from project participants was very positive. Tilley and Webb (1994) commented that without publicity the crime problem was merely contained rather than producing more enduring change. The project reports also show the need for careful management of publicity as if adverse, it can undermine an otherwise beneficial project.

Gelders et al. (2007) analysed differences between police departments in Belgium in the way they used communications with the public concerning the prevention of home burglary. They discovered quite large differences between departments. Their findings suggest that effective information campaigns require use of a "richer media mix", containing a variety of forms of communication and targeted to different audiences.

#### 11.5.3.5 Car Theft

Monaghan (1988) outlined a media campaign in Australia designed to make the public more aware of risks of car theft. The campaign involved distribution of leaflets and press releases, resulting in over 350 newspaper articles and coverage by all television channels operating at that time. The campaign was tracked using a series of telephone contacts with a large community sample.

#### 11.5.3.6 Alcohol Consumption

In itself this is of course not illegal in most countries, but given its association with many types of offending in addition to its associated health risks, many initiatives in both health and criminal justice have been focused on seeking to reduce it or help control its effects.

Gebhart et al. (2000) described a collaboration between a university and its surrounding community to reduce off-campus drinking. This drew on the concept of environmental management but also involved the use of a safety-awareness campaign for students going off campus. The programme led to a reduction in the number of reported alcohol-related incidents.

Jones-Webb et al. (2014) describe the implementation of new laws restricting the sale of high-alcohol liquors in three US cities, a change accompanied by a public awareness and education process. This was considered a vital component of making any alcohol control policy effective, and the authors identify the stakeholders who should be targets of such a campaign.

Recognizing the extent in some countries of unregistered production and unrecorded consumption of alcohol, Lachenmeier et al. (2011) proposed amongst other actions the need for education campaigns simply to make people more aware of the existence of the problem.

Johnston et al. (2018) conducted a before-and-after evaluation of a public education campaign in Western Australia designed to increase parents' awareness of the risks of alcohol consumption for adolescents in the 12–17 age range. There were two phases of mass advertising across multiple media outlets, accompanied by guidance issued by the National Health and Medical Research Council. Parents' knowledge, attitudes and behaviour, the latter, for example, in the form of providing alcohol to their children, were measured at three time points: before the campaign commenced and at post-test and follow-up points, respectively, 6 and 27 months later.

The campaign attained a fairly high public profile and achieved some successes. Parental knowledge increased consistently and significantly across the three time points, reaching a level where knowledge of the key issues was "almost universal" (p. 593). Attitudes showed a similar positive course, with some increasing consistently but others waning slightly from the second to the third measurement point. Results related to behaviour were also mixed, with no consistent pattern, though at the end of the study more parents said they had discussed with children the dangers of alcohol than did so at the beginning.

#### 11.5.3.7 Drug Use

McCaffrey (1999) reported on the use of media campaigns to reduce drug use amongst teenagers in a study carried out in 12 American cities. This involved television advertisements on the dangers of drugs and testing the extent to which young people had viewed them. There was a significant, but not large, growth in awareness of drug risks in experimental as compared to control sites. However, changes in reporting of having tried drugs were only marginal. The United States Office of National Drug Control Policy has produced several reports on its investment over a 5-year period of $1 billion to reduce drug use in the USA (Office of National Drug Control Policy, 2000). This involved extensive use of media campaigns, and the agency's reports indicate positive outcomes from this investment. There was evidence, for example, that young people who watched advertisements on the dangers of methamphetamine adopted stronger attitudes against it. However, there were difficulties in reaching a wide audience, as only a proportion of the intended audience saw the advertisements (Office of National Drug Control Policy, 2011).

#### 11.5.3.8 Drink-Driving

In the USA this is referred to as driving under the influence or driving while intoxicated or "DWI". Beck and Moser (2006) reported a survey asking respondents about their response to the introduction of police "sobriety checkpoints" (breath tests) in the state of Maryland. A media campaign had been launched to make the public aware of these checkpoints. However, in a later evaluation, Beck (2009) found no evidence of a positive impact. One reason given for this was inadequate publicity having been given to the initiative. This accords with the results obtained by Elder et al. (2004) based on their systematic review. Given heterogeneity within any population to whom media campaigns are likely to be addressed, there might also be differential effects within it, as found by Flexon and Guerette (2009) in a study of an offender-focused drink-driving awareness campaign.

#### 11.5.3.9 Violence

Attempting to influence alcohol use is often aimed towards reducing fighting and other assault, as we saw in relation to policing the Night Time Economy initiatives described in Chap. 2. But there have also been efforts to address violence directly through awareness campaigns. Spivak et al. (1989) described a project in Boston, Massachusetts, designed to reduce violence amongst adolescents, part of which involved a public-health, mass media campaign to heighten awareness of the problem of violence in the community. This included posters, billboards, tee-shirts and radio and television announcements, alongside the introduction of a violence prevention curriculum in secondary schools and a range of community support services.

On an even more ambitious level, Matzopoulous and Myers (2014) describe the inception of an *Integrated Provincial Violence Prevention Policy Framework* in the Western Cape province of South Africa. They involved a large-scale, multifaceted departure from what is described as a traditional security-centred approach. The framework entailed several levels, with the overarching aim of "engaging the whole of society" in violence reduction. It also incorporated a focus on alcohol given its links to aggression. This study was an early report on its implementation, highlighting some initial successes and also problems arising from conflicts between the numerous agencies involved.

In a global survey, Hughes et al. (2014) found that although there has been a steady increase in the output of evaluations of violence prevention programmes, only a small proportion of this entails media education programmes, with only a small number of studies having been published.

#### 11.5.3.10 Violence Towards Women

Potter et al. (2009) evaluated the effects of a poster campaign in raising awareness of sexual violence towards women on a college campus. Results were encouraging, indicating that those who had seen the posters were more likely to say they would intervene.

On a larger scale, one of the macro-level policies of the World Health Organization (2014) is a global campaign to reduce levels of all forms of violence in society, with particular attention being focused on violence against women. To this end, the World Health Organization has encouraged governments to formulate and enact multi-level *National Actions Plans* to address this and other forms of violence, using media and public information campaigns as a core element of the strategy. This approach is firmly embedded within the public health model but views criminal justice policy as an integral part of any effective process. Whittington and McGuire (2020) describe details of some of the initiatives emanating from this and summarize preliminary evidence of their impact.

#### 11.5.3.11 Domestic or Intimate Partner Violence

Salazar et al. (2003) described a project with the objective of making communities more aware of norms regarding domestic violence. In a large-scale survey, they found that official policies on intimate partner violence had an impact on public attitudes towards it. This appeared to have a particular effect in reducing victim blaming and was thought to illustrate how criminal justice responses can influence social norms and the tacit acceptance of intimate partner violence. In a review of research on this question, Campbell and Manganello (2006) note that, despite the impact of other kinds of campaigns being inconclusive, there is support for developing and delivering media campaigns to change attitudes and ultimately behaviour in relation to domestic abuse.

#### 11.5.3.12 Rape

In a parallel type of investigation, concerned with drug- or alcohol-facilitated rape, Walsh et al. (2016) considered that changing public definitions of rape through public service campaigns could have an impact on attitudes. This had a particular focus in trying to increase the extent of reporting of such rapes and of seeking help after their occurrence. Rates of doing so are lower for this than for other types of rape, following from perceptions of the stereotyping of rape victims.

#### 11.5.3.13 Child Abuse

Cardazone et al. (2014) described a community campaign in Hawaii designed to increase public awareness of the problem of child maltreatment. This centres mainly on the networking processes in coordinating the work of 24 member organizations involved in a coalition to raise this awareness, part of which was the conduct of a large-scale telephone survey to gauge awareness of risk factors for child abuse.

#### 11.5.3.14 Hate Crimes

In a document produced on behalf of Community Oriented Policing Services, part of the US Department of Justice, Whalen et al. (2013) set out details of partnerships between police and other agencies in targeting hate crime. This does not report outcome evidence but discusses many aspects of how to operate such partnerships created to address this problem. There is some evidence that it is possible to increase knowledge of, and reduce prejudicial perceptions towards, groups that are often the subject of racial discrimination. This was found by Hill and Augoustinos (2001) in a study of attitudes towards Australian aboriginal people. It is possible that by promoting intercultural awareness, there could be an effect on the volume of hate crimes.

#### 11.5.3.15 Human Trafficking

A study by Cunningham and Cromer (2016) addressed the question of whether the reporting of human trafficking in the media may be associated with the acceptance of myths concerning it, extrapolated from other myths concerning rape, child sexual abuse and prostitution. They suggested there is a need for clear public education concerning the nature and extent of human sexual trafficking.

The importance of this was recognized by Sekhon (2020) who took as a starting point the United Nations *Protocol to Prevent, Suppress, and Punish Trafficking in Persons* which came into force in December 2003 (United Nations Office on Drugs and Crime, 2018). Amongst many other objectives, this set standards for the development of public awareness of the problem. Focusing on India where this exists on a significant scale, Sekhon (2020, p. 732) suggested that the escalating levels of the problem were in part a consequence of the fact that "people simply do not know about the dangers and realities of this crime". A range of stakeholders and "duty bearers", including the police, have collective responsibility for remedying this, and Sekhon specifies the issues to be addressed if such campaigns are to be launched and are to be effective. Establishment of *Anti-Human Trafficking Units* with specially trained staff has resulted in a sharp increase in the number of offenders apprehended. Many methods of campaigning have been adopted, including public awareness films made by non-governmental organizations and the use of illustrated comics for child audiences. The effectiveness of these has not however been evaluated.

#### 11.5.3.16 Terrorism

In the present context, this type of offence differs considerably from others that have been discussed, in that those who perpetrate it do so for a wide variety of motives (Silke, 2019). What such acts have in common is the attempt to cause death, injury, damage and other harm and by doing so to attract attention or gain publicity in the most dramatic way. The unpredictability of the event is designed to instil fear and thereby put pressure on authorities responsible for public protection. Alongside detection and law enforcement, the police and other security agency response is therefore often the reverse, to calm and reassure the public and to maintain safety while enabling and encouraging citizens to remain alert as to possible risks.

The United States Federal Emergency Management Agency working in conjunction with the International Association of Chiefs of Police has reported a large-scale, multi-method study designed to develop an understanding of the public's perception of suspicious activity that might be associated with terrorist behaviour (Federal Emergency Management Agency, 2012a). This led to the production of a *Resource Guide* describing a range of strategies to improve community awareness and to make provision of appropriate resources to support local efforts in relation to this (Federal Emergency Management Agency, 2012b).

## 11.6 Discussion

The research identified in this scoping review addresses a very extensive range of problems. Portions of it focus on the general challenge of enabling the public to become more aware of crime risks and precautions that can be taken to reduce them. Other projects target a selected area of criminal activity and attempt to reduce it. Some research has reported encouraging results, whereas elsewhere they are disappointing. Without a more in-depth systematic review of studies, conclusions regarding relative effectiveness cannot be drawn, but even were that attempted, there are insufficient numbers of studies on any single area to allow any clear pattern to be identified.

Some researchers suggest that the effectiveness of policing and criminal justice campaigns could be enhanced if they adopted more of the strategies used in public health mass media campaigns. There are many of these and there are also numerous evaluations of them. However, the caveats noted earlier about discerning cause-effect relationships often still apply. Even where several studies have been published, outcomes are often mixed due to variations between them. Examples include the work of Chodzko-Zajko and Schwingel (2009) on worldwide efforts to raise public awareness of the importance of physical activity for lasting health or that of Clement et al. (2013) on reducing stigma, prejudice and discrimination against people with mental health problems. Thus, there is an ongoing debate on whether or to what extent policing can make use of similar strategies to those used in public health campaigns. While some emphasize the similarities between them (van Dijk & Crofts, 2017), others take note of the differences and explore what needs to be taken account of, if introducing a “culture of health” into policing (Anderson & Burris, 2017).

Anyone planning to embark on a public awareness campaign should perhaps also keep in mind the suggestions of Toch and Maguire (2014) who point towards changes in public opinion over time and the fact that there are diverse views within any community in how crime and the criminal justice system are viewed. At the early stages of planning a public awareness campaign, it may be valuable to locate the proposed work in the type of evidence-based policing and crime prevention matrix forwarded by Lum et al. (2011), to make decisions regarding its specificity and scope.

Meanwhile, the results of this review had some influence in research subsequently carried out by the commissioning police forces on the challenging issue of public awareness of the incidents in which someone is killed or seriously injured. A research team carried this out examining which combination of interventions, engineering, education and enforcement had the greatest beneficial impact. The public awareness element was a key component and included drink-driving and anti-speeding publicity campaigns, speed awareness courses and other elements. Based on this research, there was some redesign of the awareness campaigns.

### *11.6.1 Strengths and Limitations of the Research*

The volume of research found relevant to this review question is slightly larger than was expected, but given its disparate nature, it is still unlikely to be enough to permit any clear conclusions to be drawn. As a scoping review, the present objective was simply to map out in general terms the kinds of work reported in the area. Any review work in this field is likely to be subject to some limitations. For example, there may be internal reports prepared by police research departments that are not accessible on external databases, and they may contain valuable information. That might apply also to unpublished conference contributions and degree dissertations and to studies not published in English.

## References

Anderson, E., & Burris, S. (2017). Policing and public health: Not quite the right analogy. *Policing and Society: An International Journal of Research and Policy, 27*, 300–313.

Anderson, P., Chisholm, D., & Fuhr, D. C. (2009). Effectiveness and cost-effectiveness of policies and programmes to reduce the harm caused by alcohol. *Lancet, 373*, 2234–2246.

Arksey, H., & O'Malley, L. (2005). Scoping studies: Towards a methodological framework. *International Journal of Social Research, 8*, 19–32.

Barthe, E. (2006). *Crime prevention publicity campaigns*. Policy Guide No. 5. Center for Problem-Oriented Policing, State University of New York at Albany. http://www.popcenter.org/Responses/crime_prevention/print/

Beck, K. H. (2009). Lessons learned from evaluating Maryland's anti-drunk driving campaign: Assessing the evidence for cognitive, behavioral and public health impact. *Health Promotion Practice, 10*, 370–377.

Beck, K. H., & Moser, M. L. (2006). Does the type of exposure to a roadside sobriety checkpoint influence driver perceptions regarding drunk driving? *American Journal of Health Behaviour, 30*, 268–277.

Bullock, K., & Sindall, K. (2014). Examining the nature and extent of public participation in neighbourhood policing. *Policing and Society; An International Journal of research and Policy, 24*, 385–404.

Campbell, J. C., & Manganello, J. (2006). Changing public attitudes as a prevention strategy to reduce intimate partner violence. *Journal of Aggression, Maltreatment and Trauma, 13*, 13–39.

Cardazone, G., Sy, A. U., Chik, I., & Corlew, L. K. (2014). Mapping one strong 'Ohana: Using network analysis and GIS to enhance the effectiveness of a statewide coalition to prevent child abuse and neglect. *American Journal of Community Psychology, 53*, 346–356.

Chodzko-Zajko, W., & Schwingel, A. (2009). Transnational strategies for the promotion of physical activity and active aging: The World Health Organization model of consensus building in international public health. *Quest, 61*, 25–38. https://doi.org/10.1080/00336297.2009.10483598

Choi, J., Yim, H., & Hiks, R. D. (2020). Direct and indirect effects of crime-related media consumption on public confidence in the police. *International Journal of Police Science & Management, 22*(1), 38–49.

Clement, S., Lassman, F., Barley, E., Evans-Lacko, S., Williams, P., Yamaguchi, S., Slade, M., Rüsch, N., & Thornicroft, G. (2013). Mass media interventions for reducing mental health-related stigma. *Cochrane Database of Systematic Reviews*, (7), CD009453. https://doi.org/10.1092/14651858.CD009453.pub2

Cordner, G. (2010). *Reducing fear of crime: Strategies for police*. Office of Community Oriented Policing Services, United States Department of Justice.

Cunningham, K. C., & Cromer, L. D. (2016). Attitudes about human trafficking: Individual differences related to belief and victim blame. *Journal of Interpersonal Violence, 31*, 228–244.

Development Services Group, Inc. (2009). *Community awareness/mobilization. Literature review*. Office of Juvenile Justice and Delinquency Prevention. http://www.ojjdp.gov/mpg/litreviews/Community_Awareness.pdf

Development Services Group, Inc. (2010). *Truancy prevention: Literature review*. Office of Juvenile Justice and Delinquency Prevention. http://www.ojjdp.gov/mpg/litreviews/Truancy_Prevention.pdf

Elder, R. W., Shults, R. A., Sleet, D. A., Nichols, J. L., Thompson, R. S., Rajab, W., & Task Force on Community Preventive Services. (2004). Effectiveness of mass media campaigns for reducing drinking and driving and alcohol-involved crashes: A systematic review. *American Journal of Preventive Medicine, 27*, 57–65.

Federal Emergency Management Agency. (2012a). *Improving the public's awareness and reporting of suspicious activity: Key research findings from literature review, household surveys, focus groups and interviews*. United States Department of Homeland Security, Federal Emergency Management Agency, National Preparedness Directorate.

Federal Emergency Management Agency. (2012b). *A resource improve your community's awareness and reporting activity for law enforcement and community partners*. United States Department of Homeland Security, Federal Emergency Management Agency, National Preparedness Directorate.

Flexon, J. L., & Guerette, R. T. (2009). Differential effects of an offender-focused crime prevention media campaign. *Journal of Criminal Justice, 37*, 608–616.

Forrester, D., Chatterton, M., & Pease, K. (1988). *The Kirkholt burglary prevention project, Rochdale. Crime Prevention Unit Paper 13*. Home Office.

Forrester, D., Frenz, S., Chatterton, M., & Pease, K. (1990). *The Kirkholt burglary prevention project: Phase II. Crime Prevention Unit Paper 23*. Home Office.

Gebhart, T. L., Kaphingst, K., & DeJong, W. (2000). A campus-community coalition to control alcohol-related problems off campus: An environmental management case study. *Journal of American College Health, 48*, 211–215.

Gelders, D., Peeraer, H., & Gossens, J. (2007). Public communication about home burglary prevention in Belgium: Strengths and weaknesses tested by content analysis and focus group interviews. *Policing: An International Journal of Police Strategies and Management, 40*, 567–586.

Hamilton-Smith, N. (Ed.). (2004). *The Reducing Burglary Initiative: design, development and delivery. Home Office Research Study 287*. Home Office Research, Development and Statistics Directorate..

Hill, M. E., & Augoustinos, M. (2001). Stereotype change and prejudice reduction: Short- and long-term evaluation of a cross-cultural awareness programme. *Journal of Community & Applied Social Psychology, 11*, 243–262.

Hughes, K., Bellis, M. A., Hardcastle, K. A., Butchart, A., Dahlbertg, L. L., Mercy, J. A., & Mikton, C. (2014). Global development and diffusion of outcome evaluation research for interpersonal and self-directed violence prevention from 2007 to 2013: A systematic review. *Aggression and Violent Behavior, 19*, 655–662.

Huybers, S., Fenerty, L., Kureshi, N., Thibauly-Halman, G., LeBlanc, J. C., Clarke, D. B., & Walling, S. (2017). Long-term effects of education and legislation enforcement on all-age bicycle helmet use: A longitudinal study. *Journal of Community Health, 42*, 83–89.

Johnston, R. B., Stafford, J., Jongenelis, M. I., Shaw, T., Samsa, H., Costello, E., & Kirby, G. (2018). Evaluation of a public education campaign to support parents to reduce adolescent alcohol use. *Drug and Alcohol Review, 37*, 588–598.

Jones-Webb, R., Nelson, T., McKee, P., & Toomey, T. (2014). An implementation model to increase the effectiveness of alcohol control policies. *American Journal of Health Promotion, 28*, 328–335.

Kemshall, H., & Moulden, H. M. (2017). Communicating about child sexual abuse with the public: Learning the lessons from public awareness campaigns. *Journal of Sexual Aggression, 23*(2), 124–138.

Kuttschreuter, M., & Wiegman, O. (1998). Crime prevention and the attitude toward the criminal justice system: The effects of a multimedia campaign. *Journal of Criminal Justice, 26*, 441–452.

Lachenmeier, D. W., Taylor, B. J., & Rehm, J. (2011). Alcohol under the radar: Do we have policy options regarding unrecorded alcohol? *International Journal of Drug Policy, 22*, 153–160.

Lovbakke, J. (2007). Public perceptions. In S. Nicholas, C. Kershaw, & A. Walker (Eds.), *Crime in England and Wales 2006/07*. Home Office Research, Development and Statistics Directorate.

Lum, C., Koper, C. S., & Telep, C. W. (2011). The evidence-based policing matrix. *Journal of Experimental Criminology, 7*, 3–26.

Matzopoulous, R., & Myers, J. E. (2014). The Western Cape government's new integrated provincial violence prevention policy framework: Successes and challenges. *Aggression and Violent Behavior, 19*, 649–654.

McCaffrey, B. R. (1999). *Testing the Anti-Drug Message in 12 American Cities: National Youth Ant-Drug Media Campaign. Phase 1 (Report No. 2)*. Office of National Drug Control Policy.

McNees, M. P., Egli, D. S., Marshall, R. S., Schelle, J. F., & Risley, T. R. (1976). Shoplifting prevention: Providing information through signs. *Journal of Applied Behavior Analysis, 9*, 399–405.

Mendelsohn, H., Liu, J., Spetnagel, H. T., Venglar, C., Wilson, D., Wirth, M. O., & Nash, K. (1982). *Media campaigns and crime prevention: An executive summary*. United States Department of Justice, National Institute of Justice.

Mendelsohn, H., O'Keefe, G. J., Liu, J., Spetnagel, H. T., Wilson, D., Wirth, M. D., & Nash, K. (1981). *Public communication and the prevention of crime: Strategies for Control. Volume 1: A Narrative Report*. National Institute of Justice, Law Enforcement Assistance Administration.

Mendelsohn, H., & Wilson, D. (1978). *A mass communication strategy for generating citizen action against crime*. Center for Mass Communications Research and Policy, University of Denver.

Monaghan, L. (1988). Anatomy of a crime prevention publicity campaign. In D. Challinger (Ed.), *Preventing property crime* (Seminar Proceedings No. 23) (pp. 85–93). Australian Institute of Criminology.

Myhill, A., & Bradford, B. (2012). Can police enhance public confidence by improving quality of service? Results from two surveys in England and Wales. *Policing and Society: An International Journal of Research and Policy, 22*, 397–425.

Office of National Drug Control Policy. (2000). *Anti-drug media campaign: ONDCP met most mandates, but evaluations of impact are inconclusive*. United States General Accounting Office.

Office of National Drug Control Policy. (2011). *Progress report on the national youth anti-drug media campaign for fiscal year 2010*. Executive Office of the President of the United States.

O'Keefe, G. J., Mendelsohn, H., Reid-Nash, K., Henry, E., Rosenzweig, B., & Spetnagel, H. T. (1985). *"Taking a bite out of crime": The impact of a mass media crime prevention campaign*. Center for Mass Communications Research and Policy, University of Denver.

Peters, M. D. J., Godfrey, C. M., Khalil, H., McInerney, P., Parker, D., & Soares, C. B. (2015). Guidance for conducting systematic scoping reviews. *International Journal of Evidence-Based Healthcare, 13*, 141–146.

Pham, M. T., Rajic, A., Greig, J. D., Sargeant, J. M., Papadopoulous, A., & McEwan, S. A. (2014). A scoping review of scoping reviews: Advancing the approach and enhancing the consistency. *Research Synthesis Methods, 5*, 371–385.

Potter, S. J., Moynihan, M. M., Stapleton, J. G., & Banyard, V. L. (2009). Empowering bystanders to prevent campus violence against women: A preliminary evaluation of a poster campaign. *Violence Against Women, 15*, 106–121.

Power, N., McManus, M. A., Lynch, R., & Boworth, J. (2016). Fear of crime on the rail networks: Perceptions of the UK public and British Transport Police. *Crime Prevention and Community Safety, 18*, 91–104.

Ridgeway, G., Braga, A. A., Tita, G., & Pierce, G. L. (2011). Intervening in gun markets: An experiment to assess the impact of targeted gun-law messaging. *Journal of Experimental Criminology, 7*, 103–109.

Sacco, V. F., & Silverman, R. A. (1982). Crime prevention through mass media: Prospects and problems. *Journal of Criminal Justice, 10*, 257–269.

Salazar, L. F., Baker, C. K., Price, A. W., & Carlin, K. (2003). Moving beyond the individual: Examining the effect of domestic violence policies on social norms. *American Journal of Community Psychology, 32*, 253–264.

Sekhon, G. (2020). Combating trafficking in persons through public awareness and legal education of duty bearers in India. In J. Winterdyk & J. Jones (Eds.), *The Palgrave international handbook of human trafficking* (pp. 725–744). Palgrave Macmillan.

Silke, A. (Ed.). (2019). *The Routledge handbook of terrorism and counter terrorism*. Routledge.

Spivak, H., Hausman, A. J., & Prowthrow-Stith, D. (1989). Practitioners' forum: Public health and the primary prevention of adolescent violence – The violence prevention project. *Violence and Victims, 4*, 203–212.

Sturgeon-Adams, L., Adamson, S., & Davidson, N. (2005). *Hartlepool: A case study in burglary reduction*. Centre for Criminology and Criminal Justice, University of Hull.

Tilley, N., & Webb, J. (1994). *Burglary reduction: Findings from safer cities schemes* (Police Research Group, Crime Prevention Unit Paper no. 51). Home Office.

Toch, H., & Maguire, K. (2014). Public opinion regarding crime, criminal justice, and related topics: A retrospect. *Journal of Research in Crime and Delinquency, 51*, 424–444.

United Nations Office on Drugs and Crime. (2018). *Global report on trafficking in persons 2018*. UNODC. GLOTiP_2018_BOOK_web_small.pdf (unodc.org)

van Dijk, A., & Crofts, N. (2017). Law enforcement and public health as an emerging field. *Policing and Society; An International Journal of Research and Policy, 27*, 261–275.

Velasco, J. G. (2000). Ventura County district Attorney's senior crime prevention program. *Journal of Elder Abuse & Neglect, 12*, 103–106.

Walsh, K., Zinzow, H. M., Badour, C. L., Ruggiero, K. J., Kilpatrick, D. G., & Resnick, H. S. (2016). Understanding disparities in service seeking following forcible versus drug- or alcohol-facilitated/incapacitated rape. *Journal of Interpersonal Violence, 31*, 2475–2491.

Weatherburn, D., & Grabosky, P. (1999). Strategic approaches to property crime control. *Policing and Society: An International Journal of Research and Policy, 9*, 77–96.

Whalen, K., Alqadi, N., & McInerny, L. (2013). *Building stronger, safer communities: A guide for law enforcement and community partners to prevent and respond to hate crimes*. United States Department of Justice, Office of Community Oriented Policing Services.

Whittington, R., & McGuire, J. (2020). *Violence rewired: Evidence and strategies for public health action*. Cambridge University Press.

World Health Organization (WHO). (2014). *Global status report on violence prevention*. World Health Organization.

# Chapter 12
# Lessons Learned: Ways Forward and Next Steps

## 12.1 Introduction

This concluding chapter has two main objectives. First, we draw together what we consider to be the accumulated lessons from the reviews of various areas of research covered in previous chapters. Second, we suggest or anticipate some possible next steps for taking this kind of work further, discussing that in the context of numerous changes that are already ongoing or reportedly in preparation. Along the way we will take note of several other recent developments and issues that are interesting in themselves, but which also raise wider issues for the future directions policing might take.

Reflecting on the wide range of research summarized in preceding chapters, while many issues remain unresolved, we believe there is enough evidence to justify the conclusion that the actions of police, either by themselves or in coordination with the work of other community agencies, can have a significant impact in several areas of crime control. Pursued in the ways that have been discovered as effective in the reviews we have assembled and reported, for the most part these actions also locate the police in a network of partnerships. Working in that way, while they still retain unique attributes and powers, the police are perceived as less insular than if they worked alone and kept themselves remote from other types of public service.

As we noted at the outset, a great deal of writing on police roles and practices over the past two decades, some of it touched upon in the opening chapter, has heralded the arrival of a new era in modes of policing, a shift from the long-standing reactive model to one that is more proactive. Potentially, this provides a direction of travel for policing that holds out the prospect of higher level of achievement of some of its stated aims, including more effective crime control and improved public appreciation, and potentially greater rewards for officers through task enrichment within the law enforcement role. That represents a significant shift away from a former position of maintaining distance from the public, too often bridging that

 
J. McGuire et al., *Evidence-Based Policing and Community Crime Prevention*, Advances in Preventing and Treating Violence and Aggression,
https://doi.org/10.1007/978-3-030-76363-3_12

chasm via the use of force, sometimes implacably alienating the communities who could in principle have the greatest to gain from a more constructive, collaborative approach.

Yet, the real extent of implementation of such a change remains variable and sometimes doubtful. Koper et al. (2020) carried out a survey of 180 police agencies from diverse parts of the USA to inquire into the level of use of proactive policing. Part of this was designed to assess the extent to which police areas followed guidelines on proactive policing issued by the National Academy of Sciences. Results showed that the proportion of time spent in activities that are regarded as proactive rather than reactive was often not monitored, and where that was done, the amount of it was considerably lower than expected. Officers often lacked direction as to how to engage in proactive work, and the picture pertaining to this was very mixed across police departments, and "many agencies have limited infrastructure to track, manage and evaluate proactive policing… nor is there a strong managerial emphasis on proactivity" (Koper et al., 2020, p. 871).

Another modernizing step recommended as long ago as 1919 by August Vollmer, who, as noted in Chap. 1, is regarded as the instigator of modern American policing, was that police officers should build close working collaborations with social service agencies, though he recognized their basic unwillingness to adopt such a role. Patterson and Swann (2019) reported a systematic review of the extent to which, if at all, US police had adjusted their remit in this kind of direction and engaged in "police social work". They located 81 relevant studies, examples of collaborations between police and 12 other professional groups, from a total of 18 countries, just over half based in the USA. They covered a wide spectrum of problems, with interpersonal violence the most frequently found. Several of the specific areas of focus were of the sorts discussed in the present volume, including mental illness, partner violence and work with vulnerable adults. A key finding was that the majority of the arrangements were based on "unique models" (p. 879). That is, they lacked a number of features, such as staff training, technical assistance, resource allocation, organizational support and research and evaluation that can make services sustainable. This kind of provision too therefore is one that could gain greater momentum from more coherent coordination.

## 12.2 The Big Picture

Based on the key findings noted in the preceding chapters, we consider it justifiable to conclude that there are approaches to crime prevention that are effective in addressing several of the problems addressed here and in securing reductions in crime levels as a result. That emerged, for example, in reducing violence in the night-time economy, where there are some clear indications of strategies, appearing with a relatively good degree of consistency that can effectively reduce it. What is regarded as amongst the most intractable of social problems, domestic abuse and intimate partner violence, is not irremediable, and there are approaches such as the actions of specialist police domestic violence units that have been found to be moderately effective. In relation to mental health problems, there are several positive indicators from outcome evidence of beneficial effects in relation to a range of outcomes, when police officers work in collaborative ways with mental health professionals. The delivery of the methods that will work for these challenges is often dependent on context, and on the differential identification of subgroups, necessitating careful assessment of those variables when deciding what actions to implement. Put another way, often there are no one-size-fits-all solutions for problems the police are asked to address. Potentially viable ideas need to be adapted to circumstances, integrated with local intelligence and crime analysis.

Evidence reviews, allowing multiple comparisons to be made, can nevertheless supply valuable positioning data. Table 12.1 therefore presents summary statements on the ten issues or areas covered in this book, highlighting the methods that emerged as the most effective or that in some respects demonstrated added value in addressing what are extremely challenging problems. Gloomily but not surprisingly, there are a few areas where the record stays blank or where all that has been discovered is a virtual cul-de-sac.

Results obtained in some areas are very complex. In others it has been difficult to draw clear conclusions or to make firm recommendations, and it is likely to remain so until more and better research has been carried out. But concerning how to reduce victim and witness retraction and disengagement, for example, several steps have become identifiable that appear to be conducive to reducing attrition, and most are linked to more methodical pursuit of thorough and transparent investigative processes and improved communication with those involved. The complexities are such that no single change by itself is likely to present a solution. But by introducing marginal changes in several dimensions of a problem, the net effect can be a significant gain in effectiveness or quality of response.

Those conclusions are based on research of variable quality, but there is a sizeable proportion of it that meets relatively high standards of methodological robustness as field experiments, given the intricacies of the situations in which the work was done. There are, probably almost inevitably, some areas where the picture to date remains confusing and more research is needed. The challenges of supervising convicted sex offenders on licence from prison have been vividly highlighted by the studies examined here, but no specific approach to managing those difficulties has a demonstrable record of success. Equally for working with vulnerable adults, only tentative suggestions can be drawn from the research reviewed. But there is some evidence that the adoption by police of a more proactive regulatory and monitoring role could have an impact on the working of the system and the avoidance of negligent or abusive outcomes. Regarding services for crime victims, while it may not be a part of traditional core policing roles to provide counselling and support beyond some brief initial encounters, police could nevertheless perform a vital triage function in advising on allocation to other services according to need.

The areas considered in the book are obviously only a sample of the plethora of issues that police departments face. Many more could be added. Even within the research project that gave rise to this book, there were several areas considered for

**Table 12.1** A summary of some key findings from evidence reviews in Chaps. 2, 3, 4, 5, 6, 7, 8, 9, 10, and 11

| Issue | Principal findings |
|---|---|
| Policing the night-time economy | *Good evidence:*<br>Three main kinds of interventions were found most likely to be effective:<br>(1) Restriction of alcohol sales, through reducing hours of opening or limiting access during lockout periods<br>(2) Data exchange procedures involving collaboration between the police force and hospital emergency departments, focusing police attention on high-risk venues<br>(3) Various combinations of multi-level community interventions, including different types of components. There is no fixed formula for doing this; it needs to be adapted to context. Such interventions work better when there is also enforcement of licensing laws<br>*Some evidence, but weaker or more mixed:*<br>There was also some supportive evidence for local information campaigns, types of training for bar and door staff and police engagement of licensees in risk management inside bars |
| Managing sex offenders on license: effectiveness of registration and notification procedures | *Mixed results:*<br>Few studies have found a significant impact of registration or notification in terms of specific deterrence. A majority have found no difference between these and other procedures<br>Community notification, accessed by only a small proportion of the public, can increase as well as lower fear and can have adverse consequences for offenders and non-offending relatives. Residence restrictions for the most part have unanticipated negative consequences<br>Overall, the findings highlight the need for multi-agency liaison and collaboration in sex offender management, to enable police to respond to public expectations in this area, while balancing and responding to possible adverse effects |

(continued)

**Table 12.1** (continued)

| Issue | Principal findings |
|---|---|
| Domestic abuse and intimate partner violence | *Fairly clear evidence, though findings not positive:*<br>For arrest, after an early reportedly successful experiment, later studies found more mixed effects. The majority showed no effects though there may be an impact on a subgroup of perpetrators if they can be successfully identified via risk assessment. The latter would require additional police training<br>*No evidence* was found that dual arrest is ineffective<br>*Better evidence was found for:*<br>Domestic Violence Response Teams or Units, either police-led or based in multi-agency teams<br>Multi-agency coordinated responses including individual work, risk assessment, victim support and safeguarding showed some of the best results. But not all models produced the same outcomes consistently. There were less consistent results for coordinated community response as a public awareness or education campaign.<br>Women's police stations or women's justice services in which police provide easier access to the range of services likely to be required by victims of IPV. Several large-scale studies show promising effects of this strategy, though others indicate a need for detailed attention to structural factors in deciding how it is implemented<br>*Mixed results with some positive effects:*<br>Therapeutic interventions for DA/IPV perpetrators showed a wide range in quality of evaluation studies and in effects. The most widely used and longest established intervention (the Duluth programme) did not yield reliable positive effects. However, several other approaches involving multi-modal interventions have produced more positive outcomes (e.g. CBT, IDAP, CDVP and DVPP programmes)<br>There is preliminary evidence supporting the use of awareness and training sessions in secondary schools for long-term prevention of relational violence<br>There is promising evidence from a review of structural interventions to reduce IPV in low- and middle-income countries<br>The limited impact of many individually focused interventions supports the argument that further work is necessary at structural levels of the ecological model of partner violence discussed in the chapter |

(continued)

**Table 12.1** (continued)

| Issue | Principal findings |
|---|---|
| What works in school-based interventions? | *Mixed but generally promising evidence:*<br>While outcomes are varied, a sizeable number of studies show positive outcomes for programmes to reduce different types of antisocial behaviour in schools, including alcohol and drug misuse, aggression and violence.<br>There is also inconsistent but on balance positive evidence supporting the use of anti-bullying programmes, but better evidence when they are provided on a universal/school-wide basis within a supportive environment<br>Though based on a small number of studies, but of higher quality, there is evidence of positive outcomes from school-based programmes to reduce relational violence<br>*Evidence was not supportive of:*<br>Placement of police personnel (School Resources Officers) in schools as security officers is generally ineffective and may have counterproductive effects<br>The use of punitive sanctions, controls and enhanced security measures showed almost no beneficial effects in enhancing school safety |
| Preventing young people from involvement in violence, gangs and organized crime | *Best-supported interventions:*<br>Interventions combining law enforcement principles with service provision, sometimes incorporating multi-level components, attained firmly positive outcomes across several studies in different sites, employing strategies known as *pulling levers* and *Project Safe Neighborhoods* and in a separate initiative working with high-risk cases<br>*Mixed evidence with some positive outcomes:*<br>Skills-based interventions, mentoring programmes<br>*No evidence available:*<br>No reliable evidence base was found relating to the question of how to prevent young people from becoming involved in organized crime in adulthood |
| Multi-agency safeguarding for vulnerable and at-risk adults | *Very mixed and unclear outcomes:*<br>Clear conclusions were difficult to draw regarding this area due to the very varied nature of the located research, only a small portion of which used standard evaluation methods. Many retained items consisted of analyses of case files, reports on serious case reviews or qualitative/thematic analysis studies<br>*Moderate level of support:*<br>For the effectiveness of some forms of multidisciplinary team working in reducing abuse of older adults<br>There was good support for Elder Abuse Forensic Centers in the USA<br>Qualitative research indicated a higher level of support for a *law-* or *justice-oriented* rather than a *social-work-oriented* model of working in achieving greater protection for vulnerable persons<br>The outcomes of many investigations indicate that problems would have been avoided and safety maintained if pre-arranged procedures had been adequately followed<br>There are suggestions that police services could play a key role in coordinating other agencies in adherence to and maintenance of legal standards of care, in collaboration with Protection of Vulnerable Adults teams<br>Studies indicate a need for additional training in this area for police officers involved in investigative or monitoring roles |

(continued)

**Table 12.1** (continued)

| Issue | Principal findings |
|---|---|
| People with mental health problems | *Best evidence shows:*<br>When three types of policing response were compared, a clear trend emerged:<br>Liaison and diversion schemes: some positive results were found but not consistently<br>Street triage: showed generally more positive outcomes<br>However, crisis intervention teams showed generally the best outcomes, but officer training is essential and needs to be sustained and refreshed over time<br>In comparisons between the approaches, there was evidence of the value of (a) existence of a psychiatric triage or drop-off centre where police can transport individuals in crisis and (b) community partnerships in which the police worked alongside other relevant agencies<br>Research remains limited but to date the crisis intervention team approach stands out as more effective than the other models of service |
| Victim and witness retraction and disengagement | *Mixed results, complex evidence:*<br>For factors thought to influence retraction or withdrawal, there were no consistent associations between demographic variables and likelihood of participation in or withdrawal from the criminal justice process as a victim or witness<br>In partner violence cases, there was evidence that some relationships variables and victim responses were more likely to be associated with disengagement<br>In sexual assault cases, fear of not being believed and of being cross-examined in court were significantly associated with disengagement<br>Some specific history, individual and relational factors were also reliably associated with decisions to continue with prosecution<br>*Moderately good evidence that:*<br>Criminal investigations that use clear procedures and involve helpful initial police contacts, explicit evidence gathering, taking photographs, use of video-recorded and victim impact statements and timely contact with support services are more likely to result in cases being followed through to prosecution.<br>Coordinated work between police officers in dedicated roles or with specialist training, and prosecution services, from early stages of investigations can reduce rates of retraction and withdrawal, though this is based on one study |

(continued)

**Table 12.1** (continued)

| Issue | Principal findings |
|---|---|
| Victim counselling and support | *In previous reviews moderate to strong evidence was found for:*<br>The effectiveness of psychological therapies for assisting victims of rape, sexual assault and domestic violence<br>The value of Sexual Assault Nurse Examiners with victims of rape or other sexual assault<br>The effectiveness of domestic violence shelters<br>*Good evidence that:*<br>Provision of counselling or therapeutic services to victims of more serious crimes has beneficial effects and can result in meaningful change but is unlikely to be done in a few brief sessions only and should be delivered by trained professionals<br>There is also evidence that advocacy, hotline and other community services are valued by victims, but outcomes were not wholly consistent<br>By contrasts post-incident debriefing for crime victims has not been found to be effective<br>*At present it remains uncertain* as to which recommendations to make concerning the commissioning of victim support and counselling services |
| What works in public awareness campaigns? | *A scoping review found mainly mixed evidence in three categories*<br>(1) There is evidence that public information campaigns on crime-related issues have been helpful, but the effects of some have been comparatively weak. Results suggest messages conveyed by mass media need to be consistent with police behaviour in encounters with the public to secure reliable effects<br>(2) Studies of campaigns focused on specific police actions (neighbourhood policing, transport safety measures, weapon availability) found only weak effects of publicity and awareness efforts<br>(3) Offence-specific campaigns (shop theft, car theft, burglary, drug use, violence, violence against women, rape, child abuse, hate crimes, human trafficking, terrorism) by contrast have in many cases produced meaningful results and achieved significant levels of success, though again results are not uniform and are affected by a wide variety of factors |

review where there was very little evidence despite the importance of the topic. Three areas that were reviewed did not generate sufficient material to have formed a book chapter. There is no doubt that with reference to some issues, the position is one that Thornton et al. (2019, p. 278) characterized as an "evidence drought" where more research is urgently needed.

The issues that were raised in our project reflected the priorities of two police areas in England. In other areas with a different demographic composition, the list may well have been different, especially in larger urban centres. The UK has only one really big city, London, and several medium-sized conurbations. Many countries have far larger population hubs, while others have highly dispersed settlement patterns. These fundamental contrasts and the numerous other variations associated with them mean that the concerns and preoccupations of police will diverge markedly between places and over time.

As just mentioned, within the timescale of the project that gave the impetus to this book, three other topic areas were reviewed that were not included in the text. One dealt with the question of finding better ways to manage the level of demand on the police's *contact control room*, obviously a pivotal link with the public. For example, in the first 10 months of this research, the two police areas which commissioned the project (Norfolk and Suffolk) received a formidable 630,000+ calls for service. Despite searching 18 databases and discovering numerous attempts to address this problem (including establishment of non-emergency call lines, devising frameworks for call classification and allocation, and staff training schemes), no empirical studies were found on how to compare and choose between systems. The state of knowledge had not yet reached even a minimal critical mass. In the few years since we carried out preliminary searches on this however, the position may have significantly altered.

Another area contemplated for review was that of *talent management*. Police today perform a wider range of tasks than at any time in their history; sustaining this requires a prodigious range of skillsets. There is a large literature on police recruitment, selection, training and promotion (Cox et al., 2016), but until not long ago, the concept of talent management represented a departure from traditional models of undertaking those processes, especially at the higher levels of organizations. However, searches of eight databases and of five leading police journals over a 17-year period located relatively little material that could form an evidence base. Several police departments had produced discussion documents on this issue, but none carried any empirical weight, in the sense of providing evidence why one approach to the problem might be preferable to another. It may also be that in a workplace where there is often a need for collective action and an ethos of interdependence, the identification of individual talent is more difficult than elsewhere (Gold et al., 2016).

A third area considered, one that was in part reflexive in relation to the project itself and connected to some of the questions raised in the next section of this chapter, was that of how best to translate the findings of research into practice. As this was to some extent overtaken by parallel developments, we discuss it more fully below. While for both this and the two preceding questions there was relevant research in adjacent fields, the amount of it that could be suitably applied to policing was limited; hence the net result was inconclusive.

That position too might have changed in recent years. The number of other areas that it would be useful to review is large, and the size of the gap in applicable knowledge is hard to estimate. It is likely that in some, there will already be sizeable quantities of research studies available and results that could prove useful in policing. Many areas of criminological research, such as the operation of drug sales and markets, the investigation of child sexual abuse or responses to terrorism and security issues, have generated so much information that the analysis, evaluation and application of them have become specialisms in themselves.

Police forces increasingly give active consideration to new ways of working and to questions previously outside the familiar remit of the role as traditionally conceived, in order to increase the effectiveness of preventive efforts. If that can be made to work, pursuing it makes sense with respect to results at all levels, in terms of safety and harm reduction, efficient use of resources and relations with the public. There are examples of the extension of police interest to areas that were formerly outside the boundaries of policing.

One is the possibility of early intervention and of being involved in what is called *primary prevention* of the development of problems in individuals' lives. This entails involvement with local authorities, children's services and health agencies concerned with children whose well-being is impaired by *adverse childhood experiences* and who are at risk of later involvement, for example, with "county lines" trafficking gangs in drug sales and distribution. The College of Policing in England and Wales has made research funding available for studies in this realm. Police officers work with relevant partners in efforts to prevent both temporary involvement in crime and longer-lasting ensnarement in it, due to the convergence of adverse events and circumstances. Several initiatives related to young people who may be vulnerable in these respects have been proposed by police forces themselves, including family-centred approaches and enhanced community provision, with police playing a pivotal role.

Another area, this time concerned with adults, is that of *offender management*, in which police have sought to enlarge the range of groups they work with. Decisions regarding areas of responsibility are usually based on an assessment of the harm individuals cause underpinned by the use of an algorithm (of varying quality and sophistication). This has been a development from the Ministry of Justice's *Integrated Offender Management* process initially centred on acquisitive offenders, moving later to focus on those who may be less prolific but pose greater risk of causing serious harm, such as intimate partner violence offenders or sexual recidivists. Both this and the preceding departure are indicative of the fresh perspectives being adopted on the role of the police and their relation to the public, to other public bodies and to government.

## 12.3 Next Steps for Evidence-Based Policing

Now that the concept of evidence-based policing (EBP) has been widely discussed and much work has already been done in alignment with the approach, we might expect that it is firmly implanted in the ethos of policing. Although from a historical vantage point it is not long since it was first proposed, it has already demonstrated its value, and given its almost axiomatic soundness, it is difficult to see how it can ever be discarded. But it could become marginalized or remain an issue to which lip service is paid, rather than achieving a status in which most police officers regard it as an inherent part of their practice.

In the UK, Fleming and Wingrove (2017) obtained feedback from 90 police officers or other staff from four constabularies attending an EBP pilot training programme. While in principle the participants regarded research as useful to their roles, they described several barriers to applying it in practice, including "a lack of organizational clarity, support, and resources" (p. 209), and there was a cynical view of it as something only done by senior officers as a device to gain promotion. Palmer et al. (2019) surveyed the views of 625 police staff from a single police force on their attitudes towards EBP. While the term was widely recognized, there were differences between the ranks, with constables significantly less likely to be aware of its meaning than those of higher ranks and more likely to attach value to on-the-job experience than to scientific training or expert knowledge. At a more fundamental level, it may be that there are gaps in how well the concept is understood. In a survey conducted in 2011–2014 in the USA, of over 1300 staff, including a large number of patrol officers, Telep and Somers (2019) found multiple definitions of what EBP was believed to mean.

Another risk is that it comes to be perceived as not having delivered what it supposedly promised. As the originator of the concept of EBP, Sherman (2015) has himself expressed such a concern: "The smothering claim of the 'police craft' paradigm is that evidence has nothing to offer police… the biggest risk is *high expectations for immediate results* and that EBP 'works'" (pp. 17, 19). In reviewing the extent of its adoption and implementation by police agencies, Sherman made a series of suggestions for guiding a "tipping point", supplemented with many detailed possibilities. Amongst other ideas they include the following. One is a proposal for the establishment of evidence-based policing units within police departments and services, serving as a resource to the agency as a whole, collating and communicating research results relevant to operational tasks. Second, there is the suggested provision of a comprehensive training programme, with several levels of activity including in-service events, or sponsoring police personnel in the pursuit of degrees that incorporate a research component. Third, police departments should generate and energize closer links with universities through the dissemination of research training and the production of project reports. Fourth, it is recommended that police services collaborate to create a permanent *Central Registry of EBP Projects*, subject to a peer review process. To work well, that would involve longer-term maintenance of a dedicated EBP website.

Essentially, these innovations represent different dimensions of a process of fostering closer connections between research and practice, for example, between universities with departments that specialize in this field and the cultivation of a research culture within police services. There are several ways to carry this into practice and monitor and sustain it. Fortunately, there already are central registries of EBP projects on both sides of the Atlantic. In the UK this takes the form of the College of Policing's (2017) research map. There have been invitations to submit applications for further projects, also promoted by the College of Policing (2020a) within its *Vulnerability and Violent Crime Programme*, which includes a series of projects launched in 2019. To maintain the momentum, this has been accompanied by the establishment of a website acting as a Knowledge Hub for evidence-based projects and allied activity (College of Policing, 2020b).

There are other dimensions within these initiatives. As an integral part of sustaining the usefulness of EBP, there needs to be an accessible mechanism for summarizing and communicating the findings of research to senior officers and operational commanders of police forces. As part of the *Crime Reduction Toolkit* developed by the What Works Centre for Crime Reduction originally based in University College London (now housed in the College of Policing), Thornton et al. (2019) have constructed a tool known as *Effect, Mechanism, Moderator, Implementation, Economics* (EMMIE) designed to "act as a framework to effectively communicate research evidence to those with a responsibility for and competency to deal with crime" (2019, p. 269). It comprises an on-screen display which, based on the findings of systematic reviews, provides summary ratings on five key aspects of an intervention: its impact on crime, the mechanism by which it works, the contexts in which it works best, how to implement it and its costs. The synoptic landing page enables comparisons to be made between different interventions for a given problem, with detailed information on each then accessed through menu-driven selections.

Other steps in the translational process have been suggested or amplified by Telep and Shader (2019), who describe the creation of a *What works in policing?* website by the Office of the City Auditor in Seattle in 2014, in conjunction with George Mason and Arizona State universities, and by Santos and Santos (2019) who advocated adapting the *knowledge to action* (KTA) framework, one of many approaches used in the field of medicine, for policing purposes. Aspects of these suggestions closely parallel those made by Sherman (2015) and the crime reduction toolkit elucidated by Thornton et al. (2019).

Evidence that these proposals are at the very least on the right track comes from a study by Boulton et al. (2020) of the impact of a set of 29 research studies undertaken within a single police constabulary, where a dedicated EBP unit had been created. Once completed, the level of dissemination of the projects varied markedly, but just over half (52%) were judged to have been implemented in some way and to have led to changes in practice. Features that were associated with greater likelihood of having a practical impact were the use of mixed methods of research, and *transferability*, that the findings were perceived as relevant for "current knowledge, policy, or practice" (p. 4) such that they could be used in multiple contexts.

## 12.4 Predictive Policing

Some of these successes and related proposals might however be surpassed by the widespread adoption of what has been acclaimed as possibly the most advanced form of intelligence-led policing to date, *predictive policing*. In some ways this carries the shared aspirations of problem-oriented, intelligence-led and hotspot policing to their logical conclusion. That is, if a way can be found to predict where or when crimes are likely to occur, police can take pre-emptive action accordingly. Such geospatial or spatiotemporal analysis can be extended to help identify those who might be most likely to be involved in, or affected by, criminal acts, including both offenders and victims. Thus, analysis of past patterns can focus on predicting future crime events, or on identifying places that are at increased risk of them; on forecasting who is at risk of involvement in crime, or at heightened risk of becoming a victim of it; and even on determining who is likely to be guilty of specific past crimes and then taking appropriate preventive action (Perry et al., 2013).

There is not yet a consensus on how to define predictive policing. At its inception it was viewed as primarily place-based (Hunt, 2019), whereas later discussions reached towards the idea that its targets included persons as well as places. Meijer and Wessels (2019, p. 1033) have proposed a definition as follows: "Predictive policing is the collection and analysis of data about previous crimes for identification and statistical prediction of individuals or geospatial areas with an increased probability of criminal activity to help developing policing intervention and prevention strategies and tactics".

The concepts that underpin this type of analysis emerged from the process of crime mapping and the study of repeat victimization. This was first put into practice from 1994 onwards by the New York Police Department, using *Computerized Crime Comparison Statistics* (COMPSTAT), a data-analytic program for predicting crime events and appraising police performance (Bureau of Justice Assistance, 2013). This generated reports for weekly strategy meetings focused on crime control and the focus of police activity. From an academic standpoint, related concepts were formulated by Bowers et al. (2004), who forwarded proposals concerning the use of *prospective* hotspot mapping techniques. But the initial application of the idea is usually traced to the work of Police Commissioner William J. Bratton, who worked at different times in both New York and Los Angeles police departments.

In New York City in the 1990s, there were annual recorded falls in many types of offence, including a substantial drop in homicide rates. These changes were attributed by many commentators to the introduction of COMPSTAT, which was made central to police practice, alongside the pre-existing broken windows model, also championed by Police Chief Bratton. The method was disseminated more widely following more refined development of the techniques of *predictive analytics* by the Los Angeles Police Department. These became more broadly known through a symposium held there in 2008, linked to community-oriented and intelligence-led policing. The techniques have numerous potential applications, from mapping the likelihood of volume crimes such as theft or burglary to the more daunting task of countering political insurgency (Perry et al., 2013).

However, in an analysis comparing crime rates in different US cities over time, Levitt (2004) showed that the observed trends in New York were similar to those seen from the late 1980s onwards in other US cities where no such system was in use. On those and other grounds, Levitt (2004) expressed scepticism over the causes of the observed changes, suggesting there were other explanations than innovations in policing strategies. Since then, revelations by 1770 retired NYPD officers of how data were manipulated have also raised questions over the genuine effectiveness of the methods (Eterno et al., 2016).

Since that time, there have been varying outcomes from research studies designed to evaluate predictive policing. Fitterer et al. (2015) reported a pilot study of the use of geographic information systems for predicting the occurrence of break-and-entry and other property crimes in Vancouver. Analysis showed the system was successful in doing this, yielding automatically updated predictive maps of residential and commercial burglaries. Mohler et al. (2015) reported the results of two randomized controlled field trials, one conducted in the USA and the other in the UK. In each, a data-analytic technique was used to predict crime frequency at specific locations, and police patrol activity and crime levels were then evaluated. Both experiments showed significant drops in crime, an average of 7.4%, a better result than if predictions had been made by crime analysts.

Other studies, however, cast doubts on the efficacy of the techniques. Hunt et al. (2014) evaluated a predictive policing experiment in Shreveport, Louisiana, but found no significant evidence of impact on the targeted outcomes of residential and business property crimes. There were, however, some reported improvements in community relations. Saunders et al. (2016) devised statistical procedures for predicting gun violence in Chicago, by developing a *Strategic Subjects List* identifying high-risk persons, but this did not prove successful for predicting homicide or shooting incidents. Moreover, when Ratcliffe et al. (2020) examined how predictive policing and the use of algorithms linked to the patrol task and how officers on those duties in Philadelphia perceived it, there was a sizeable gap in interpretations. Officers considered that their own experience and knowledge of local areas was marginalized, and the prescribed task in some respects "got in the way" of the real work of policing; "the technology conflicted directly with the whole notion of police patrolling as a craft" (pp. 649, 651).

Meijer and Wessels (2019) reported a systematic review of research on predictive policing, locating 37 relevant bodies of literature, the earliest dating to 2010, and including 24 research articles published in the period from then until 2017. The number of studies that reported evaluations of the effectiveness of predictive policing was found to be somewhat limited. Overall while there were some positive results, there were also some disappointing ones and others that were ambiguous. At the same time, studies specifically designed to examine the claimed drawbacks of the approach found little clear evidence of them. At present therefore, the position regarding its value remains unclear, with on the one hand "little support for the claimed benefits" (p. 1031) but on the other hand no firm demonstration of the supposed drawbacks.

A more serious kind of objection to predictive policing however came from its alleged discriminatory effects in leading towards the targeting of local areas with high proportions of residents from ethnic minority populations. The scale of this problem was such that a joint statement was issued by a collection of 17 community agencies, coordinated by the American Civil Liberties Union (2019), stating that the net result of its arrival was a further concentration of policing in communities that were already over-policed, raising significant civil rights concerns. Data which form the basis of predictive policing were not neutral but reinforced pre-existing biases in how the police operate. The method focused exclusively on the crime rate, thus neglecting other community needs, and resulted in higher rates of stop and search or of arrest in deprived areas which often have had higher proportions of minorities. Placing that in a broader context, very few if any of the problems addressed in the chapters of this book found more forceful solutions to be the most effective ones. The same dangers have been warned against by the United Nations Committee on the Elimination of Racial Discrimination (2020). This notes that "rapid advances in technological development mean that increasingly, the actions of law enforcement officials are determined or informed by algorithmic profiling, which may include big data, automated decision-making and artificial intelligence tools and methods", creating a great risk that reliance on such methods "may also reproduce and reinforce biases and aggravate or lead to discriminatory practices" (p. 7).

Addressing the question of discriminatory effects, Brantingham et al. (2018) reanalysed data from the controlled experiments on the use of predictive policing in Los Angeles reported by Mohler et al. (2015, as briefly outlined above). They tested whether there were indications of bias in terms of differential arrest rates amongst minority communities. This study found no differences between racial-ethnic groups or any evidence of discriminatory outcomes. The authors acknowledge nevertheless that arrests are an "imperfect proxy" for police contacts overall. They concluded that there remains a need to "guard against bias in predictive policing and ensure fairness in outcomes" (p. 5).

By contrast a more in-depth study of police practices in locations where predictive models were being applied suggested high levels of caution were needed. From a set of 13 locations where data were available, Richardson et al. (2019) undertook detailed case studies of this in Chicago, New Orleans and Maricopa County, Arizona. In each of these locations, there was a known history of police acting unlawfully or in biased ways in the usage of data that had been subject to external investigations. They found extensive evidence that the predictive policing models being employed were using what they termed "dirty data", that is, there were inbuilt biases in the information used to construct predictive models, such that the net result was one of "runaway feedback loops, where police are repeatedly sent back to the same neighborhoods regardless of the actual crime rate" (Richardson et al., 2019, p. 41).

In principle, it is not unreasonable to expect that ideas of this nature, if implemented carefully, ought to prove useful. Considering the future applications of it, some researchers have expressed optimism and confidence in the potential of predictive policing for forestalling acts of crime (Egbert & Krasmann, 2018). But there remains "legitimate concern that the use of algorithms may replicate or amplify the disparities inherent in police-recorded data" (Babuta & Oswald, 2020, p. viii). If one of the main sequelae is to replicate the injustices or give rise to the same grievances that are familiar from other forms of forceful policing, the improvements come at considerable cost. Discussion of this once again poses basic questions about the objectives of policing.

Drawing on an interview and focus-group study with 26 respondents from police forces or advisory and expert bodies in the UK, Babuta and Oswald (2020) recognized how growing emphasis on data analytics driven by information demand, diminishing resources and increased focus on prevention means that methods such as predictive policing have important potential. They considered too however that "the development of policing algorithms is often not underpinned by a robust empirical evidence base regarding their claimed benefits" (Babuta & Oswald, 2020, p. 9). Hence there are problems of data quality and reliability. In addition, the approach is data-heavy, and although based on a blend of routine activity theory, rational choice theory and crime pattern theory, each an important strand within criminology, there is an absence of theory of cause and effect in the approach. In practice the use of the techniques depends on the availability of the requisite skills and expertise.

Taking a balanced approach, Babuta and Oswald (2020, pp. 47–48) suggest that "many deployments of police algorithms and automation will not impact significantly on citizens' human rights or civil liberties", but given that there can be "profound implications" in criminal justice settings, police forces should undertake regular review of whether any algorithm "is still being used for the purposes and interventions for which it was developed". The UN Committee on the Elimination of Racial Discrimination (2020, p. 11) also recommended that "States should adopt measures to ensure that public information from the police and other law enforcement agencies is based on reliable and objective statistics and does not perpetuate stereotypes and bias against ethnic groups that are victims of discrimination".

## 12.5 Conclusion

As we commented at the outset, reflecting on the brief look backwards that was given in Chap. 1, almost from the moment the role first appeared in ancient times and throughout its history since then, policing appears to have been in an almost constant state of transition and flux. Police serve vital and indispensable functions in present-day, highly complex societies, yet defining their role with precision remains challenging because different sectors of the populace have differing expectations of them. In a sense policing has been a mirror of some of the main preoccupations of society, most importantly its concerns with crime and disorder, but also power relations between different groups. Their historical role as agents of one social group tasked with controlling other groups remains a troubling backdrop to current debates on police accountability.

Clearly police forces can best achieve their appointed objectives when they are trusted by the public, and all relevant stakeholders recognize the importance of this. Succeeding in that is partly dependent on the quality of their everyday interactions with the public, when they respond to calls and provide the kinds of protection citizens want. But it is also likely to be influenced by reputational factors. In relation to this, police have been beset by a series of scandals of different kinds, often of an extremely serious and damaging nature. In the UK they have included the corruption of the notorious West Midlands Serious Crime Squad, which operated from 1974 to 1989, where officers were found to have "systematically fabricated evidence, tortured suspects, and written false confessions to obtain convictions for serious crime" so causing "literally dozens of abortions of justice" (Naughton, 2013, p. 42). Subsequently a judge-led inquiry into the 1993 murder in London of a young black man, Stephen Lawrence, by a group of white youths, and the profoundly flawed investigation than ensued, led to the Metropolitan Police being infamously portrayed as manifesting *institutional racism* (Home Office, 1999; the *MacPherson Report*). Some years later, further revelations of a different kind showed how, over a 40-year period, undercover police officers infiltrated community organizations and pressure groups very few of which posed any threat to the rest of society, maintaining false identities, establishing relationships and even fathering children with members of those groups (Evans & Lewis, 2013).

In the USA, where reportedly "cops think that everyone is an asshole" (Stinson, 2020, p. 5), the problem of police violence is so extensive that criminologists have applied the same kinds of theoretical explanation to it as they have used to understand criminal violence in general. In Australia, there was what became known as the "Lawyer X" scandal, in which a defense attorney passed confidential information on her clients to police, who covertly relied on her as an "intelligence gold mine" for many years. It is thought that more than 1,000 convictions arising from this were unlawfully obtained, compromising the position of staff up to the most senior levels (Dowsley & Carylon, 2021).

Problems of these and related kinds are by no means confined to the world's most affluent societies. They can also be found in countries lower down the scale of economic development (Hope, 2015). According to the *Global Corruption Barometer* surveys conducted by the Berlin-based Transparency International, the police, nominally the principal upholders of law in society, are often viewed as either the most corrupt public institution or as running closely behind elected representatives in that respect (Hardoon & Heinrich, 2013).

Returning to the central theme of this book, of whether it is feasible to achieve crime reduction through the methods of community policing, guided by a systematic evidence base, we offer the conclusion that there is an expanding body of research that supports this as a viable direction of movement for police services. Is the advent of predictive policing a technological fix for the problem of effectiveness? It may be a significant addition to policing methods, but outcome studies show somewhat mixed results, and potentially it further undermines trust in police in those locations where it most urgently needs to be built.

For many problems, algorithm-driven patrols and checks also leave unresolved the question of what exactly police could or should do, what type of intervention to employ. We consider that the kinds of evidence amassed in this book, if put into application, would enhance perceptions of the police by better integrating their work with that of other agencies, while also producing better results. We suggest that acting on some of the research reviewed here could make a valuable contribution to solving those problems: of taking forward, in synchrony, the agendas of police effectiveness in protecting the public while also establishing better police-community relations.

## References


American Civil Liberties Union and 16 other organizations. (2019). *Joint statement: Predictive policing today: A shared statement of civil rights concerns*. https://www.aclu.org/other/statement-concern-about-predictive-policing-aclu-and-16-civil-rights-privacy-racial-justice

Babuta, A., & Oswald, M. (2020). *Data analytics and algorithms in policing in England and Wales towards a new policy framework*. Occasional Paper. London: Royal United Services Institute for Defence and Security Studies.

Boulton, L., Pythian, R., Kirby, S., & Dawson, I. (2020). Taking an evidence-based approach to evidence-based policing research. *Policing*. https://doi.org/10.1093/police/paaa057

Bowers, K. J., Johnson, S. D., & Pease, K. (2004). Prospective hot-spotting: The future of crime mapping? *British Journal of Criminology, 44*(5), 641–658.

Brantingham, P. J., Valasik, M., & Mohler, G. O. (2018). Does predictive policing lead to biased arrests? Results from a randomized controlled trial. *Statistics and Public Policy, 5*(1), 1–6.

Bureau of Justice Assistance. (2013). *COMPSTAT: Its origins, evolution, and future in law enforcement agencies*. Bureau of Justice Assistance, Police Executive Research Forum.

College of Policing. (2017). https://whatworks.college.police.uk/Research/Research-Map/Pages/Research-Map.aspx

College of Policing. (2020a). https://www.college.police.uk/What-we-do/Development/leadership-development-choices/Pages/Knowledge-hub-professional-communities.aspx

College of Policing. (2020b). Knowledge hub professional communities | College of Policing

Cox, S. M., Marchionna, S., & Fitch, B. D. (2016). *Introduction to policing* (3rd ed.). Sage Publications.

Dowsley, A., & Carylon, P. (2021). *Lawyer X: The Scandalous Story of how Melbourne's Gangland War was really 'won'*. Sydney: HarperCollins.

Egbert, S., & Krasmann, S. (2018). Predictive policing: Not yet, but soon preemptive? *Policing and Society, 30*(8), 905–919.

Eterno, J. A., Verma, A., & Silverman, E. B. (2016). Police manipulations of crime reporting: Insiders' revelations. *Justice Quarterly, 33*(5), 811–835.

Evans, B., & Lewis, P. (2013). *Undercover: The true story of Britain's secret police*. Guardian Books.

Fitterer, J., Nelson, T. A., & Nathoo, F. (2015). Predictive crime mapping. *Police Practice and Research: An International Journal, 16*(2), 121–135.

Fleming, J., & Wingrove, J. (2017). 'We would if we could … but not sure if we can': Implementing evidence-based practice: The evidence-based practice agenda in the UK. *Policing, 11*(2), 202–213.

Gold, J., Oldroyd, T., Chesters, E., Booth, A., & Waugh, A. (2016). Exploring talenting: Talent management as a collective Endeavour. *European Journal of Training and Development, 40*, 513–533. https://doi.org/10.1108/EJTD-11-2015-0091

Hardoon, D., & Heinrich, F. (2013). *Global corruption barometer 2013*. Transparency International.

Home Office. (1999). *The Stephen Lawrence Inquiry: Report of an Inquiry by Sir William Macpherson of Cluny. Cm 4262*. The Stationery Office.

Hope, K. R. (2015). An analytical perspective on police corruption and police reforms in developing societies. In K. R. Hope Sr. (Ed.), *Police corruption and police reforms in developing societies* (pp. 3–32). CRC Press.

Hunt, J. (2019). From crime mapping to crime forecasting: The evolution of place-based policing. *National Institute of Justice Journal, 281*, https:// nij.ojp.gov/topics/articles/crime-mapping-crime-forecasting-evolution-place-based-policing

Hunt, P., Saunders, J., & Hollywood, J. S. (2014). *Evaluation of the Shreveport predictive policing experiment*. RAND Corporation.

Koper, C. S., Lum, C., Wu, X., & Fritz, N. (2020). Proactive policing in the United States: A national survey. *Policing: An International Journal, 43*(5), 861–876.

Levitt, S. D. (2004). Understanding why crime fell in the 1990s: Four factors that explain the decline and six that do not. *Journal of Economic Perspectives, 18*(1), 163–190.

Meijer, A., & Wessels, M. (2019). Predictive policing: Review of benefits and drawbacks. *International Journal of Public Administration, 42*(12), 1031–1039.

Mohler, G. O., Short, M. B., Malinowski, S., Johnson, M., Tita, G. E., Bertozzi, A. L., & Brantingham, P. K. (2015). Randomized controlled field trials of predictive policing. *Journal of the American Statistical Association, 110*(512), 1399–1411.

Naughton, M. (2013). *The innocent & the criminal justice system: A sociological analysis of miscarriages of justice*. Palgrave Macmillan.

Palmer, I., Kirby, S., & Coleman, R. (2019). Assessing the appetite for evidence based policing: A UK based study. *International Journal of Police Science & Management, 21*(2), 91–100.

Patterson, G. T., & Swann, P. G. (2019). Police social work and social service collaboration strategies one hundred years after Vollmer: A systematic review. *Policing: An International Journal, 42*(5), 863–886.

Perry, W. L., McInnis, B., Price, C. C., Smith, S. C., & Hollywood, J. S. (2013). *Predictive policing: The role of crime forecasting in law enforcement operations*. RAND Corporation.

Ratcliffe, J. H., Taylor, R. B., & Fisher, R. (2020). Conflicts and congruencies between predictive policing and the patrol officer's craft. *Policing and Society: An International Journal of Research and Policy, 30*(6), 639–655.

Richardson, R., Schultz, J. M., & Crawford, K. (2019). Dirty data, bad predictions: How civil rights violations impact police data, predictive policing systems, and justice. *New York University Law Review, 94*(15), 15–55.

Santos, R. G., & Santos, R. B. (2019). A four-phase process for translating research into police practice. *Police Practice and Research: An International Journal, 20*(6), 585–602.

Saunders, J., Hunt, P., & Hollywood, J. S. (2016). Predictions put into practice: A quasi-experimental evaluation of Chicago's predictive policing pilot. *Journal of Experimental Criminology, 12*, 247–371.

Sherman, L. W. (2015). A tipping point for "totally evidenced policing": Ten ideas for building an evidence-based police agency. *International Criminal Justice Review, 25*(1), 11–29.

Stinson, P. M. (2020). *Criminology explains police violence*. University of California Press.

Telep, C. W., & Shader, C. G. (2019). Creating a 'what works' translational tool for police: A researcher-city government partnership. *Police Practice and Research: An International Journal, 20*(6), 603–616.

Telep, C. W., & Somers, L. J. (2019). Examining police officer definitions of evidence-based policing: Are we speaking the same language? *Policing and Society: An International Journal of Research and Policy, 29*(2), 171–187.

Thornton, A., Sidebottom, A., Belur, J., Tompson, L., & Bowers, K. (2019). On the development and application of EMMIE: Insights from the What Works Centre for Crime Reduction. *Policing and Society, 29*(3), 266–282.

United Nations Committee on the Elimination of Racial Discrimination. (2020). *General recommendation no. 36 on preventing and combating racial profiling by law enforcement officials*. Office of the United Nations High Commissioner of Human Rights.

# Index





J. McGuire et al., *Evidence-Based Policing and Community Crime Prevention*, Advances in Preventing and Treating Violence and Aggression,
https://doi.org/10.1007/978-3-030-76363-3